Pediatric Digestive Surgery

Mario Lima
Editor

Pediatric Digestive Surgery

Springer

Editor
Mario Lima
Pediatric Surgery
S. Orsola-Malpighi Hospital
Bologna University
Bologna
Italy

ISBN 978-3-319-40523-0 ISBN 978-3-319-40525-4 (eBook)
DOI 10.1007/978-3-319-40525-4

Library of Congress Control Number: 2016960035

Printed on acid-free paper

This Springer imprint is published by Springer Nature
The registered company is Springer International Publishing AG
The registered company address is Gewerbestrasse 11, 6330 Cham, Switzerland

Dedicated to Pascal de Lagausie,
great friend,
talented surgeon,
and magnificent teacher

Preface

In recent decades, pediatric surgery has been enriched by new knowledge in the field of surgical diseases, and the development of new technologies has allowed the application of the most advanced surgical techniques also to the pediatric patient. After publication of the previous volumes on thoracic surgery and urology, this third volume comes from the need to create a focus on digestive surgical pathology.

For its implementation, collaboration of leading experts in the international scenario was sought in order to provide readers with an updated tool for their knowledge.

The Symposium on Pediatric Digestive Surgery that was held in November 2015 in Bologna was the occasion to invite the best international pediatric surgeons to offer their contribution.

This volume contains an assessment on prenatal, radiological, and anesthesiologic aspects of the main digestive disorders and chapters on the management of each topic.

This volume concludes with the treatment of pediatric cancer and with a chapter on the use of augmented reality in digestive surgery.

I wish to thank all those who have actively collaborated on the creation of this book, and all the authors, who for friendship and desire to pass on their knowledge, agreed to provide their contribution.

I also thank all the staff of Springer for their long and patient work.

Bologna, Italy — Mario Lima

Contents

Contributors

Daniele Alberti, MD Department of Pediatric Surgery, "Spedali Civili" Children's Hospital, University of Brescia, Brescia, Italy

Emanuela Angeli Department of Pediatric Cardiac Surgery and GUCH Unit, Azienda Ospedaliero-Universitaria S. Orsola-Malpighi, Bologna, Italy

Michelangelo Baldazzi Pediatric Radiology, S. Orsola-Malpighi Hospital, Bologna, Italy

Luca Bertelli Pediatric Unit, S Orsola-Malpighi Hospital, Bologna, Italy

Adrian Bianchi, MD, FRCS, FRCSEd Neonatal and Paediatric Reconstructive Surgeon, Manchester, UK

Arnaud Bonnard, MD, PhD Department of Pediatric Surgery, Robert Debré Children University Hospital, APHP, Paris, France

Giovanni Boroni, MD Department of Pediatric Surgery, "Spedali Civili" Children's Hospital, Brescia, Italy

Steven W. Bruch, MD C.S. Mott Children's Hospital, University of Michigan, Ann Arbor, MI, USA

Nasser Bustangi Department of Pediatric Surgery, Centre Hospitalier Universitaire, Saint-Etienne, France

Noemi Cantone Pediatric Surgery, S. Orsola-Malpighi Hospital, Bologna University, Bologna, Italy

Teresa Capriati Artificial Nutrition Unit, Bambino Gesù Children's Hospital, Rome, Italy

Filomena Carfagnini Pediatric Radiology, S. Orsola Malpighi Hospital, Bologna, Italy

Arnold G. Coran C.S. Mott Children's Hospital, University of Michigan Hospital and Health Systems, Ann Arbor, MI, USA

Rita Cozzali Pediatric Gastroenterology Unit, Foligno Hospital, Foligno (PG), Italy

Pascal de Lagausie, MD, PhD Department of Pediatric Surgery, Hôpital Timone-Enfant, Marseille, France

Rosina De Rose Department of Pediatric Anaesthesia and Intensive Care, S. Orsola-Malpighi University Hospital, Bologna, Italy

Francesca Destro Pediatric Surgery, S. Orsola-Malpighi Hospital, Bologna University, Bologna, Italy

Antonella Diamanti, MD Hepatology, Gastroenterology and Nutrition Unit, Bambino Gesù "Children Hospital", Rome, Italy

Giovanni Di Nardo Pediatric Gastroenterology Unit, International Hospital Salvator Mundi, Rome, Italy

Neil Di Salvo Pediatric Surgery, S. Orsola-Malpighi Hospital, Bologna University, Bologna, Italy

Gabriele Egidy Assenza Department of Pediatric Cardiac Surgery and GUCH Unit, Azienda Ospedaliero-Universitaria S. Orsola-Malpighi, Bologna, Italy

Tommaso Gargano Pediatric Surgery, S. Orsola-Malpighi Hospital, Bologna University, Bologna, Italy

Gaetano Domenico Gargiulo Department of Pediatric Cardiac Surgery and GUCH Unit, Azienda Ospedaliero-Universitaria S. Orsola-Malpighi, Bologna, Italy

Andrea Gentili Department of Pediatric Anaesthesia and Intensive Care, S. Orsola-Malpighi University Hospital, Bologna, Italy

Daniela Giorgio Artificial Nutrition Unit, Bambino Gesù Children's Hospital, Rome, Italy

Florent Guerin, MD, PhD Department of Pediatric Surgery, Kremlin Bicetre Children University Hospital, APHP, Paris, France

Elisa Iannella Department of Pediatric Anaesthesia and Intensive Care, S. Orsola-Malpighi University Hospital, Bologna, Italy

Sara Isoldi Pediatric Gastroenterology Unit, Sapienza – University of Rome, Rome, Italy

Shaun M. Kunisaki, MD C.S. Mott Children's Hospital, University of Michigan, Ann Arbor, MI, USA

Valeria Landuzzi Department of Pediatric Anaesthesia and Intensive Care, S. Orsola-Malpighi University Hospital, Bologna, Italy

Mario Lima Pediatric Surgery, S. Orsola-Malpighi Hospital, Bologna University, Bologna, Italy

Manuel Lopez Department of Pediatric Surgery, Centre Hospitalier Universitaire, Saint-Etienne, France

Michela Maffi Pediatric Surgery, S. Orsola-Malpighi Hospital, Bologna University, Bologna, Italy

Jacques Marescaux IHU Strasbourg, IRCAD, Strasbourg, France

Reva Matta Clinical Surgery, University of Balamand, El-Koura, Lebanon

Division of Pediatric Surgery, Department of Surgery, Saint George Hospital University Medical Center, Beirut, Lebanon

Girolamo Mattioli Pediatric Surgery Unit, Istituto Giannina Gaslini, DINOGMI University of Genoa, Genoa, Italy

Anastasia Mentessidou, MD Department of Pediatric Surgery, Chelsea Children's Hospital, Chelsea and Westminster Hospital NHS Fdn Trust, Imperial College London, London, UK

Maria Cristina Mondardini Department of Pediatric Anaesthesia and Intensive Care, S. Orsola-Malpighi University Hospital, Bologna, Italy

Philippe Montupet Hôpitaux Universitaires Paris-Sud, Bicêtre Hospital, Université Paris XI, Le Kremlin-Bicêtre Cedex, France

Didier Mutter IHU Strasbourg, IRCAD, Strasbourg, France

Stéphane Nicolau IRCAD, Strasbourg, France

Lluís Nisa Department of Clinical Research, University of Bern, Bern, Switzerland

Giuseppe Pagliaro Pediatric Gastroenterology Unit, Sapienza, University of Rome, Rome, Italy

Filippo Parolini, MD Department of Pediatric Surgery, "Spedali Civili" Children's Hospital, Brescia, Italy

Patrick Pessaux IHU Strasbourg, IRCAD, Strasbourg, France

Andrea Pession Pediatric Units, S Orsola-Malpighi Hospital, University of Bologna, Bologna, Italy

Francesco Petridis Department of Pediatric Cardiac Surgery and GUCH Unit, Azienda Ospedaliero-Universitaria S. Orsola-Malpighi, Bologna, Italy

Gianluigi Pilu Department of Obstetrics and Gynecology, Bologna University, Bologna, Italy

Alessio Pini Prato Pediatric Surgery Unit, Istituto Giannina Gaslini, DINOGMI University of Genoa, Genoa, Italy

Luca Pio Pediatric Surgery Unit, Istituto Giannina Gaslini, DINOGMI University of Genoa, Genoa, Italy

Antonio Poerio Pediatric Radiology, S. Orsola Malpighi Hospital, Bologna, Italy

Matthew W. Ralls C.S. Mott Children's Hospital, University of Michigan Hospital and Health Systems, Ann Arbor, MI, USA

Olivier Reinberg Pediatric Surgery, Pully, Switzerland

Kishore Sandu Department of Otorhinolaryngology – Head and Neck Surgery, Lausanne University Hospital, Lausanne, Switzerland

Amulya K. Saxena, MD, PhD, DSc(hon), FRCS(Glasg) Department of Pediatric Surgery, Chelsea Children's Hospital, Chelsea and Westminster Hospital NHS Fdn Trust, Imperial College London, London, UK

Aurélien Scalabre Department of Pediatric Surgery, Centre Hospitalier Universitaire, Saint-Etienne, France

Luc Soler IRCAD, Strasbourg, France

Daniel H. Teitelbaum C.S. Mott Children's Hospital, University of Michigan Hospital and Health Systems, Ann Arbor, MI, USA

David C. van der Zee Department of Pediatric Surgery, Wilhelmina Children's Hospital, University Medical Center, Utrecht, The Netherlands

François Varlet Department of Pediatric Surgery, Centre Hospitalier Universitaire, Saint-Etienne, France

Sophie Vermersch Department of Pediatric Surgery, Centre Hospitalier Universitaire, Saint-Etienne, France

Prenatal Diagnosis and Obstetric Management

1

Gianluigi Pilu

In Europe ultrasound examinations are commonly performed in virtually all pregnancies, usually between 11 and 13 weeks' gestation and around 20 weeks' gestation [1]. One of the main objectives of these investigations is the detection of fetal anomalies. The uptake of anomalies is variable in different studies, and indeed, the value of universal screening for anatomic malformations is debated [1–3]. The detection rate much varies depending upon different factors and the affected organs in particular. Sonographic investigation of the fetal gastrointestinal tract suffers from many limitations mostly because the fetal bowel is almost completely empty in early gestation. Furthermore, the esophagus and anorectal tract are incompletely seen. As a consequence of this, most intestinal obstructions are not identified until late in gestation or even after birth (Fig. 1.1).

Nevertheless, the identification of abnormal fetal sonographic findings of the gastrointestinal tract does occur, and in these cases, pediatric specialists are usually consulted to discuss the management strategy in the perinatal period and the prognosis. Such consultations have a particular relevance when the diagnosis is made in early gestation and the couples are considering the option of a pregnancy termination. It seems important to stress that caution is necessary when discussing the implications of antenatal diagnosis. The accuracy of sonography is limited, and anomalies identified in utero tend to have a different outcome than those that are identified after birth. Ancillary methods are now available for prenatal diagnosis in selected cases, including genetic testing and magnetic resonance, and multidisciplinary discussion is certainly indicated.

In the following pages, we will briefly review the state of the art of prenatal diagnosis of the anomalies of the gastrointestinal tract, focusing upon the information that seem relevant for the pediatric surgeons who work in close contact with obstetric departments.

1.1 Normal Sonographic Appearance of the Fetal Gastrointestinal Tract

Fetuses start swallowing amniotic fluid early in gestation, and the fluid-filled stomach is visible as early as 9 weeks of gestation as a C-shaped sonolucent structure in the upper left quadrant of the abdomen. The bowel has normally a uniform echogenic appearance until the third trimester of pregnancy when meconium-filled loops of large bowel are commonly seen. The liver is large prenatally and comprises most of the upper abdomen. The gallbladder is usually seen since midgestation as an ovoid cystic structure to the right and below the intrahepatic portion of the

G. Pilu
Department of Obstetrics and Gynecology,
Bologna University, Via Massarenti 13,
40138 Bologna, Italy
e-mail: gianluigi.pilu@aosp.bo.it

M. Lima (ed.), *Pediatric Digestive Surgery*, DOI 10.1007/978-3-319-40525-4_1

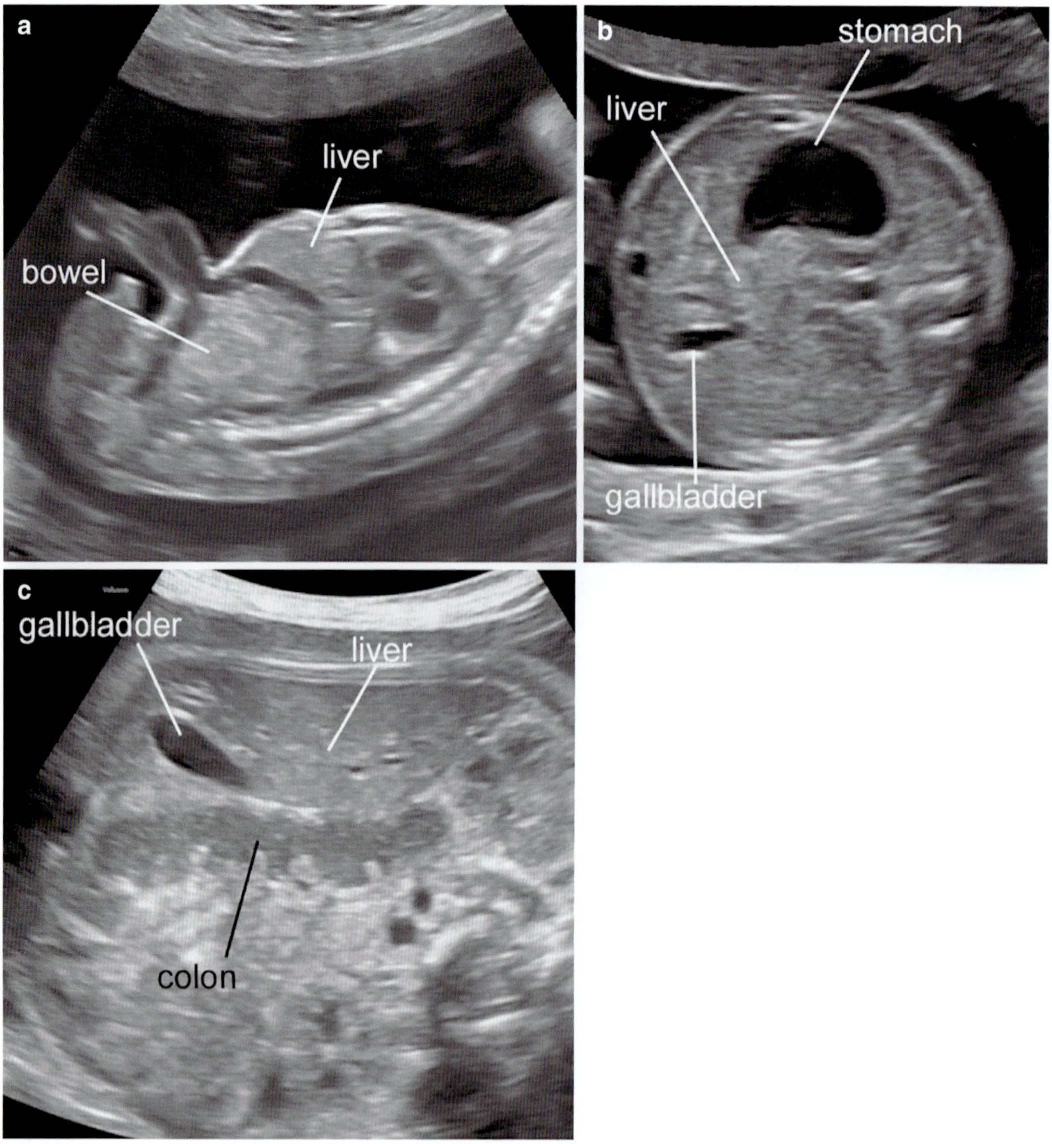

Fig. 1.1 The normal appearance of the fetal gastrointestinal system at 20 weeks (**a**, **b**) and close to term gestation (**c**); at 20 weeks the liver is large and occupies the entire upper abdomen, and the stomach and gallbladder are fluid filled and easily visible; the bowel is empty and appears sonographically homogeneous; in advanced gestation, the meconium-filled large bowel can be seen

umbilical vein. The spleen may also be visualized posterior and to the left of the fetal stomach. The proximal and distal esophagus can be at times visualized, when the fetus is in a favorable position and particularly in the course of swallowing. However, it is impossible to visualize the entire length. The anal complex can also be seen although usually only in late gestation (Fig. 1.2).

1.2 Esophageal Atresia

As the esophagus is poorly and anyhow incompletely visualized with fetal sonography, most cases of atresia escape antenatal detection [4]. The majority of cases are associated with a tracheoesophageal fistula that allows distal transit of fluid and filling of the stomach. In

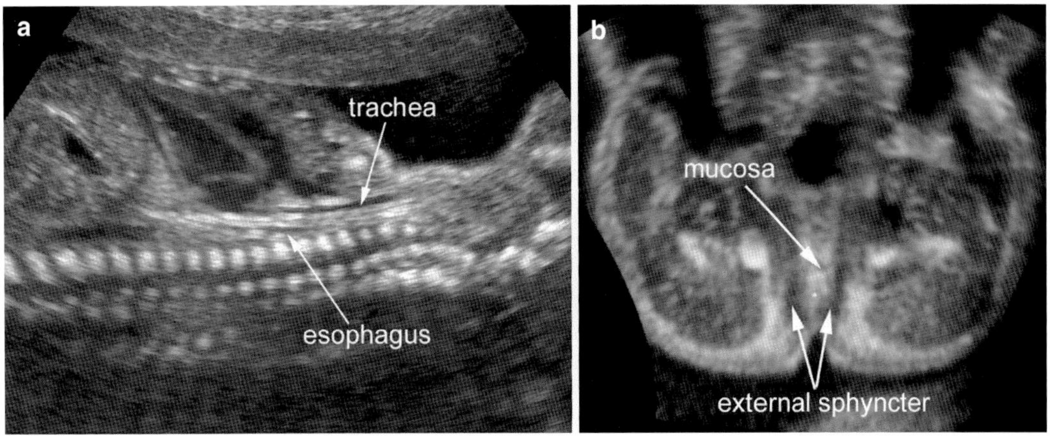

Fig. 1.2 It is difficult to demonstrate sonographically the fetal esophagus and the anorectal complex. When the fetus is in a favorable position and the quality of the images is adequate, at least the distal esophagus coursing posterior to the trachea (**a**), and the echogenic anorectal mucosa, surrounded by the sonolucent external sphincter (**b**) may be seen

late gestation, however, the size of the fistula does not allow adequate transit and as a consequence of this fluid accumulated into the amniotic cavity, and the stomach appears minimally distended.

The diagnosis of esophageal atresia is suspected when, in the presence of polyhydramnios (usually only in the third trimester), repeated ultrasonographic examinations demonstrate a small stomach bubble. In most cases the condition can only be suspected and the final diagnosis is only possible after birth. The only exception is in cases in which during swallowing the dilated proximal esophageal pouch is seen, as an elongated upper mediastinal and retrocardiac anechoic structure. This finding however is present only after 28 weeks and transiently [4].

The differential diagnosis for the combination of a small stomach bubble and polyhydramnios includes intrathoracic compression, by conditions such as diaphragmatic hernia, and muscular-skeletal anomalies causing inability of the fetus to swallow. Fetal magnetic resonance has also been reported to be of help in these cases [4].

In one of the largest available series, polyhydramnios was present in 50 % of cases, and the atresia was suspected or diagnosed antenatally in about one-third of cases, at a median gestational age of 31 weeks. As expected type 1 atresia was more frequently suspected (polyhydramnios in 100 % of cases, small gastric bubble in over 80 % of cases) than cases with a tracheal fistula (polyhydramnios 50 % of cases, small gastric bubble in 25 %) [4].

Esophageal atresia and tracheoesophageal fistula are often associated with other major defects, including chromosomal anomalies, malformations, and syndromic associations, that are not always obvious on prenatal examinations (Fig. 1.3).

1.3 Duodenal Atresia

Prenatal diagnosis is based on the demonstration of the characteristic "double bubble" appearance of the dilated stomach and proximal duodenum, commonly associated with polyhydramnios. Although the characteristic "double bubble" can be seen as early as 20 weeks, it is usually not diagnosed until after 25 weeks suggesting that the fetus is unable to swallow sufficient volume of amniotic fluid for bowel dilatation to occur before the end of the second trimester of pregnancy.

In a review of the literature, prenatal diagnosis was made in 77 % of cases. Other malformations were often present and trisomy 21 was found in about one-third of cases [5] (Fig. 1.4).

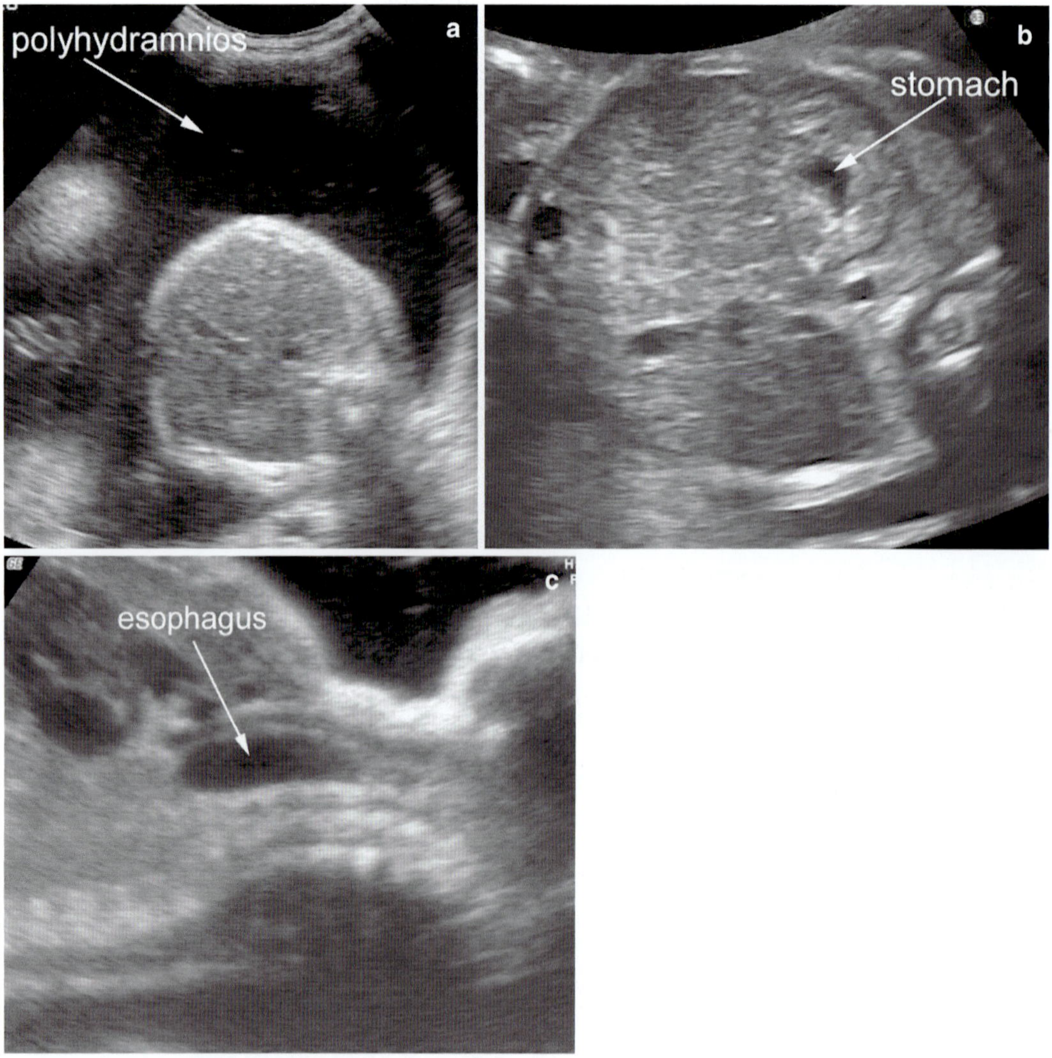

Fig. 1.3 Esophageal atresia. The amniotic fluid is much increased (**a**), the stomach bubble is small (**b**), and the proximal esophagus forms a pouch when the fetus swallows (**c**)

1.4 Pyloric Atresia

Few cases of pyloric atresia, often in association with other malformations, have been described. The typical finding includes polyhydramnios and a large stomach that usually appear only in the third trimester of gestation. The index of suspicion is increased when dilatation of the esophagus is also seen [5].

1.5 Intestinal Obstruction

In early gestation the bowel is virtually empty and it has a homogeneous echogenic texture. Only in the third trimester of gestation it becomes possible to visualize the large bowel, distended by echogenic meconium. The appearance is very variable and the size of the colon has been reported to vary between 7 and 20 mm. Individual

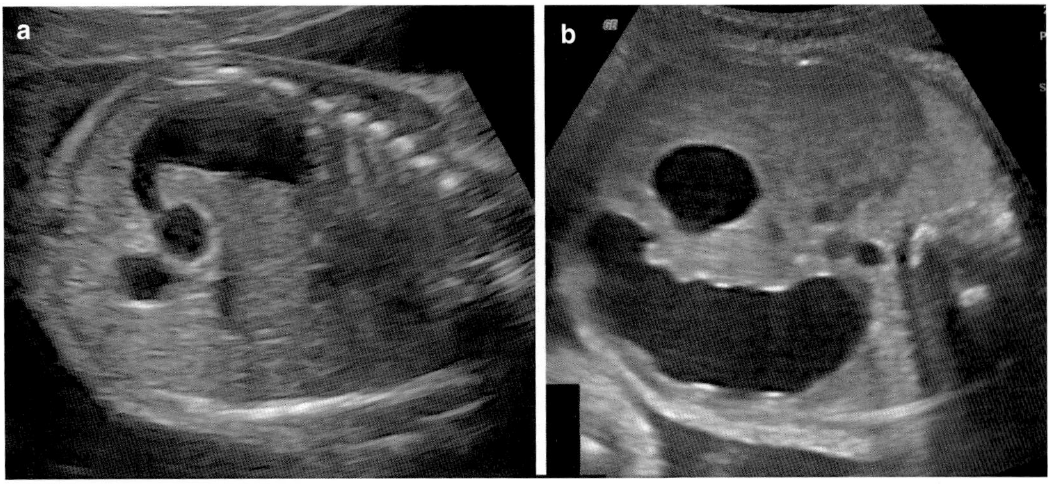

Fig. 1.4 Duodenal atresia; double bubble sign in the second (**a**) and third trimester (**b**)

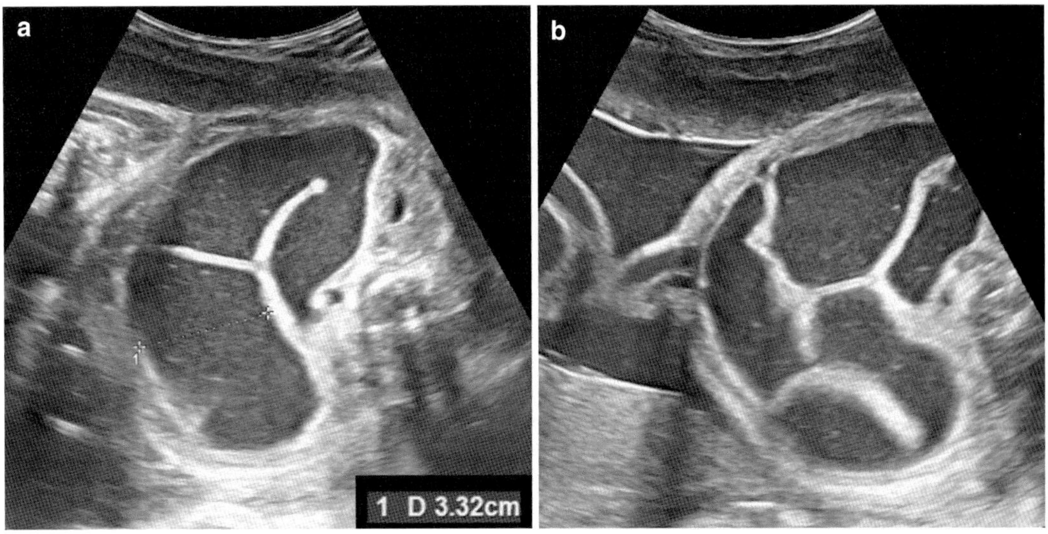

Fig. 1.5 Ileal atresia; gross dilatation of bowel loops. During real-time examination, increased perystalsis (**a, b**) was seen.

small bowel loops may be seen at times, usually with a maximum diameter of few mm.

Small bowel obstruction is usually visible only late in pregnancy and almost invariably after 25 weeks of gestation. The diagnosis is easy when distended, fluid-filled, and peristaltic bowel loops are seen. The presence of polyhydramnios increases the index of suspicion. However, at times it may be difficult to differentiate bowel obstruction from normally prominent large bowel. It is not rare that the final diagnosis can only be made after birth. The whirlpool sign suggesting the presence of a volvulus has been described in fetuses.

In a review of the literature, about 50% of small bowel obstruction were detected antenatally, and false-positive diagnosis was frequent (the specificity was as low as 30%). The detection rate was greater with jejunal than ileal obstruction (60% and 25%, respectively). Cystic fibrosis has been reported in up to 13% of cases [5] (Fig. 1.5).

1.6 Meconium Peritonitis

Intrauterine perforation of the bowel may lead to a local sterile chemical peritonitis, with the development of a dense calcified mass of fibrous tissue sealing off the perforation. Bowel perforation usually occurs proximal to some form of obstruction, although this cannot always be demonstrated. In many cases of meconium peritonitis, ultrasound will only reveal findings of intestinal obstruction. However, a specific diagnosis can be made if dilated bowel loops are found in association with ascites and calcium deposit. It may also be possible to document at times a typical sequence of events: ascites associated with segmental dilatation of bowel loops, followed by disappearance of the fluid and progression of bowel enlargement, usually in the presence of intra-abdominal calcifications. Cystic fibrosis has been reported in up to 20 % of these cases [5].

1.7 Abdominal Cysts

Abdominal cysts are frequent findings at ultrasound examination. Renal tract anomalies or dilated bowel are the most common explanations, although cystic structures may arise from the biliary tree, ovaries, mesentery, or uterus. The correct diagnosis of these abnormalities may not be possible by ultrasound examination, but the most likely diagnosis is usually suggested by the position of the cyst, its relationship with other structures, and the normality of other organs [6].

1.7.1 Choledochal Cysts

Choledochal cysts represent cystic dilatation of the common biliary duct. They are uncommon and their etiology is unknown. Prenatally, the diagnosis may be made ultrasonographically by the demonstration of a cyst in the upper right side of the fetal abdomen. The differential diagnosis includes enteric duplication cyst, liver cysts, situs inversus, or duodenal atresia. The absence of polyhydramnios or peristalsis may help differentiate the condition from bowel disorders.

1.7.2 Ovarian Cysts

Ovarian cysts are common, and they may be found in up to one-third of newborns at autopsy, although they are usually small and asymptomatic. Fetal ovarian cysts are hormone sensitive (hCG from the placenta) and tend to occur after 25 weeks of gestation; they are more common in diabetic or rhesus-isoimmunized mothers as a result of placental hyperplasia. The majority of cysts are benign and resolve spontaneously in the neonatal period. Potential complications include the development of ascites, torsion, infarction, or rupture. Prenatally, the cysts are usually unilateral and unilocular although if the cyst undergoes torsion or hemorrhage, the appearance is complex or solid. Large ovarian cysts can be found in association with polyhydramnios possibly as a consequence of compression on the bowel. Obstetric management should not be changed, unless an enormous or rapidly enlarging cyst is detected or there is associated polyhydramnios; in these cases, prenatal aspiration may be considered. A difficult differential diagnosis is from hydrometrocolpos, which also presents as a cystic or solid mass arising from the pelvis of a female fetus. Other genitourinary or gastrointestinal anomalies are common and include renal agenesis, polycystic kidneys, esophageal atresia, duodenal atresia, and imperforate anus. Most cases are sporadic, although few cases are genetic, such as the autosomal recessive McKusick-Kaufman syndrome with hydrometrocolpos, polydactyly, and congenital heart disease (Fig. 1.6).

1.7.3 Mesenteric or Omental Cysts

Mesenteric or omental cysts may represent obstructed lymphatic drainage or lymphatic hamartomas. The fluid contents may be serous, chylous, or hemorrhagic. Antenatally, the diagnosis is suggested by the finding of a multiseptate or unilocular, usually in the midline, cystic lesion of variable size; a solid appearance may be secondary to hemorrhage.

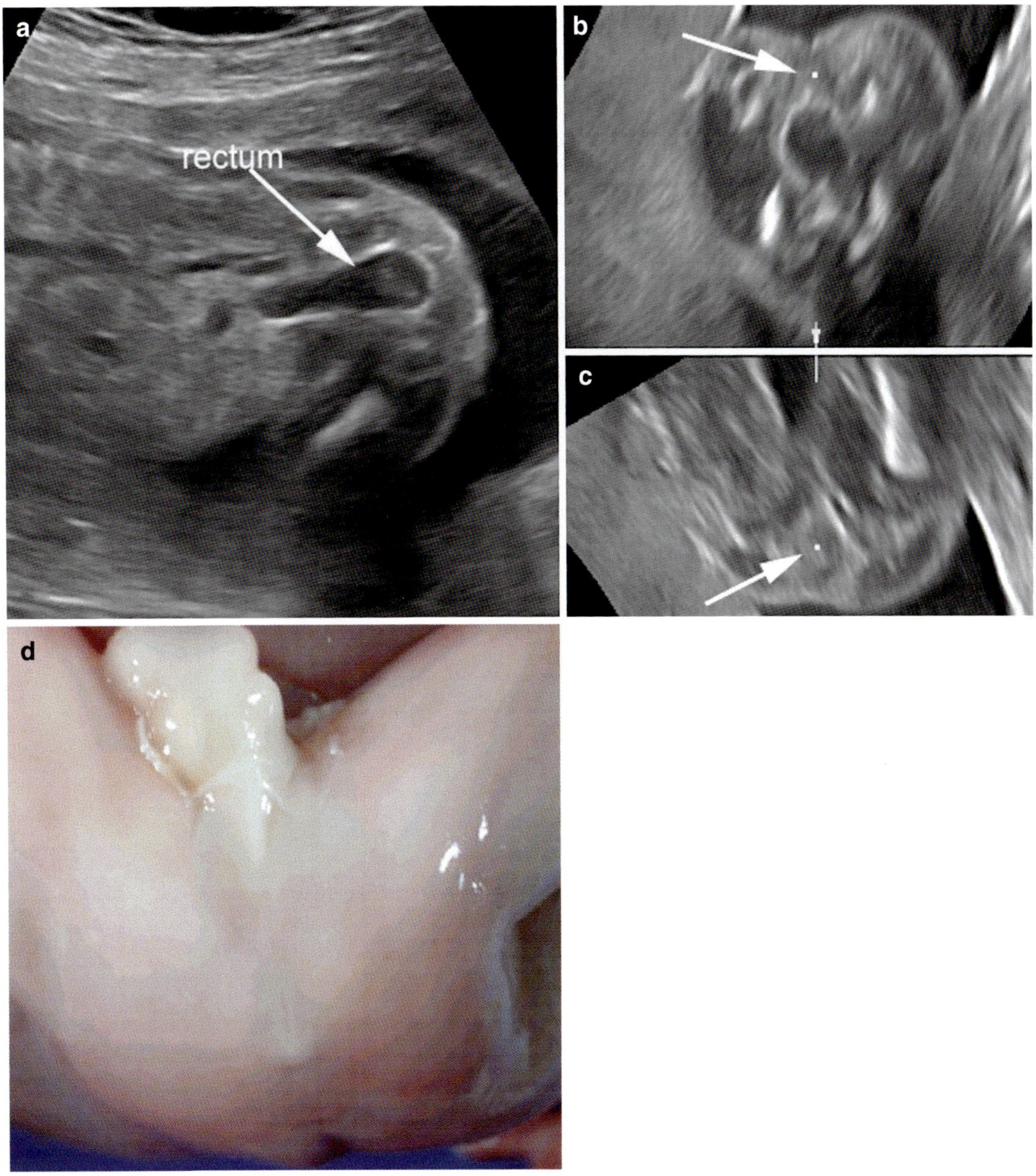

Fig. 1.6 Imperforate anus. In this fetus at 20 weeks of gestation with multiple anomalies, the diagnosis was suggested by the enlargement of the rectum (**a**) in association with the failure to demonstrate the echogenic anal mucosa (**b**, **c**); the diagnosis was confirmed at the time of autopsy (**d**)

1.7.4 Intestinal Duplication Cysts

They are quite rare and may be located along the entire gastrointestinal tract. They sonographically appear as tubular or cystic structures of variable size. They may be isolated or associated with other gastrointestinal malformations. Differential diagnosis includes other intra-abdominal cystic structures and also bronchogenic cysts, adenomatoid cystic malformation of the lung, and pulmonary sequestration. The thickness of the muscular wall of the cysts and the presence of peristalsis may facilitate the diagnosis. Postnatally surgical removal is carried out.

1.8 Anorectal Malformation

The fetal anus and rectum are poorly demonstrated by ultrasound and are not a part of the standard examination of fetal anatomy. As a general rule, anorectal malformations are not amenable to antenatal diagnosis. In a handful of cases, however, anorectal atresia has been suspected antenatally, usually by the observation of a dilatation of the upper rectum and failure to demonstrate the anorectal complex that is normally formed by the anechoic ring of the external sphincter muscle surrounding the echogenic mucosa (Fig. 1.6) [7].

1.9 Obstetrical Management of Fetal Intestinal Anomalies

Intestinal anomalies are invariably treated after birth, and standard obstetric management is usually not changed. As a general rule, delivery may occur at the term and vaginally. A possible exception is represented by the presence of polyhydramnios that is frequently found with esophageal and duodenal atresia, less frequently with small bowel obstruction. An excessive amount of amniotic fluid may result in overdistension of the uterus and trigger premature labor or rupture of the membranes. The administration of tocolytic drugs in these cases is of limited efficacy, and in the presence of severe polyhydramnios, most perinatologists would favor serial evacuative amniocenteses. When there is potential for prematurity, maternal administration of steroids should also be considered to prevent neonatal respiratory distress.

Of special concern is the issue of fetal pain. It is difficult for perinatologists to observe with ultrasound fetuses with obstructed bowel that demonstrate gross intestinal dilatation with intense peristalsis and overdistension of the abdomen and vomit incessantly and not to think the agony they are experiencing. Little is known about fetal pain, and the ultimate psychological consequence of long-enduring distress, but studies on premature infants do suggest that this may have a major impact [8]. Unfortunately, an effective approach to pain therapy in utero is not available yet, but certainly this problem will have to be addressed in the future.

Conclusions

In most cases, intestinal anomalies will escape prenatal detection and will be recognized only postnatally. The pediatric surgeon may however be consulted prior to birth in the presence of abnormal fetal sonographic findings. At times the diagnosis will be clear-cut (double bubble sign and polyhydramnios indicating duodenal atresia, grossly dilated and peristaltic bowel loops suggesting small bowel obstruction, a whirlpool sign suggesting a volvulus). In other cases, there will be many uncertainties. It is important to stress that the accuracy of antenatal imaging technique in the identification and differentiation of gastrointestinal anomalies is limited. In many cases, a definitive diagnosis will only be possible after birth.

References

1. Salomon LJ, Alfirevic Z, Berghella V, Bilardo C, Hernandez-Andrade E, Johnsen SL, Kalache K, Leung KY, Malinger G, Munoz H, Prefumo F, Toi A, Lee W, Committee ICS (2011) Practice guidelines for performance of the routine mid-trimester fetal ultrasound scan. Ultrasound Obstet Gynecol Off J Inter Soc Ultrasound Obstet Gynecol 37(1):116–126
2. Ewigman BG, Crane JP, Frigoletto FD, LeFevre ML, Bain RP, McNellis D (1993) Effect of prenatal ultrasound screening on perinatal outcome. RADIUS Study Group. N Engl J Med 329(12):821–827
3. Grandjean H, Larroque D, Levi S (1999) The performance of routine ultrasonographic screening of pregnancies in the Eurofetus Study. Am J Obstet Gynecol 181(2):446–454
4. Spaggiari E, Faure G, Rousseau V, Sonigo P, Millischer-Bellaiche AE, Kermorvant-Duchemin E, Muller F, Czerkiewicz I, Ville Y, Salomon LJ (2015) Performance of prenatal diagnosis in esophageal atresia. Prenat Diagn 35(9):888–893
5. Tonni G, Grisolia G, Granese R, Giacobbe A, Napolitano M, Passos JP, Araujo E Jr (2015) Prenatal

diagnosis of gastric and small bowel atresia: a case series and review of the literature. J Matern Fetal Neonatal Med Off J Eur Assoc Perinatal Med Federation Asia Oceania Perinatal Soc Inter Soc Perinatal Obstet 23:1–9
6. Catania VD, Briganti V, Di Giacomo V, Miele V, Signore F, de Waure C, Calabro GE, Calisti A (2016) Fetal intra-abdominal cysts: accuracy and predictive value of prenatal ultrasound. J Matern Fetal Neonatal Med Off J Eur Assoc Perinatal Med Federation Asia Oceania Perinatal Soc Inter Soc Perinatal Obstet 29(10):1691–1699
7. Perlman S, Bilik R, Leibovitch L, Katorza E, Achiron R, Gilboa Y (2014) More than a gut feeling – sonographic prenatal diagnosis of imperforate anus in a high-risk population. Prenat Diagn 34(13):1307–1311
8. Valeri BO, Holsti L, Linhares MB (2015) Neonatal pain and developmental outcomes in children born preterm: a systematic review. Clin J Pain 31(4):355–362

2 Gastro-Intestinal Tract Radiology

Filomena Carfagnini, Michelangelo Baldazzi, and Antonio Poerio

The main diagnostic techniques for gastrointestinal pathology in childhood have always been and still are plain abdominal radiographs and conventional contrast studies. However, gastrointestinal imaging has continued to evolve over time, with new techniques and methods gradually being added to the diagnostic procedures, particularly ultrasound (US), magnetic resonance imaging (MRI), and computed tomography (CT).

For gastrointestinal studies in children, it is important to know the indications for the different imaging techniques, to understand the relationship between the techniques, and to consider the use of these newer techniques rather than conventional radiological studies, also considering the role of prenatal diagnosis and how this has, in some cases, changed the diagnostic process.

The different diagnostic techniques for gastrointestinal tract studies in children are described here, noting for each the main indications and specific characteristics, bearing in mind that a diagnosis can be determined by a single investigation or can be the result of one or more studies.

The indications for each imaging modality, and the order in which examinations must be conducted, should be considered carefully to avoid unnecessary examinations. In the radiological examination of children, the problem of radiation protection should be addressed first and foremost, regardless of the part of the anatomy being imaged.

2.1 Imaging Techniques

2.1.1 Plain Abdominal Radiograph

The *plain abdominal radiograph* uses the natural contrast agent of air, and in the neonatal period is the examination most frequently used; in some cases it is the only one required for the diagnosis. In a healthy neonate, air can usually be identified in the stomach within minutes of birth, and within 3 h the entire small bowel usually contains gas. After 8–9 h, healthy neonates demonstrate sigmoid gas.

Delayed passage of gas through the neonatal gut may occur as a result of traumatic delivery, hypoglycemia, septicemia, or brain damage. Absence of gas in the bowel may be noted in neonates with severe respiratory distress who are undergoing mechanical ventilation, and in neonates undergoing continuous nasogastric suction.

The diagnosis of obstruction is based on some interruption of this dispersion of air. Radiography

F. Carfagnini (✉) • M. Baldazzi • A. Poerio
Pediatric Radiology, S. Orsola-Malpighi Hospital, Via Albertoni 15, Bologna, Italy
e-mail: filomena.carfagnini@aosp.bo.it; michelangelo.baldazzi@aosp.bo.it; antonio.poerio@studio.unibo.it

M. Lima (ed.), *Pediatric Digestive Surgery*, DOI 10.1007/978-3-319-40525-4_2

is the most valuable means of determining whether obstruction is present. This modality is often diagnostic; even if it is not, however, it may help to determine the next most useful diagnostic procedure [1–5].

Congenital anomalies causing incomplete obstruction (e.g., stenoses, webs, duplications, malrotations, peritoneal bands, aganglionosis) may not manifest until later in life, and other types of examinations (e.g., US and barium enema studies) are generally needed for diagnosis.

Abdominal radiography is often performed only in the supine antero-posterior (AP) view, especially in the neonatal period; only if required is the trans-lateral view with a horizontal beam added, and this allows the recognition of air-fluid levels and facilitates the visualization of pneumoperitoneum (Fig. 2.1). In pneumoperitoneum, in equivocal cases, the study can be completed by an additional view in the left lateral (LL) decubitus position, with a horizontal beam.

All cases of *pneumoperitoneum*, however determined, and *upper-obstructive conditions* have an exclusively radiographic diagnosis – duodenal atresia with a double-bubble sign; less frequently pyloric atresia, with a single-bubble sign; and jejunal atresia, with a few dilated loops causing upstream obstruction and complete absence of air downstream (Fig. 2.2). None of these conditions usually require further radiological evaluation after radiography: contrast studies are usually contraindicated, and additional procedures are not usually helpful and may even delay surgery, resulting in death.

The role of the plain abdominal radiograph combined with a chest radiograph in the diagnosis of *esophageal atresia* should be mentioned; this disease is suspected at prenatal US by the combination of polyhydramnios, reduced intraluminal liquid in the fetal gut, and inability to detect the fetal stomach.

Radiological confirmation of esophageal atresia is based on findings on AP and lateral chest radiographs, which show a blind pouch of the proximal esophagus, which is distended with air. Radiographic evaluation should always include the abdomen to assess the presence of gastrointestinal air due to the existence of the fistula, allowing the classification of tracheo-esophageal

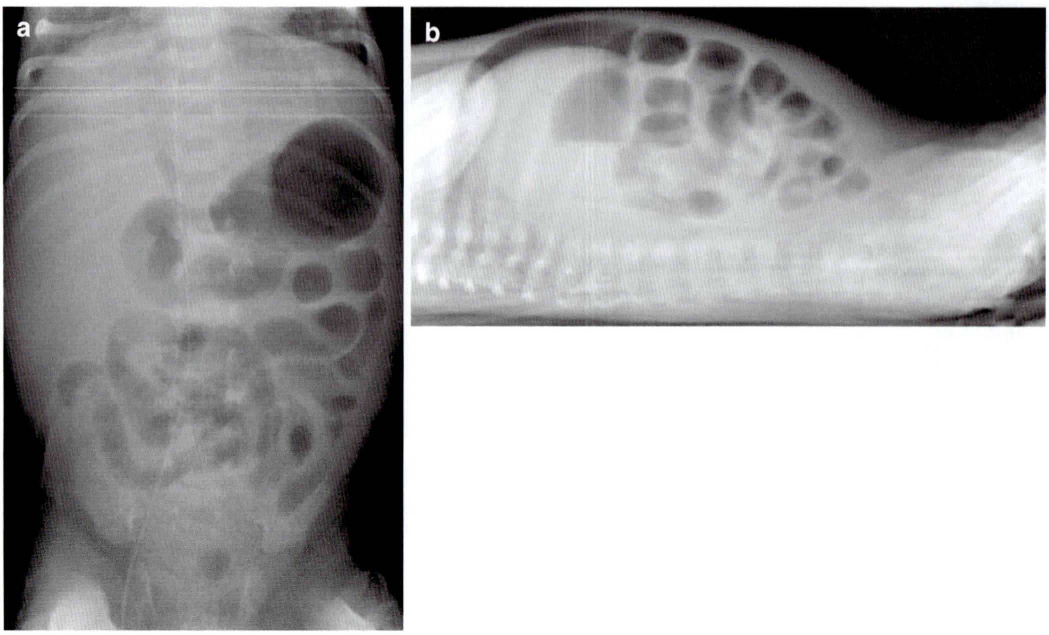

Fig. 2.1 Plain abdominal radiographs: supine antero-posterior view (**a**) and trans-lateral view (**b**) show the presence of pneumoperitoneum

atresia. In types I and II there is a complete absence of air in the stomach and bowel, whereas in types III and IV, air is commonly present.

When an H-shaped fistula without atresia is suspected, an esophagogram with low-osmolality water-soluble non-ionic contrast media can show the fistula [6].

The plain abdominal radiograph also has a role in the early diagnostic phase of *anorectal malformations*; in such cases, you need to perform, with classification intent, a plain abdominal radiograph in the trans-lateral prone view for the evaluation of the rectal cul-de-sac and its distance from the perineum.

Furthermore, this study allows you to detect the sacrococcygeal anomalies that are often found in caudal regression syndrome or other skeletal abnormalities in a more syndromic context (VACTERL association; vertebral defects, anal atresia, cardiac defects, tracheo-esophageal fistula, renal anomalies, and limb abnormalities).

2.1.2 Contrast Studies

Contrast studies remain as key to the demonstration of many diseases, both congenital and acquired. Their use, however, is slowly declining, thanks to the increased availability and dissemination of endoscopic techniques and video capsule endoscopy (VCE).

The aim of the modern radiologist is to work in close collaboration with the gastroenterologist and surgeon, to perform contrast studies only in selected patients, using the correct technique, at the lowest radiation dose possible to meet specific diagnostic questions.

Many diseases are also studied exclusively by a continuous fluoroscopy technique, by the last image-capture technique, or by pulsed fluoroscopy with capture of the acquired series. High-dose standard full exposures are reserved for cases of difficult diagnosis or when more definite anatomical detail is essential (e.g., in thin tracheo-esophageal fistulas).

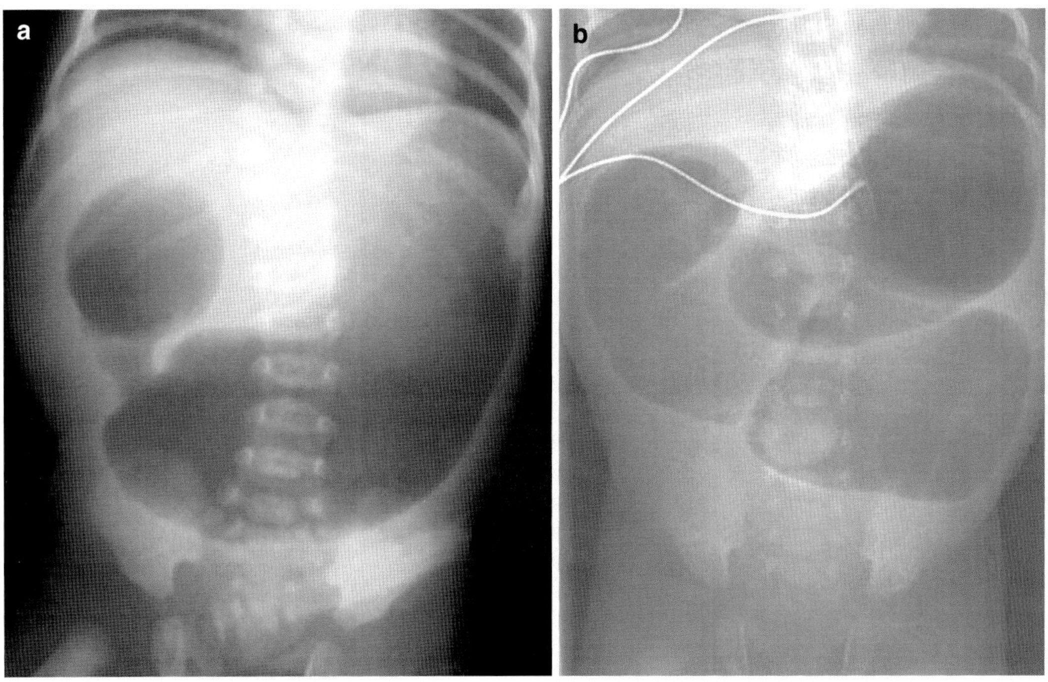

Fig. 2.2 Plain abdominal radiographs: duodenal atresia with the double-bubble sign, due to distension of the stomach and proximal duodenum (**a**) and jejunal atresia (**b**), with a few dilated loops and absence of air in the lower portion of the abdomen. Note the presence of thoracic right-side hemivertebra (**a**)

2.1.2.1 Contrast Studies of the Upper Gastrointestinal Tract

Contrast studies of the upper gastrointestinal tract are *upper gastrointestinal (UGI) series*, small bowel follow through (SBFT), and small bowel enema.

Upper Gastrointestinal (UGI) Series

In well infants or children, barium is the preferred contrast medium for UGI series.

For imaging of the esophagus, stomach, and duodenum there is a choice of barium formulations and the choice of preparation is at the discretion of the radiologist.

As mucosal detail is rarely required, or indeed obtainable in children, preparations with a lower density are used; these can be successfully diluted, do not settle out and set while in suspension, and do not flocculate in the time taken to perform the test.

In neonates, especially premature infants, and in circumstances where aspiration is a risk or a perforation of the gastrointestinal tract is suspected, a low-osmolality water-soluble non-ionic contrast medium is ideally used (Fig. 2.3).

The child should be starved for approximately 3–4 h before the study, or for the maximum gap between feeds if still breast-fed.

High-density high-osmolality water-soluble non-ionic contrast media should never be used because of the risk of aspiration and consequent possible serious complications, such as acute pulmonary edema [1, 3–5].

Although the 24-h pH probe is now the mainstay for making or confirming the diagnosis of reflux in children, UGI series are still used in many centers to confirm that the underlying gastrointestinal anatomy is normal. Conversely, the presence or absence of reflux during a routine UGI series should be noted, as this may be an important incidental finding.

Reflux often occurs immediately after the passage of the bolus (liquid or solid) through fractionally delayed closure of the gastro-esophageal junction (GEJ). Thus, if water is given (two or three consecutive mouthfuls are sufficient) even small amounts of reflux of barium at the GEJ may be captured. Beaking of the GEJ is a cardinal sign that reflux is likely to occur imminently, and if the radiologist sees this he/she should wait for a few more moments to see whether this is confirmed. If reflux does not occur after two or three episodes of drinking water then the child should be turned to the left lateral (LL) position and then slowly returned to supine. This encourages barium to wash over the GEJ, which may cause reflex relaxation of the GEJ with subsequent reflux. If after these two maneuvers reflux has not been demonstrated, then the study

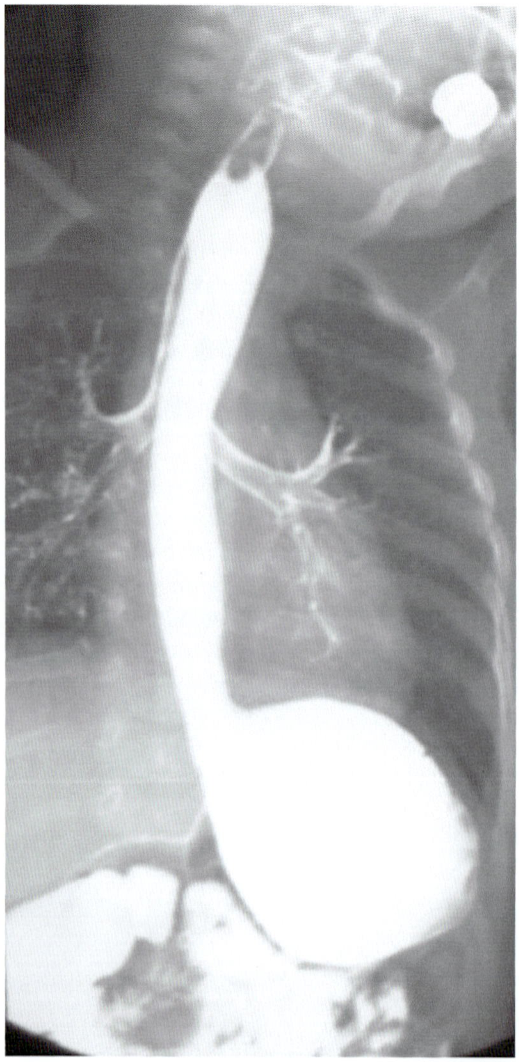

Fig. 2.3 Upper gastrointestinal series: gastroesophageal reflux with massive aspiration

should be ended. There is no indication for tilting the child head down or for performing any other non-physiological reflux- or vomit-inducing maneuvers [3–5].

Although tube *esophagram* has traditionally been the gold standard examination for H-type tracheo-esophageal fistula, a contrast swallow (performed in the correct way) can be sufficient for making the diagnosis. However, a normal contrast swallow does not absolutely rule out the presence of a tracheo-esophageal fistula, and if high clinical concern remains, then a tube esophagram is still indicated.

The tube esophagram (as part of a UGI series) remains the test of choice in those children known to have a risk of aspiration or those being ventilated at the time of the study. UGI series may be performed for no other reason than to reveal an alternative explanation for the child's symptoms, such as significant reflux.

It is worth noting that even a contrast swallow followed by a high-quality tube esophagram does not always demonstrate an occult fistula, and in occasional cases bronchoscopy may also have to be performed. Similarly, bronchoscopy may miss a fistula revealed by a contrast study. The tests are therefore complementary [6].

SBFT and Small Bowel Enema

Both SBFT and small bowel enema examinations are in precipitous, and probably terminal, decline with the advent of VCE, MRI of the bowel, and the use of US in examining the bowel.

The SBFT may still be performed in specific circumstances, including the following: in preparation for elective gut resection for surgical planning, when information regarding small bowel transit is required (such as in pseudo-obstruction and dysmotility states); in suspected subacute obstruction, or obstruction (noting that in adults CT is now routinely used for this indication, but this is not standard practice in pediatrics due to radiation dose concerns); in confirming patency in anticipation of VCE in patients at high risk of stricture (including patients with *Crohn's disease*); in children who cannot tolerate VCE; and to assess complications of inflammatory bowel disease (IBD) if other modalities are not suitable.

The first part of the study is as for a UGI series, and the child can then sit outside the fluoroscopy room for another 20 min. The child should continue to slowly but steadily drink more contrast media during this time to ensure that there is a continuous column of contrast passing through the gut during the study. Serial images are then acquired at appropriate intervals to answer the clinical question [1–5].

2.1.2.2 Contrast Studies of the Lower Gastrointestinal Tract

Imaging of the lower gastrointestinal tract has not changed substantially over recent years, and a water-soluble contrast enema (for neonatal conditions) and, less frequently, a barium enema for older infants and children remain the mainstay of imaging [1–5, 7–11].

Loopograms have an important role in children who have a stoma. Low-density water-soluble contrast media is generally used, with the benefit that as more is instilled it does not become excessively dense and cause technical problems with exposure factors. However, there are a few instances, such as when trying to demonstrate a subtle fistula in an anorectal malformation, in which the limited use of denser water-soluble contrast media may be necessary to achieve sufficient definition. This will largely be at the discretion of the radiologist.

In neonates, enema studies are indicated in cases of bowel obstruction, especially lower intestinal obstruction.

Upper intestinal obstruction in neonates is characterized by bilious vomiting (which frequently occurs after the first feeding) and abdominal distension at clinical examination. Specific common causes of upper intestinal obstruction include atresia of the jejunum or proximal ileum and peritoneal bands. Partial obstruction can be caused by jejunal stenosis, peritoneal bands, duplication cyst, malrotation, and Meckel's diverticulum.

The generic diagnosis of upper intestinal obstruction is usually straightforward at radiography, which demonstrates a few dilated bowel loops, more than would be seen in duodenal atresia and fewer than in ileal atresia or other causes of lower bowel obstruction. There is no gas in the lower portion of the abdomen in jejunal atresia. The patient usually requires no further radiological investigation, although barium enema examinations are still performed in attempts to exclude second and third areas of atresia lower in the bowel. In isolated proximal atresia of the jejunum, the colon is normal in size, because the remaining small bowel distal to the atresia produces sufficient intestinal secretions to produce a normal-caliber colon [1–5].

Lower intestinal obstruction is defined as an obstruction that occurs in the distal ileum or colon. Signs include large bowel obstruction with vomiting, abdominal distension, and failure to pass meconium. The differential diagnosis includes ileal and colonic atresia, meconium ileus or peritonitis, Hirschsprung disease, and functional immaturity of the colon. Anorectal malformations are also an important cause of lower intestinal obstruction, but are almost always evident at physical examination.

The diagnosis of lower intestinal obstruction is usually apparent at abdominal radiography because of the presence of many dilated intestinal loops, but radiographic differentiation between ileal and colonic obstruction is difficult, if not impossible. This distinction can readily be made with a barium enema study, which helps to determine the presence of microcolon (Fig. 2.4), indicates the position of the cecum with regard to possible malrotation, and shows the level of the obstruction in colonic atresia [1–4].

Ileal atresia is an important cause of lower intestinal obstruction. Plain radiographs (AP and LL views) show numerous dilated loops of bowel occupying the entire abdominal cavity and multiple air-fluid levels. When this degree of distension is reached, the mucosal pattern of the small bowel is effaced and it may be impossible to differentiate small bowel from colon. In such a case, a barium enema study is mandatory to determine the presence of a colonic lesion. In ileal atresia, the colon has a normal location but a minute caliber (functional microcolon).

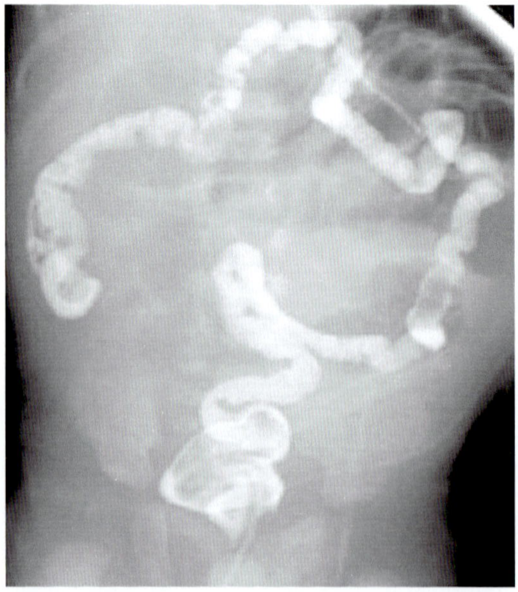

Fig. 2.4 Barium enema study shows severe functional microcolon

Colonic atresia is less common than ileal atresia. It is often indistinguishable from obstruction of the distal ileum, especially when the atresia is located in the ascending colon. The colon proximal to the point of atresia is often massively dilated, and a mottled pattern of gas and feces may be identified. Barium enema examination usually reveals a distal microcolon with obstruction to the retrograde flow of barium at the site of the atresia [2–5, 8].

Meconium ileus is the result of intraluminal obstruction of the colon and lower small bowel, due to the impaction of meconium, and represents the earliest clinical manifestation of cystic fibrosis. Mechanical obstruction occurs when desiccated meconium pellets occlude the distal small bowel and the more proximal small bowel loops are distended with tenacious meconium paste. The abdomen is filled with gas-distended loops and occasionally there is a relative absence of air-fluid levels due to abnormally thick intraluminal meconium. The admixture of gas with meconium may give rise to a soap-bubble appearance similar to the fecal pattern in the colon in older patients.

Contrast enema examination will show a functional microcolon, involving the entire large bowel, and may show impacted meconium pellets, particularly in the right colon or in the distal ileum, caused by retained meconium (Fig. 2.5). Meconium ileus is among the few pediatric conditions for which an enema is used, with high-osmolality water-soluble iodinated contrast, because of its therapeutic effects. Advantage is taken of the high osmotic pressure of the contrast medium: the surrounding tissue is forced to release considerable amounts of fluid, which then flows into the gut and dissolves the inspissated meconium. Therefore, the enema is both diagnostic and therapeutic, and can be followed by the expulsion of meconium during or after the procedure.

Meconium ileus may be complicated by volvulus of a distal intestinal loop, perforation, atresia, or peritonitis [2–4, 8, 9, 12].

Meconium peritonitis is a chemical peritonitis resulting from intrauterine bowel perforation. Common underlying disorders include small bowel atresia, meconium ileus, volvulus, and

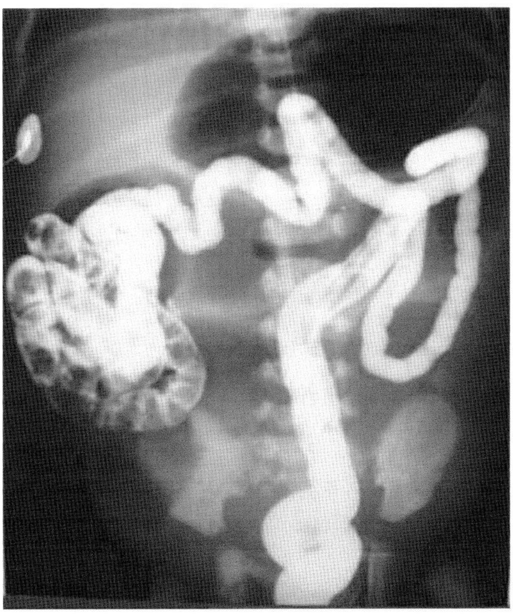

Fig. 2.5 Contrast enema with high-osmolality water-soluble contrast in meconium ileus

intussusception, although some cases are idiopathic. The extruded bowel contents provoke an intense peritoneal inflammatory reaction, leading to the formation of dense fibrotic tissue. This tissue often calcifies, resulting in the characteristic intraperitoneal calcifications identified prior to birth with US and after birth with abdominal radiography and US. The calcifications of meconium peritonitis may extend into the scrotum through a patent vaginal process to produce a calcified mass in the scrotum [2–5, 8, 9, 12].

Hirschsprung disease is a form of lower intestinal obstruction caused by the absence of normal myenteric ganglion cells in a segment of the colon. The aganglionosis varies in length but always extends proximally from the anal canal, and the rectosigmoid area is involved in most cases. Ultrashort segment disease (in which aganglionosis is essentially limited to the region of the internal sphincter) is very rare, as is aganglionosis involving the entire alimentary tract. In children with Hirschsprung disease, the absence of ganglion cells results in the failure of the distal intestine to relax normally. Peristaltic waves do not pass through the aganglionic segment and there is no normal defecation, leading to functional obstruction. Abdominal distension, constipation, and bilious vomiting are the predominant signs and symptoms of obstruction and appear within a few days after birth.

Radiography performed in children with Hirschsprung disease yields findings similar to those in other forms of lower small bowel obstruction: variable gaseous distension of the colon and small bowel, often with air-fluid levels. The colon is usually difficult to identify accurately, and gas is usually absent in the rectum.

Barium enema studies demonstrate patency of the colon, which is short but usually normal in caliber. A transition zone between the narrow and dilated portions of the colon, in the shape of an inverted cone, is the most characteristic radiological finding. When this transition zone is observed, the examination should be discontinued, because filling of the more proximal dilated bowel beyond the transition zone may lead to impaction (Fig. 2.6). However, the distension of

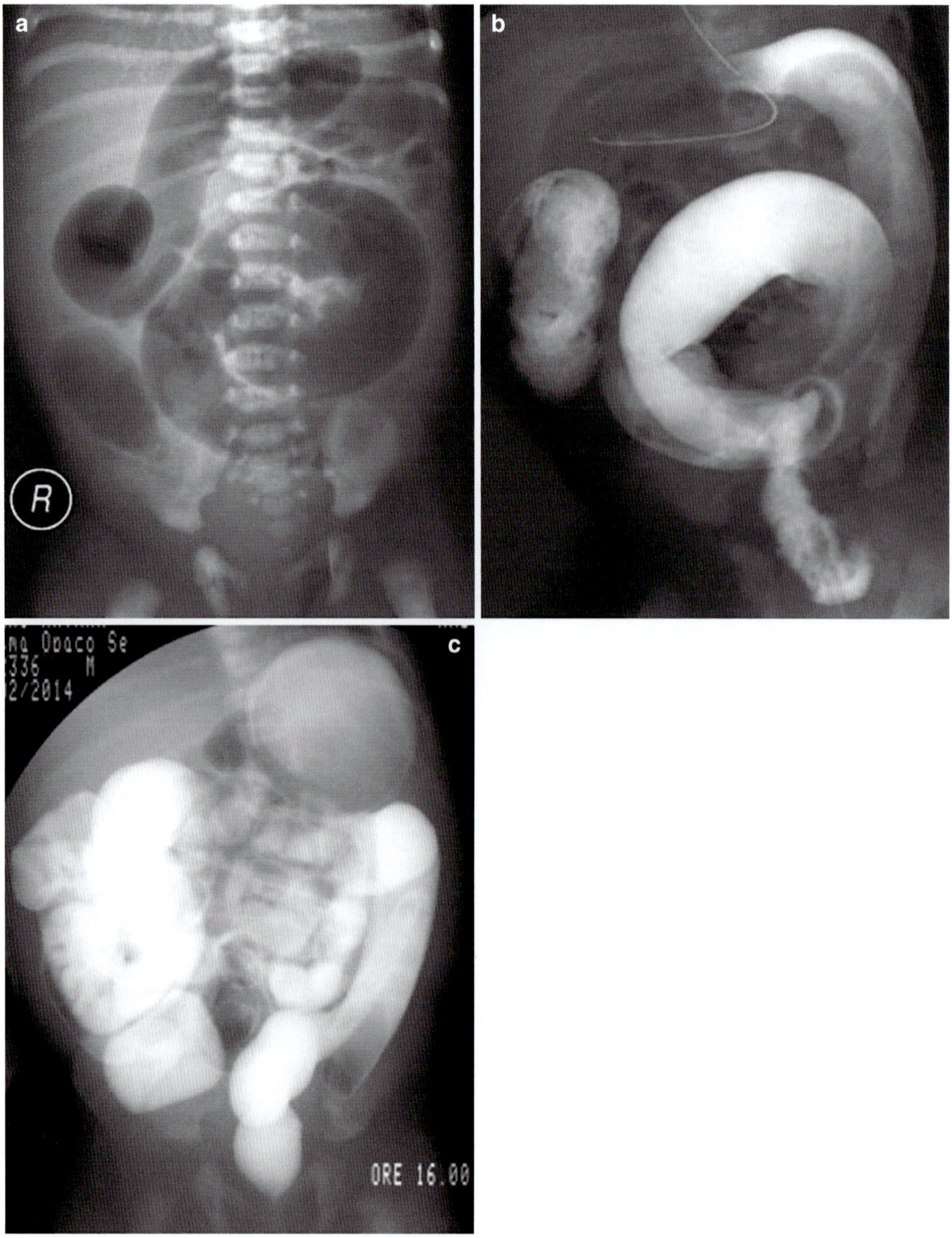

Fig. 2.6 Hirschsprung disease. Plain abdominal radiograph (**a**) and barium enema (**b**, **c**). Note in **c** the ascent of the contrast to the stomach in the late study, due to complete aganglionosis

the bowel proximal to the segment of deficient innervation is gradual, and a transition zone is seen in only 50% of neonates with Hirschsprung disease during the first week of life. Abnormal contractions and irregular peristaltic activity of the aganglionic portion of the colon may be useful indicators of the disease, although they are nonspecific findings that are also seen in colitis.

Twelve-hour-delayed postevacuation images are useful in dubious cases.

The radiological diagnosis of total colonic aganglionosis is difficult. Findings at barium enema examination may be normal or may include a short colon of normal caliber, microcolon, or a transition zone in the ileum [2–4, 10, 11].

Functional immaturity of the colon is a common cause of neonatal obstruction, particularly in premature neonates and in those whose mothers were treated during labor with magnesium preparations or sedatives; the condition also occurs in neonates with diabetic mothers. The condition has also been encountered in children with septicemia, hypothyroidism, or hypoglycemia. Functional immaturity of the colon comprises several entities, most notably small left colon syndrome and meconium plug syndrome. Affected patients have abdominal distension, difficulty in initiating evacuation, and sometimes vomiting; typically, however, the bowel distension is less severe than that seen with an organic obstruction. The condition is both diagnosed and treated with a contrast enema.

In *small left colon syndrome*, barium enema examination demonstrates a distended right and transverse colon with a transition to a very small-diameter descending and rectosigmoid colon near the splenic flexure. The rectum is usually quite distensible.

In *meconium plug syndrome*, barium enema examination with high-osmolality water-soluble contrast shows a small caliber of the left colon with a large meconium plug. The rectum is usually normal in size, unlike findings in Hirschsprung disease. The enema can be both diagnostic and therapeutic and is usually accompanied by the passage of meconium during or after the procedure [10, 11].

Typically, there is clinical improvement following the enema, and over the course of hours to days the radiographic and clinical signs of obstruction subside.

In older children the main indication for a barium enema is intestinal intussusception, with the enema used exclusively for therapeutic purposes, since the diagnosis is made by sonography.

The role of the enema in reducing intestinal intussusception is well known and recognized, but in the literature there are many differing reports about the contrast medium to be used; namely, air or liquid. An air enema is considered to be better at reduction, cleaner (appearance of peritoneal cavity at surgery when perforation occurs), safer, and faster, with less radiation when compared with a liquid enema. Reported perforation rates are not significantly different. The recurrence rates for air versus liquid enema reductions do not differ (approximately 10%). However, while the air enema may be preferred in experienced hands, the liquid enema is also safe and effective. Barium is no longer the liquid contrast medium of choice, due to the risk of barium peritonitis, infection, and adhesions when perforation occurs during the enema procedure. Neither sedation nor medications increase the enema success rate. More recent reports of air enema intussusception reduction show better results than liquid enema intussusception reduction. The air enema may use higher intraluminal pressure, which results in a higher reduction rate.

To avoid ionizing radiation exposure to children, the use of US with either water or air reduction techniques has been reported, showing intussusception reduction rates equivalent to those using *fluoroscopy*.

The use of delayed attempts (reports vary between 30 min and 1 day) after the initial attempt have shown further success in enema reductions of intussusceptions. Delayed enema should not be performed if the child is clinically unstable or if the initial enema does not partially reduce the intussusception.

The most important potential complication of enema use is bowel perforation (the mean perforation rate was 0.8%). There are no statistically significant differences between air and liquid enema perforation rates. This risk depends on each radiologist's patient population and technique, as well as on the duration of symptoms. Because of this small but real risk of barium peritonitis, infection, and adhesions when perforation occurs during the enema procedure, iodinated contrast is preferred over barium when using liquid enema reduction.

Children with evidence of peritonitis, shock, sepsis, or free air on abdominal radiographs are not candidates for enema use [4, 5].

2.1.3 Ultrasound (US)

Ultrasound (US) is an excellent imaging modality for the evaluation of the gastrointestinal tract in pediatric patients, so that it is now considered as an extension of the clinical evaluation, both in emergency conditions and for elective studies [13, 14].

In addition to the well established primary role of US in specific diseases, such as in hypertrophic pyloric stenosis and intestinal intussusception, the diagnostic reliability of US has been widely demonstrated in many other pathological conditions, such as in acute *appendicitis*, chronic intestinal inflammatory diseases (IBD), necrotizing enterocolitis (NEC), gastro-esophageal reflux, neonatal intestinal obstruction, intestinal malrotation, and acute volvulus in intestinal malrotation. Furthermore, US is successfully used even in less conventional applications, such as in esophageal atresia and anorectal malformations.

The well known advantages of US, particularly its lack of ionizing radiation and easy access, makes this imaging technique an ideal one for the evaluation of the pediatric patient with gastrointestinal tract diseases. Major drawbacks include its operator-dependency and reproducibility, apart from factors related to the patient, such as non-collaboration, obesity, and the interposition of a large amount of gas. Most of these limitations can be overcome with a comprehensive, careful, and dedicated examination technique using modern US capabilities.

US is also an excellent bedside high-yield imaging tool in intensive care units and it can also be used to guide therapeutic maneuvers, such as in the reduction of intussusception or in enema for meconium ileus.

In the past few decades, advances in US technology have greatly improved the quality of gastrointestinal US imaging, with a consequent positive impact on its diagnostic yield. Improvements in US probes, particularly high-resolution linear probes, permit better spatial resolution and better penetration in the far field, whereas improvements in contrast resolution can now be achieved with recent US modes such as image compounding, speckle/noise reduction filters, and (tissue) harmonic imaging.

Likewise, progress in Doppler techniques allows better depiction and quantification of even the slow flow of small vessels within normal and pathological gastrointestinal structures.

For any US examination the choice of adequate transducers, adjustment of basic parameters, and the choice of US modality is fundamental to obtain a proper image quality.

In general, the optimal transducer must have the highest possible frequency that is still able to penetrate the anatomical area of interest, providing the best spatial resolution.

The initial evaluation of the entire abdominal cavity is performed with a curved array transducer; then the individual structures of the gastrointestinal tract are specifically examined with a *high-resolution linear probe*, which allows detailed visualization of the esophageal wall, gastric wall, and bowel wall, as well as detailed visualization of the relevant surrounding structures. Not infrequently, curved array probes may also be needed in order to obtain a better access window to image deeper structures in older children (e.g., the esophago-gastric junction, the sigmoid colon, and the rectum) or to allow for a broader field of view.

In addition to the conventional trans-abdominal approach, other less common types of approaches might be necessary, and should be included in specific disease conditions, such as the suprasternal and mediastinal US approach to visualize the upper esophagus in tracheo-esophageal atresia or the *perineal US* approach to evaluate the anal canal or the distal rectal pouch location and its distance to the skin surface in anorectal or in cloacal malformations.

A well known limitation of US examinations is bowel gas interposition, but with a careful and proper bowel US technique this obstacle can often be partially overcome. Gentle graded compression is the essential technique in US of the gastrointestinal tract, as it displaces undesirable gas, shortens the distance to the skin surface, and isolates the bowel loops, while displacing adjacent ones. Furthermore, it helps to localize the origin of pain ("sonopalpation") and to assess the bowel compressibility.

In small patients and particularly in critically ill neonates, SBFT can be performed and followed by US.

Filling techniques are the basis for therapeutic maneuvers under US guidance, such as in the nonsurgical reduction of an ileo-colic intussusception or in the attempt to resolve meconium ileus.

2.1.3.1 Upper Gastrointestinal Tract US

In neonates *esophageal atresia* is usually diagnosed with frontal and lateral radiograms, but US can provide additional precious information to the surgeon. Besides the role of abdominal and cardiac US in searching for associated abnormalities, mediastinal US allows the characterization of the length, morphology, and structure of the wall in a blind upper esophageal pouch; this condition can be improved by the administration of a small amount of saline fluid through the esophageal tube. Rarely, even a tracheo-esophageal fistula may be recognized by US [13].

With a superior abdominal US approach, the cardia and the adjacent distal esophagus are often easily depicted, although visualization of the entire distal esophageal length behind the heart is difficult and restricted.

In neonates and infants with suspected *gastroesophageal reflux disease (GERD)*, US is a widely available, non-invasive, and sensitive method that can provide useful anatomical and functional information, although its role in GERD is still controversial and debated. The complex issue of GER and GERD is related to many factors, including the nonspecific nature of symptoms in young children, the difficult distinction between physiological and pathological GER, and the impasse in establishing a cause-effect relationship between GER and symptoms or complications related to GERD.

Nevertheless, US is considered by many authors as the primary non-invasive imaging tool in a child with vomiting, particularly in patients younger than 2 years of age, as it can provide alternative diagnoses other than GER and rule out gastric outlet obstruction.

More important than the US detection of GER, per se, is the fact that one can correlate the US findings with the occurrence of clinical symptoms. Furthermore, US can provide information on functional aspects such as the esophageal clearance of the refluxed gastric content, the opening of the gastroesophageal junction (GEJ), and gastric emptying, and US can potentially detect an associated hiatal hernia. Anatomical details of the gastroesophageal structure, such as the length of the abdominal esophagus and the gastroesophageal angle (angle of His), can be assessed, and these features seem to have high sensitivity and high positive predictive value for GER.

US is generally considered the modality of choice to confirm or exclude the diagnosis of *hypertrophic pyloric stenosis (HPS),* as both the lumen and the surrounding musculature are directly visualized [15–17]. The diagnosis of HPS is based on US morphological and dynamic findings: the most significant criteria are a thickened pyloric muscle (greater than 3 mm), a pyloric length greater than 18 mm, and the lack of luminal opening of the pyloric channel (Fig. 2.7). The usually distended stomach, seen as an indirect sign of gastric outlet obstruction, must be interpreted according to the time of the last meal. Changing the patient position may be necessary to improve visualization of the pyloric channel hidden by a distended stomach.

It is also important to evaluate the pyloric canal over time, to differentiate HPS from pylorospasm, a transient phenomenon that can have morphological features and measurements simi-

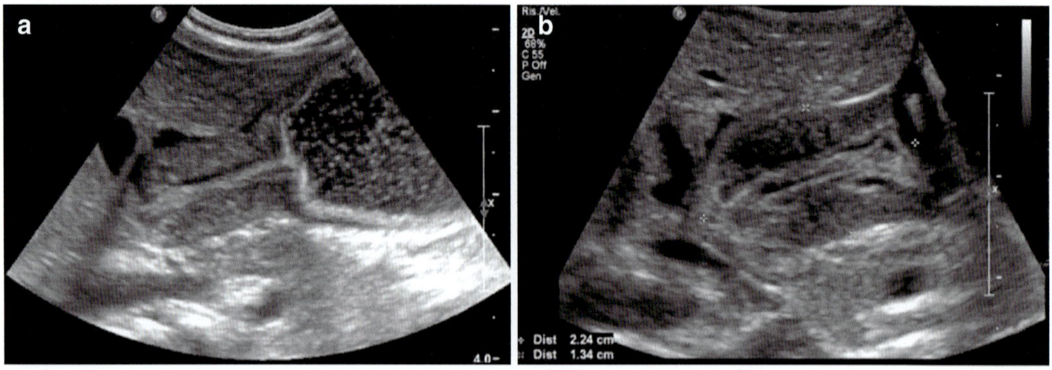

Fig. 2.7 (**a**, **b**) Hypertrophic pyloric stenosis. Ultrasound (US) study (**a**, **b**) shows a thickened pyloric muscle (greater than 3 mm), increase of pyloric length (greater than 18 mm), and distended stomach due to the lack of luminal opening of the pyloric channel

lar to those of HPS. In doubtful cases a repeated US after some time can clarify the diagnosis.

Gastric duplication cysts are usually easily recognized when they have the classic US appearance of localized fluid formations with a thick layered wall. Gastric emptying may be used to highlight the close relationship of the cyst with the gastric wall [18].

Other gastric pathologies can be suspected in abdominal US examinations performed in a child with vomiting, epigastric pain, or other nonspecific abdominal discomfort. Such pathologies may be a cause of focal or diffuse thickening of the stomach wall (e.g., eosinophilic gastritis, chronic granulomatous disease, tumoral diseases such as polyps and lymphoma), but also of intraluminal anomalies (e.g., bezoar, ingested foreign bodies).

After the US evaluation of the esophageal-gastric junction, stomach, and pylorus, the next step is to follow the duodenum to check the third duodenal portion, which normally passes between the abdominal aorta and the superior mesenteric artery; the normal position of the duodenojejunal junction can also be identified, on the left side of the aorta.

2.1.3.2 Small and Large Bowel US

US can also be used to recognize *intestinal malrotations* [12, 19–22]. The diagnosis of these abnormalities has been modified in the past few years. Barium enema and radiographic study of the upper gastrointestinal tract has been used to evaluate the duodenum morphology, duodenal-jejunum junction position, and cecum position, and this study is still considered the standard criterion. Actually, in addition to these invasive examinations that use X-rays, US examination with color Doppler is used to identify intestinal anomalies of rotation and fixation. The best known US finding is an abnormal relationship between the superior mesenteric artery (SMA) and the superior mesenteric vein (SMV), although a normal position does not exclude the presence of abnormal midgut rotation. In addition, the normal position of the third duodenal portion is believed to be a more reliable marker than the position of the mesenteric vessels to exclude intestinal malrotation (Fig. 2.8).

The finding of an abnormal relationship between the SMA and the SMV may be demonstrated either incidentally or on specific examination. The SMA/SMV relationship should be considered part of abdominal US screening in infants and children with abdominal pain or in asymptomatic pediatric patients to prevent future obstructive or ischemic complications.

Midgut volvulus is the most frequent cause of acute abdomen in newborns, and it is a common consequence of intestinal malrotation. However, it can affect children also. It is a life-threatening emergency; early diagnosis is important in this disease, to avoid the risk of intestinal infarct and necrosis. If not promptly diagnosed and treated, midgut volvulus leads to death or a lifelong

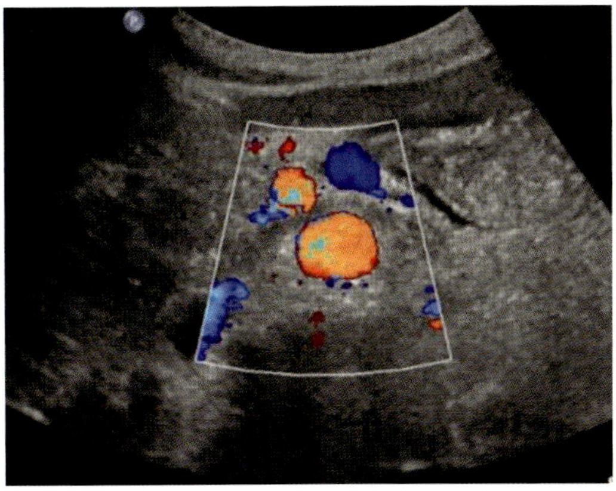

Fig. 2.8 Intestinal malrotation. US study shows abnormal relationship between the superior mesenteric artery and superior mesenteric vein, the latter seen to the left of the artery

dependence on total parenteral nutrition in survivors with short bowel syndrome.

Therefore, learning to recognize the US findings of midgut volvulus is imperative: the volvulus is responsible for a whirlpool-like appearance on cross-sectional images, created when the SMV and the mesentery wrap around the SMA in a clockwise direction. Visualization is enhanced by the vascular signal on color Doppler flow US [23–25] (Fig. 2.9).

For the neonate with the classic appearance of a whirlpool sign, additional imaging investigation is often unnecessary, and the surgeon should be alerted to plan for emergency surgery. The advantages of US for this age group are apparent, since it can be performed at the bedside in intensive care units and lacks the adverse effects of ionizing radiation.

The diagnosis of *neonatal bowel obstruction* or the confirmation of the prenatal diagnosis is based on clinical and radiological signs on a plain abdominal radiograph, occurring with a delay of 12–24 h; in very distal obstruction the signs may appear even later.

US can contribute to the diagnosis of neonatal bowel obstruction with important additional information; first of all, it can document the obstruction, showing severe distension of the proximal bowel loops (diameter from 16 to 40 mm) with thin walls and increased peristalsis, filled with fluid, and punctuated with echodense particles of gas. The distal bowel is small in size (3–4 mm) with echodense or target-like meconial content [19].

Furthermore, US allows the assessment of colon size and its content, a main marker to suggest the probable location of the obstruction, thus indicating the need to perform a contrast enema in case of lower bowel obstruction. The colon is of normal caliber (9–14 mm) in very proximal small bowel atresia, while microcolon (3–5 mm) is easily recognized in distal small bowel atresia and in meconium ileus. In meconium ileus, severe microcolon is present, but the small bowel is less dilated and less peristaltic than in other small bowel atresias. The most important finding is the characteristic appearance of the dilated bowel loops, which contain abnormal meconium: the thick meconium sticks to the bowel walls, resulting in a pseudo-thickening. The distal bowel loops, in the right lower quadrant, are small (3–4 mm), with a target-like appearance due to impacted meconial pellets.

Hydrocolon is present in *meconium plug syndrome* and *small left colon syndrome* [2, 3, 19].

Besides being observed in small bowel obstruction, hepatic, splenic, scrotal, and peritoneal calcifications are observed in *meconium peritonitis* with single or multiple meconium pseudo-cysts and free intraperitoneal fluid [2, 3, 7, 8].

Occasionally US study highlights the cause of obstruction, either intrinsic (e.g., duodenal web) or extrinsic (e.g., gastrointestinal duplication cyst or annular pancreas).

In *anorectal malformations*, the distance between the rectal cul-de-sac and the perineum can be reliably measured with perineal US [13, 26, 27]. Furthermore, US study can show associated genito-urinary tract and dysraphic abnormalities; therefore, all patients with congenital anorectal malformations should have a genito-renal tract and spinal US examination as a screening test in the early newborn period (Fig. 2.10).

US is still not routinely used for the diagnosis and follow up of *NEC*, but it can provide information that is not provided by plain abdominal radiography and that may affect the management of NEC. Like radiography, US can depict intramural gas, portal venous gas, and free intraperito-

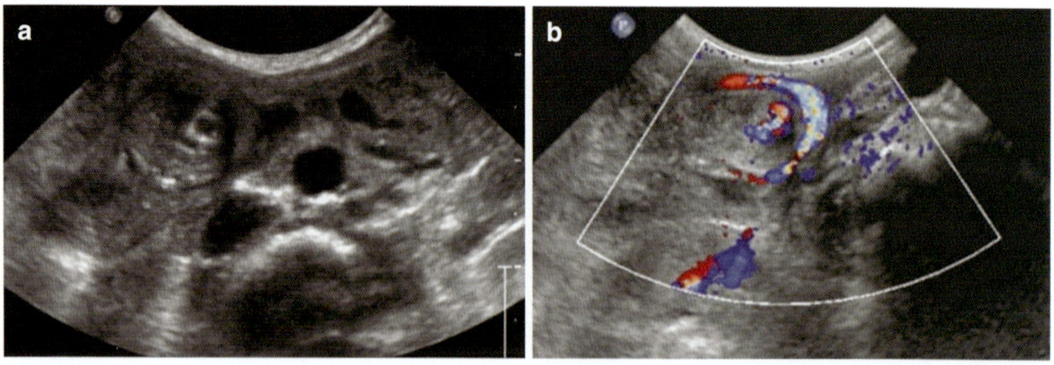

Fig. 2.9 US study (**a**) with color Doppler (**b**) showing the whirlpool sign, with the superior mesenteric vein and mesentery wrapped around the superior mesenteric artery in a clockwise direction

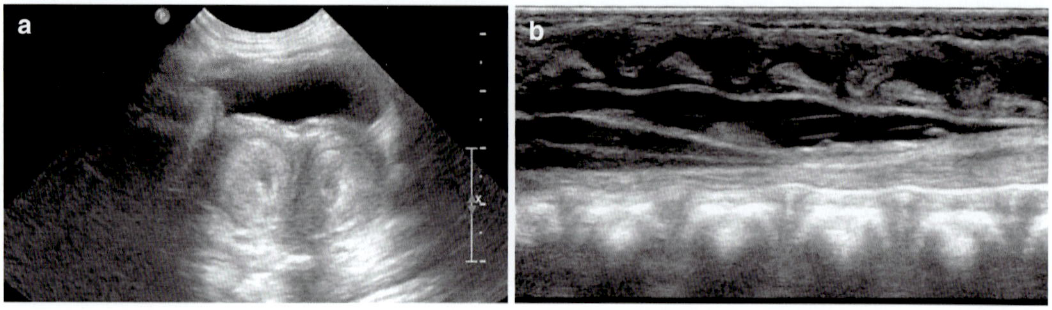

Fig. 2.10 Anorectal malformations. US of genital tract shows an associated didelphys uterus (**a**), while normal anatomy of the spinal cord on US spinal study (**b**) rules out occult myelodysplasia

neal gas; however, the main advantage of abdominal US over plain abdominal radiography, including color Doppler US, is that abdominal US can show intraabdominal fluid, bowel wall thickness, and bowel wall perfusion [28–31].

In NEC, the ability to depict abdominal fluid is the first major advantage of US study over plain abdominal radiography, showing whether the fluid is intraluminal or extraluminal and whether it is free in the peritoneal cavity or is a more localized fluid collection.

The second major advantage of abdominal US in NEC is its ability to visualize the bowel wall directly and to assess bowel wall thickness, echogenicity, and peristalsis.

With both bowel wall thickening and thinning the normal echogenicity of the wall (so-called gut signature) is lost and it may be difficult to differentiate the bowel wall from the echogenic intraluminal content in severely affected loops. Bowel wall thickening is accompanied by increased echogenicity of the full wall thickness; however, this is a nonspecific sign, as it is also seen in other causes of diffuse edema in the absence of inflammation or ischemia.

The third major advantage of abdominal US, including color Doppler, in NEC is the ability to directly assess arterial perfusion of the bowel wall, to infer the viability of individual loops.

Three categories of flow are recognized on color Doppler: normal, increased, and absent. The hyperemia is the result of the vasodilation of mural and mesenteric vessels secondary to intestinal inflammation, with specific flow patterns ("zebra" pattern, "Y" pattern, and "ring" pattern).

Flow is absent when no color Doppler signals are identified in the bowel wall.

Thinning of the bowel wall and lack of perfusion are highly suggestive of non-viable bowel and may be seen before visualization of pneumoperitoneum on plain abdominal radiography. As mortality is higher after perforation, earlier detection of severely ischemic or necrotic loops, before perforation occurs, could reduce morbidity and mortality in NEC (Fig. 2.11).

US is the modality of choice to accurately diagnose or exclude *intestinal intussusception*, determining the location (ileo-ileal or ileo-colic) and the type (idiopathic or secondary to the presence of a lead point), with a decisive impact on the therapeutic approach [13].

Typical signs of intussusception are the "target" and the "pseudo-kidney" signs, respectively, on transverse and longitudinal planes. A small amount of intraperitoneal free fluid can often be seen and should not preclude a non-surgical reduction attempt. The lower success rates of non-surgical reductions are related to the presence of trapped fluid within the intussusception and the absence of flow on color Doppler in the intussusception wall, indicative of vascular impairment of the bowel (Fig. 2.12). When these signs are present enema reduction should be performed with extreme caution, due to the high risk of perforation.

Small bowel intussusceptions, in contrast to intussusceptions of the large bowel, are transient, asymptomatic, and relatively common. They are usually encountered around the periumbilical region, are small in diameter (less than 2 cm), and tend to resolve spontaneously within a few minutes.

The diagnostic role of US in *IBD* in children, and particularly in Crohn's disease, continues to increase, as it has several advantages over other imaging techniques. Abdominal US is easily performed, readily available, and less expensive than other imaging modalities, and obviously it does not use ionizing radiation; the fact that ionizing radiation is not used is essential in pediatric patients with IBD, who are at higher risk of increased diagnostic radiation exposure than the general population, owing to repetitive imaging. Unlike with MRI, sedation, oral contrast, or bowel cleansing are not required with US.

Most published studies have found bowel US to be a valuable tool in children with suspected or known IBD [32–35]. Bowel wall thickening is the hallmark of intestinal disease: in the pediatric age group, thicknesses greater than 2.5 mm and 2 mm, respectively, for the small and the large bowel are considered abnormal. A careful and attentive US examination also reveals the location and extension of the involved segments, their vascular features on color Doppler, and the extramural signs of disease, such as hyperechogenicity of the surrounding fat planes, regional lymphadenopathy, abscesses, and fistulas; abnormal wall stratification and abnormal peristalsis can also be noted (Fig. 2.13).

The correlation of these findings with the clinical history and the laboratory data often permits us to narrow the differential diagnosis, thus directing further additional imaging.

Another important application of US in IBD is in the follow-up of patients with known disease to monitor treatment and to ensure early detection of intra-abdominal complications in relapse.

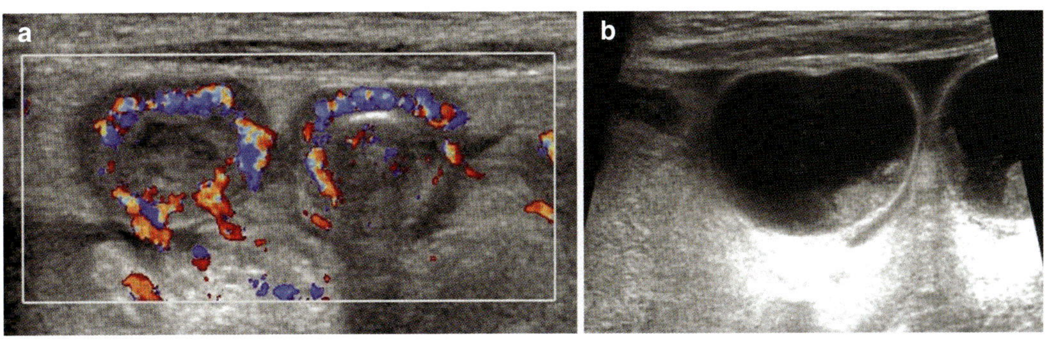

Fig. 2.11 Necrotizing enterocolitis (NEC). Color Doppler sonography (**a**) shows two loops with a thickened bowel wall and ring pattern with increased perfusion. Thinning bowel walls (**b**) are seen in a patient with a poor outcome

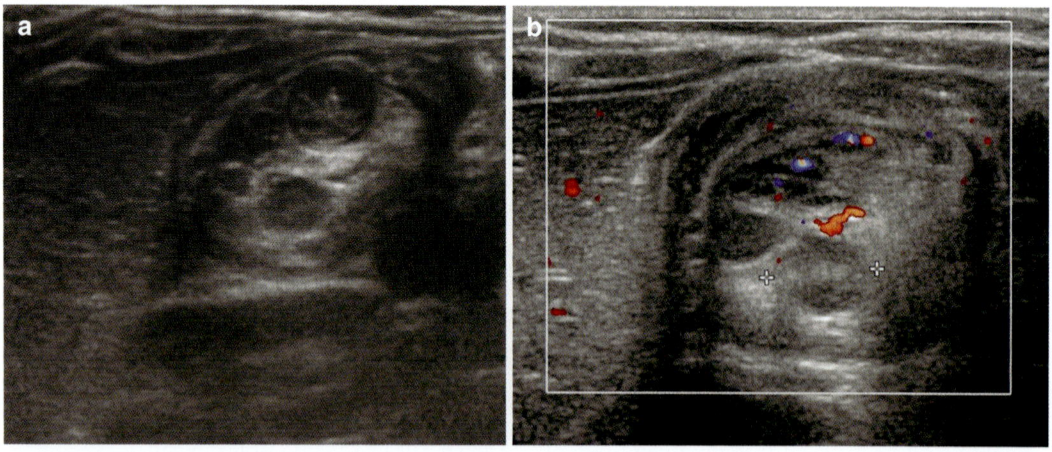

Fig. 2.12 US study with color Doppler. Intestinal intussusception with target appearance on tranverse plane. Note the presence of lymph nodes within the intussusception (**a**), with preserved vascular signal of the loop on color Doppler US (**b**)

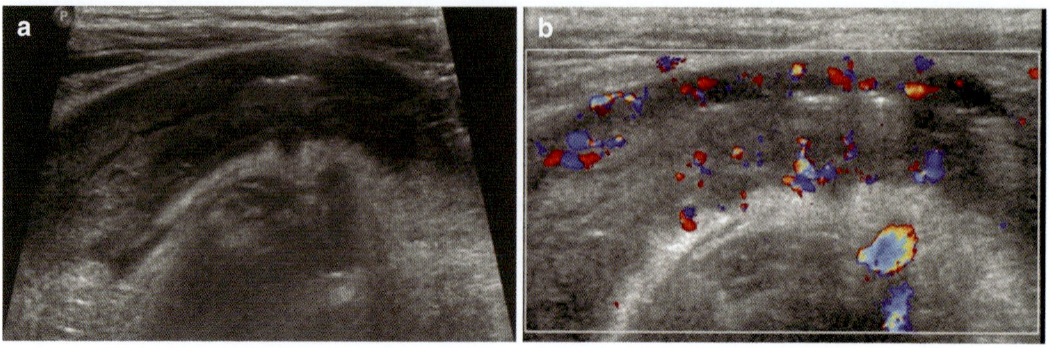

Fig. 2.13 Crohn's disease: bowel wall thickening with narrowed lumen (**a**) and hyperemia on color Doppler (**b**) of the terminal ileum

Color Doppler US provides additional information about disease activity and it may help to distinguish between inflammatory and fibrotic bowel stenosis.

Appendicitis is the most common pediatric surgical emergency. US often provides a reliable contribution to the diagnosis by supporting or excluding appendicitis; it is helpful in the differential diagnosis, thus avoiding unnecessary radiation exposure when imaging is needed.

Typical signs of appendicitis include an aperistaltic, noncompressible, dilated appendix (outer diameter greater than 6 mm) and white target appearance in axial section, sometimes with appendicolith; other secondary changes include echogenic prominent pericecal fat and peri-appendicular free fluid and/or fluid collection. On color Doppler US, increased vascularity of the appendicular wall is observed in early inflammatory phases, whereas no flow can be detected if the appendix is necrotic or perforated.

Imaging is not necessary in every child suspected of having appendicitis, particularly in boys with a clear clinical picture. Conversely, US is especially valuable in girls, in whom ovarian conditions must be considered in the differential diagnosis, which is difficult to achieve clinically.

Mesenteric lymphadenitis is a self-limiting disorder showing inflammation of mesenteric lymph nodes, caused by various types of bacteria, mycobacteria, and viruses. It is a common cause of abdominal pain in children, sometimes mimicking acute appendicitis. It should be noted that some mesenteric lymph nodes are commonly seen on abdominal US in pediatric patients, even in those who are asymptomatic, and the nodes are not necessarily related to any pathological process.

Except for lymphoma, tumors of the small and large colon are rare in children. The most frequent subtype of non-Hodgkin lymphoma occurring in children is *Burkitt's lymphoma*, and it frequently affects the gastrointestinal tract, most commonly the ileocecal region and mesentery.

Burkitt's lymphoma has a rapid growth and can present with intestinal obstruction owing to secondary intussusception. On US it is seen as a mass with low or heterogeneous echogenicity, with low vascularity on color Doppler.

Several other diseases may first come to attention during an abdominal US examination, including intraluminal conditions, such as polyps or abnormal content (such as in cystic fibrosis); bowel wall involvement in various inflammatory (e.g., benign lymphoid hyperplasia), infectious (e.g., viral or bacterial enterocolitis), infiltrative, and hematological (e.g. Henoch-Schonlein purpura, graft versus host disease, neutropenic colitis) conditions; or traumatic disorders. US may also disclose other conditions, such as hernias, Meckel's diverticulum, duplication cysts, and other tumor and tumor-like conditions.

2.1.4 Magnetic Resonance Imaging (MRI)

Gastrointestinal study is a relatively recent *MRI* application. For several years, in fact, the long acquisition times have limited the use of MRI in the abdominal area, in which the study of structures with peristalsis led to low-quality diagnostic images because of the presence of motion artifacts. The continuous technological development of MRI, with a coil system gradient that currently allows us to capture images more quickly, is best suited to gastrointestinal study [35]; however, the duration of the investigation is still likely to require sedation in young children and/or in those who are non-cooperative.

The primary characteristic of MRI must also be emphasized – this is the obtaining of multiplanar images with high-resolution tissue contrast, without the use of *ionizing radiation*.

MRI for the study of the gastrointestinal tract sees continuous innovations, but the clinical indications are not always well defined. From this point of view, the study of certain diseases of the bowel, in particular chronic inflammatory diseases, can be carried out with MRI, with its diagnostic performance already established in the literature, while MRI studies of the esophagus, stomach, and colon are currently considered to be experimental [36] (Fig. 2.14).

MRI imaging is now used for the study of extraluminal pathologies and for the study of oncological diseases.

The use of MRI in the study of *anorectal abnormalities* deserves special mention, particularly in the preoperative evaluation of the newborn or infant prior to definitive pull-through repair surgery, and in the postoperative review of the older pediatric patient with continuing problems [27, 37]. Furthermore, when the radiographic or US examination is abnormal, MRI can be used also to accurately depict the likely associated intraspinal pathology, such as tethered cord, caudal regression syndrome, hydromyelia, or a lipoma of the terminal filum.

Examination during sedation or spontaneous sleep may provide more accurate estimation of the true level of an elevator sling.

MRI allows direct visualization of the distal rectum and related musculature (levator ani muscle, puborectal muscle, external sphincter) without additional ionizing radiation, but with multiplanar capabilities (Fig. 2.15). Associated lesions such as *sacrococcygeal hypoplasia* and lumbar spine or renal anomalies can be evaluated [27, 39].

2.1.4.1 Entero-MRI

MRI has good sensitivity and specificity for *IBD* in children. It is used to study the entire intestine, especially the small intestine, which still remains largely out of the range of the endoscope (Fig. 2.16).

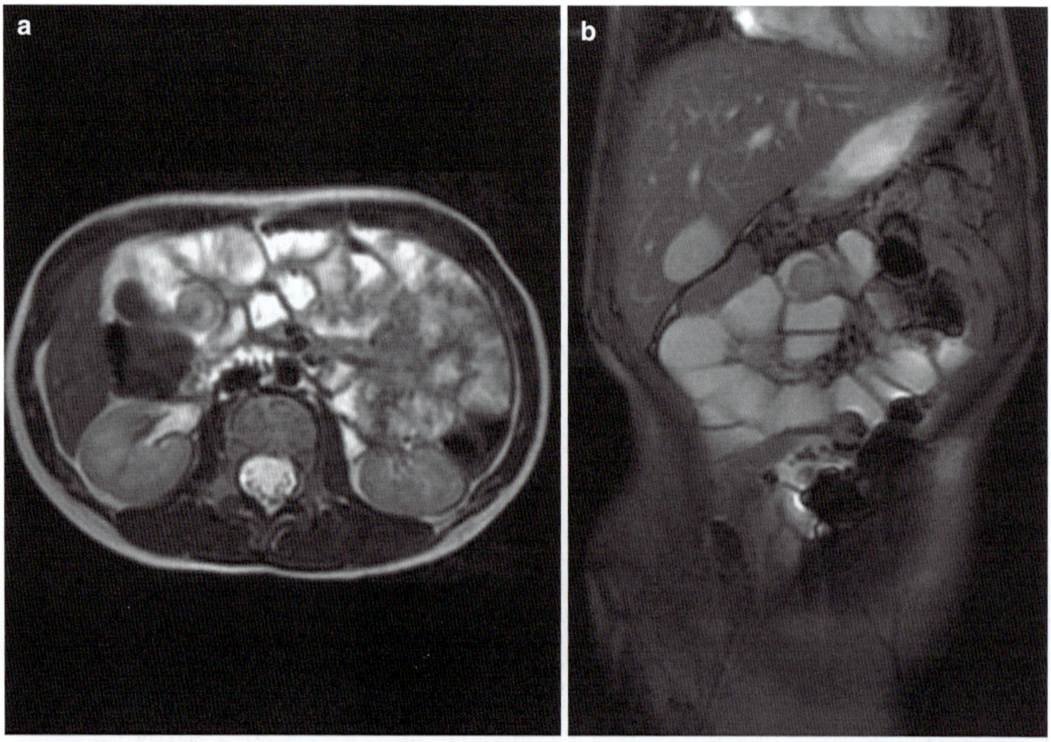

Fig. 2.14 Magnetic resonance imaging (MRI): axial T2-weighted image (**a**) and coronal T2-weighted image (**b**) show an ileal intraluminal filling defect (polypoid mass)

The survey preparation includes fasting from the night before the study in larger children, and exclusive intake of clear liquids on the day of the examination.

Entero-MRI also requires adequate bowel distension, obtained through the oral administration of contrast medium. The contrast medium used may be negative, positive, or biphasic. Biphasic media are preferred for better visualization of the bowel wall; they consist of aqueous solutions containing isoosmolar substances (polyethylene glycol) that possess the same intensity as the water signal, providing a high signal on T2-weighted sequences and a low signal on T1-weighted sequences. These characteristics make such media ideal in a digestive study, creating ideal conditions for contrast resolution between the lumen and wall. Positive contrast media, which were those used in the past, have poor contrast resolution, and negative media are used for a better definition of the wall signal.

The first acquisitions are possible after approximately 45 min from initiation of the contrast agent [40, 38].

Pharmacologically-induced hypotonia (with intravenous injection of hyoscine butylbromide) is performed to reduce possible artifacts from the intestinal peristalsis and prolong the relaxation time of the small bowel.

The use of MRI in the study of *anorectal abnormalities* deserves special mention, particularly in the preoperative evaluation of the newborn or infant prior to definitive pull-through repair surgery, and in the postoperative review of the older pediatric patient with continuing problems [27, 37]. When the radiographic or US examination is abnormal, then MRI can be used to accurately depict the likely associated intraspinal pathology, such as tethered cord, caudal regression syndrome,

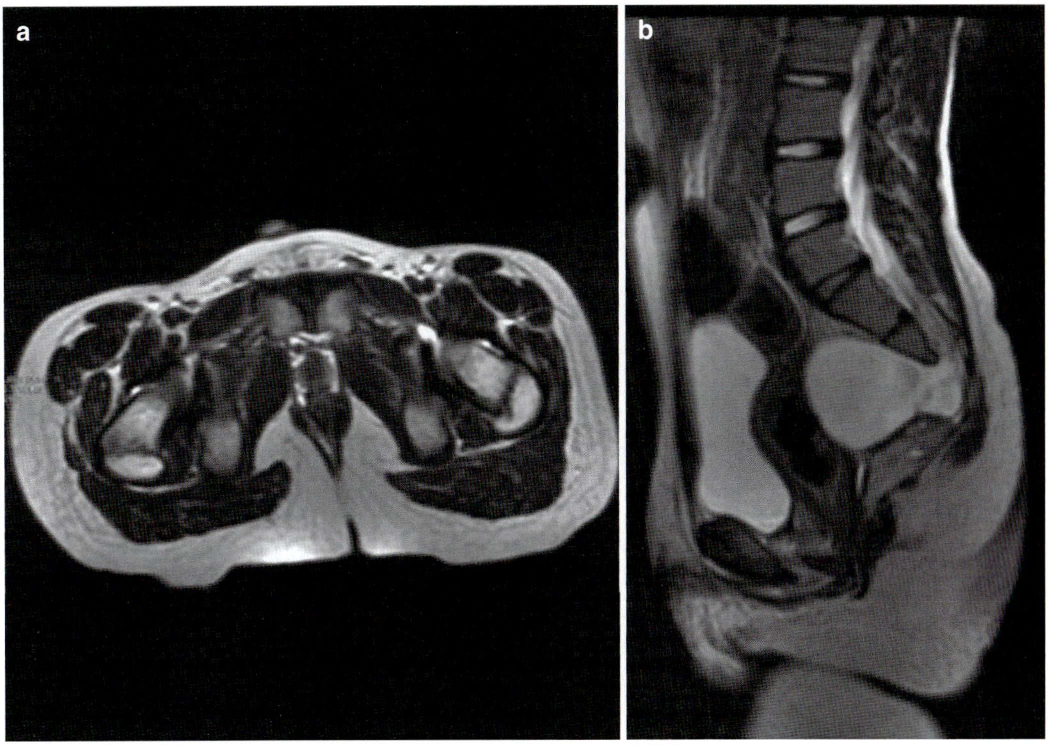

Fig. 2.15 Axial (**a**) and sagittal (**b**) T2-weighted MRI: postsurgical evaluation. Axial image shows *left-sided* puborectalis muscle that appears as a triangle with the apex directed posteriorly. Sagittal T2-weighted image (**b**) shows the presence of an associated sacral anterior meningocele

hydromyelia, or a lipoma of the terminal filum. Examination during sedation or spontaneous sleep may provide more accurate estimation of the true level of an elevator sling. MRI allows direct visualization of the distal rectum and related musculature (levator ani muscle, puborectal muscle, external sphincter) without additional ionizing radiation, but with multiplanar capabilities (Fig. 2.16). Associated lesions such as *sacrococcygeal hypoplasia* and lumbar spine or renal anomalies can be evaluated [27, 38].

The administration of paramagnetic contrast material by injection allows for proper evaluation of the intestinal walls; the enhancement following injection of the contrast agent provides information on the activity of the disease and indicates whether there is any hypervascularization of the intestinal wall, as well as helping to distinguish inflammatory processes by showing fibrotic aspects of thickened walls. The administration of paramagnetic contrast material with MRI can provide information about the wall thickness and the presence of fixed bowel loops, and can detect superficial mucosal abnormalities, creases and ulcerations, abnormal wall morphology, and extraluminal abnormalities (lymphadenopathy, increased mesenteric vasculature, abscesses, and fistulas) [37, 40].

2.1.5 Computed Tomography (CT)

CT investigation involves high doses of ionizing radiation, and in young patients it is therefore reserved for cases in which it can be valuable for diagnostic and therapeutic purposes and for management, taking into account the *ALARA (As Low As Reasonably Achievable) principle*, according to which the administration of the lowest possible radiation dose for the diagnostic purpose is planned.

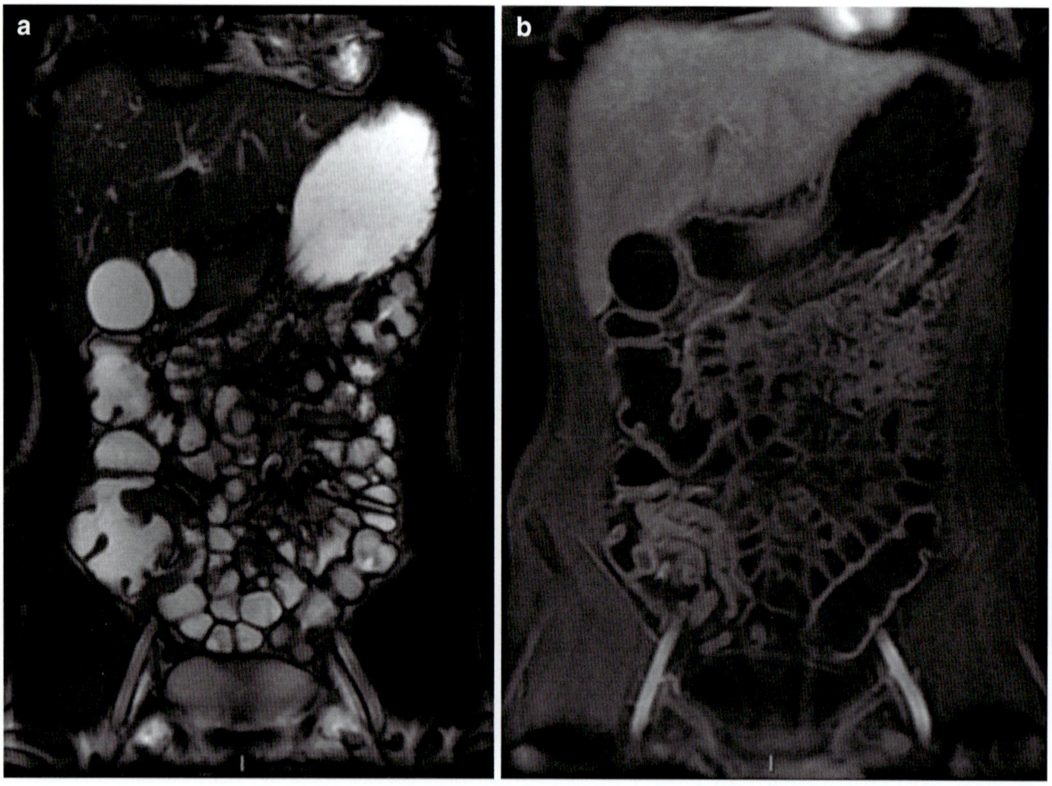

Fig. 2.16 Coronal MRI: T2-weighted dynamic FIESTA (**a**) and T1-weighted post-contrast image (**b**) show thickening of the terminal ileum, with important contrast enhancement

Because of the relative poverty of intra-abdominal adipose tissue, which greatly affects contrast between different structures, we do not routinely acquire CT scans without contrast medium, as these would lack diagnostic sensitivity. Thus, the CT scan is usually acquired only in the portal-venous phase, with considerable saving of the radiation dose administered to the patient.

Image acquisition during the arterial phase is reserved for cases where it is important to evaluate the arterial vascular anatomy or where it is necessary to typify extensive pathologies and their relationships with vascular structures.

The images are acquired with a 5-mm layer thickness, and are subsequently reconstructed in the thinnest layer (1–2 mm), with the possibility of multiplanar and three-dimensional (3D) reconstructions.

CT is therefore a level II methodology, and is used exclusively to further elucidate radiographic findings and US doubts, or where more accurate morphological and anatomical assessment is required, especially in settings of urgency, such as for the study of acute abdominal conditions (complications of appendicitis or cecal Meckel's diverticula) or acute complications of chronic inflammatory conditions (bowel perforation, fistulas, or bleeding in *Crohn's disease*) [41].

In common clinical practice, CT angiography is frequently used for the evaluation of vascular thoracic and abdominal anatomy. A typical example is that of research of abnormal vessels, one of the most frequently represented being an aberrant right subclavian artery (lusoria) originating directly from the medial aortic arch profile; in these cases CT-depth investigation is performed after a pathological esophagogram shows the classic compression sign, caused by the abnormal blood vessel, on the rear profile of the proximal esophagus (Fig. 2.17).

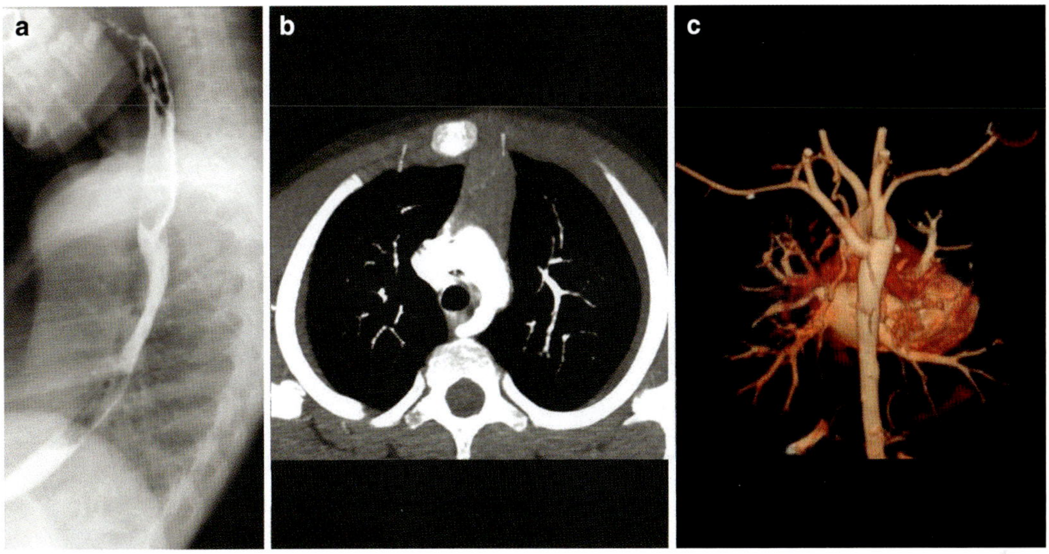

Fig. 2.17 Upper gastrointestinal (UGI) lateral view (**a**) of the esophagus shows a pathological compression of the rear profile of the proximal esophagus, confirmed by axial (**b**) and three-dimensional (3D) (**c**) images on computed tomography (CT) study

Another characteristic indication for CT angiography is in the study of suspected stenosis of mesenteric vessels or other pathological conditions that produce decisive changes in the normal vascular anatomy. Examples are portal cavernoma, a condition of pre-hepatic portal hypertension in the pediatric age group, where portal vein thrombosis occurs with subsequent arterialization of the hepatic blood flow and the progressive development of portal systemic shunt in typical locations (Fig. 2.18).

CT scans are also used in the evaluation of masses, especially in the thoracic region, and for the staging of tumors (Fig. 2.19); the most common form of tumor in children is undoubtedly Burkitt's lymphoma.

Finally, *entero-CT* deserves particular mention. This is the investigation used in the evaluation of the extension and complications of IBD, particularly Crohn's disease, and which allows us to obtain a simultaneous display of both luminal and extraluminal pathology, such as the presence of fistulae or abscesses. Adequate opacification and distension of the bowel loops with an oral contrast medium (most commonly water or oral low-density barium contrast medium) is important to avoid the misinterpretation of normal collapsed segments for masses or wall abnormalities [41–43].

The intravenous administration of iodinated contrast medium for entero-CT helps in the subsequent evaluation of the extension of tumor and inflammatory disease of the intestinal walls, and also helps in the evaluation of blood vessels and abdominal organs (Fig. 2.20).

Pharmacologically-induced hypotonia of the bowel to prevent movement artifacts is not indicated beacuse of the high speed of scanning of modern CT equipment.

In adult patients, entero-CT is used in both the acute setting of acute small bowel obstruction and in the elective situation with respect to IBD and the investigation of small bowel tumors. However, its use in children has remained limited due to the *radiation burden*, and MRI of the small bowel is now the preferred technique in children.

The benefits of CT when compared with MRI include better spatial resolution, fewer motion-related artifacts, increased availability, reduced cost, and shorter examination time. The benefits

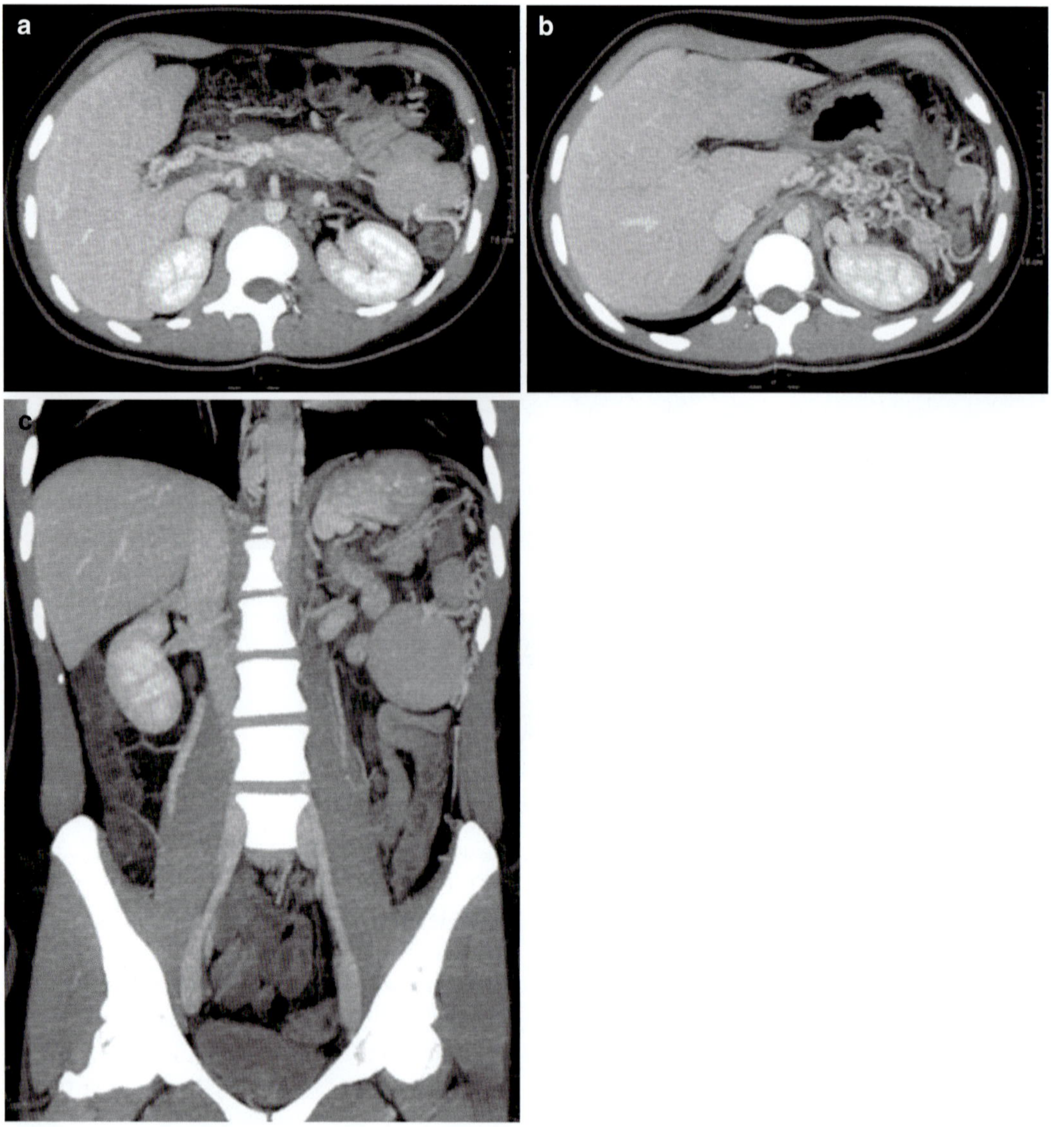

Fig. 2.18 Axial and coronal CT images show the presence of portal cavernoma (**a**) and collateral venous vessels due to a portal systemic shunt (**b**, **c**)

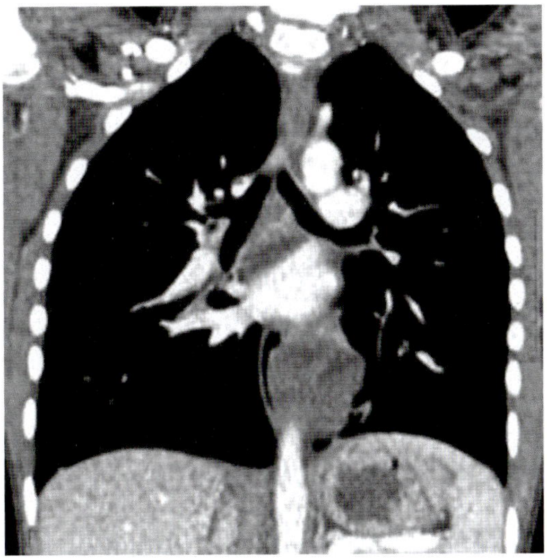

Fig. 2.19 Coronal CT image shows an esophageal duplication

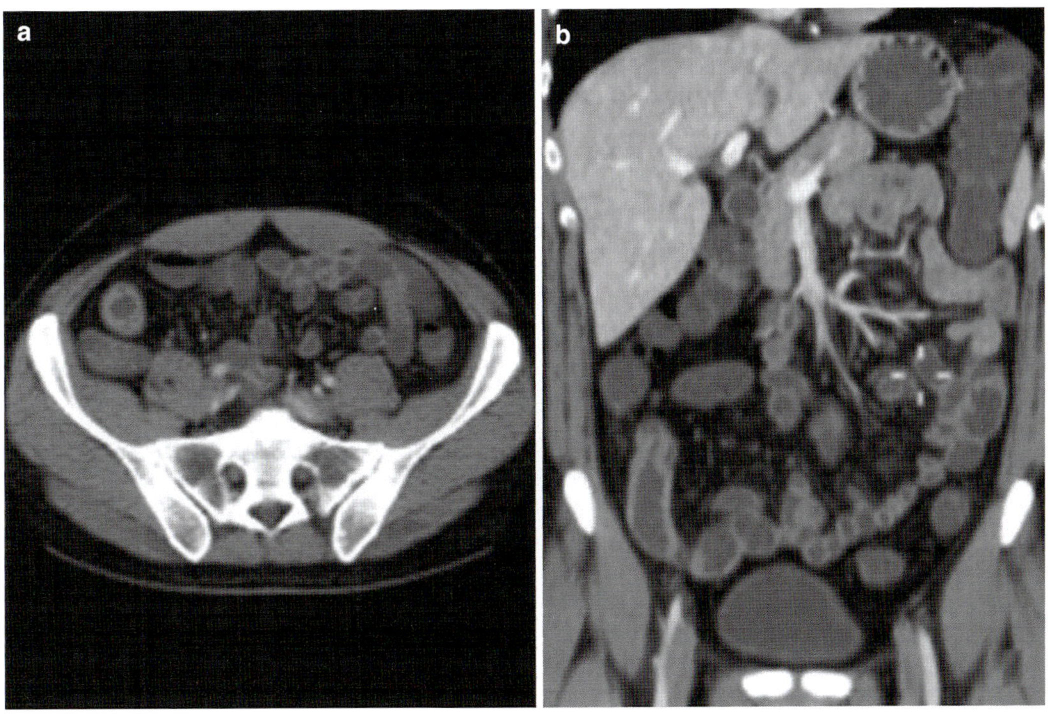

Fig. 2.20 Axial (**a**) and coronal (**b**) CT images show a pathological thickening of the terminal ileum

of MRI include better contrast resolution and the lack of ionizing radiation. It should be remembered that Crohn's disease is a chronic disease and any such patient is likely to be imaged more than once, so the cumulative radiation dose must be considered by the pediatric radiologist in this context. Recent studies have demonstrated similar sensitivities for CT and MRI in the detection of small bowel Crohn's disease [41–45].

References

1. Berrocal T, Torres I, Gutieerrez J et al (1999) Congenital anomalies of the upper gastro-intestinal tract. Radiographics 19:855–872
2. Berrocal T, Lamas M, Gutieerrez J et al (1999) Congenital anomalies of the small intestine, colon, and rectum. Radiographics 19:1219–1236
3. Ryan S, Donoghue V (2010) Gastrointestinal pathology in neonates: new imaging strategies. Pediatr Radiol 40:927–931
4. Hiorns MP (2011) Gastrointestinal tract imaging in children: current techniques. Pediatr Radiol 41:42–54, 53
5. Leighton JA, Wallace MB (2007) Update on small bowel imaging. Gastroenterology 132:1651–1654
6. Laffan EE, Daneman A, Ein SH et al (2006) Tracheoesophageal fistula without esophageal atresia: are pull-back tube esophagograms needed for diagnosis? Pediatr Radiol 36:1141–1147
7. Saleh N, Geipel A, Gembruch U et al (2009) Prenatal diagnosis and postnatal management of meconium peritonitis. J Perinat Med 37:535–538
8. Chan KL, Tang MH, Tse HY et al (2005) Meconium peritonitis: prenatal diagnosis, postnatal management and outcome. Prenat Diagn 25:676–682
9. Khan NA, Rea D, Hayes R et al (2005) Nonoperative management of uncomplicated meconium ileus with gastrografin enema factors that contribute to successful reduction. Pediatr Radiol 35:S97–S98
10. Jamieson DH, Dundas SE, Belushi SA et al (2004) Does the transition zone reliably delineate aganglionic bowel in Hirschsprung's disease? Pediatr Radiol 34:811–815
11. Jester I, Holland-Cunz S, Loff S et al (2009) Transanal pull-through procedure for Hirschsprung's disease: a 5-year experience. Eur J Pediatr Surg 19:68–71
12. Sizemore AW, Rabbani KZ, Ladd A et al (2008) Diagnostic performance of the upper gastrointestinal series in the evaluation of children with clinically suspected malrotation. Pediatr Radiol 38:518–528
13. Lobo ML, Roque M (2014) Gastrointestinal ultrasound in neonates, infants and children. Eur J Radiol 83:1592–1600
14. Fonio P, Coppolino F, Russo A et al (2013) Ultrasonography (US) in the assessment of pediatric non traumatic gastrointestinal emergencies. Crit Ultrasound J 5(suppl 1):S12
15. Hernanz-Schulman M (2009) Pyloric stenosis: role of imaging. Pediatr Radiol 39:S134–S139
16. Leaphart CL, Borland K, Kane TD et al (2008) Hypertrophic pyloric stenosis in newborns younger than 21 days: remodeling the path of surgical intervention. J Pediatr Surg 43:998–1001
17. Huang YL, Lee HC, Yeung CY et al (2009) Sonogram before and after pyloromyotomy: the pyloric ratio in infantile hypertrophic pyloric stenosis. Pediatr Neonatol 50:117–120
18. Hur J, Yoon CS, Kim MJ et al (2007) Imaging features of gastrointestinal tract duplications in infants and children: from oesophagus to rectum. Pediatr Radiol 37:691–699
19. Veyrac C, Baud C, Prodhomme O et al (2012) US assessment of neonatal bowel (necrotizing enterocolitis excluded). Pediatr Radiol 42(Suppl 1):S107–S114
20. Nagdeve NG, Qureshi AM, Bhingare PD et al (2012) Malrotation beyond infancy. J Pediatr Surg 47:2026–2032
21. Ashley LM, Allen S, Teel RL (2001) A normal sonogram does not exclude malrotation. Pediatr Radiol 31:354–356
22. Yousefzadeh DK (2009) The position of the duodenojejunal junction: the wrong horse to bet on in diagnosing or excluding malrotation. Pediatr Radiol 39:S172–S177
23. Applegate KE (2009) Evidence-based diagnosis of malrotation and volvulus. Pediatr Radiol 39: S161–S163
24. Pracros JP, Sann L, Genin G et al (1992) Ultrasound diagnosis of midgut volvulus: the "whirlpool" sign. Pediatr Radiol 22:18–20
25. Epelman M (2006) The whirlpool sign. Radiology 240:910–911
26. Haber HP, Seitz G, Warmann SW et al (2007) Transperineal sonography for determination of the type of imperforate anus. AJR 189:1525–1529
27. McHugh K (1998) The role of radiology in children with anorectal anomalies; with particular emphasis on MRI. Eur J Radiol 26:194–199
28. Kim WY, Kim WS, Kim IO et al (2005) Sonographic evaluation of neonates with early-stage necrotizing enterocolitis. Pediatr Radiol 35:1056–1061
29. Epelman M, Daneman A, Navarro OM et al (2007) Necrotizing enterocolitis: review of state-of-the-art imaging findings with pathologic correlation. Radiographics 27:285–305
30. Silva CT, Daneman A, Navarro OM et al (2007) Correlation of sonographic findings and outcome in necrotizing enterocolitis. Pediatr Radiol 37:274–282
31. Faingold R, Daneman A, Tomlinson G et al (2005) Necrotizing enterocolitis: assessment of bowel viability with color doppler US. Radiology 235:587–594

32. Horsthuis K, Stokkers PC, Stoker J (2007) Detection of inflammatory bowel disease: diagnostic performance of cross-sectional imaging modalities. Abdom Imaging 33:407–416
33. Spalinger J, Patriquin H, Miron MC et al (2000) Doppler US in patients with Crohn disease: vessel density in the diseased bowel reflects disease activity. Radiology 217:787–791
34. Di Mizio R, Maconi G, Romano S et al (2004) Small bowel Crohn disease: sonographic features. Abdom Imaging 29:23–35
35. Rufo PA, Bousvaros A (2007) Challenges and progress in pediatric inflammatory bowel disease. Curr Opin Gastroenterol 23:406–412
36. Hiorns MP (2008) Imaging of inflammatory bowel disease. How? Pediatr Radiol 38:S512–S517
37. Paolantonio P, Ferrari R, Vecchietti F et al (2009) Current status of MR imaging in the evaluation of IBD in a pediatric population of patients. Eur J Radiol 69:418–424
38. Eltomey MA, Donnelly LF, Emery KH et al (2008) Postoperative pelvic MRI of anorectal malformations. AJR 191:1469–1476
39. Borthne AS, Abdelnoor M, Rugtveit J et al (2006) Bowel magnetic resonance imaging of pediatric patients with oral mannitol MRI compared to endoscopy and intestinal ultrasound. Eur Radiol 16:207–214
40. Lohan D, Cronin C, Meehan C et al (2007) MR small bowel enterography: optimization of imaging timing. Clin Radiol 62:804–807
41. Paulsen SR, Huprich JE, Hara AK (2007) CT enterography: noninvasive evaluation of Crohn's disease and obscure gastrointestinal bleed. Radiol Clin North Am 45:303–315
42. Dillman JR, Adler J, Zimmermann EM et al (2010) CT enterography of pediatric Crohn disease. Pediatr Radiol 40:97–105
43. Gaca AM, Jaffe TA, Delaney S et al (2008) Radiation doses from small-bowel follow-through and abdomen/pelvis MDCT in pediatric Crohn disease. Pediatr Radiol 38:285–291
44. Rajesh A, Maglinte DD (2006) Multislice CT enteroclysis: technique and clinical applications. Clin Radiol 61:31–39
45. Rogalla P (2005) CT of the small intestine. Eur Radiol 15:D142–D148

3 Diagnostic and Therapeutic Endoscopy

Giovanni Di Nardo, Giuseppe Pagliaro, and Andrea Pession

3.1 Introduction

3.1.1 Pre-procedure Preparation

Physiologic issues (the emotional and psychosocial well-being of both patients and their caregivers) have an important role in preparation for endoscopy in pediatric patients. Informed consent should be obtained from a parent or guardian or from older children when appropriate. According to the American Academy of Pediatrics (AAP), a pre-procedure health evaluation specific to elective procedures should be obtained, and it includes a health history, American Society of Anesthesiology score of physical status, medication history, allergy assessment, age, weight, and baseline vital signs. A physical examination including a focused assessment of the heart, circulation, lungs, head, neck, and airway should be performed. Laboratory tests are not required in the pre-procedure assessment and need only be performed for clinical indications.

Endocarditis prophylaxis should be considered in patients with congenital heart disease; in particular, those with significant valve lesions and those with surgically placed shunts or artificial material in their circulation. Routine endoscopy with or without biopsy does not warrant antibiotic prophylaxis.

The AAP guideline on sedation in pediatric patients, with presumed normal gastric emptying, advises fasting for a minimum of 2 h after ingesting clear liquids, from breast milk for 4 h and from formula, nonhuman milk, and solids for 6 h before elective sedation. The risks of sedation without appropriate fasting in emergent cases must be weighed against the necessity for the procedure and the expected benefit.

3.1.2 Intra-procedural Sedation and Monitoring

Almost all gastrointestinal (GI) procedures in children are performed using endoscopist-administered moderate sedation or anesthesiologist-administered deep sedation and general anesthesia to ensure patient safety and comfort. Premedication with either oral (0.5 mg/kg) or intranasal (0.2 mg/kg) midazolam allows easier intravenous line

G. Di Nardo (✉)
Pediatric Gastroenterology Unit, International Hospital Salvator Mundi, Rome, Italy
e-mail: giovanni.dinardo3@alice.it

A. Pession
Pediatric Units, S. Orsola-Malpighi Hospital, University of Bologna, Bologna, Italy

G. Pagliaro
Pediatric Gastroenterology Unit, Sapienza, University of Rome, Rome, Italy

M. Lima (ed.), *Pediatric Digestive Surgery*, DOI 10.1007/978-3-319-40525-4_3

placement and division from parents particularly in selected group of children with a high level of anxiety before sedation.

Routine oxygen supply is a low-cost, high-benefit practice because data suggest that a significant number of children could have transient apnea and oxygen desaturation during sedation for endoscopy.

Although the short duration of most endoscopic procedures does not contribute to dehydration or hypothermia, children should be well draped, and room temperatures should be appropriately adjusted to avoid these possibilities.

Neurologically impaired patients can be particularly susceptible to benzodiazepines and opiate/benzodiazepine associations. Administration of sedation in children should always be weight based and usually titrated by response, allowing adequate time between doses to assess effects and the need for additional medication. Higher relative doses may be finally required in the preschool, elementary, and pre-teenage groups compared with teenage patients.

The AAP guidelines recommend continuous pulse oximetry and heart rate monitoring at all levels of sedation by a dedicated trained attendant who is specifically assigned to monitor the patient's vital signs. Most pediatric gastroenterologists are well trained and certified to provide moderate sedation, and most procedures can be safely performed outside the operating room. However, because the high frequency of progression to deep sedation, personnel trained specifically in pediatric rescue maneuvers including airway management and pediatric advanced life support should be readily available.

All supplies necessary to rescue any child experiencing cardiovascular complications during a procedure should be readily available in any unit performing pediatric procedures.

3.1.3 Post-procedure Monitoring and Discharge

After conclusion of endoscopic procedures, children should be monitored for adverse effects of the endoscopy or sedation. Vital signs and oxygen saturation should be monitored at specific intervals. The child should be easily awake, protective reflexes should be intact, and speech and ambulation appropriate for age should have returned to pre-sedation levels. Patients who have received reversal agents (e.g., flumazenil, naloxone) may require longer periods of observation as the half-life of the sedative may exceed that of the reversal medication leading to resedation.

Before discharge, specific written and verbal instructions and information should be given to a parent, legal guardian, or other responsible adults. This should include signs and symptoms of potential adverse events, steps to follow in the event of an adverse event, and a phone number at which 24-h coverage is available. Special instructions to observe the child's head position to prevent airway occlusion should be given in cases in which the child will travel in a car seat. In such cases, it may be preferable to have more than one adult who accompanies the child on the day of the procedure.

In this chapter, we will describe technique, indication, and potential complications of the main diagnostic and therapeutic endoscopic procedures available for pediatric population [1–3].

3.2 Esophagogastroduodenoscopy

3.2.1 Indications and Contraindications

Common indications for esophagogastroduodenoscopy (EGDS) in children are summarized in Table 3.1. Diagnostic EGDS may be specifically indicated to evaluate common pediatric conditions such as allergic, infectious, or peptic esophagitis, infectious or inflammatory gastritis, and celiac disease. Infants and children are unlikely to localize their symptoms to the upper GI tract; a number of nonspecific signs and symptoms (failure to thrive, unexplained irritability, and anorexia) may motivate upper endoscopy in young children.

Two other common pediatric diseases that may require endoscopy are the ingestion of

Table 3.1 Common indications for upper endoscopy in children

Diagnostic
Dysphagia
Odynophagia
Intractable or chronic symptoms of GERD
Vomiting/hematemesis
Persistent epigastric pain
Unexplained irritability
Anorexia
Weight loss/failure to thrive
Anemia (unexplained)
Diarrhea/malabsorption (chronic)
Gastrointestinal bleeding
Caustic ingestion
Therapeutic
Foreign-body removal
Stricture dilation
Esophageal variceal ligation
Upper GI bleeding control

Adapted by Ref. [1]

foreign bodies and caustic substances. The protocol for endoscopic evaluation of foreign body ingestion is similar to that in adults and has been well described elsewhere. Compared with standard practice in adults, it is generally recommended that foreign body removal in children should be done while they are under general anesthesia with endotracheal intubation to protect the airway from aspiration. Emergent foreign body removal in children is indicated for any symptomatic esophageal foreign body and for asymptomatic esophageal button batteries because of the high risk of esophageal tissue necrosis and risk of fistula formation. Another increasingly common indication for emergent foreign body removal in children is ingestion of powerful magnets, often manufactured as toys. Ingestion of two or more magnets has been associated with significant risks of obstruction, perforation, and fistula development of the upper and lower GI tracts, necessitating surgical intervention and even bowel resection. An algorithm to assist emergency department physicians and gastroenterologists in providing timely care, including endoscopic removal of magnets, was recently published and endorsed by the North American Society of Pediatric Gastroenterology, Hepatology, and Nutrition.

In cases of witnessed ingestion of caustic substances in which patients are manifesting symptoms, upper endoscopy should be performed to assess for esophageal, gastric, and duodenal injury. Universal performance of EGD in the setting of unwitnessed caustic ingestion without evidence of oropharyngeal injury is controversial, especially in asymptomatic patients. However, there is a well-recognized lack of correlation between symptoms of caustic ingestion and degree of esophageal injury. Endoscopy within 24 h of caustic ingestion is usually considered safe and provides important prognostic information.

EGDS is usually not recommended in infants for the evaluation of uncomplicated gastroesophageal reflux disease (GERD) or congenital hypertrophic pyloric stenosis. It is also generally not indicated in older children for evaluation of functional GI disorders, including self-limited abdominal pain.

Upper endoscopy is a safe procedure in otherwise healthy children 1 year of age and older, although discharge instructions should address sore throat and hoarseness, which may occur after the procedure in as many as one third of patients.

There are few contraindications to perform endoscopic procedures in children. The size of the patient is rarely a contraindication, and upper endoscopic examinations can be performed safely in neonates as small as 1.5–2 kg. Relative contraindications include coagulopathy, neutropenia, and unstable cardiopulmonary disease. In patients with these conditions, it is important to ascertain whether the benefits of performing the procedure outweigh its risks.

3.2.2 Equipment Requirements

The technical aspects of performing upper endoscopy are essentially the same in children and adults. The main difference is the smaller endoscopy equipment necessary to evaluate the smaller and more angulated anatomy of infants

Table 3.2 Neonatal and pediatric gastroscopes

Manufacturer	Model	Insertion tube (length/diameter, mm)	Definition/magnification/color enhancement	Biopsy channel (diameter, mm)
Olympus	GIF-N180	1100/4.9	Standard/none/NBI	1/2.0
	GIF-XP 180N	1100/5.5	Standard/none/NBI	1/2.0
Fujinon	EG530N	1100/5.9	High-definition/zoom/	1/2.0
	EG530NP	1100/4.9	High-definition/zoom/	1/2.0
Pentax	EG1690K	1100/5.4	Standard/zoom/iSCAN	1/2.0
	EG1870K	1050/6.0	Standard/zoom/iSCAN	1/2.0

Adapted by Ref. [2]
NBI narrow-band imaging

Table 3.3 Equipment compatible with pediatric endoscopes

Small biopsy forceps
Small polyp snare
Pediatric roth net
Small alligator forceps
Small rat-tooth forceps
Small injection needle
Small argon plasma coagulator probe
Two-prong graspers

Adapted by Ref. [2]

and young children. The newborn esophagus measures 8–10 cm in length and approximately 5 mm in diameter. In addition, the antrum and proximal duodenum may be more angulated in young children. Although standard adult endoscopes are generally safe in children weighing more than 25 kg, there are a number of commercially available endoscopes less than 6 mm in diameter with the necessary tip deflection that should be used in infants and children weighting less than 10 kg (Table 3.2). Gastroscopes ≤6 mm are recommended in children below 2.5 kg and preferred in children below 10 kg. Standard adult gastroscopes may be considered in children of 2.5–10 kg only if endotherapy is required. In children above 10 kg, standard adult gastroscopes can be tolerated. The main limiting factor with all pediatric endoscopes is the small working channel (2.0 mm) that makes suctioning more difficult and limits their use for therapeutic maneuvers. Table 3.3 lists equipment compatible with most of pediatric endoscopes.

3.2.3 Technique

The patient lies on the left side with the chin tucked against the chest and the bite guard placed between the teeth. Several methods can be used to insert the endoscope. The safe way is under direct vision.

Under direct vision (Fig. 3.1a, b), the instrument tip is advanced to the larynx, and the open glottic aperture is visualized (Fig. 3.1c). A slit can be recognized between the posterior wall of the hypopharynx and the cuneiform and corniculate tubercles (Fig. 3.1d). This slit leads to the upper esophageal sphincter, which curves gently around the posterior side of the cricoid cartilage. The instrument tip should pass a little to the left or right of the midline (Fig. 3.1e), taking care not to deviate into either piriform recess. The esophageal lumen becomes visible for a brief moment, and the tip is advanced into the esophagus (Fig. 3.1f).

In the blind insertion method, the endoscope is first passed over the base of the tongue toward the hypopharynx under external visual control. Care is taken that the endoscope tip is not retroflexed toward the nasopharynx and does not deviate to the left or right into the piriform recess. The instrument tip can be gently advanced just to the introitus of the upper esophageal sphincter. Following initial resistance, a distinct "give" is felt as the endoscope slips into the upper esophagus. Once the instrument tip is within the esophagus, the insertion is continued under endoscopic vision.

In both methods (blind and direct vision insertion), there is always a short segment of the esophagus that must be traversed without vision.

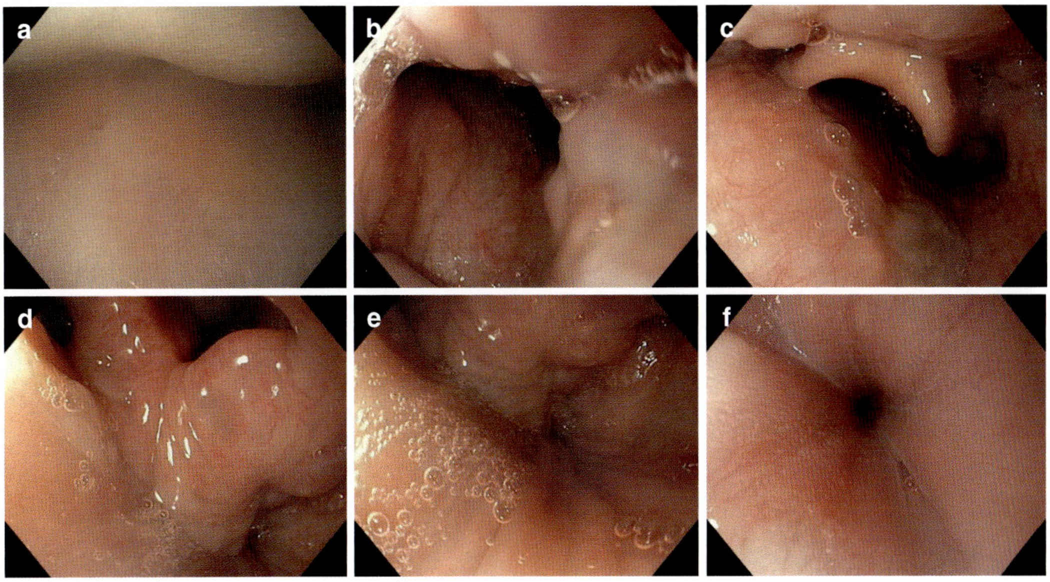

Fig. 3.1 Endoscopic view showing the different phases of the under vision insertion method

The upper esophageal sphincter appears as a lip-shaped eminence surrounding a transversely oriented, slit-like lumen. The cervical esophagus is a straight, collapsed tube that appears largely featureless at endoscopy. Air insufflation distends it to a round, symmetrical lumen that is affected very little by respiratory movements.

The aorta indents the middle esophagus from the lateral side and runs almost horizontally as it crosses the esophagus. The left main bronchus indents the esophagus from the anterior side just below the aortic arch. In the endoscopic image, it runs obliquely downward in a counterclockwise direction. The aorta and bronchus could not be always recognized. Unusual shapes are occasionally noted in thin patients.

The retrocardiac esophagus appeared just below the middle esophageal constriction. This portion of the esophagus is compressed anteriorly by the left atrium and posteriorly by the aorta, resulting in an elliptical lumen. Distinct pulsations could be documented.

The lumen of the distal esophagus again appears round and symmetrical. The lower esophageal constriction is visible in the distance. The muscular contraction and accompanying venous plexus create a typical endoscopic picture of longitudinal folds with concentric luminal narrowing.

Endoscopy is the best procedure to evaluate the gastroesophageal junction. The endoscopist identifies and evaluates the sphincter itself, the diaphragmatic hiatus in relation to the incisor teeth, and the transitional region between the squamous epithelium of the esophagus and the columnar epithelium of the stomach, which are separated by a visible junction called the Z-line. It has an important role to assess whether the lower esophageal sphincter is competent or incompetent, although this assessment varies considerably among different examiners.

The first region that is seen after entry is the junction of the fundus and body of the stomach. To improve vision, air is insufflated, the lesser curvature being on the right and the angulus in distance. When liquids are present, suction is used to reduce aspiration risk. At this point, it is better to rapidly progress in the duodenum to avoid traumatic lesions and the overinflation required for retrovision. Progression is made with a clockwise rotation of 90°, bending the tip upward (Fig. 3.2a). This double maneuver brings the pylorus into view. To put the pylorus in the antrum axis, the tip is angled down. The shaft is then advanced toward the pylorus, which will open with the help of air insufflation. The intubation of the pylorus is achieved with the tip slightly bent down and right. A view of pale mucosa of

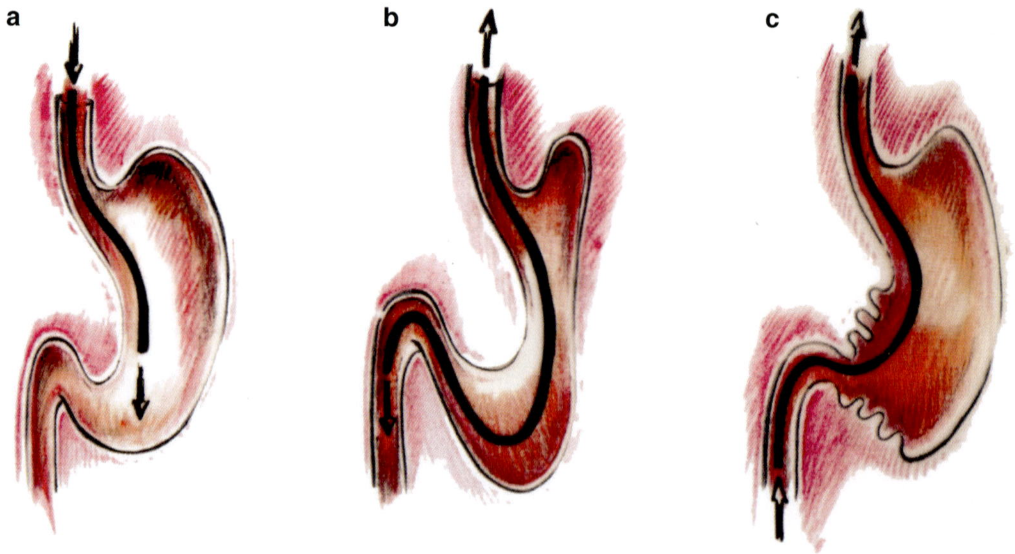

Fig. 3.2 Schematic view of the endoscopic maneuvers required for advancing the endoscope in the stomach and duodenum. (**a**) Progression is made with a clockwise rotation of 90°, bending the tip upward; (**b**) pushing will bring the tip in front of the duodenal angle; it is then bent to the right and up; (**c**) withdrawal is necessary to obtain an optimal view, because of the paradoxically progression of the endoscope owing to the straightening of the gastric loop

the bulb is achieved by withdrawal and air insufflation, the anterior wall placed to the left and the posterior wall to the right. The superior duodenal angle is visualized before passage to the second portion of the duodenum. This progression is usually carried out blindly because of the sharp angle and needs to be made with care. Pushing will bring the tip in front of the duodenal angle; it is then bent to the right and up (Fig. 3.2b). At last, withdrawal is normally necessary to obtain an optimal view, because of the paradoxically progression of the endoscope owing to the straightening of the gastric loop (Fig. 3.2c). Sometimes, rectification of the last maneuver is needed with deflection of the tip upward and to the left.

During the withdrawal, a careful mucosal examination is performed using circumferential movements with air insufflation to provide a well-distended mucosa and to improve visualization of possible small lesions. A retrovision maneuver in the stomach is the best way to fully visualize the fundus, the lesser curvature, and the cardia (Fig. 3.3). While it is in the back portion of the proximal antrum, a 180–210° angulation is necessary to bring into the view the angulus and the lesser curvature (Fig. 3.3a). Keeping the angulation, a 180° rotation around the shaft's axis will permit visualization of the greater curve and the fundus (Fig. 3.3b–e). A key difference between pediatric and adult diagnostic procedures is that routine tissue sampling (usually performed during the withdrawal phase) is performed in children from at least the duodenum, stomach, and esophagus during EGDS. It is standard pediatric endoscopy practice to obtain biopsy specimens, even in the absence of gross abnormalities, because the risks of sedation and performing repeat endoscopy in pediatric populations are considered to outweigh the risks of obtaining biopsy specimens. Several studies have also shown that it may be particularly difficult to rule out clinically significant disease based only on endoscopic appearance of the upper GI tract in children, and biopsies during pediatric EGDS are generally considered necessary even in the absence of any macroscopic endoscopic findings.

3.2.4 Complications

Although about one third of pediatric patients presented sore throat or hoarseness after EGDS under general anesthesia, all other reported complications are uncommon particularly (less than

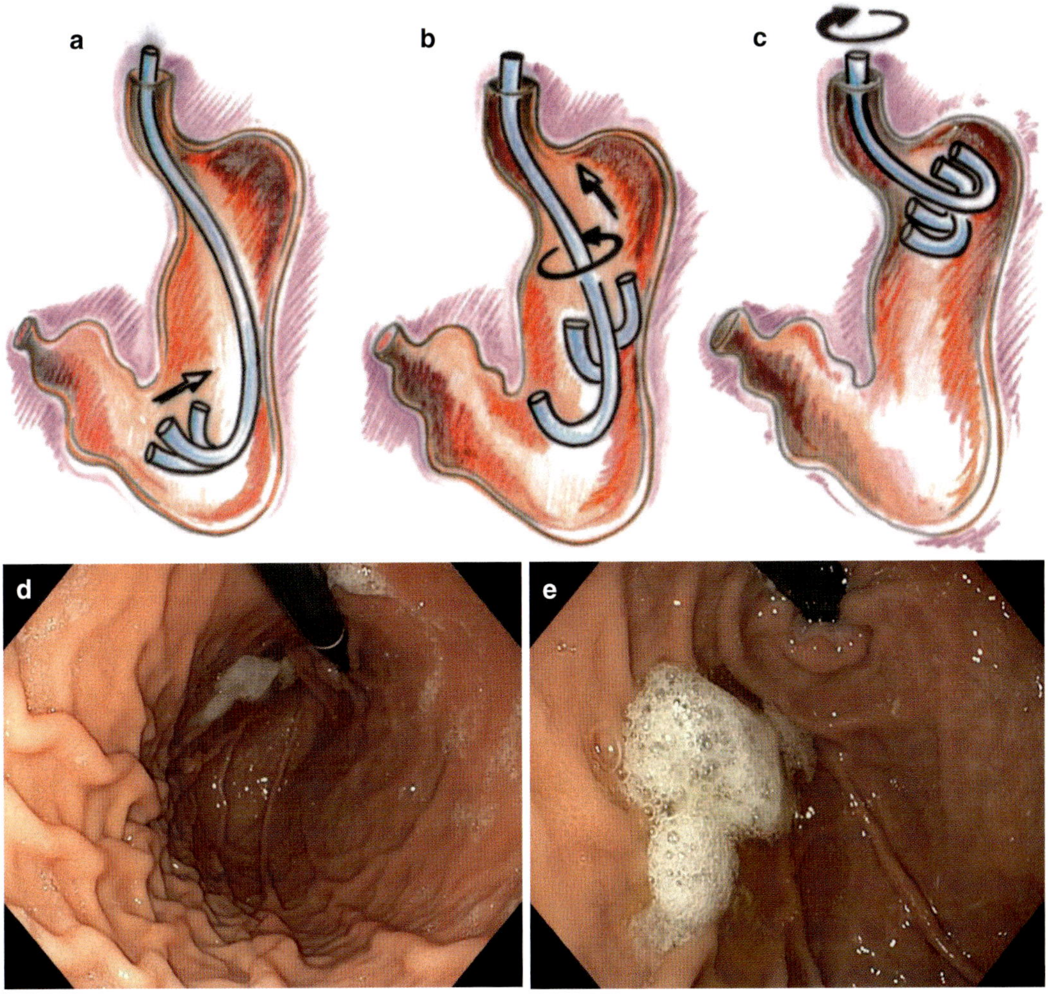

Fig. 3.3 Schematic (**a**, **b**, **c**) and endoscopic view (**d**, **e**) of the retrovision maneuver

1 %) when performed by well-trained pediatric equip. They are mostly related to the anesthesia and infrequently to the procedure itself. Hypoxic episodes and aspiration are always possible under deep sedation. Allergic patients could react to the medications or to the latex. Finally, rare complications are hypotension, arrhythmia, and malignant hyperthermia.

Complications related to the endoscopic procedure include perforation, parietal hematoma, embolism, and infection. Perforation principally involves the esophagus; it is due to therapeutic endoscopy and its signs could appear with some delay. To minimize this risk, it is mandatory to never push forward without vision. In case of suspected perforation, surgical referral is urgent to choose a conservative or a surgical approach. Intramural duodenal hematoma has been described after endoscopic biopsies and occurs more frequently in children than in adults. The clinical presentation mimics abdominal occlusion, it is frequently associated with pancreatitis and always resolves spontaneously between 4 days and 2 weeks with fasting nasogastric suction and fluid replacement. Surgical drainage is unnecessary and therefore contraindicated. Fatal massive embolism has been reported in two children with Kasai procedure because of potential vessel leakage. Infectious complications can result from the patient's own flora, from patient to patient by the endoscope and between the patient and the staff. This seems rare and can be seen in cardiac-risk patients; therefore, prophylactic antibiotics are suggested only to selected patients [4, 5].

3.3 Colonoscopy

3.3.1 Indications and Contraindications

In the last years, colonoscopy has become a routine procedure also for pediatric patients. It is safely used in all groups of children, including newborns. Common indications for colonoscopy are shown in Table 3.4. There is no pediatric colon cancer screening guideline, and therefore patient volume of pediatric colonoscopies at the population level is far lower than that of adults. Uncommon, but nevertheless critically important, indications for colonoscopy in children include surveillance for neoplasia in children with long-standing inflammatory bowel disease and hereditary polyposis syndromes as well as for graft-versus-host disease.

Colonoscopy is not recommended in children with acute self-limited diarrhea, stable recognized irritable bowel syndrome, chronic nonspecific abdominal pain, constipation with or without impaction, and inflammatory bowel disease that is responding to treatment.

There are few contraindications to perform colonoscopy in children. The size of the patient is rarely a contraindication, and lower endoscopic examinations can be performed safely in neonates as small as 1.5 to 2 kg. Diagnostic colonoscopy is absolutely contraindicated in anyone with fulminant colitis, toxic megacolon, or suspected perforated bowel. Recent intestinal resection represents a possible contraindication to the examination. Relative contraindications include coagulopathy, neutropenia, and unstable cardiopulmonary disease. In patients with these conditions, it is important to ascertain whether the benefits of performing the procedure outweigh its risks.

Table 3.4 Common indications for colonoscopy in children

Diagnostic
Chronic or profuse diarrhea
Lower GI bleeding
Polyposis syndrome (diagnose and surveillance)
Failure to thrive/weight loss
Lower GI tract lesions seen on imaging studies
Rejection of intestinal transplant
Abdominal pain (clinically significant)
Therapeutic
Polipectomy
Stricture dilation
Hemostasis
Foreign-body removal

Adapted by Ref. [1]

3.3.2 Equipment Requirements

Although the instruments are similar, pediatric colonoscopy is different from adults in many aspects such as preparation, sedation, technique, and spectrum of therapeutic manipulations. First at all, in contrast to adults, endoscopic examinations in children are usually performed under deep sedation or general anesthesia to reduce emotional stress caused by separation from parents and the preparation for the procedure itself. Moreover, in children, colonoscopy is usually performed by specialized pediatric gastroenterologists. However, surgeons or adult gastroenterologists may be consulted for advanced or therapeutic endoscopy in pediatric patients. Knowledge of the equipment available for use in smaller patients, primarily those weighing less than 10–15 kg, is required.

Pediatric colonoscopes have variable insertion tube lengths (133–170 cm), shaft diameters (9.8–11.8 mm), and channel size (2.8–3.8 mm). Pediatric colonoscopes with a shaft that can be stiffened as needed are also available. These variable-stiffness colonoscopes were designed to improve the ease of insertion by reducing looping in more mobile sections of bowel with the ability to maintain flexibility in more fixed sections. There are no published data to support colonoscope choice in children, but recommendations based on experience state that the lower weight limit for the use of a standard adult or pediatric colonoscope is 12–15 kg. In children weighing between 5 and 12 kg, colonoscopy can be performed by using infant or standard adult gastroscopes. Children weighting less than 5 kg may undergo successful ileocolonoscopy with ultrathin gastroscopes, although this can be technically challenging because of the flexibility of the insertion tube. Pediatric colonoscopes with a working channel of 2.8 mm will not accommodate larger accessories (e.g., jumbo biopsy forceps).

3.3.3 Bowel Preparation

Bowel cleansing for colonoscopy in pediatric patients must prioritize safety and compliance and should take into account patient's age, clinical status, and anticipated willingness or ability to comply. To date, bowel preparation regimens for children have not been standardized and vary greatly among medical centers and individual practitioners. Ingestion of clear liquids for 24 h and a normal saline solution enema (5 mL/kg) may be sufficient for infants younger than 2 years of age. For children older than 2 years of age, cleansing can be accomplished with intestinal lavage by using osmotic agents, such as polyethylene glycol solutions with and without electrolytes, dietary restrictions, and stimulant laxatives, such as senna and bisacodyl, and/or enemas.

Polyethylene glycol with electrolytes is used as the primary agent for bowel cleansing; most children will require approximately 80 mL/kg of the solution. Most will also be unlikely to ingest sufficient volume because of its noxious taste. Administration of polyethylene glycol with electrolytes via a nasogastric tube in a hospital setting for 24 h before the procedure is a safe and appropriate treatment, especially in children younger than 6 years of age. PEG-3350 without electrolytes in doses as much as 10 times higher than those recommended for standard treatment of constipation is emerging as the preparation of choice in many pediatric units. Several studies have reported on the safety and efficacy of 4-day bowel preparations by using PEG-3350 without electrolytes in children.

We have recently confirmed that low-volume PEG preparations and sodium picosulphate plus magnesium oxide plus citric acid preparations (NaPico+MgCit) are a good alternative to the standard PEG solutions for bowel preparation in children due to their comparable safety and efficacy profile. Moreover, NaPico+MgCit-based preparations appeared to be more tolerated, representing a promising regimen for bowel preparation in children [6, 7].

3.3.4 Technique

Patient is placed in the left lateral decubitus position. Complete colonoscopy can be performed successfully in the majority of children. Many factors can influence and complicate the procedure, e.g., redundant large intestine, improper preparation, or previous surgeries. General principles of a safe and effective colonoscopy include:

- The intubated colon adopts configuration and shape according to manipulations and movements with the colonoscope, and the pattern of these changes are predictable, as well as the direction in which the colonoscope tip should be moved.
- Rotation, twisting, withdrawal, deflation, and simultaneous to and from movements of the shaft will prevent formation of big loops (Fig. 3.4), mesenteric stretching, and related abdominal pain and discomfort.
- Excessive insufflation leads to overdistension and diminishes ability to telescope the bowel.
- Excessive pushing forward creates more problems than benefits.

The principles of pediatric colonoscopy are similar to those in adults, but should be more acute because of the child's small stature and angulations. In the child, it is frequently possible to palpate a loop of the scope in the abdomen, a clue that instrument withdrawal and straightening are needed. Meticulous attention to technique

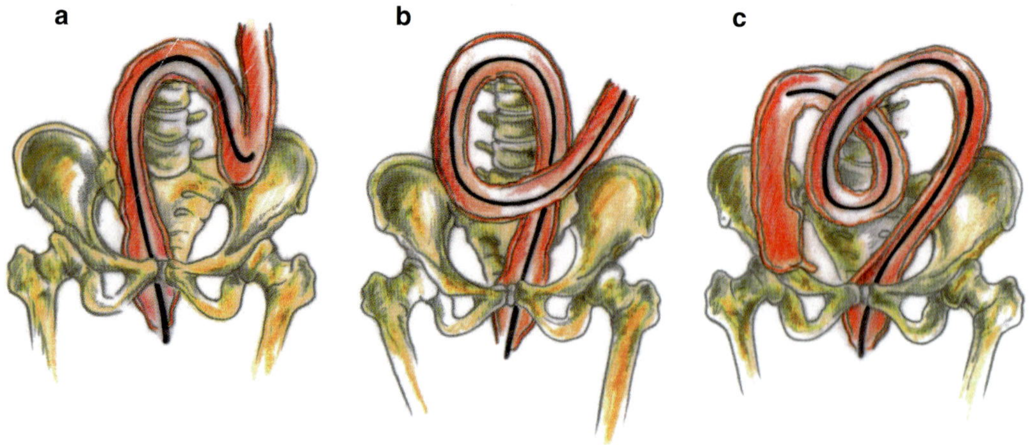

Fig. 3.4 Schematic view of the loops that may form during colonoscopy. N-loop (**a**), alpha-loop (**b**) and gammaloop (**c**)

is required in children because the colon wall is thin, and, in the presence of anesthesia using propofol, there should not be any noticeable feedback from the patient that would provide a clue as to pain or discomfort from an overstretched mesentery or overdistended bowel.

The key to effective colonoscopy is to minimize pain and discomfort. It is critical to try and keep the lumen of the bowel in sight knowing where the tip of the colonoscope is and trying to keep the colonoscope straight with avoidance of loops.

The mucosal pattern of the colon is best studied as the instrument is slowly withdrawn. However, we believe that it is important to carefully pay attention at the mucosa while advancing forward, since trauma could sometimes occur to the mucosa with the passage of the instrument, and, if abnormalities are not identified beforehand, one is always left wondering whether what one sees is due to colonoscopy vs. the underlying pathology.

An additional difference between pediatric and adult diagnostic procedures is that routine tissue sampling is performed in children from at least from the colon and terminal ileum.

3.3.5 Complications

The potential risks and complications of colonoscopy include bleeding, perforation, infection, and difficulties with sedation (such as paradoxical reaction to the agent used).

Bowel perforation and hemorrhage related to pediatric colonoscopy are serious but rare complications. During diagnostic colonoscopy, the estimated frequency of colonic perforation, most commonly in the sigmoid, is in the range of 0.2–0.8 %. The frequency is higher with therapeutic colonoscopy procedures such as polypectomy but is still comparatively rare ranging from 0.5 to 3 %. Mortality is extremely low and should be substantially less than 0.2 %.

3.4 Capsule Endoscopy

3.4.1 Introduction

Since 2001, when it was introduced, capsule endoscopy (CE) has become widely adopted as a clinical tool in the evaluation of small bowel disease. Though the first pediatric studies were initiated in that year, marketing clearance for CE in pediatric patients 10 years of age and older by the US Food and Drug Administration, the Health Canada, and the European Medical Agency did not occur until 2003. Supported by additional experience in children as young as the age of 10 months, the Food and Drug Administration

(FDA) expanded the role for CE for the use in children ages 2 years and older in 2009, approved the use of a patency capsule for this same age group, and has now approved mucosal healing as an additional indication.

Because CE avoids ionizing radiation, deep sedation, or general anesthesia required by other imaging methods, CE has the potential to be particularly valuable in pediatrics. Most of the small bowel has been inaccessible for mucosal evaluation, and much of our knowledge of small bowel disorders has been dependent on laboratory manifestations which are often surrogate markers, radiographic studies which provide indications of more advanced disease and surgical/pathological teachings that provide much information about severe conditions but a limited understanding of their prelude and potential for medical treatment. The recent developments with deep enteroscopy are difficult and invasive in children and as yet insufficiently evaluated with the indication for their use often abnormalities that are initially seen on the less invasive CE.

In many ways, this first decade of small intestinal CE has presented the equivalent of the expansion of knowledge that occurred when traditional endoscopy was introduced. Then, clinicians began to realize the different visual manifestations of gastroduodenal and colonic diseases that could not be appreciated radiologically or pathologically. Additionally, visual findings were gradually able to be explained and then associated with known conditions. The same appears true now for capsule endoscopy. Suspicious nonspecific lesions and bulges seen with CE are being further explained when pathologic samples are obtained with biopsy or surgical removal.

3.4.2 Small Bowel Capsule

3.4.2.1 Indications and Contraindications

Guidelines have been promulgated regarding the indications for CE use by societies such as the American Society for Gastrointestinal Endoscopy.

In pediatrics, the suspicion of CD and evaluation of existing inflammatory bowel disease (IBD) are the most common indications, followed by obscure/occult gastrointestinal bleeding (OGIB), abdominal pain/diarrhea, and polyposis (Fig. 3.5). Even within the pediatric population, clinical indications are age-stratified (Table 3.5). The approved indications for the pediatric and adult populations may expand as the broader utility of the capsule is recognized. Already, the capsule is useful to diagnose allergic disorders, a newly recognized enteropathy in cystic fibrosis, and to evaluate unrecognized causes of abdominal pain. The capsule could be used in monitoring medical therapy in Crohn's disease and graft-versus-host disease. The finding of jejunal lesions in ulcerative colitis and the use of the capsule to differentiate patients thought to have indeterminate colitis (IBD-U) and nonspecific colitis prove to be valid uses of CE especially before a colectomy is performed. Though

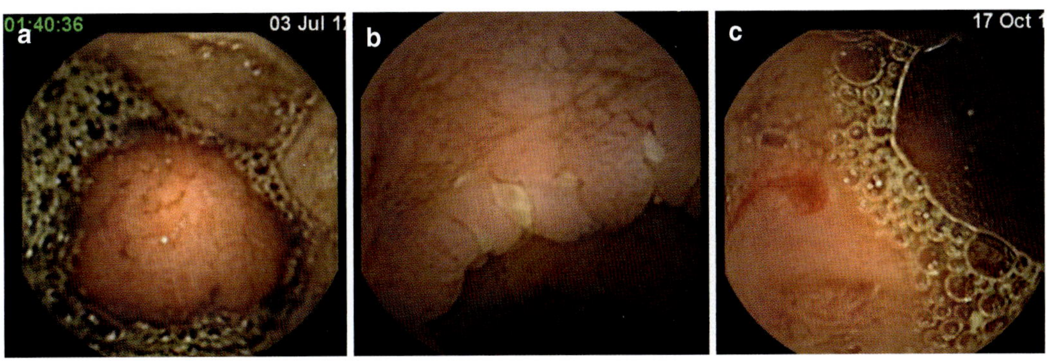

Fig. 3.5 Capsule endoscopic findings of small bowel polyp (**a**), ulcers (**b**) and active bleeding from Angiodysplasia (**c**)

Table 3.5 Clinical indications for CE by age

	Adult	Pediatric	Age <8 years
Procedures (*n*)	22,840	1013	83
OGIB + IDA (%)	66	15	36
CD/UC/IC (%)	10	63	24
Abdominal pain (%)	11	10	14
Polyps/neoplasms (%)	3	8	-
Others (%)	10	4	25

CD Crohn's disease, *IDA* iron deficiency anemia, *OGIB* obscure gastrointestinal bleeding, *IC* indeterminant colitis, *UC* ulcerative colitis

CE may not change the decision regarding surgery (though it has done that), CE may alter the type of surgery that is performed. Additionally, diagnostic algorithms based on CE results have been employed in selected intestinal motility disorders and suggest that wider application of CE are likely, expanding the thoughtful use of this modality.

CE is contraindicated in pregnancy, patients with known or suspected gastrointestinal obstructions, strictures or fistulas, Zenker's diverticula, small bowel motility abnormality, documented surgical ending blinding loop, cardiac pacemakers, or other implantable electromedical devices. Despite this last indication, recent studies have shown that the clinical use of capsule endoscopy is safe in patients with implantable cardioverter defibrillators (ICDs), and even when the capsules were in closest proximity to the ICDs, no interference was observed.

The main limitations of CE include its lack of therapeutic capabilities (including biopsy), the inability to control its movement, its high rate of incidental findings, difficulty in localizing identified lesions (because of the impossibility to wash out the lesion or reexamined it), and the potential to miss single-mass lesions. Certain segments of the SB, such as the second portion of the duodenum or the terminal ileum, may not be seen well by the capsule and therefore have limited diagnostic accuracy. Accuracy can be also decreased by the obscuration of the lens by food, bile, or stools. Moreover, despite the expected life span of ~8 h, the capsule battery may run out before the entire small bowel is visualized, particularly in cases of delayed small bowel transit time.

3.4.2.2 Technical Aspects

CE is a painless noninvasive diagnostic procedure that is performed by swallowing a capsule.

The original mouth to anus (M2A) capsule endoscope (PillCam SB, Given Imaging) has three components: a capsule "endoscope" an external receiving antenna with attached portable hard drive, and a customized PC workstation with a dedicated software for review and interpretation of images M2A capsule which weights 3.7 g and measures 11 mm in diameter × 26 mm in length. The slippery coating of the capsule allows easy ingestion and prevents adhesion of lumen contents, whereas the capsule moves via peristalsis from the mouth to the anus. The capsule includes a complimentary metal oxide silicon (CMOS) chip camera of 256 × 256 pixels, a short focal length lens, 4–6 white light-emitting diode (LED) illumination sources, two silver oxide batteries, and a UHF band radio telemetry transmitter.

Image features include a 140° field of view, a 1:8 magnification, a 1–30 mm depth of view, and a minimum size of detection of about 0.1 mm. The activated M2A capsule provides images at a frequency of two frames per second until the battery expires after 7 ± 1 h, which enables the device to take up to 55,000 .jpg images during 8-h procedure. The pictures are transmitted via an eight-lead sensor array, arranged in a specific fashion on the patient's belly, to a recorder, which is worn on a belt. The recorder is downloaded into a Reporting and Processing of Images and Data computer workstation and seen as a continuous video film.

Now in its second generation, PillCam SB 2 has the same dimension as the previous PillCam, but it has an angle of view of 156°. The wider angle of view permits to cover more than double the visualized mucosal surface area; therefore, the entire circumferences of the intestinal folds can be visualized.

Moreover, the second-generation capsule includes a three-lens system, an automatic light exposure sensor to improve the optics. An improved method to process the digital information produces images with uniform exposure to light with a higher image resolution and a better sharpness of the mucosal detail, as well as an increase in the depth of view. The software also has additional support systems as a localization system, a blood detector, a double and quadri picture viewer, a quick viewer, a single picture adjustment mode, an inflammation (Lewis) scoring system, and an atlas to assist the interpreter. By now, there are five CE systems: the PillCam SB2 (Given Imaging, Yokneam, Israel), the Endo Capsule (Olympus America, Center Valley, PA), the OMOM capsule (Jinshan Science and Technology, Chongqing, China), the MiroCam (IntroMedic, Seoul, Korea) and CapsoCam Plus (CapsoVision, Saratoga, CA, USA).

The patient fasts overnight, and, on the morning of the procedure, a comfortable belt containing sensors is fitted at the patient's waist, with easy-fasten straps for quick adjustments and removal. The camera is activated by the removal of the capsule from its magnetic holder, and it is given to the patient with a glass of water. After the patient has successfully swallowed the capsule, then the capsule is passively moved along by peristalsis. Two hours after ingestion, the patient is allowed to drink, while eating is allowed after 4 h. During the procedure the patient may carry on with his daily activities. After 8 h, the patient will return to the physician's office to return the sensor belt and data recorder. The PillCam video capsule passes naturally with a bowel movement, usually within 24 h. The physician will then download images from the data recorder for review.

The data recorder is a small portable recording device that communicates with the capsules as the capsule passes through the GI tract. The data recorder is placed in the recorder pouch which is attached to the belt around the patient's waist. Actually there is a RAPID real-time device that enables real-time viewing during a PillCam procedure.

In patients who are unable to swallow the capsule as younger children, or patients with difficulty in swallowing, the examination is carried out placing the capsule with the endoscope directly in the duodenum. Many different techniques to deliver the capsule have been described even for the pediatric population with different device as a foreign body retrieval net alone, a retrieval net and translucent cap or translucent ligation adaptor, a polypectomy snare, and the others with or without an overtube.

Before the procedures, all parents or legal guardians have to give informed consent for their children, and this consent was given in full oral explanation and in writing, above all for the risk of retention.

Upper and lower endoscopies are necessary before performing capsule endoscopy, to exclude lesions from the upper and lower gastrointestinal tract.

3.4.2.3 Patient Preparation

The presence of intestinal contents or a delayed gastric or intestinal transit may cause the failure of the complete visualization of the intestinal mucosa. Despite several studies have examined the possibilities of improving bowel cleanliness and shortening transit time with different medication, small bowel preparation is still a controversial issue. Capsule manufacturer recommend a bowel preparation with a 12-h fast. From European guidelines, there is evidence for a benefit from bowel preparation for capsule endoscopy, but there is so far no consensus on the preparation regimen.

3.4.2.4 Adverse Events

Capsule retention is defined as having a capsule that remains in the digestive tract for more than 2 weeks. Causes of retention cited in the literature include: NSAID strictures, Crohn's disease, small bowel tumors, intestinal adhesions, ulcerations, and radiation enteritis. The frequency of this problem varies: in some studies in adults, it has been reported in less than two percent of all capsule endoscopy in adults. In a recent pediatric review, the percentage of capsule retention was reported to be variable from 0 % up to 20 %. Prior to the development of the patency capsule, gastroenterologists were dependent on clinical history and radiographic studies to determine the safety and utility of CE. Radiographic studies to evaluate the potential safety for CE have been misleading because capsule retention has been documented in patients with normal small bowel radiography, and conversely safe capsule passage has been described in patients with strictures identified radiographically (see section "Patency Capsule"). It is important to underline that in some circumstances, capsule retention is permitted to identify the exact localization of lesions that needed surgery anyway. In our experience, this happened in a patient in whom the capsule was retained in a blinding surgical ending loop with multiple mucosal ulcerations and a gut wall dilatation. The surgeon found immediately the lesions because of the capsule retention. It appears that the risk of retention is dependent upon the clinical indication and not on the age difference. The highest risk factors for capsule retention include known IBD, previous SBFT demonstrating small bowel CD, and a BMI <5th percentile combined with known IBD, though retention occurred despite the absence of stricture on SBFT. Rare cases of perforation, aspiration, or small bowel obstruction have been reported in adults with none reported in children. However, children have suffered mucosal trauma when capsules have been placed with the Roth net. As a result, specific capsule placement devices are now being used.

3.4.3 Patency Capsule

The majority of capsule retentions have occurred in patients with normal small bowel radiological studies, yet functional patency may be present in patients with radiologically documented strictures. To avoid this concern, an identically sized patency capsule (PC) containing a mixture of barium, lactose and a radiofrequency identity tag was developed. The currently available version has dual timer plugs that gradually implodes if passage does not occur within 30 h. The PC can serve as a useful guide and may lessen the likelihood of CE retention, particularly in known CD where the risk of retention is greatest.

3.4.4 Colon Capsule

Colon capsule endoscopy represents an innovative noninvasive, painless, swallowed "colonoscope" that is able to explore the colon without requiring sedation and air insufflation. The US FDA did not approve it yet, but it is available in Israel and in part of Europe.

Theoretically, all patients with suspected or known colonic disease, referred for conventional colonoscopy are potentially candidates for a colon capsule examination including suspected lesions detected at a previous exam, gastrointestinal bleeding, unexplained iron deficiency anemia, positive fecal occult blood test, clinically significant diarrhea of unknown origin, surveillance for colonic neoplasia, colorectal cancer screening, chronic inflammatory bowel disease, etc.

But we know from adults study that colon capsule should not be considered alternative to conventional colonoscopy but complementary to traditional colonoscopy in case of incomplete colonoscopy, when conventional colonoscopy is contraindicated or in patients who are unwilling to undergo colonoscopy. There are also several studies for the utilization of the colon capsule for screening of colorectal cancer, but to date there are not reasonable results because of the low sensitivity in identifying patients with colonic polyps as compared with standard colonoscopy. Although colon capsule endoscopy represents a reliable system that is not invasive and well tolerated, there are no studies in children.

3.4.4.1 Technical Aspects

There are some differences between the small bowel and colon that make the evaluation of the colon more difficult. First of all, the colon has a much wider diameter. This allows the capsule to flip around its own axis and change directions preventing, full visualization of the mucosal surface.

This problem has been partially solved by adding another camera, allowing both ends of the capsule transmit images. The first generation of the colonic capsule had two cameras on both heads, taking four frames per second. It is 5 mm longer than the small bowel capsule (dimension 11 × 32 mm).

Moreover, the angle of view from each imager is 156°, and it permits greater imaging coverage of the larger cross-sectional diameter of the colon. The second problem is that the capsule has to travel through the stomach and the small bowel to reach the colon and this journey is time consuming. Two changes were made to solve this problem. First of all, a third battery and a sleep mode were added to economize on energy. The transmission of images ceases for an hour and a half after ingestion to allow travel to the target area. With increased energy stores (third battery) and decreased energy consumption (sleep mode), the capsule transmits images from the entire colon. It acquires images at a rate of four frames per second (two for each imager) and has a total operating time of 10 h, approximately. Images transmitted by CCE are recorded in a portable, external recorder (DR2C) specifically developed for colon capsule, and then the images are downloaded in a workstation and visualized.

Recently a second-generation colon capsule has been developed to improve the sensibility of the examination. The new colon capsule is slightly longer than the previous (31.5 mm versus 31 mm), and the angle of view has been increased from 156° up to 172° for each camera, thus offering a panoramic view of the colon (360°). In order to conserve battery energy, the capsule is equipped with an adaptive frame rate, and it captures 35 images per second when in motion and four images per second when it is virtually stationary.

This specific image rate is controlled in real time by the new data recorder which both stores the images and analyzes the capsule images. The data recorder is able to recognize the localization of the capsule, and to save more battery, colon capsule 2 works at a low rate of images per minute during its journey into the stomach and the small bowel, and then when images from small bowel are not anymore detected, then it switches into the adaptive frame rate.

The possibility to identify the site of the capsule permits to notify at the patient by a sounding signal and by a vibration that the capsule is still into the stomach, and the preparation protocol needs to be continued with prokinetic agents. In the small bowel, a beeping sound, a vibration, and a message on the display inform the patients to finish the preparation with a laxative to accelerate the small bowel transit. Transfer of the recorded images to the workstation and review of the videos with rapid software are similar to small bowel capsule. The new rapid software does however now include a simple graphic interface tool for polyp size estimation.

Another difference between the small bowel and colon is that the colonic surface is covered by fecal material and the mucosa of the colon will not be visualized by the capsule. The bowel cleansing has to be superior to the cleansing process applied for conventional colonoscopy since no suction of liquid is possible during capsule endoscopy so if colon is unclear the bowel mucosa may not be seen by CCE. Therefore, novel colon preparation regimens were developed to provide a clean colon and to promote CCE propulsion through the entire colon to the rectum.

By now, there is not any study to determinate the optimal bowel preparation for children, and also for adults, the optimal bowel preparation has yet to be determined. For adults, the most widely used preparation regimen includes an oral preparation of polyethylene glycol (PEG) osmotic solution, boost doses of sodium phosphate solutions, and prokinetic agents.

With this regimen, colonic preparation was judged adequate in a median of 77 % (range 35–89 %) of cases, and the rate of complete examination appears to be very close to the ≥95 % rate recommended for screening colonoscopy.

In children, the preparation protocol is similar to adults, including for three days before the examination patients take a diet without fibers, the day before a clear liquid diet with or without a small breakfast (only milk), and 2–4 L (50 ml/kg) of split dose polyethylene glycol (PEG), half on the previous evening and half in the morning until 2 h prior to capsule ingestion.

A written informed permission is signed by parents' patients to carry out the procedure. Twenty minutes before capsule ingestion, patients take prokinetic agents as domperidone at the dose of 10–20 mg, and the capsule is then swallowed with water. By real-time modalities, it is possible to check when the capsule reaches the duodenum. If, after an hour from ingestion, the capsule is still in the stomach intramuscular prokinetic is administered. Once the capsule arrives to duodenum, the physician activates the capsule and the patient can go home.

Patients or their parents were asked to inform the physician when the capsule was passed in the stools [8–11].

3.5 Enteroscopy

3.5.1 Introduction

Evaluation of small intestinal mucosa has an important role in the treatment of children with different gastrointestinal disorders. Although, for many years small bowel contrast studies were the only practical and effective diagnostic tools on the basis of the length and tortuosity of the small intestine.

Complete visualization of the small bowel mucosa has been obtainable since the introduction of capsule endoscopy (CE) in 2001. Whereas CE has revolutionized diagnostic approach to small bowel disorders, inherent limitations of CE exist. The main limitations of capsule endoscopy include an inability to control the capsule and direct the viewing in real time, as well as inability to perform biopsies or therapeutic intervention and the possible risk of retention. In addition, for some children, voluntary ingestion of the CE can be daunting or impossible, and the capsule should be endoscopically inserted with dedicated device.

Historically, push enteroscopy or surgically assisted enteroscopy was used to further evaluate or treat detected lesions. However, the lack of efficacy and the invasive nature of these procedures, respectively, indicated a need for new methods.

Device assisted enteroscopy (DAE) has recently been reported as an effective method to achieve deep small bowel intubation allowing histologic evaluation and therapeutic intervention and has replaced push and surgically assisted enteroscopy. This advancement has assisted in the care of not only adults but also children and adolescents, although indications and number of application of these techniques may differ because of disease frequencies.

3.5.2 Indications and Contraindications

Indications for enteroscopy are well known in adults. International societies have published algorithms for the different clinical indications clarifying the role of this invasive and potentially dangerous technique in each clinical setting. Main indications and contraindications in children are listed in Table 3.6.

Table 3.6 Common indications and contraindications for enteroscopy in children

Indications
Obscure gastrointestinal bleeding
Suspected or known Crohn's disease
Polyps
Altered intestinal anatomy (e.g., Roux-en-Y)
Eosinophilic gastroenteropathies
Contraindications
Absolute Intestinal perforation Peritonitis Patient toxicity Cardiovascular instability
Relative Patient size/age Severe neutropenia Severe thrombocytopenia or coagulopathy Recent digestive surgery Partial or complete bowel obstruction Extensive intra-abdominal adhesions Toxic megacolon Connective tissue disorders Intra-abdominal vascular aneurysm Pregnancy

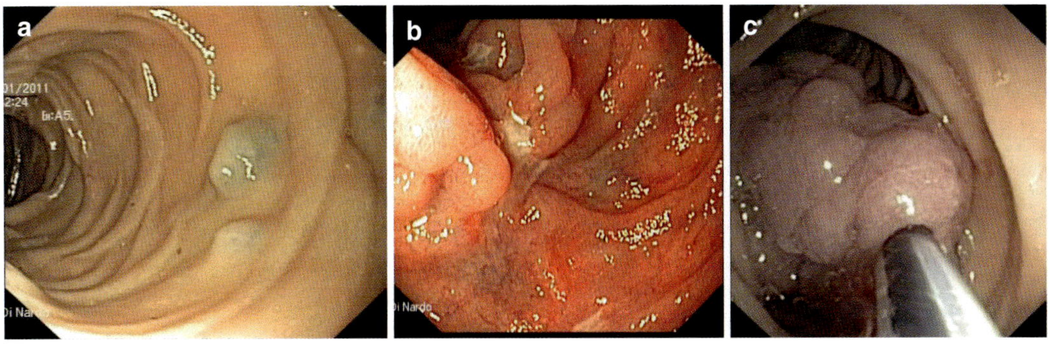

Fig. 3.6 Vascular malformation (**a**), deep ulcer (**b**) and giant jejunal polyp (**c**) detected during Single Balloon Enteroscopy

OGIB is the most common indication for enteroscopy in children. To date, considering the published pediatric case series, a total of 84 patients were studied for OGIB, and it was diagnostic in 62 patients (73.8 %). Diagnoses were Meckel's diverticulum (16.6 %), vascular lesions (15.4 %) (Fig. 3.6a), Crohn's disease (13 %) (Fig. 3.6b), ulcer (5.9 %), and polyps (5.9 %) (Fig. 3.6c). Endoscopic therapeutic procedures were described in 11 patients (13 %), although the published data did not evaluate the outcome.

Only in our recent study, CE has been systematically performed (including second look with CCE-2) before enteroscopy in children with OGIB, and this combined approach significantly increased the overall diagnostic yield (86 %) as compared to previous pediatric data.

In conclusion, enteroscopy has a high diagnostic yield in diagnosing the cause of OGIB in children with the advantage of therapeutic intervention and histologic diagnosis. Nevertheless, future prospective studies are needed to establish the correct place of enteroscopy in the diagnostic algorithm of children with OGIB.

In children with suspected Crohn's disease (CD), DAE is recommended when conventional studies including EGDS, ileocolonoscopy, imaging of small bowel, and CE have been undetermined and histological diagnosis and/or therapeutic procedure would alter disease management (Fig. 3.7). In the setting of established CD, DAE is indicated when endoscopic visualization and biopsies of the small intestine beyond the reach of EGDS or ileoscopy is necessary in order to exclude an alternative diagnosis (lymphoma, tuberculosis, or carcinoma) or undertake a therapeutic procedure including dilation of small bowel stricture, removal of retained capsule, and treatment of bleeding lesions (Fig. 3.8).

Small bowel polyps may cause intermittent bleeding, obstruction, intussusception, or progression to malignancy. Polypectomy might reduce the risk of multiple or urgent laparotomies with intestinal resection, which can result in morbidity and mortality. In published pediatric case series, 50 pediatric patients underwent enteroscopy for surveillance and treatment of small bowel polyps; 98 procedures and at least 318 polypectomies were performed. Not all the procedures allowed a complete evaluation of the small bowel. Although further studies are needed to assess the role of enteroscopy in the management algorithm of children with suspected or established small bowel polyps, it is an effective and safe alternative to surgery for the treatment of isolated and easy accessible small bowel polyps in children.

Contraindications for DAE are listed in Table 3.6.

3.5.3 Equipment

DAE was introduced for the first time in 2001 with double-balloon enteroscopy (DBE). Subsequently, single-balloon enteroscopy (SBE) and spiral enteroscopy have become available during the follow years. Unfortunately, no data reporting the use of spiral enteroscopy in children have been published to date, and the 16 mm outer diameter of the

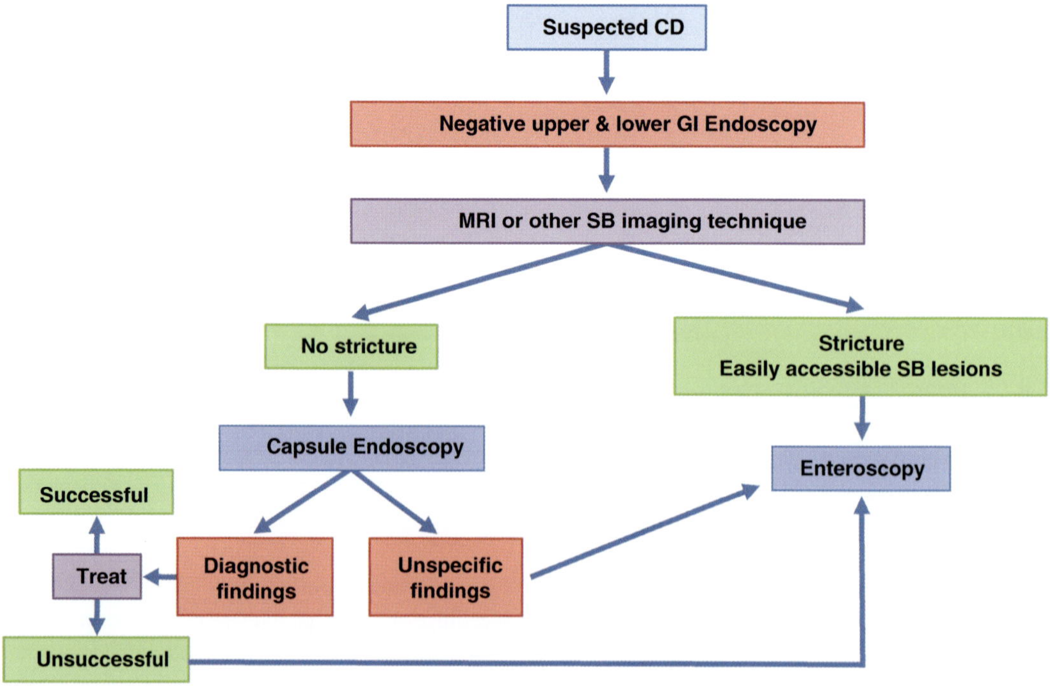

Fig. 3.7 Proposed algorithm in patients with suspected small bowel Crohn's disease. (Adapted by ref 16)

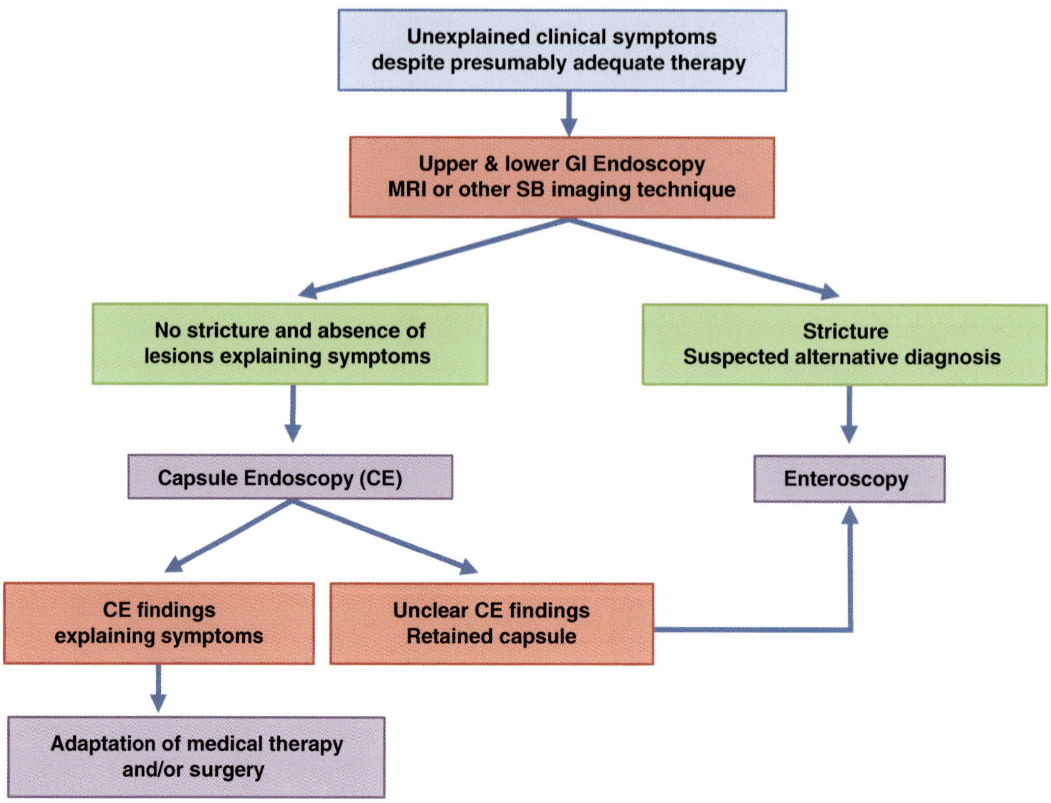

Fig. 3.8 Proposed algorithm in patients with established small bowel Crohn's disease. (Adapted by ref 16)

overtube currently makes this technique impractical for the majority of pediatric patients.

Commercially available since 2003, DBE (Fujinon Inc., Saitama, Japan) utilizes two primary models of endoscopes both with a working length of 200 cm (but with different outer diameters and channel diameters, 8.5 mm/2.2 mm and 9.8 mm/2.8 mm, respectively) plus a soft overtube, measuring either 12.2 or 13.2 mm in the outer diameter with a balloon located at the distal tip, and a length from 105 cm to 145 cm. The second balloon of the double-balloon system is located on the tip of the enteroscope and is inflated during overtube advancement to anchor the scope and prevent slippage.

Single-balloon enteroscopy (Olympus America Inc.) includes an enteroscope (outer diameter of 9.2 mm, channel diameter of 2.8 mm, working length of 200 cm) and a soft 13.2 mm outer diameter overtube (length of 140 cm) with a distal balloon designed to deeply intubate the small bowel. The overtube and the distal tip balloon are made of silicone rubber.

3.5.4 Technique

Balloon-assisted enteroscopy (BAE) including SBE and DBE is performed in children with the same technique described in adults. Obviously, there are some special considerations to take into account in performing BAE in children. The patient size could be the greatest limitation to the use of BAE in pediatric age. On data, DBE has successfully been performed from 2 years of age and SBE from 3 years of age, with a weight at least of 14 kg for both procedures. A smaller abdominal cavity, thinner intestinal walls, and a narrower intestinal lumen make BAE technically more difficult in younger children; thus, it requires a higher level of skill by the endoscopists. DBE is performed inflating the balloon that facilitates anchoring and shortening of the intestine, thus leading to straightening of the bowel yet to be examined and allowing deep advancement of the enteroscope. The bowel that has already been examined is "telescoped" onto the overtube during retraction. In this way, repeated advancement and retraction, or "pushing and pulling," ultimately leads to successful advancement throughout the small bowel. Complete small bowel viewing, from duodenum to cecum, is feasible although difficult. A combined antegrade and retrograde approach is often used to increase the amount of small bowel examined.

Regarding SBE, the primary difference with DBE is that there is no balloon on the tip of the enteroscope, which some feel makes it less complex to perform. In the past, DBE seemed to be able to achieve a greater depth of insertion compared to SBE. However, a recent randomized multicenter trial showed a similar depth of insertion and diagnostic yield in both techniques.

For both DBE and SBE, the patients need only to fast before the oral examination (approximately 12 h for solid food and 4 h for clear liquids). For retrograde examinations, a standard colonoscopy preparation is necessary. BAE in adults is usually performed either with conventional conscious sedation or with propofol based on local attitudes. General anesthesia with intubation is strongly recommended in children.

Depending on experience, radiologic fluoroscopy can be used as an aid in BAE, especially early on in the learning curve (Fig. 3.9); it can also be of usefulness when adhesions are expected because of prior abdominal surgery or massive SB involvement in children with Crohn's disease.

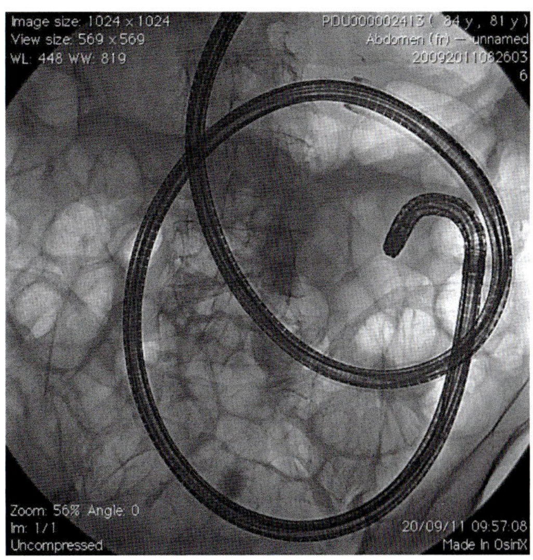

Fig. 3.9 Fluoroscopic view during oral enteroscopic approach

When stenosis is expected, radiology is certainly useful to assess stricture complexity.

Choice of oral versus anal approach is guided by the location of suspected disease. Several tools, including CE, MRI, and US, may be used to assist in localizing the lesion and direct the choice of the enteroscopic approach. In cases in which lesions are difficult or unable to be previous identified and located, both approaches can be considered. Complete small bowel assessment may at times be desired but in many cases is not necessary (e.g., primary lesion is encountered, obviating the need for complete examination) or unachievable. In many cases, the oral approach is chosen first due to the lower technical difficulty and consequently the greater depth of insertion when compared with the anal approach. Indeed, published series for DBE and SBE in adults and children have noted technical challenges to consistent passage through and beyond (proximally) the ileocecal valve. This can be explained by several factors inherent to normal anatomy, patient disease characteristics, and procedural difficulties. Total enteroscopy with BAE is defined as a complete evaluation of the small bowel, with either a single approach or a combined oral (anterograde)-anal (retrograde) approach. However, it may not be feasible in all patients; the reported success rate is 16–86%. If the lesion is not reached with a single approach, an Indian ink tattoo performed at the deepest point of insertion is used to document a complete SB examination.

All therapeutic procedures available for traditional endoscopy can be performed during BAE using dedicated devices. On data, there are not specific and well-established learning programs for enteroscopy, especially for pediatric endoscopists.

3.5.5 Complications

In adult population, the rate of complications ranged from 1.2 to 1.6%. Self-limited and mild post-procedure throat pain, abdominal pain, and discomfort were frequently described in both adult and pediatric patients. To date, only three major complications have been reported in the pediatric literature when endoscopic therapy has been performed. A laparoscopic-assisted DBE with the resection of several polyps was complicated by a pelvic abscess in the absence of perforation. One bleeding that was effectively treated endoscopically in a patient who had multiple resected polyps over a span of several endoscopic procedures. Finally, a jejunal perforation occurred in a child with Peutz-Jeghers syndrome who underwent two consecutive therapeutic DBE procedures within 18 days. The limited number of major complications in children would suggest a highly favorable safety profile. However, given the small number of patients studied, it may be premature to make definitive conclusions [12–16].

3.6 Cholangiopancreatography and Endoscopic Ultrasound

3.6.1 Introduction

Diseases requiring endoscopic retrograde cholangiopancreatography (ERCP) and/or endoscopic ultrasound (EUS) in children have a low incidence, thus limiting the experience and giving the impression that these procedures are more difficult in children. There is also lack of consensus about the indications to these procedures in the pediatric population. Generally, patients are referred to a tertiary care facility, and often the procedure is performed by an adult endoscopist.

3.6.2 Indications

ERCP is important in the evaluation of neonatal cholestasis to support a diagnosis of biliary atresia and other causes of biliary obstruction including choledocholithiasis. In recent years, indication to ERCP is mainly limited to therapeutic purposes, on the basis of the evolution of diagnostic imaging technique. During ERCP, a variety of therapeutic maneuvers could be achieved including sphincterotomy, sphincteroplasty, stones extraction, stricture dilation, and stent placement. Most common indications to ERCP in the pediatric age are discussed below.

ERCP can be a less invasive approach to obtain a cholangiogram in children with suspected biliary atresia. According to several studies, ERCP could avoid unnecessary surgery by distinguishing biliary atresia from other causes of neonatal cholestasis. In one report of 140 infants with suspected biliary atresia, ERCP was successfully performed in 87 %. ERCP findings were confirmed by intraoperative cholangiogram in 80 % of the cases. In another series, ERCP was 86 % sensitive and 94 % specific for detecting biliary atresia and 100 % sensitive and 90 % specific for detecting choledochal cysts.

Biliary atresia was classified by Kasai into three main types depending on the level of biliary obstruction. In Kasai type I, the common bile duct is obliterated. In Kasai type IIa, the common hepatic duct is obliterated; in type IIb, there is atresia of the common bile duct, common hepatic duct, and cystic duct. In Kasai type III, the entire extrahepatic biliary tree is obstructed. Kasai types I, IIb, and III are indistinguishable based on ERCP findings because the obstructed common bile duct prevents visualization of the remainder of the biliary tree.

There is also a classification of ERCP findings:

- Type 1: Nonvisualization of the biliary tree
- Type 2: Visualization of the distal common duct and gallbladder
- Type 3: Visualization of the gallbladder and the complete common duct, with both hepatic ducts and visualization of biliary lakes at the porta hepatis

Caroli disease is a congenital disorder characterized by multifocal, segmental dilatation of large intrahepatic bile ducts. The condition is frequently associated with renal cystic disease of varying severity. Caroli initially described two variants, with (Caroli syndrome) or without (Caroli disease) hepatic fibrosis. ERCP is usually required only if other less invasive imaging studies, like ultrasonography or magnetic resonance cholangiography, failed to establish the diagnosis.

Cystic dilatations of biliary ducts originally were termed choledochal cysts, considering only cysts of the extrahepatic bile duct. Since 1977, a new clinical classification includes intrahepatic cysts. Biliary cysts are found by abdominal ultrasound, computed tomography (CT), or magnetic resonance cholangiopancreatography (MRCP). ERCP can be used as a supplementary test to confirm the diagnosis and categorize the type of cyst to facilitate surgical planning.

The Todani classification is based on site of the cyst or dilatation and includes five types of cysts:

- *Type I*: The most common (80–90 %), saccular, or fusiform dilatation of common bile duct (CBD)
- *Type II*: Diverticulum protruding from the CBD
- *Type III* (*choledochocele*): Dilatation of the duodenal portion of CBD
- *Type IVa*: Multiple dilatations of the intrahepatic and extrahepatic ducts
- *Type IVb*: Multiple dilatations of the extrahepatic bile ducts
- *Type V*: Cystic dilatation of intrahepatic biliary ducts, excluding Caroli disease

The Todani classification does not include type VI: An isolated cyst of the cystic duct (very rare). Only single case reports are documented in the literature.

Types I, II, and IV biliary cysts are associated with an increased risk of malignancy, and surgical excision is recommended.

Endoscopic sphincterotomy is indicated in the following types of cysts:

1. Fusiform bile duct dilation with a widely dilated common channel. In contrast to cystic dilation, fusiform dilation is more commonly associated with low-grade, short strictures located at or distal to the pancreaticobiliary junction.
2. Distal bile duct stricture, which typically occurs at the point of connection with the pancreatic duct. Up to 8 % of such patients

develop cystolithiasis (which may be multiple) involving intrahepatic and extrahepatic ducts.
3. Choledochocele (type III cyst).

Noteworthy, an anomalous pancreaticobiliary junction (APBJ) can present in up to 70 % of patients with biliary cysts. It is characterized by a junction of the bile duct and pancreatic duct outside the duodenal wall with a long common duct channel. According to the Kimura classification, there are three types of APBJ:

1. Type B-P – Common bile duct joining the main pancreatic duct.
2. Type P-B – Pancreatic duct joining the common bile duct; this type is more likely to be associated with recurrent pancreatitis than the B-P type.
3. Long Y type – A long common channel, without common bile duct dilatation.

Sclerosing cholangitis in children is usually related with an underlying disorder, and approximately 14 % of children with sclerosing cholangitis have underlying inflammatory bowel disease. The diagnosis of sclerosing cholangitis is usually established by magnetic resonance MRCP. The typical finding is pruning of the peripheral biliary tree with stenosis and dilation.

ERCP allows cytological sampling of the stenosis and therapeutic intervention in case of obstructive symptoms (Fig. 3.10). In case of dominant ductal strictures, according to the data of literature in the adult population, there is indication to endoscopic treatment with sphincterotomy and balloon dilation to relieve the obstruction.

Choledocholithiasis is rare in the pediatric population, and it is typically related with hemolysis, infection, chronic liver disease, or choledochal cyst. A review including 382 pediatric patients with gallstones found sickle cell disease, parenteral nutrition, and cardiac surgery as the most common risk factors with the highest frequency in infants, often without symptoms. The incidence of gallstones rises in girls during puberty. Ultrasonography does not always identify small stones in the biliary system. Thus, magnetic resonance cholangiopancreatography (MRCP) or endoscopic ultrasound (EUS) are often required to evaluate patients with a clinical suspicion.

The role of ERCP and the benefit of endoscopic sphincterotomy in children with choledocholithiasis have not been confirmed. Infants and children who presented no symptoms but have small common bile duct stones on an imaging study should usually be managed conservatively, since the stones (or sludge) are likely to pass spontaneously. Sphincterotomy generally should be reserved for symptomatic patients or those with underlying lithogenic disorders.

Malignant strictures of extrahepatic ducts are rare in children. There are few cases described in literature in which stenting successfully relieved the obstruction.

Bile duct complications after liver transplantation include bile duct strictures, leaks, and bile casts. The onset can be early or late (within or after 4 weeks from transplant). Diagnosis relies on MRCP, with ERCP playing only a therapeutic role.

The role of EUS is well established in adult GI and pancreatobiliary diseases. There is, instead, poor literature regarding the use of EUS in pediatric patients because usefulness of EUS in children has been only recently appreciated, and published papers often report few patients and single center experiences. Even if the pathology may differ between the two populations, EUS indications in children are similar to those described in adults. Also the reported results show a great impact of EUS in the management of disease in the pediatric population, in particular for what concerns pancreatobiliary disease (Fig. 3.11).

EUS could be used as a diagnostic tool to avoid more invasive procedure as ERCP in the evaluation of the common bile duct or the pancreatic duct. In children with clinical signs of CBD obstruction, EUS avoided diagnostic ERCP in the majority of cases. Also in pancreatic disease, EUS altered patient management or was used as a therapeutic tool in EUS-guided treatment.

There are few reports on interventional diagnostic or therapeutic pancreaticobiliary EUS in

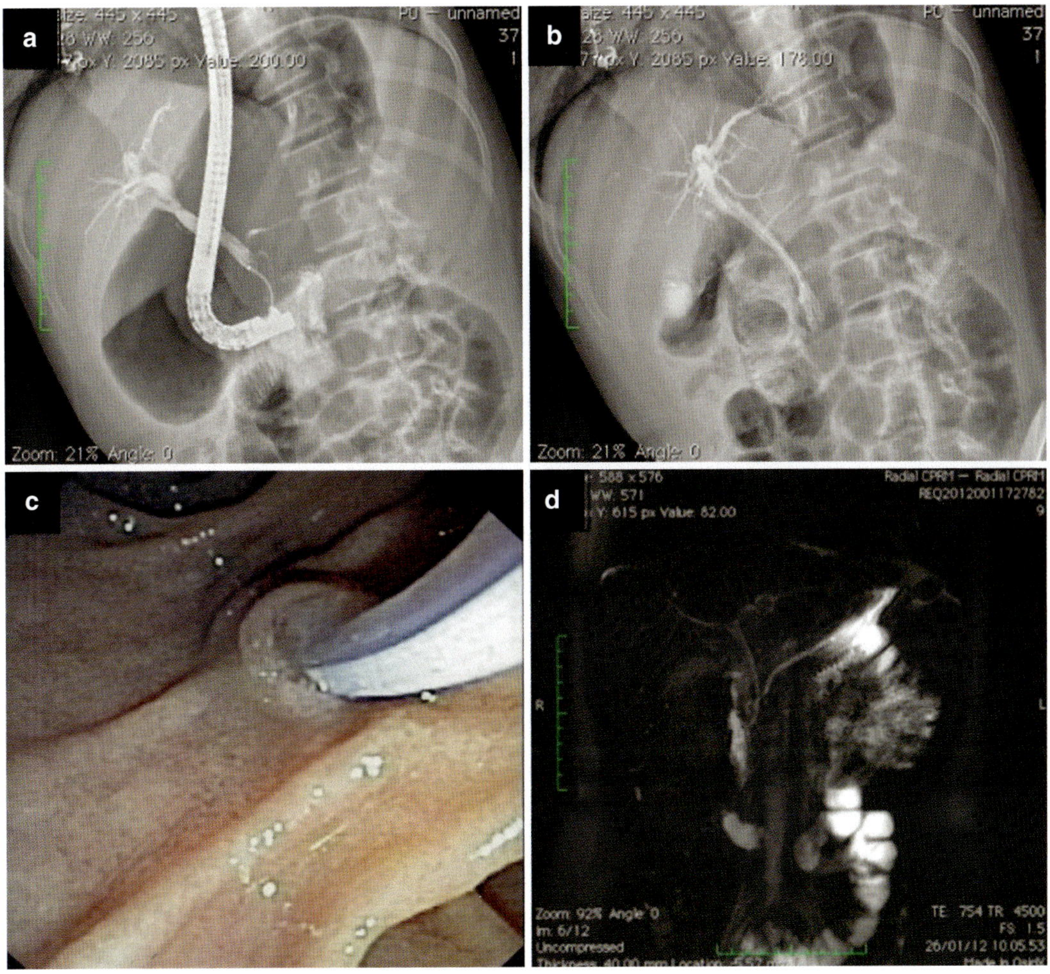

Fig. 3.10 Radiological (**a**, **b**) endoscopic (**c**) and MRI (**d**) findings of plastic biliary stents placed in a child with chronic pancreatitis associated to jaundice and choledochal dilation

the pediatric population. The principal described indications have been EUS-FNA and pancreatic fluid collection drainage. Despite the small sample size, in the pediatric population results of fine needle aspiration were similar to those achieved in adults in terms of success rate and diagnostic accuracy. In particular, the use of EUS-FNA could diagnose an autoimmune pancreatitis or could be useful in case of chronic fibrosing pancreatitis for a differential diagnosis from malignant masses. EUS-guided pseudocyst drainage has been used with high success rate in the pediatric population. In a case series published in 2013, a total of seven children underwent EUS-guided drainage of PFCs. The etiology was blunt abdominal trauma in five, hereditary pancreatitis in one, and idiopathic pancreatitis in one. Both technical and treatment success rates were 100 %. Two patients underwent repeat EUS-guided drainage due to lack of adequate resolution of pancreatic fluid collection on follow-up computed tomography. No immediate or delayed complications were reported. At a median follow-up of 1033 days, all of the children were doing well with no recurrence of the collections. EUS-guided rendezvous or ductal drainage has been occasionally reported. A case of pancreatic duct drainage by the rendezvous technique has been reported in a child and EUS-guided biliary drainage in a 13-year-old patient

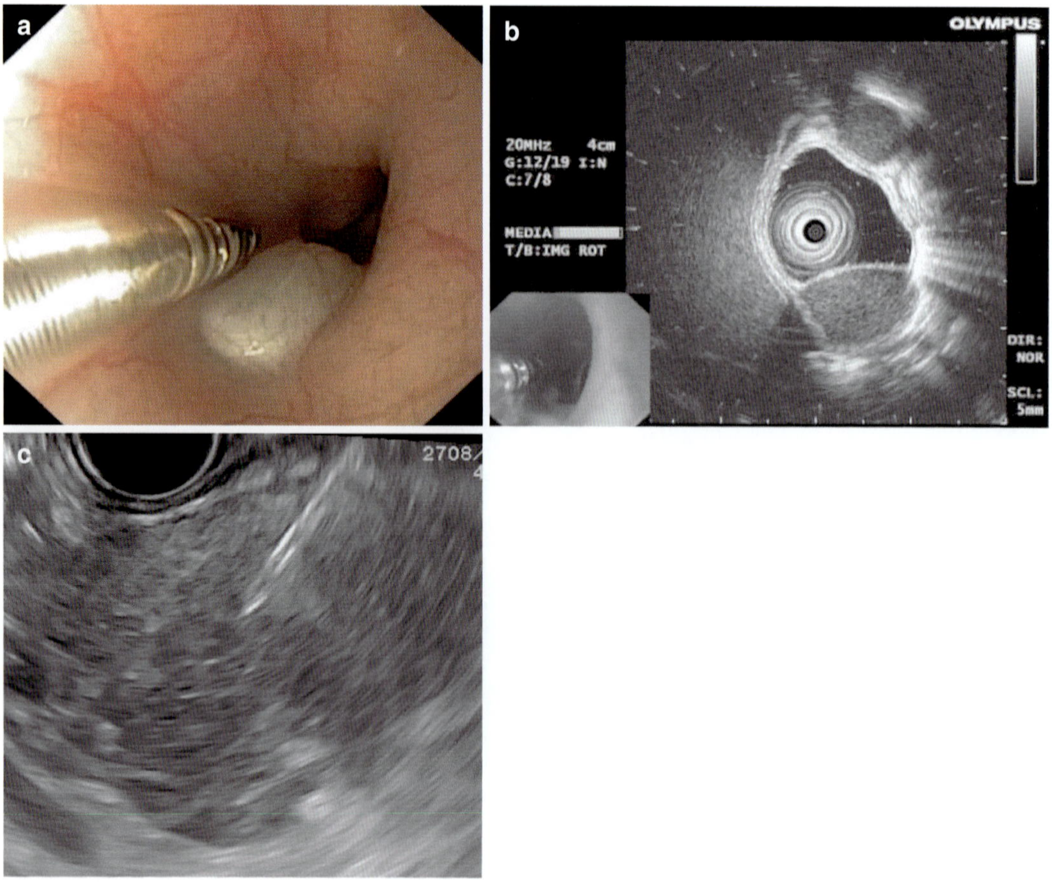

Fig. 3.11 Endoscopic (**a**) and EUS (**b**) appearance of esophageal duplication cyst. EUS-guided FNA of a pancreatic mass (**c**)

with metastatic rhabdomyosarcoma obstructing the biliary tract and involving the duodenum. This technique is rarely used even in the adult population.

Pediatric mediastinal masses represent a diagnostic and therapeutic challenge. They are a heterogeneous group of potentially life-threatening diseases. Transesophageal EUS with FNA allows assessment and biopsy of posterior and middle mediastinal lesions. The reported cases in literature are principally mediastinal nodes in which EUS-FNA was used for cytological diagnosis.

There are several reports about the use of EUS for the evaluation of esophageal, gastric, duodenal, or rectal disease. The technique and results are comparable to the ones in the adult population with a significant impact of EUS on the management of the patients. In the differential diagnosis of esophageal stenosis, EUS with miniprobes can diagnose the nature of the stenosis, thus guiding the further treatment. Subepithelial lesions or duplication cyst can be distinguished in the upper gastrointestinal tract by endoscopic ultrasound. Rectal ultrasound has been used in patients with anal fistulas and underlying Crohn's disease.

3.6.3 Patient Preparation and Sedation

The preparation and sedation of a patient undergoing ERCP/EUS is similar to that used for upper gastrointestinal endoscopy. In the case of pediatric setting, an adequate explanation of the procedure should be provided to the little patient and parents. If an adult endoscopist is performing the procedure, a close collaboration with a pediatric team should be implemented in order to provide an adequate care. Deep sedation with an anesthesiologist is highly recommended, since children cannot fully cooperate during procedures performed under conscious sedation. Post-procedure monitoring is not different than other endoscopic procedures requiring sedation. ERCP and EUS can be performed on an ambulatory basis when performed for diagnosis only. Therapeutic ERCP has a greater potential risk for serious complications, and overnight observation in the hospital may be indicated. Because ERCP is associated with a higher risk for bacteremia than diagnostic endoscopy, in selected cases, an antibiotic prophylaxis should be considered.

3.6.4 Equipment

For ERCP, a pediatric duodenoscope, with a diameter of 7.5 mm is mandatory in neonate and infants younger than 12 months and is preferred for children younger than 3 years. In older children and adolescents, a standard adult duodenoscope with a diameter of 11 mm can be used.

For EUS, thinner instruments are preferred in small patients. In children, 3 years of age or older a standard EUS equipment can be used.

3.6.5 Technique

ERCP is usually performed with the patient in the prone or semiprone position. The duodenoscope is inserted into the second portion of the duodenum and then is straightened in "short route" with a slow withdrawn. When it is not possible to perform this maneuver, the approach to cannulation of the papilla is performed with the "long route." In this case, the instrument stands along the greater curvature of the stomach. Cannulation technique in children is the same as in adults, but it is necessary to consider the narrower lumen of the children's duodenum that can add some difficulty. In neonates, deep selective cannulation of the bile duct is generally impossible because of the small duct diameter.

In children older than 1 year and adolescents, the rate of successful cannulation is more than 95 %, comparable to reports in adults. In neonates and young infants, the rate of successful cannulation of the common bile duct is often lower than in adults.

In EUS examination, the maneuvers are similar with the exploration of pancreatic head and uncinate accomplished from the duodenum while pancreatic body and tail visualized from the stomach. The experience of the endoscopists may account for a large part of the variability.

3.6.6 Complications

Complications of ERCP are pancreatitis, infection, hemorrhage, and perforation. A series of 329 ERCP for biliary or pancreatic indication reported a total of 32 complications (10 %), mostly pancreatitis with no deaths. The rate of post-ERCP pancreatitis seems to be higher in the patients undergoing pancreatic duct stent placement (7 of 28 procedures, 25 %). There is a very limited experience with EUS in the pediatric population. The complication rate not seems to differ from the adult series being very low especially for diagnostic examination [17–20].

3.7 Polypectomy

3.7.1 Introduction

Polypectomy is the most common endoscopic therapeutic intervention performed in children. In more recent decades, endoscopic polypectomy has endorsed continuous advances because of improvements in the endoscopic technology and techniques.

Polypectomy is difficult to learn, requiring a baseline level of skills in instrument handling including the ability to precisely and efficiently control the instrument tip and therapeutic devices.

3.7.2 Technique

Polyp shape and location both influence the success and technique of endoscopic polypectomy. Pedunculated polyps are much easier to remove than sessile and flat polyps, although they are still associated with a risk of postpolypectomy hemorrhage. The right colon, especially the cecum, is thinner walled than the left with consequent higher rates of complications after removing polyps from this colonic region. Polyps draped over the ileocecal valve are the most difficult to remove and are associated with the highest need for surgery. Rectal polyps are probably the easiest to resect, particularly if located in the lower half of the rectum that is extraperitoneal, minimizing the consequences of full-thickness electrocautery.

Different polypectomy snares are available with variable shape (oval, crescent, hexagonal), size (standard, mini, macro), and reusable vs. disposable. Before polypectomy, the snare should always be checked to make certain that the tip closes at least 1.5 cm into the plastic sheath. The point on the handle at which the snare has closed so that the snare has just entered the plastic sheath should also be marked, as this indicates when mechanical closure is complete and approximately the amount of tissue enclosed in the snare.

All kind of polyps should be captured in the "six o'clock position" because the snare enters the field roughly at this orientation; this can usually be accomplished by rotation of the colonoscope relative to the polyp or changing the patient's position. Because the optical element is located above the working channel of the endoscope, attempting to capture polyps at other orientations may result in losing the visual field against a fold prior to capture of the polyp. It is often easier to remove a polyp during the withdrawal phase of the examination because in this phase loops are removed and the polyp may be more easily snared because both torque and tip deflection are more responsive when the colonoscope is straightened. Additionally, advancing proximal to the lesion, deploying the snare, and dragging it over the polyp often facilitate placement of the snare.

Pedunculated polyps should be sufficiently manipulated to assure the colonoscopist that the snare is near the polyp's head but not around a portion of the head or normal tissue in order to leave a sufficient stalk for regrasping if immediate bleeding occurs. Once snared, the lesion should be lifted away from the colonic wall to minimize contact with the opposing colonic wall avoiding contralateral electrocautery injury. After transection, the stalk should be observed briefly to ensure that no immediate bleeding is occurring. In such a case, bleeding can be treated by regrasping the stalk and holding it for 5–10 min. Alternatively, injection of diluted adrenalin or application of clips has been reported as useful methods to stop immediate postpolypectomy bleeding. For large pedunculated lesions, additional strategies such as epinephrine injection (1:10,000) and attachment of a detachable loop snare (Fig. 3.12a, b) or of a metal endoclip (Fig. 3.12c–e) to the stalk prior to polypectomy should be considered to prevent postpolypectomy bleeding.

Sessile polyps can be removed by standard monopolar electrocautery using principles similar to those for pedunculated polyps. Transection in a single piece is generally feasible even for large polyps with a diameter within 2 or 3 cm. After grasping, the polyp is lifted or tented into the lumen in order to create an artificial stalk. In the right colon, it is advisable to partially deflate the lumen. Large sessile polyps represent a particular challenge to endoscopists because of the risks of hemorrhage, perforation, and inadequate polypectomy.

The submucosal injection technique has been proposed to make removal of large sessile colonic polyps easier and safer. Injection of fluids into the submucosa under the polyp increases the distance between the base of the polyp and the serosa, thus reducing the risk of bleeding, thermal injury, and perforation. The most commonly used fluid is saline (normal or hypertonic), with or without epinephrine. With time, this fluid will be reabsorbed; thus, other fluids have been used in an attempt to prolong the effect, including 10 % glycerol/5 % fructose, 50 % dextrose, sodium hyaluronate, and hydroxypropyl methylcellulose. Sometimes

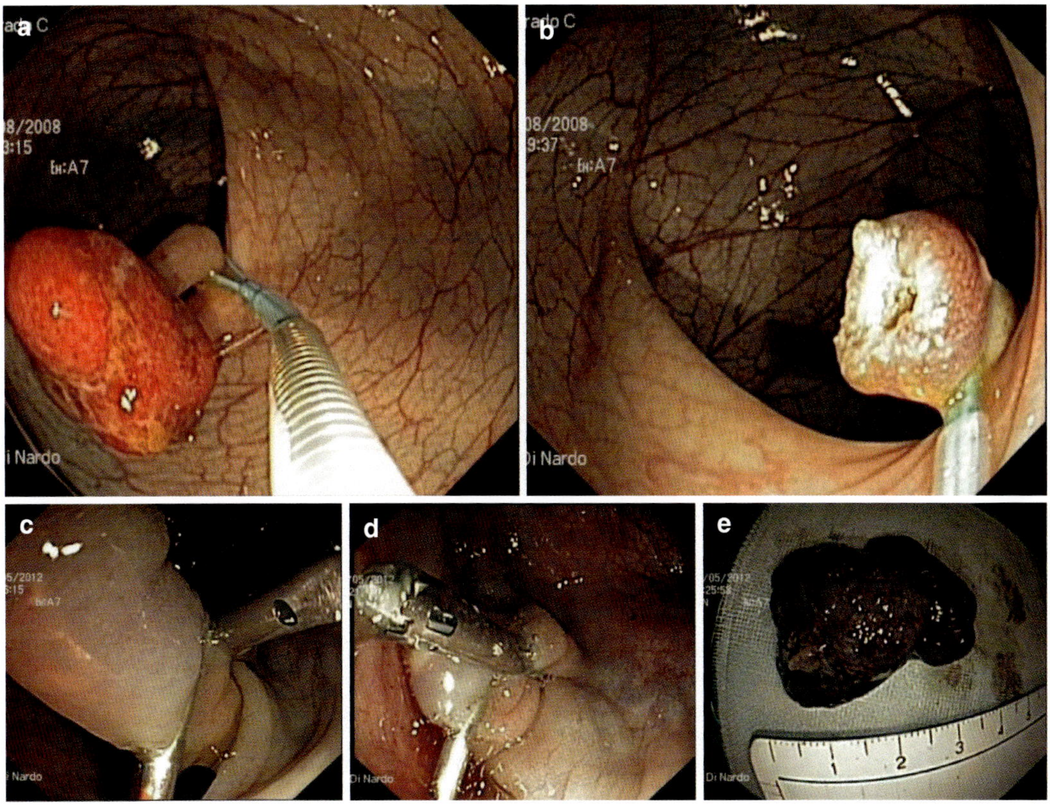

Fig. 3.12 Detachable loop snare (**a**, **b**) and metal endoclip (**c**–**e**) applied to the stalk of two giant pedunculated polyps to prevent postpolypectomy bleeding

few drops of methylene blue can be added to enhance visualization of polyp margins. Fluid is injected using a standard sclerotherapy needle. The needle may be placed into the submucosa at the edge of a polyp, or if the polyp is large and flat, multiple injections may be given around the periphery and directly into the center of the polyp. The desired elevation may require 3–4 mL of solution, although larger volumes can be injected safely. It is preferable to inject the proximal (far) aspect of the polyp first. If the distal aspect is injected first, the polyp can be tilted away from the colonoscope, making subsequent resection more difficult. If a bleb does not immediately form, slowly withdraw and lift the needle slightly while injecting until bleb formation is observed. However, if the polyp fails to elevate (the "non-lifting sign"), it may be an indication of infiltration of the lesion into the submucosa and muscularis propria. Alternatively, this phenomenon may also be caused by a prior attempt at polypectomy with healing and scarring of the layers, preventing this separation by fluid injection or by the needle penetration out of the colon wall, and so the fluid is being injected into the peritoneum.

Most (over 80–90 %) of the polyps encountered during routine endoscopy are less than 10 mm; therefore, techniques to remove these lesions must be optimized due to its important clinical consequences. These polyps can be resected using a number of different techniques, including hot or cold biopsy (with or without cautery), hot or cold minisnare, or cold biopsy followed by fulguration with a bipolar electrode. Cold snaring is the best technique for virtually all small (<10 mm) and most diminutive (<5 mm) polyps. Cold snaring allows efficient resection of polyp tissue in a single piece, with a margin of normal tissue to ensure complete eradication. Occasionally, polyps less than 10 mm are narrow-based and bulky or pedunculated. In these occasional situations, hot snare resection may be warranted because of the higher risk of immediate bleeding with a more vascular pedicle.

The technique of cold snaring is fundamentally different from snaring with electrocautery. With cold snaring, the endoscopist advances the snare sheath, opens the snare, and encircles the polyp. The snare is then slowly and progressively closed, with the aim of capturing 1–2 mm of normal tissue around the polyp, until complete closure is achieved and the polyp is guillotined. Suction can help the snare to capture the polyp and surrounding tissue. The polyp can then be readily suctioned and retrieved.

3.7.3 Retrieval of Multiple Polyps

Retrieval of multiple polyps or multiple fragments of a big polyp could be a difficult challenge. A single snared polyp could be retrieved with the standard polypectomy snare; alternatively, a prolonged grasping device or wire basket may be used. In addition, dedicated Roth Net snare with a special net has been introduced for the removal of multiple fragments in one shot and has been proved to be safe and useful. The retrieval net could be particularly useful after piecemeal resection of large polyps in the proximal colon to avoid repeated introduction. Polyps as large as 7–8 mm in diameter could be aspirated and retrieved through the colonoscope using the commercially available filtered polyp suction trap. A useful trick for forced aspiration of larger polyp fragments is to remove the suction bottom valve, cover the opening with a finger, and wait.

3.7.4 Complications

Endoscopic polypectomy could be associated with complications, such as bleeding, perforation, and postpolypectomy coagulation syndrome. Most of these complications are self-limiting or could be readily managed conservatively and/or endoscopically. More rarely, they could be life threatening and/or require surgery. Risk factors for complications in this setting include multiple polypectomies, increased size, right colon location, and inexperienced endoscopist.

Bleeding, either immediate or delayed (usually within 1 week, but possible in up to 3–4 weeks), is the most frequently observed complication.

For small polyps, the immediate bleeding rate is 0.5–2.2 %, while delayed bleeding is rare (0.3–0.6 %). Most of the bleeding discovered in this setting is either self-limiting or easily treated in the same endoscopic session, with clip placement or adrenaline injection (1:10,000). Some of the proposed methods of preventing bleeding, such as prophylactic use of hemostatic clips or prophylactic argon plasma coagulation, on the polypectomy scar do not seem to be useful for preventing delayed bleeding in this setting.

Pedunculated polyps have an increased risk of bleeding. Epinephrine injection to both the stalk and the polyp head, as well as looping and clipping techniques, has been successfully deployed to prevent the risk of bleeding after hot snare polypectomy. Even though injection of epinephrine may only prevent immediate but not delayed bleeding, this is the most widely used preventive method.

Perforation (immediate or delayed) is the second most common complication of polypectomy. For small and diminutive polyps, the risk of perforation is nil when cold polypectomy is performed. Perforation in polypectomy has in fact been mostly associated with electrocautery, so this technique is no longer advisable. On the other hand, removal of large lesions is associated with higher perforation rates (0–1.5 %). Lesions larger than 50 mm, located at the proximal colon especially the cecum, are other important risk factors for perforation, since the colonic wall is thin, while rectal location is a protective factor against perforation since the wall is thicker and retroperitoneal. Patients suffering from severe persistent pain that is not diminished by the passage of flatus should undergo X-ray examination to seek the presence of extraluminal air. A CT scan should also be considered. When the endoscopist is sure that perforation has occurred by virtue of seeing the peritoneal cavity or other organ, then immediate surgical exploration is required.

Postpolypectomy coagulation syndrome is a rare manifestation of peritoneal irritation because of electrocautery but without evidence of perforation on computed tomography scan. It occurs in 1.3–3.7 % of patients undergoing excision of large lesions (usually >2 cm), but requires hospitalization in only 0.07 %. Fever, abdominal pain, and increased inflammation markers characterize it. Symptoms may occur up to 5 days after polypectomy, but this syndrome has an excellent prognosis and is managed conservatively with medical therapy [21–23].

3.8 Hemostasis Techniques

3.8.1 Introduction

Therapeutic endoscopy is indicated for patients with active bleeding at the time of endoscopy and for patients with high-risk stigmata or lesions associated with a high rebleeding rate identified at endoscopy. High-risk stigmata associated with ulcers include an evidence of active bleeding, an oozing from beneath an overlying clot, and a nonbleeding visible vessel at its base. A visible vessel usually appears as a red, blue, or white plug or mound.

Gastroduodenal vascular malformations and Dieulafoy lesions (an isolated blood vessel protruding through a small nonulcer mucosal defect), although are a rare source of upper gastrointestinal bleeding, have a high risk of bleeding with a high complication rate if left untreated. The complication and rebleeding rates of these lesions significantly decrease with effective endoscopic therapy.

Diffused mucosal bleeding from duodenitis or gastritis is usually not responsive to endoscopic intervention, except for portal hypertensive gastropathy. Esophageal and gastric varices could also have endoscopic characteristics that are associated with a high rebleeding rate and will be discussed in a dedicated section. Colonic lesions amenable to endoscopic therapy include bleeding ulcers, vascular malformations, polyps, and bleeding polyp stalks. Colonic varices, either caused by portal hypertension or hereditary, are less amenable to endoscopic therapy than their upper tract counterparts because of their diffuse nature unless a discrete bleeding point is identified at the time of endoscopy.

3.8.2 Nonvariceal Gastrointestinal Bleeding

Three endoscopic techniques could be used to control nonvariceal gastrointestinal bleeding: injective, thermal, and mechanical. The specific technique used depends on equipment availability, site and type of bleeding lesion, and experience of the endoscopist.

Standard pediatric gastroduodenoscopes have a 2.0-mm operative channel, and consequently they will accommodate needles for injection therapy but will not allow the use of thermal and mechanical devices. Standard adult gastroduodenoscopes have a 2.8-mm operative channel sufficient for all devices; however, the outer diameter (8.6–9.8 mm) of these endoscopes cannot be used in children below 10 kg. Adult therapeutic gastroduodenoscopes have either one or two operative channels ranging in sizes from 2.8 to 3.8 mm, but their outer diameter (11.3–12.9 mm) usually precludes their use in children below 20–25 kg.

Pediatric colonoscopes have a 2.8–3.8-mm channel allowing the use of all hemostatic devices.

3.8.2.1 Injection Technique

This is an inexpensive and easy-to-learn method usually performed by injection of a liquid agent at three or four sites around an exposed bleeding vessel and then directly at the site of the vessel. The rationale for this technique is that a visible vessel is not an end artery and that for effective

Table 3.7 Selected endoscopic accessories for injective hemostasis

Type	Diameter/size	Min endoscopic channel required (mm)	Representative products and manufacturers
Injection needle	23G, 25G 21G	2.0 2.8	Various
Injection-coagulation catheter	7 F (25G) 10 F (25G)	2.8 3.7	Injection gold probe/Boston Scientific
Injection-polypectomy snare	3.0 mm (25G)	3.7	iSnare/US Endoscopy

Adapted by Ref. [24]

Table 3.8 Sclerosant agents for nonvariceal bleeding

Solution	Concentration	Volume/number of injections/location	Max total volume	Comments
Hypertonic saline-epinephrine combination	3.6 % saline + 1:20,000 epinephrine or 7.2 % saline + 1:20,000 epinephrine	3 mL 3–4 injections at base of bleeding vessel	9–12 mL	Repeat prophylactic injections if visible vessel present 24–48 h after first hemostasis
Epinephrine with normal saline	1 mL 1:1000 epinephrine + 9 mL normal saline	0.5–2.0 mL injected in multiple sites around bleeding vessel and into bleeding point itself	10 mL	Larger volumes in range for spurting vessels
Epinephrine followed by polidocanol	5–10 mL epinephrine 1:10,000 Polidocanol 1 % 5 mL	Inject epinephrine into submucosa directly around blood vessel to achieve hemostasis by compression/vasocostriction, then obliterate vessel with polidocanol	Epinephrine 5–10 mL Polidocanol 5 mL	May substitute bipolar coagulation for polidocanol
Thrombin in normal saline	100 IU thrombin in 3 mL normal saline	Inject into bleeding vessel 10–15 mL total volume	10–15 mL	
Epinephrine with normal saline for polypectomy	1 mL 1:1000 epinephrine + 9 mL normal saline	1.0–2.0 mL per injection injected in multiple sites (3–4) around polyp to be raised up	30 mL	Goal is lack of vascular markings within injection site

Adapted by Ref. [24]

hemostasis tamponade of the feeding vessel is required. Injection is most easily performed by injection of the proximal site of the lesion first and distally thereafter; this avoids that injection over the distal site of the lesion as creation of the submucosal bleb may lift the bleeding site away from the view. Hemostasis results from a combination of vasoconstriction, mechanical tamponade, and cytochemical mechanisms.

Injection needles consist of an outer sheath (plastic, Teflon, or stainless steel) and inner hollow-core needle (19–25 gauge). Using a handle on the end of the needle sheath, the operator can retract the needle into the sheath for safe passage through the working channel of the endoscope. When the catheter is placed near the target lesion, the needle can be extended out of the end of the sheath to a preset distance, and a syringe attached to the handle is used to inject liquid agents. A combined injection needle/multipolar probe and a combined injection needle/snare are available to allow for sequential injection and coagulation (Table 3.7).

Table 3.8 lists the most commonly used solutions, their concentrations, appropriate volumes, and recommended injection site. Except under unusual circumstances, injection therapy should be confined to a single solution (single agent or a combination agent) during an injection episode to minimize the risk of ulcer extension or perforation.

The main criticism of injective technique is that it may only provide temporary control of hemorrhage. For this reason, it is generally used to stop or slow down active bleeding prior to application of conclusive therapy such as thermal or mechanical technique.

Complications are usually related to the substance injected (e.g., arrhythmias and hypertension after adrenaline, bowel ischemia, and perforation after sclerosing agent injection in the thinner walled duodenum or right colon) and rarely to inappropriate technique (e.g., increased bleeding, rebleeding).

3.8.2.2 Thermal Techniques

Thermal devices generate heat either directly (e.g., heater probe [HP]) or indirectly by passage of electrical current through tissue (e.g., multipolar electrocautery [MPEC] probes, argon plasma coagulator [APC]).

Heater probe consists of a Teflon-coated hollow aluminum cylinder with an inner heating coil. A thermocoupling device at the tip of the probe maintains a constant temperature. Probe activation results in delivery of a preselected amount of energy in joules to the probe tip. Once the pulse has been initiated, the duration of activation is predetermined. The probe is water perfused to prevent tissue adherence. Coagulation should be around the bleeding point or stigmata first and then directly upon it. If a twin-channel instrument is used, the endoscopist is able to tamponade the bleeding with the probe while simultaneously suctioning in the region of the ulcer base. The number of joules per pulse should be reduced, especially in right-sided colonic lesions. In 1–3 % of cases, perforation may occur after heater probe application for gastrointestinal bleeding because of the variable depth and extent of tissue injury after application. Precipitation of bleeding has been reported in up to 5 % of cases after heater probe application.

Because of these limitations, the bipolar probe or MPEC is more commonly used. In these devices, current is transmitted from one electrode on the probe to another electrode. Energy is delivered when any pair of electrodes is in contact with the bleeding target. MPEC probes may have six points through which current can be passed; contact between any two is sufficient, allowing for tangential contact. The maximal temperature achieved with this method is significantly less than that of monopolar coagulation, resulting in less tissue injury and also greater efficacy for vessels <2 mm. As with the heater probe, the correct technique is to compress the bleeding vessel first and then to coagulate. Pulses should be applied as short, multiple pulses (2 s long) or a single pulse as long as 6–10 s. In adults, up to 40 s total of electrocoagulation may be required.

Increased bleeding after bipolar coagulation has been reported in cases with a visible vessel; usually this bleeding is controllable with further bipolar coagulation, but on occasion surgery has been required. MPEC seems to be equally effective to heater probe in terms of hemostasis, incidence of rebleeding, transfusion requirement, and need for emergency surgery.

In addition to sequential combination therapy, a combination probe is available that allows for sequential injection and coagulation without the use of a dual-channel endoscope or catheter exchange.

The APC is a noncontact electrocoagulation device that uses high-frequency monopolar alternating current conducted to target tissues through ionized argon gas (argon plasma).

The probes, consisting of a Teflon tube with a tungsten monopolar electrode contained in a ceramic nozzle close to the distal end of the probe, are 2.3 or 3.2 mm in outer diameter and are available in lengths of 220 or 440 cm. Probes are available to direct plasma either parallel or perpendicular to the axis of the catheter (Fig. 3.13). Gas flow rates can be varied from 0.5 to 7.0 L/min, the power settings vary from 0 to 155 W, and the generator voltage ranges from 5000 to 6500 V. Argon gas passes through the coagulation probe with an electrode at its tip. The foot switch activates the electrode, resulting in a flow of electrically activated ionized gas from the probe to the tissue causing tissue desiccation at the interface.

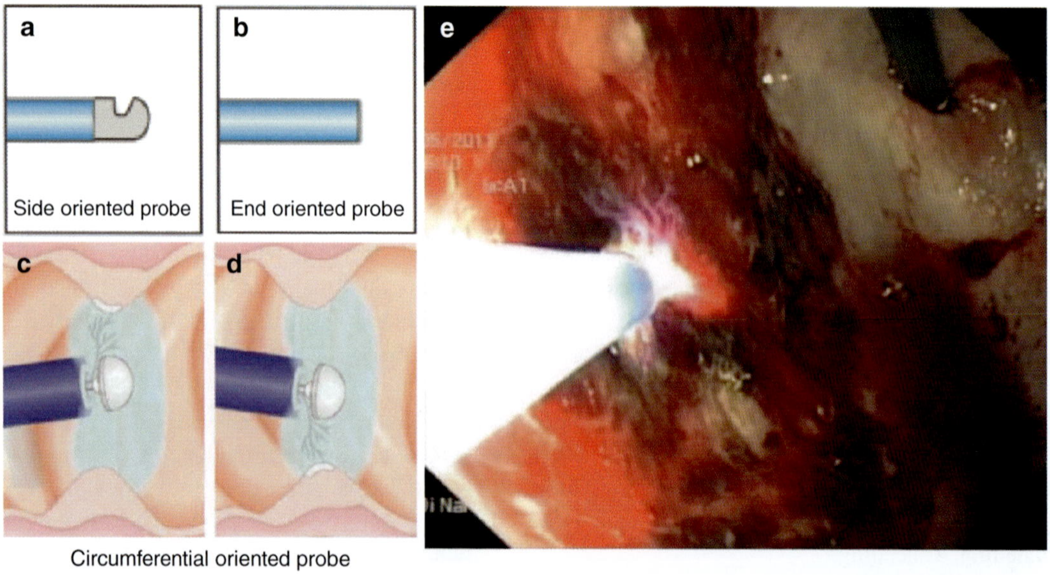

Fig. 3.13 Schematic representation of the available different oriented probe for Argon Plasma Coagulator (APC) application (**a–d**). Endoscopic view of APC treatment of a diffuse gastric bleeding (**e**)

If the catheter is not near target tissue (2–8 mm), there is no ignition of the gas, and depression of the foot pedal results only in flow of inert argon gas. After desiccation, the electrical resistance of the treated area increases, prompting the current to move to the untreated area of lower resistance. The depth of coagulation is dependent on the power setting, the gas flow rate, the duration of application, and the distance between the probe tip and the target tissue. The surface to be treated should be cleared of fluids, limiting the usefulness of the APC in cases of active bleeding. If the overlying surface is not clear, then a coagulated film may develop and the tissue beneath the surface may not be adequately treated. The correct technique is to put the probe to an optimal operating distance and to move the endoscope shaft to paint the confluent area to be coagulated. The noncontact nature of the technique makes it possible to treat large areas rapidly, in comparison with the heater probe or MPEC. The probe tip should not contact the tissue because this is a monopolar probe and deep tissue injury may occur with contact, although the safety of the technique is not forfeited by occasional inadvertent tissue contact. Care must also be taken to continuously aspirate the argon gas, which is flowing under steady pressure whenever the foot switch is activated during the procedure, because failure to do so can result in overdistension of the stomach or bowel, especially in smaller patients. Appropriate modifications will be required in pediatric patients, with current generators having minimum gas flow rates of 0.5 L/min and in right-sided colonic lesions that could be elevated with a saline cushion before treatment to reduce the risk of perforation.

Applications for the APC include hemostasis of vascular ectasias, treatment of bleeding ulcers, treatment of residual adenomatous tissue, and ablative therapy. The primary pediatric indication is likely to be treatment of symptomatic gastrointestinal vascular lesions (Fig. 3.13).

Complications have been reported in 0–24 % of patients in various adult series and include gaseous distension, pneumatosis intestinalis, pneumoperitoneum, pneumomediastinum, subcutaneous emphysema, pain at the treatment site, chronic ulceration, stricture, bleeding, transmural burn, and perforation.

3.8.2.3 Mechanical Techniques

Endoscopic clips consist of a metal double- or triple-pronged preloaded clip, a delivery deployment catheter, and a handle used to operate and deploy the clip. Clips are available in a variety of jaw lengths and opening angles, they require a 2.8-mm endoscope channel for deployment, and triple-pronged clip requires a 3.2-mm endoscopic channel. A double-pronged clip with reopening and repositioning capability up to five times before deployment is available.

The preferred technique is to identify and clip the bleeding point first and then to apply additional clips around the bleeding point if necessary. Because this is a mechanical technique, secure clip deployment is achieved with maximal capture of tissue around the bleeding vessel. Optimal clip positioning is best achieved with the clip extended a relatively short distance from the endoscope tip. This allows for more precise clip application and allows for exertion of downward force on the clip during its placement. The correct technique is to position the clip slightly away from the arterial base, allowing for an en face or tangential approach, and to push the open clip downward while simultaneously applying suction. The clip should be slowly closed and, if optimally positioned, deployed. Reopening clips can be repositioned before deployment if required. The limitations of clip application relate to the location of the lesion and to size criteria. The proximal lesser curvature and gastric cardia may be difficult to approach for clipping directly or in the retroflexed position, and in some cases it is easier to carefully expose the clip before retroflexion. Duodenal ulcers involving the posterior wall of the duodenal bulb, fibrotic ulcers, and arterial vessel larger than 2 mm in diameter may be difficult to clip. In most cases, the clips dislodge spontaneously within 2–4 weeks and pass in the stool, although some have been in place for >1 year.

Although no adverse effects have been reported, magnetic resonance imaging may be contraindicated if clips are present. Clipping for acute nonvariceal hemostasis is associated with primary hemostasis rates in the range of 84–100 %, with low rebleeding rates, comparable with those achieved with injection, thermal, and combination therapies. As with thermal therapy, hemostatic clipping has been used as part of combination therapy in conjunction with epinephrine injection.

Clipping and other mechanical techniques have been shown to be more efficacious and are associated with a lower rebleeding rate than nonmechanical therapies for patients with Dieulafoy lesion, Mallory-Weiss tears, and colonic bleeding after biopsy, after polypectomy, from hemorrhoids, or from solitary rectal ulcer syndrome. Complications after clipping are extremely rare but include a case wherein a clip inadvertently perforated a gastric ulcer and was applied to the splenic artery, and a case of colonic perforation thought to be due to clip placement for postpolypectomy bleeding.

Detachable loops consist of a circular- or elliptical-shaped nylon loop preloaded onto a delivery system that includes a hook wire to which the loop is attached within a Teflon sheath and an opening handle. The outer diameter of 2.6 mm requires a 2.8-mm operative channel. Both reloadable and single-use preloaded devices are available. The loop is used in a manner similar to the technique of polypectomy snare placement. The maximal loop opening size is 30 mm. The loop is tightened with advancement of a silicon rubber stopper. The loop is then detached after hemostasis is achieved without transecting the lesion. The primary indication for loop placement is for the prevention or management of postpolypectomy bleeding. When the loop is applied before polypectomy snare placement, care must be taken to avoid entanglement of the loop in the polypectomy snare. Before polypectomy, detachable loop placement should result in change of the color of the polyp head without transection. If the loop is applied too tightly, amputation of the polyp may occur with resultant bleeding; if it is too loose, bleeding may occur after polypectomy. Hemostatic loop placement has also been effective in the management of bleeding Dieulafoy lesions and has been used for bleeding gastric varices.

3.8.3 Variceal Bleeding

Currently endoscopic variceal ligation (EVL) is the primary choice for the endoscopic management of variceal bleeding in children. However,

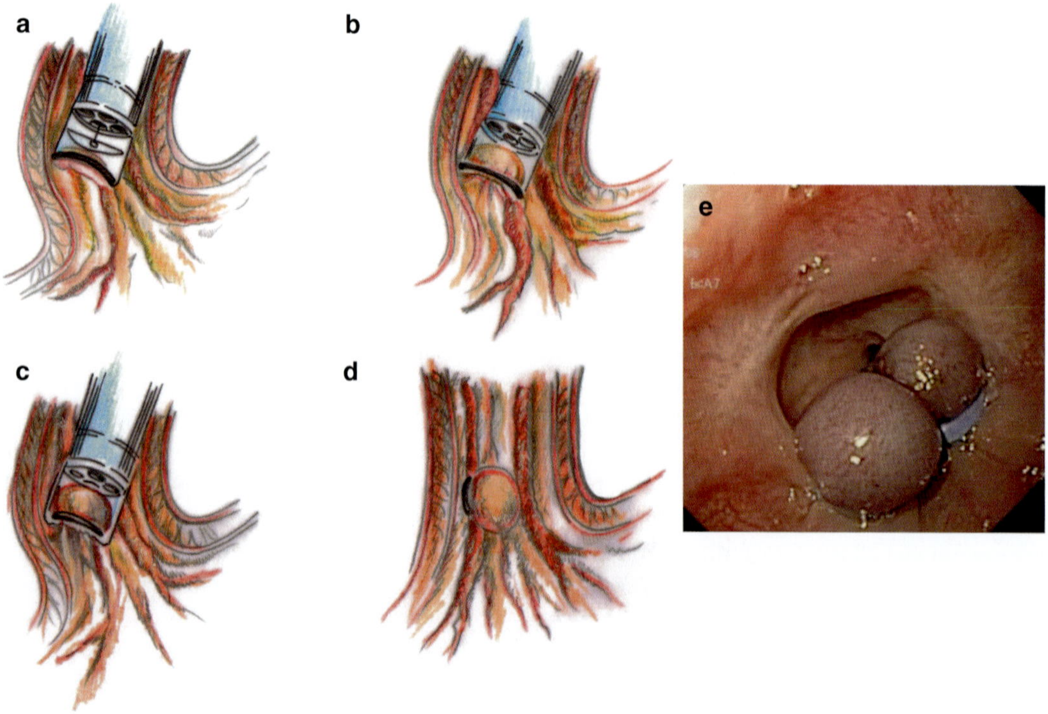

Fig. 3.14 Schematic representation of endoscopic variceal banding ligation (EVL) technique (**a**–**d**) and endoscopic view at the end of the procedure (**e**)

this treatment cannot be applied to small children due to technical limitations, and sclerotherapy is still recommended as an alternative approach in these cases. Primary endoscopic prophylaxis is only indicated in some children (i.e., patients who live in remote areas far from emergency medical care), and secondary prophylaxis is recommended for cirrhotic children, whereas a meso-Rex shunt operation is the first choice for prophylaxis in children with extrahepatic portal vein obstruction (EHPVO). Many of the current recommendations for the management of variceal bleeding have been adopted from case series in children and RCTs in adults.

An extensive experience with emergency sclerotherapy exists in children. A variety of agents have been used (sclerosants, chemically irritating compounds such as ethanolamine/tetradecyl sulfate). These sclerosants are injected either intra- or para-variceal, until bleeding has stopped. In the setting of emergency sclerotherapy, it is important to be aware of the significant incidence of associated bacteremia and to consider antibiotic prophylaxis in most patients. The effectiveness of sclerotherapy has been studied for both prevention and subsequent bleeding episodes. Considerably, whereas a band ligation device can only be used with an adult endoscope, an injection needle can be applied to every scope. Hence, sclerotherapy can be applied even to a neonate. It is also a very inexpensive method and is not technically difficult.

Although endoscopic sclerotherapy has been widely used with effective treatment of bleeding in neonates and children, side effects from the sclerosants can be significant, such as perforation, bleeding, ulceration, and stricture formation at the injection site. The range of complications associated with sclerotherapy has prompted the development of alternative endoscopic methods such as band ligation.

EVL can stop variceal bleeding through rubber band ligation of the variceal vessel and consequent mechanical strangulation (Fig. 3.14). After confirming the target varices that require ligation, the scope is advanced under direct vision until the banding cylinder is in full 360° contact with the varix (Fig. 3.14a). After full contact is made, suction is applied by depressing the endoscopic aspiration control valve, which draws the varix and surrounding mucosa into the banding chamber (Fig. 3.14b). Once the chamber is completely filled by the varix, which is evident by a complete "red out" and loss of endoscopic visibility, the trip wire is pulled (Fig. 3.14c) to push the elastic band over the varix. The engorged varix is strangulated at the mucosal junction (Fig. 3.14d, e). Treatment begins with ligation of the most distal variceal columns in the esophagus just above the gastroesophageal junction, commencing with the bleeding varix, if one is present. Subsequent ligations of the remaining varices are performed at increasingly higher levels, proceeding upward in a spiral fashion to avoid circumferential placement of bands at the same level. Large varices should have additional bands placed more proximally within the distal 10 cm of the esophagus. A 2-cm mucosal bridge between adjacent bands is essential to minimize mucosal necrosis, rebleeding, and dysphagia. After banding, patients eat soft food for 2 days. Repeated treatments are performed at intervals of 2 or 4 weeks. On average 6–9 bands are applied at the initial session and progressively fewer at subsequent session. EVL may be a preferable approach because it is easier and safer. Direct comparisons of endoscopic sclerotherapy and variceal ligation both in adult and pediatric patients demonstrated similar rate of control of active bleeding and recurrence of hemorrhage with significantly lower overall complications and mortality rate for EVL. In addition, variceal ligation appears to lead to obliteration in fewer sessions. Potential concerns of this technique in children includes the impossibility to perform this technique in small children due to the scope and associated ligature attachment size as compared to the child's size (youngest described case was 4 years old) and the possible entrapment of the full thickness of the esophageal wall (esophageal wall is thinner than adults) by the rubber band with subsequent risk of ischemic necrosis and perforation.

For the endoscopic treatment of gastric variceal bleeding in adults, vascular occlusion with N-butyl-2-cyanoacrylate injection is recommended because sclerotherapy has shown a high rate of complications and band ligation shows a lower rate of therapeutic success and higher rate of rebleeding than vascular occlusion in these cases. The intravariceal injection of N-butyl-2-cyanoacrylate causes rapid occlusion of the varices when it makes contact with blood. To prevent damage in the working channel when applying this method, the radiographic contrast agent lipiodol is mixed with the N-butyl-2-cyanoacrylate to delay permanent hardening and enable radiologic observations after the procedure. If the N-butyl-2-cyanoacrylate is too dilute to travel through the vessels due to slow hardening, there is a risk of a fatal cerebral or pulmonary embolism developing. Small aliquots are thus recommended for these injections. Even though this technique may be considered in children, only a pilot study involving eight patients younger than 2 years old and weighing less than 10 kg who had gastroesophageal varices has been performed. Although glue injection (0.5–2 mL injected) was successful in all infants with immediate control of bleeding and a low rebleeding rate of 37.5 % requiring a second treatment with cyanoacrylate, this data is too small to properly evaluate this treatment modality in pediatric cases [24–26].

3.9 Dilation Techniques

Stricture dilation may be indicated when there is associated clinical impairment or a need to access beyond the stricture for diagnosis or therapy. Dilators used in gastrointestinal endoscopy can be allocated into two categories: fixed diameter push-type dilators (bougie dilators) and balloon dilators.

Bougie dilators are available in a variety of designs, calibers, and lengths and are usually reusable. They exert both radial and longitudinal forces when advanced through a stenosis and are used primarily in the treatment of esophageal and rectal strictures. Users should refer to the manufacturer's instructions for guidance on reprocessing.

Nonwire-guided bougie dilators (Hurst and Maloney dilators) are flexible push-type dilators that do not accommodate a guidewire. They are available in a variety of diameters and are internally weighted with tungsten for gravity assistance. Hurst dilators have a blunt, rounded tip, whereas Maloney dilators have an elongated, tapered tip.

Wire-guided bougie dilators (Savary-Gilliard and America dilation system dilators) are flexible, tapered, polyvinyl chloride, and latex-free cylindrical solid tubes with a central channel to accommodate a guidewire. Tucker dilators are small (4–13.3 mm) silicone bougies tapered at each end; loops on each end can be pulled antegradely or retrogradely across strictures. A gastrostomy is required for use. These may be useful in the treatment of tortuous strictures secondary to caustic ingestion.

Balloon dilators are available in an array of designs, and lengths; calibers are marketed only for single use. They exert only radial forces when expanded within a stenosis and can be used in the treatment of all accessible strictures throughout the GI tract including small bowel strictures. They are designed to pass through the endoscope with or without wire guidance so that dilation can be observed. Balloon dilators are made of low-compliance inflatable thermoplastic polymers that allow uniform and reproducible expansion to their specified diameter at maximum inflation. The majority of balloon dilators allow for sequential expansion to multiple diameters. Dilating balloons are expanded by pressure injection of liquid (e.g., water, radiopaque contrast) by using a handheld accessory device. The hydraulic pressure of the balloon is monitored manometrically to gauge radial expansion force. Inflation with radiopaque contrast enhances fluoroscopic observation.

Achalasia balloon dilators are large-diameter (30, 35, and 40 mm) polyethylene balloon dilators specific for achalasia. All currently available achalasia balloon dilators are wire guided, single use and do not pass through the endoscope. They are positioned across the esophagogastric junction by using fluoroscopic guidance with visualization aided by the radiopaque markers on the balloon. Balloon insufflation with air is monitored manometrically.

3.9.1 Patients Preparation and Techniques

Patient preparation will depend upon the main cause and site of stricture. Patients with achalasia may require prolonged fasting and removal of food rests using a nasoesophageal tube. Adequate colon cleansing is needed for the treatment of lower GI tract stricture, and laboratory tests may be warranted in patients with blood dyscrasias or those taking anticoagulant therapy. Prior to endoscopy, all patients have to provide written informed consent, also with written information about the risk of perforation, and the possible need for surgery. General anesthesia is needed to perform dilation in children. After the procedure, patients should be observed for 24 h. Radiographic contrast examination is not performed routinely before dilation, but it is performed after dilation of achalasia or complex strictures to exclude perforation. Antibiotics are not used routinely before dilation. Anticoagulants should be discontinued. PPI therapy is recommended after esophageal dilation for peptic stricture.

Dilation can be performed with or without endoscopic, fluoroscopic, and/or wire guidance. Selection of different types of dilators depends on operator preference, type, and site of the stricture. Selection of the appropriate size is critical for safe and effective dilation. Techniques may need to be modified for complex strictures (e.g., length >2 cm, lumen diameter <12 mm, tortuous) and/or specific disease states and locations in the GI tract.

Wire-guided bougie dilators (Savary and American dilators) are passed over a guidewire endoscopically placed and subsequent endoscope removal (Fig. 3.15a). Nonwire-guided bougies (Hurst and Maloney) are passed blindly into the esophagus. These may have a higher rate of perforation in the presence of large hiatal hernias or complex strictures.

Balloon dilators in the GI tract may be passed with or without wire guidance. The balloon is positioned across the stenosis and inflated under direct endoscopic visualization. Nonwire-guided balloons are used in a similar fashion but are passed across the stenosis by using endoscopic visualization only (Fig. 3.15b).

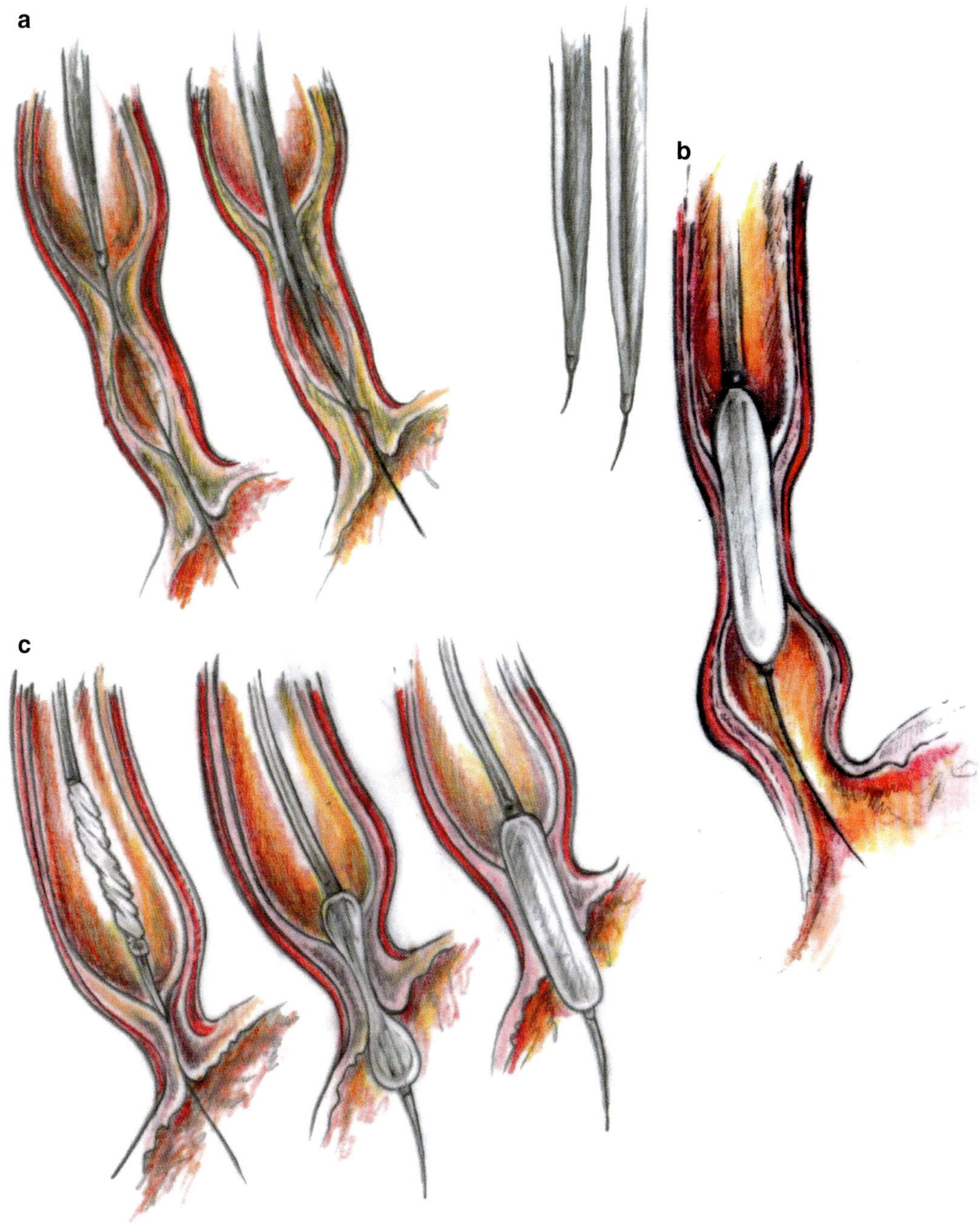

Fig. 3.15 Schematic representation of esophageal dilation performed with Wire-guided Savary dilator (**a**), with a nonwire-guided balloon (**b**) and with a large diameter wire-guided balloon in a case of Achalasia (**c**)

Pneumatic balloon dilation of the lower esophageal sphincter with a large-diameter wire-guided balloon is the mainstay of endoscopic therapy for achalasia (Fig. 3.15c). Dilation is generally performed over a wire endoscopically placed and under fluoroscopic guidance initially using a 30-mm balloon. Although nonfluoroscopically guided dilation using endoscopic visualization alone has been reported. A brief 6-s dilation, sufficient to obliterate the balloon's waist, was shown to be as effective as the standard 60-s dilation.

Although the choice of dilatation device is left to the individual endoscopist, the "rule of three" has been the standard for bougie dilation. Specifically, the initial dilator chosen should be based on the known or estimated stricture diameter; serial increases in diameter are then performed. After moderate resistance is encountered with the bougie dilator, no greater than three consecutive dilations in increments of 1 mm should be performed in a single session. Although this rule does not apply to balloon dilators, most balloons allow a three-step inflation process, each of 1 mm, practically paralleling the "rule of three."

Current AGA recommendations for management of peptic esophageal stricture include consideration that steroid injection into benign strictures immediately before or after dilation has been advocated to improve outcome by decreasing the need for repeat dilations. This technique has also been successfully used to prevent stricture recurrence after balloon dilation in children with stenotizing Crohn's disease (Fig. 3.16).

Interruption of strictures (e.g., esophageal webs, Schatzki rings) with biopsy forceps or needle-knife electrocautery, either as the sole treatment or in conjunction with dilation, has been successfully demonstrated.

3.9.2 Complications

Perforation is the major complication associated with endoscopic dilation (0.1–1 %). It appears that perforations are common using a single

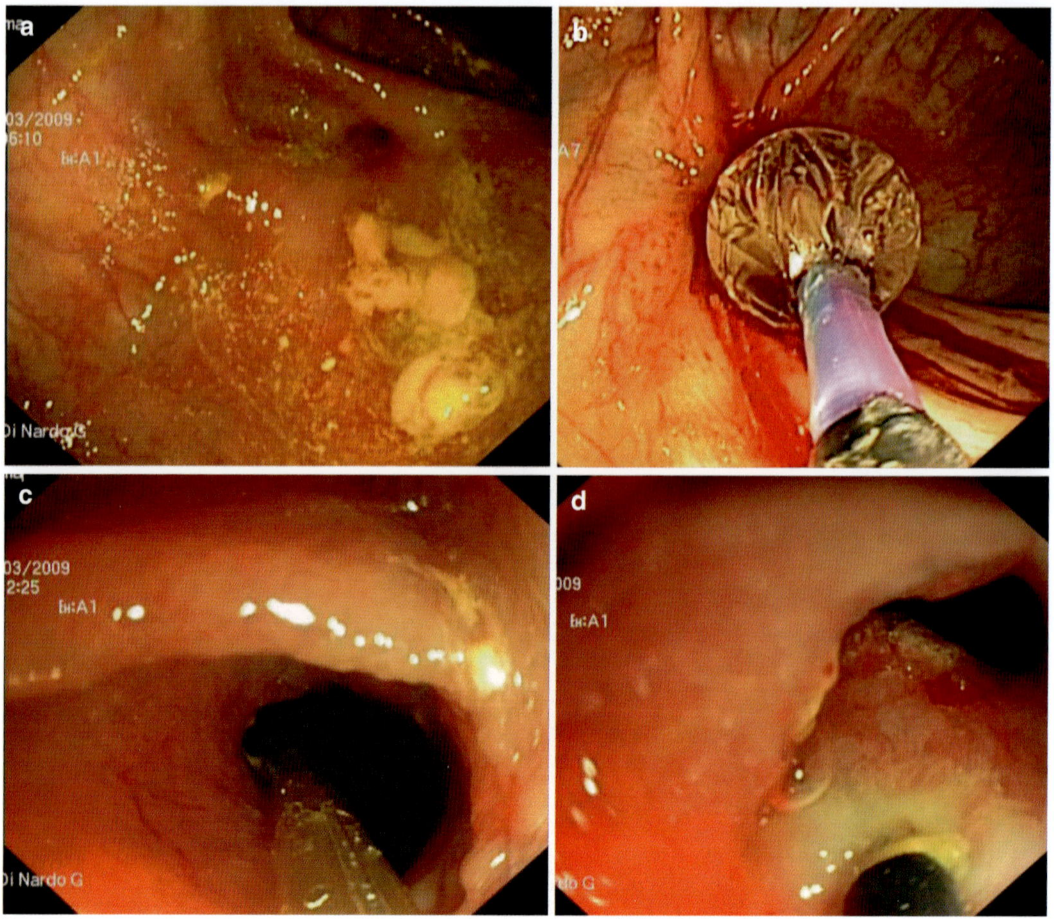

Fig. 3.16 Endoscopic view of ileocolonic stricture (**a**) balloon dilation (**b**, **c**) followed by intralesional steroid injection (**d**) in a child with Crohn's disease

nonwire-guided bougie size dilator particularly in children with complex stricture or with a large hiatal hernia. Other possible complications include chest pain, bleeding, and bacteremia.

The risk of perforation with balloon dilation in achalasia is in the range of 3–4 % with a mortality rate of <1 %. Other complications associated with achalasia dilation include prolonged pain and intramural hematomas. Open surgical repair with myotomy of early recognized endoscopic perforation offers an outcome similar to that of elective open myotomy. However, if endoscopic perforation occurs after pneumatic dilation, laparoscopic myotomy is usually not technically feasible. In patients with failed myotomy, pneumatic dilation could be safely performed.

Perforation after dilation usually occurs at the site of the stricture, but it could happen also in different site mainly related to the inappropriate use of nonwire-guided dilators and consequent creation of false track through the intestinal wall. Some experts recommend endoscopic inspection immediately upon completion of the dilatation procedure as the appearances may raise the possibility of perforation and prompt early treatment. Perforation should be suspected if severe or persistent pain, dyspnea, tachycardia, or fever develops. Physical examination may reveal subcutaneous crepitus of the chest or cervical region in cases of esophageal perforation. Although a chest or abdominal radiograph could show a perforation, a normal study result does not exclude this diagnosis and a water-soluble contrast esophagram or computed tomogram of the chest/abdomen may be necessary to disclose a perforation [27–29].

3.10 Percutaneous Endoscopic Gastrostomy

3.10.1 Indications and Contraindications

In children unable to take adequate oral nutrition reliably and safely for more than 1–3 months, placement of a gastrostomy should be considered to avoid complications of nasogastric tube feeding. Gastrostomy could be used not only as an enteral tube feeding but also for gastric decompression and/or to administrate medications.

Table 3.9 Indications and contraindications for PEG

Indications	*Underlying disorders*
Inability to swallow	Neurological disorders Multiple congenital malformations Oropharyngeal dysmotility Epidermolyis bullosa Others
Inadequate caloric intake	Cystic fibrosis Congenital heart disease Chronic respiratory failure Oncologic disease
Special feeding requirements	Unpalatable formula in multiple food allergies, metabolic diseases, or renal failure
Continuous enteral feeding	Short bowel syndrome
	Malabsorption
Contraindications	
Absolute Colonic interposition Severe and uncorrectable bleeding disorder Gastric varices Severe ascites Pharyngeal or esophageal obstruction	
Relative Hepatosplenomegaly Ascites Previous abdominal surgery Scoliosis Microgastria	

Adapted by Ref. [30]

The most common indications for percutaneous endoscopic gastrostomy (PEG) placement are listed in Table 3.9 and could be listed in four main groups: inability to swallow, inadequate caloric intake, special feeding requirements, and continuous enteral feeding.

There are a number of relative but few absolute contraindications to PEG placement (see Table 3.9). Uncorrectable coagulopathy and unfavorable anatomy resulting in lack of transillumination with inability to bring the anterior gastric wall in apposition to the abdominal wall are considered the main absolute contraindications for PEG placement. Careful patient selection and care in performing the procedure are known to reduce morbidity and mortality, which are generally higher in patients with acute states of severe illness, such as heart failure.

3.10.2 Technique

PEG placement should be carried out in an operating room under general anesthesia. Prophylactic use of antibiotics (a single dose of broad-spectrum antibiotic administered before the procedure) is recommended to prevent local or systemic infection. An endoscopist together with an appropriately trained assistant, who is responsible for skin puncture and insertion of the guidewire, is warranted for PEG placement. Available PEG placement kits typically contain a gastrostomy tube with internal and external retaining devices, a skin trocar, a guidewire, and a plug adaptor for the tube. Gastrostomy tubes are made from polyurethane or silicone rubber and are available in a range of sizes from French gauge 9–24, with sizes 12–15 being suitable for most of the children.

The most popular technique of insertion is the "pull" technique because it has many advantages over the other techniques especially in young children. The patient is placed in the supine position, and the anterior abdominal wall is cleaned using an operative skin disinfection protocol. An endoscopic examination of the esophagus and stomach is then performed. The duodenum is not examined so as to minimize intestinal air distension.

The stomach is inflated however, so as to bring the anterior gastric wall in close contact with the abdominal wall. The endoscopist's assistant now identifies the correct skin puncture site (Fig. 3.17). The best option is to enter the stomach close to the junction of the gastric antrum and body. The site is located by using endoscopic transillumination (a bright point of light should be seen on the abdominal wall). If a clear point of transillumination cannot be identified, the assistant should not proceed with the puncture because this suggests the colon lies interposed between the stomach and the abdominal wall. When a good transillumination can be identified (Fig. 3.17c), the assistant applies digital compression at the proposed insertion site, and the endoscopist confirms that this is a suitable entry point in the stomach (Fig. 3.17a, b). The correct insertion point is usually midway between the umbilicus and the junction of the costal margin and left midclavicular line.

Some operators may first insert a needle so that the endoscopist can confirm the correct location (Fig. 3.17d). The assistant now performs the puncture by holding the trocar perpendicular to the abdominal wall and pushing it through into the inflated stomach. The endoscopist confirms entry of the trocar and its overlying plastic sheath (Fig. 3.17e). The trocar is withdrawn while leaving the sheath in situ to provide a secure track for the guidewire. The guidewire is passed through the plastic sheath (Fig. 3.17f), the endoscopist grasps it with the forceps (Fig. 3.17g–i), and the sheath is then withdrawn as the guidewire is slowly drawn into the stomach. The entire assembly including endoscope, forceps, and guidewire is then withdrawn. The guidewire now passes through the abdominal puncture, into the stomach, and out through the mouth. The proximal end of the guidewire is tied to a loop on the end of the gastrostomy tube (Fig. 3.17l). The distal end of the guidewire is gently pulled, drawing the tube and its internal bolster through the mouth, down the esophagus, into the stomach, and out through the puncture site, until the internal retaining device comes to lie on the anterior gastric wall (Fig. 3.17m). Sometimes it is necessary to make a small incision at the puncture site to facilitate passage of the gastrostomy tube out through the skin.

The distal end of the tube, still attached to the guidewire, is now cut off. An outer retaining device such as a disk is passed over the external tube, and this holds the tube at the abdominal wall so that it cannot slip back into the stomach. It is important to ensure that this external retaining device is not so loose as to be ineffective or so tight as to cause pressure damage. Local anesthetic may be injected around the incision point to reduce postoperative discomfort.

The tube is now cut to the desired length and the adaptor plug is inserted. A small amount of iodinated disinfectant may be applied to the external retaining device. A dry dressing is applied to the site for removal after 24–48 h. Finally, the endoscope should be reinserted to confirm that the inner retaining device is positioned correctly and to ensure that there is no bleeding (Fig. 3.17n).

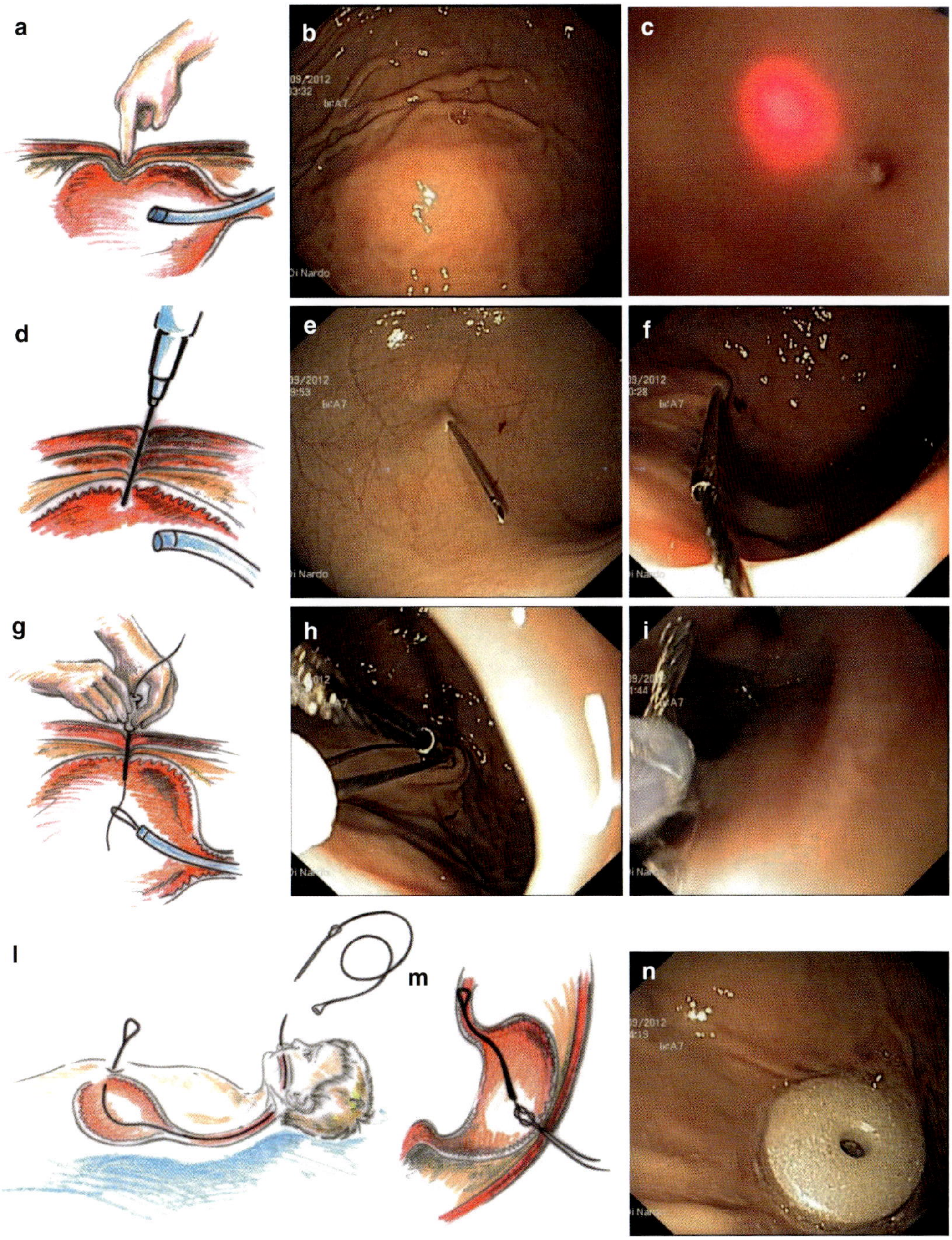

Fig. 3.17 Schematic representation and endoscopic view of the different PEG placement phases. (**a–c**) The endoscopist's assistant identifies the correct skin puncture site. (**d**) The assistant now performs the puncture by holding the trocar perpendicular to the abdominal wall and pushing it through into the inflated stomach. (**e**) The endoscopist confirms entry of the trocar and its overlying plastic sheath. (**f**) The guide wire is passed through the plastic sheath. (**g–i**) The endoscopist grasps it with the forceps and the sheath is then withdrawn as the guide wire is slowly drawn into the stomach. The entire assembly including endoscope, forceps, and guide wire is then withdrawn. (**l**) The proximal end of the guide wire is tied to a loop on the end of the gastrostomy tube. The distal end of the guide wire is gently pulled, drawing the tube and its internal bolster through the mouth, down the oesophagus, into the stomach and out through the puncture site, until the internal retaining device comes to lie on the anterior gastric wall (**m**). (**n**) Finally, the endoscope should be reinserted to confirm that the inner retaining device is positioned correctly and to ensure that there is no bleeding

Children should be admitted overnight to ensure adequate pain control and safe initiation of feeds. In the immediate postoperative period, the patient's general condition is monitored and the abdomen is examined for signs of peritonitis or significant pneumoperitoneum. Most of the children require some analgesia during the first 2 days. PEG should be used after 24 h starting with saline solution for few hours and then with designated liquid formula.

For 1 week, daily aseptic cleaning of the site is recommended and a sterile dressing can be applied. Subsequently, simple washing is sufficient and a dry dressing may be placed over the outer collar. Occlusive dressings are not recommended as they increase the risk of local infection.

After a period of 2–3 months or more, once the gastrostomy tract has healed, a more suitable device known as "gastrostomy button" can replace the gastrostomy tube. This device consists of a shorter (0.5–4.5 cm in length) and wider (e.g., 14–16 French) tube, just sufficient to traverse the fixed track, with some form of internal retaining device.

Their fixed length requires measurement of the formed track before insertion of the new device. This can be done with a graduated measuring device before selection of the correct length of device.

They can be inserted and removed quite easily, usually without need for sedation or general anesthesia. Only the first insertion of this device should be performed under endoscopic control to be sure that the balloon is correctly placed in the stomach and not in the colon as in the case of gastrocolic fistula. The only disadvantages are that they need to be changed every 4–6 months.

3.10.3 Complications

Complications may be classified as early and late.

Early complications as a direct result of PEG placement occur within 30 days of insertion and include pneumoperitoneum, colonic injury or gastrocolic fistula, small bowel injury, hepatic/splenic injury, bleeding, and stoma leak.

Pneumoperitoneum is a frequent postoperative finding identified radiologically in 5–50 % of patients. It is usually of minor clinical consequence, but could be a sign of iatrogenic bowel injury and hence should not be dismissed in the relevant clinical context.

Colonic injury or gastrocolic fistula is uncommon, but owing to the displacement of the transverse colon over the anterior gastric wall, it can lead to puncture of the colon during the blind insertion of the needle/trocar. Risk factors include under- or overdistension of the stomach, a left diaphragmatic hernia, and significant kyphoscoliosis. This complication could be detected early or late, frequently after many months, and even only during exchange of the PEG tube with gastrostomy button (Fig. 3.18). Clinical signs include the presence of undigested feed in stools, diarrhea immediately after feeding, feculent vomiting, or discharge from the gastrostomy track.

Small bowel injury is most common in children who have undergone prior abdominal surgery and occurs owing to adhesions that have fixed small bowel loops anterior to the liver, making them highly susceptible to injury during trocar insertion.

Stoma leak is common after PEG placement and may only need gentle tightening of the external fixation device to ensure close apposition of the internal bumper to the gastric wall. More persistent leaks may however lead to peritonitis.

Hemorrhage is an extremely rare complication resulting from gastric, peritoneal, retroperitoneal, and abdominal wall injuries. Hypotension without evidence of intraluminal bleeding is suggestive of parenchymal lesions (mainly liver and spleen) and should be promptly recognized and treated surgically. Puncture of abdominal wall vessels may present with bleeding from the PEG tract itself. Tightening the external and internal bumper may assist with hemostasis.

Late complications include local infection, granulation tissue, and buried bumper syndrome.

Peristomal wound infection is one of the most common complications of PEG (30–40 %). Prophylactic antibiotics are able to reduce stomal infection rates. If discharge occurs around site or erythema is present, the site could be swabbed

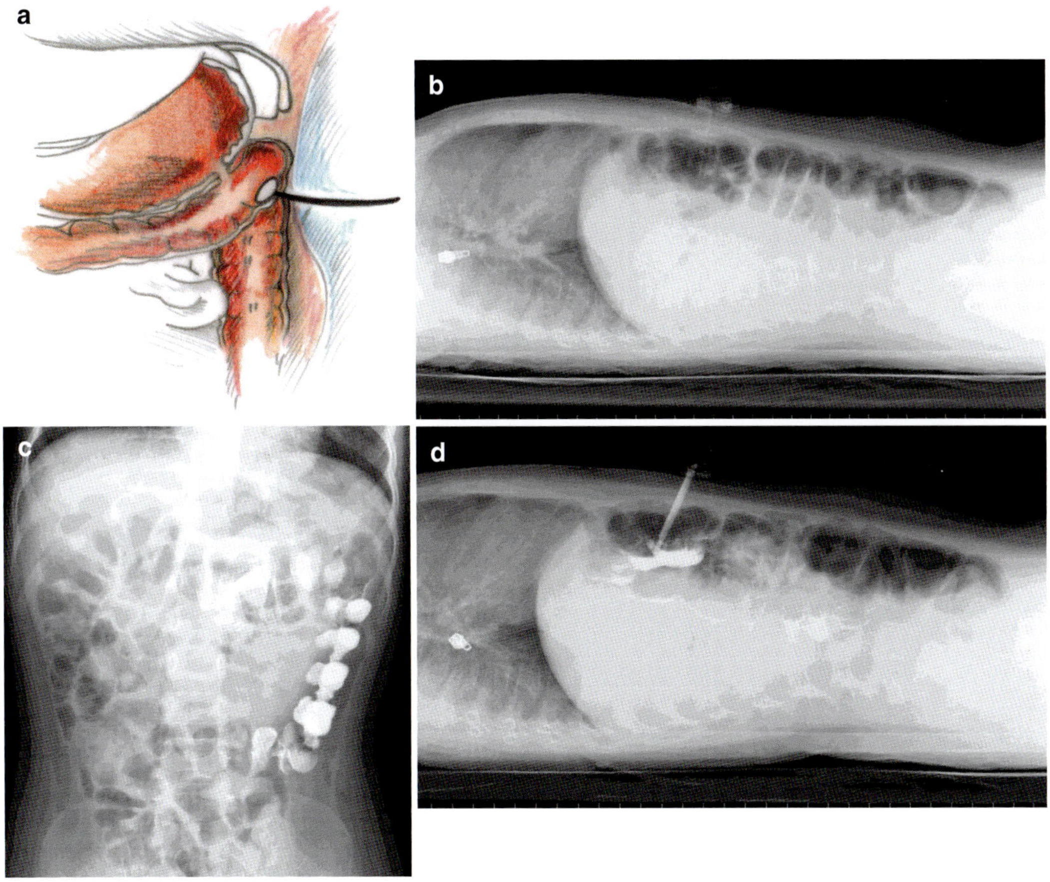

Fig. 3.18 Schematic (**a**) representation of a gastrocolic fistula as a complication of PEG. Radiographic study (**b–d**) with water-soluble contrast solution shows tip of tube in the lumen of trasverse colon

and evidence of colonization and antibiotic sensitivities obtained. The site is almost always colonized without causing tissue infection, although pain around the site and tissue swelling suggest bacterial invasion. Depending on clinical status, the child may need topical or systemic antibiotics. Less than 5 mm of erythema around the outer stoma site is common and is likely owing to local irritation by movement of the external bumper or minimal leakage.

Overgranulation at the gastrostomy site is seen as red/pink tissue at the stomal border that extends above the surrounding skin. This is a common complication that is usually owing to an ill-fitting device, wherein excessive movement or leakage leads to an excessive healing response. The granulation tissue has a tendency to bleed easily; it tends to discharge continuously and may cause local pain. Treatment options include silver nitrate, topical corticosteroids, cryotherapy, or surgical debridement. Silver nitrate does not cause any pain if applied only to the granulation tissue and is helpful to shrink down excessive granulation tissue.

Buried bumper is most common in the second year after insertion and occurs in approximately 2 % of children. The internal flange migrates through the gastric wall and potentially into the peritoneal space. Signs include difficulty in infusing fluid and feeds, with an increasing difficulty in moving and rotating the PEG during the weekly cares. This may be minimized by ensuring a correctly fitting device at regular review, particularly to ensure increasing tube length in line with weight gain.

If suspected, an upper endoscopy is warranted. Feeds should be discontinued until a diagnosis is made, as complications include sudden peritonitis and the formation of intraperitoneal or abdominal wall abscesses. In some cases, it is possible to pass a guidewire through the tube lumen under endoscopic control, gently dilate the tract with a dilator, and use the patent tract to insert a button.

3.10.3.1 PEG Care

It is quite normal to experience some clear or colored discharge from around the site for the first 7–10 days post placement while the site is healing. The site should be cleaned daily with warm soapy water; after cleaning, it is essential to ensure the area is fully dry. The use of creams and powders around the tube should be avoided as this may contribute to irritation and softening of the skin, which can lead to superficial skin infection.

In addition to the observation of the site for infection, a PEG requires daily care. One should also check and document any erythema, skin breakdown, granulation tissue, and pain, swelling, or offensive discharge.

Baths can be given once the incision site has healed. This is normally a minimum of 48 h after the gastrostomy has been placed. Swimming is permitted, but should not be encouraged for 2 weeks following gastrostomy placement. Dressings that cover, sit under, or occlude the gastrostomy are not recommended and usually not required. In specific circumstances, dressings may be helpful, such as silver dressings for the treatment of excessive granulation tissue formation and antimicrobial dressings in the presence of minor, superficial infection.

Flushing of the gastrostomy tube is essential to maintain tube patency, prevent tube blockages, and reduce bacterial overgrowth. Commonly, 20 mL of water is recommended, with smaller volumes used in certain circumstances, for example, if a child is fluid restricted and to avoid fluid volume overload. Caregivers should be instructed not to pull on the tube and to avoid any persistent tension as this may lead to progressive migration of the bumper into the abdominal wall, leading to "buried bumper syndrome." To prevent this complication, PEG should be carefully pushed into the stomach by 1–2 cm and then rotated once a week from day 7 postinsertion.

Teaching of all peoples involved in the care of the PEG begins before PEG placement and at the time of the decision to proceed to insertion. Teaching initially includes the demonstration of different devices and explanation of the planned surgical procedure. However, in addition to teaching the child and family, support for staff involved in caring for each patient in the community may be necessary. There are several key aspects of PEG use and care that should be taught. The family and caregivers should have the following competencies assessed to confidently be able to manage their child's PEG tube [30, 31].

References

1. ASGE Standards of Practice Committee; Lightdale JR et al (2014) Modifications in endoscopic practice for pediatric patients. Gastrointest Endosc 79:699–710
2. ASGE Technology Committee; Barth BA et al (2012) Equipment for pediatric endoscopy. Gastrointest Endosc 76:8–17
3. Cote CJ et al (2006) Guidelines for monitoring and management of pediatric patients during and after sedation for diagnostic and therapeutic procedures: an update. Pediatrics 118:2587–2602
4. Samer Volonaki E et al (2012) Gastrointestinal endoscopy and mucosal biopsy in the first year of life: indications and outcome. J Pediatr Gastroenterol Nutr 55:62–65
5. Leichtner AM et al (2013) NASPGHAN guidelines for training in pediatric gastroenterology. J Pediatr Gastroenterol Nutr 56(Suppl 1):S1–S8
6. Turner D et al (2010) Evidence-based recommendations for bowel cleansing before colonoscopy in children: a report from a national working group. Endoscopy 42:1063–1070
7. Di Nardo G et al (2014) Bowel preparations for colonoscopy: an RCT. Pediatrics 134:249–256
8. Di Nardo G et al (2012) Investigation of small bowel in pediatric Crohn's disease. Inflamm Bowel Dis 18:1760–1776
9. Oliva S et al (2015) Capsule endoscopy followed by single balloon enteroscopy in children with obscure gastrointestinal bleeding: a combined approach. Dig Liver Dis 47:125–130
10. Oliva S et al (2014) Small bowel cleansing for capsule endoscopy in pediatric patients: a prospective randomized single-blinded study. Dig Liver Dis 45:51–55
11. Oliva S et al (2014) Capsule endoscopy in pediatrics: a 10-years journey. World J Gastroenterol 20:16603–16608

12. Barth BA (2011) Enteroscopy in children. Curr Opin Pediatr 23:530–534
13. Annese V et al (2013) European evidence based consensus for endoscopy in inflammatory bowel disease. J Crohns Colitis 7:982–1018
14. ASGE Standards of Practice Committee; Fisher L, Lee Krinsky M, Anderson MA et al (2010) The role of endoscopy in the management of obscure GI bleeding. Gastrointest Endosc 72:471–479
15. Di Nardo G et al (2012) Usefulness of single-balloon enteroscopy in pediatric Crohn's disease. Gastrointest Endosc 75:80–86
16. Di Nardo G et al (2013) Enteroscopy in paediatric Crohn's disease. Dig Liver Dis 45:351–355
17. Vegting IL et al (2009) Is endoscopic retrograde cholangiopancreatography valuable and safe in children of all ages? J Pediatr Gastroenterol Nutr 48:66–70
18. Scheers I et al (2015) The diagnostic and therapeutic role of endoscopic ultrasound in pediatric pancreaticobiliary disorders. J Pediatr Gastroenterol Nutr 61:238–247
19. Attila T et al (2009) EUS in pediatric patients. Gastrointest Endosc 70:892–898
20. Bjerring OS et al (2008) Impact of upper gastrointestinal endoscopic ultrasound in children. J Pediatr Gastroenterol Nutr 47:110–113
21. Anderloni A et al (2014) Advances, problems, and complications of polypectomy. Clin Exp Gastroenterol 7:285–296
22. Hewett DG (2013) Colonoscopic polypectomy: current techniques and controversies. Gastroenterol Clin North Am 42:443–458
23. Carpenter S et al (2007) Polypectomy devices. ASGE Technology Status Evaluation Report. Gastrointest Endosc 65:741–749
24. Kay MH et al (2007) Therapeutic endoscopy for nonvariceal gastrointestinal bleeding. J Pediatr Gastroenterol Nutr 45:157–171
25. Conway JD et al (2009) Endoscopic hemostatic devices. ASGE Technology Status Evaluation Report. Gastrointest Endosc 69:987–996
26. Kim SJ et al (2013) Recent trends in the endoscopic management of variceal bleeding in children. Pediatr Gastroenterol Hepatol Nutr 16:1–9
27. Siddiqui UD (2013) Tools for endoscopic stricture dilation. ASGE Technology Committee. Gastrointest Endosc 78:391–404
28. Di Nardo G et al (2010) Intralesional steroid injection after endoscopic balloon dilation in pediatric Crohn's disease with stricture: a prospective, randomized, double-blind, controlled trial. Gastrointest Endosc 72:1201–1208
29. Di Nardo G et al (2012) Pneumatic balloon dilation in pediatric achalasia: efficacy and factors predicting outcome at a single tertiary pediatric gastroenterology center. Gastrointest Endosc 76:927–932
30. Frohlich T et al (2010) Review article: percutaneous endoscopic gastrostomy in infants and children. Aliment Pharmacol Ther 31:788–801
31. Heuschkel RB et al (2015) ESPGHAN position paper on management of percutaneous endoscopic gastrostomy in children and adolescents. J Pediatr Gastroenterol Nutr 60:131–141

Anesthesia in Pediatric Digestive Surgery

4

Andrea Gentili, Valeria Landuzzi, and Maria Cristina Mondardini

4.1 Introduction

Anesthesia for digestive surgery is not a subspecialty, but some aspects are typical to this type of surgery.

Abdominal surgery in the pediatric patient may be performed for a wide variety of congenital, neoplastic, traumatic, and infectious diseases. An optimal approach to the planning of anesthesia for digestive surgery requires not only a good knowledge of the technical features and an understanding of the physiological alterations associated with the anesthetic and surgical procedure but also of the patient's underlying status.

In addition some physiological modifications associated with digestive surgery are influenced by particular surgical approaches such as laparoscopy or liver resections, by the anesthetic agents administered, by the patient's underlying myocardial and respiratory function, and by the patient's age: many critical pathologies need quick surgical correction in neonatal age. Regarding the age in which the pathologies may be corrected, it is necessary to consider the potential neurotoxicity of the anesthetic drugs [1–3].

A. Gentili (✉) • V. Landuzzi • M.C. Mondardini
Department of Pediatric Anaesthesia and Intensive Care, S. Orsola-Malpighi University Hospital, Via Massarenti 9, Bologna, Italy
e-mail: andrea_gentili@libero.it; valeria.landuzzi@aosp.bo.it; mariacristina.mondardini@aosp.bo.it

Digestive surgery comprises different pathologies involving the gastrointestinal tract, liver, and abdominal wall defects and also the esophageal tract, which has characteristics of surgery and of anesthesia typical of thoracic surgery.

4.2 Anatomic and Physiological Characteristics of the Digestive System in Neonates, Infants, and Children

Major differences exist between the gastrointestinal system characteristics of preterms, neonates, infants, and very young children and those of adults. Some of them have special features useful from the point of anesthesia and intensive care:

- The esophagus has a tender thin mucous membrane, well supplied with blood vessels. Glandules of an esophagus in newborns are completely absent; muscular and elastic tissues are poorly advanced. The position of the proximal entrance of the esophagus in newborns is high, at the third to fourth cervical vertebras, while in the adult, it is at the seventh vertebra. The length of the esophagus is calculated by Bischoff's formula: 1/5 lengths of body + 6.3 cm.
- The stomach in infants is set horizontally. The cardia area of the stomach is undeveloped; therefore, regurgitation is possible. The

M. Lima (ed.), *Pediatric Digestive Surgery*, DOI 10.1007/978-3-319-40525-4_4

pyloric part is well developed, and an overdevelopment of pylorospasm is observed. The capacity of the stomach in newborns is 30–35 ml, in 1-year-olds 250–300 ml, and in 8-year-olds 1000 ml. Low production of gastric juice and low acidity are marked. The muscular layer is undeveloped, and the gastric air bubble is enlarged.

- The small intestine is long and highly mobile; therefore, invaginations are frequently possible. Secretor insufficiency and high permeability promote penetration into the blood of undigested components of nutrition, toxins, and microorganisms, causing sensitization. The immaturity of the ileocecal valve promotes the entrance of bacterial flora from the colon.
- The colon is situated higher and has a length proportional to the body height of the child. Haustration under 6 months is absent. The settling in the intestine of normal microflora begins in the first hours of life and usually comes to an end by 7–10 days; therefore, transitional dysbacteriosis is observed.
- The liver in children is quite large, 4 % of body mass in newborns, and 2 % in adults. The parenchyma of the liver is poorly differentiated, and the lobular structure is typical only by the end of the first year of life. The liver is sanguineous and easily enlarged in infectious diseases, intoxication, and circulatory insufficiency. In children hemorrhagic syndrome in liver diseases develops more often.
- The gastrointestinal tract presents the largest surface area of the body exposed to antigens and microbes. The intestine must therefore have intricate mechanisms to allow the entry of nutrients and other beneficial molecules while preventing potentially harmful microbes and other agents from gaining entry into the inner milieu. Several factors lead to a hostile gastrointestinal environment that predisposes the neonate and infant to disease. These include the introduction of feeding tubes into the stomach or more distal intestine, the routine use of broad-spectrum antibiotics that select for resistant pathogens that thrive in the unusual microbial environment of the neonatal and pediatric intensive care unit, intrinsic immaturities of the infant gastrointestinal tract, and the lack of adequate nutrition.

4.3 Preoperative Evaluation

The preoperative history and physical examination are directed at identifying acute and chronic problems and underlying medical conditions, as well as previously undiagnosed diseases that may place the child at an increased risk during the perioperative management [4].

The preoperative history must include insights about intestinal malabsorption, gastroesophageal reflux, digestive tract infections, and triggers of hepatic failure, such as infectious, toxic, metabolic, infiltrative, and ischemic/vascular problems. Clinical serious conditions may accompany such diseases and, in addition to the specific symptoms, may include fatigue and weight loss. In neonatal age, in pathologies such as esophageal atresia and abdominal wall defects, an evaluation of the prenatal and maternal history is mandatory as well as a search for undiagnosed illnesses, disorders, or anomalies, specifically genetic syndromes and congenital heart diseases.

The physical examination also focuses on the gastrointestinal and hepatobiliary system but begins with the pathology, the global assessment, and the clinical status of the child.

The preoperative examination of poor esophageal function, of a full stomach, and bowel obstruction attempts to identify previous problems, which may place the patient at increased risks during anesthesia induction, such as an inhalation syndrome.

In patients with a neurological disease, it is important to evaluate the respiratory tract, identifying phenomena of dysventilation, atelectasis, or respiratory infections. In the presence of active bronchospasm, a preoperative treatment may be necessary, and intraoperative anesthetic techniques may be required to prevent the exacerbation of bronchoconstriction of the small airways [5].

In patients with esophageal atresia, it is important to assess possible inhalation of saliva or gastric content into the respiratory tract and to evaluate the gastrointestinal distension.

When a laparoscopy is about to be performed, the respiratory system and cardiocirculatory function should be examined paying attention to all the determinants of myocardial performance. Particularly, preload evaluation is mandatory if an abdominal mass compresses the inferior vena cava.

Laboratory and instrumental evaluations are often important in the preparation of anesthesia for abdominal surgery. Among the preoperative laboratory tests, particular attention should be given to the complete blood count, which may indicate anemia as a reflection of chronic malabsorption, and the white blood cell count and the indexes of infection, which may indicate the presence of active abdominal infection, and the platelets, which can be associated with a splenic sequestration. In addition, an investigation involving tests of hepatic function and coagulation is recommended in patients with liver compromise: children who have liver diseases, portal hypertension, or splenic diseases are at increased risk for intraoperative and postoperative bleeding.

Radiological screening (chest radiographs, computed tomographic scans, magnetic resonance imaging) is essential to assess the abdominal anatomy and any additional information concerning alterations associated with findings that may influence the anesthetic and surgical management (Table 4.1).

Echocardiography is performed to check for cardiovascular anomalies, right and left ventricle performances, and pulmonary pressure.

Lung function testings have been widely used in children 6–8 years of age or greater. Simple spirometry is easiest to obtain. The results of such tests are generally used as indicators of the complexity of perioperative management.

In patients about to be submitted to digestive surgery, the following procedures are indicated:

- An effective optimization of preoperative therapy
- An appropriate assessment of the need for blood products
- An assessment of the presence and ultimate need for intravenous access with consideration of temporary or long-term central venous catheter
- A rating for antibiotic needs
- An analgesic perioperative plan

Risk evaluation and informed consent are essential elements in preoperative assessment. The American Society of Anesthesiologists developed and modified later the classification of physical status (ASA) to define a correlation of clinical condition and tolerance to surgery. The correct information about all possible anesthetic techniques (a pamphlet should be given before the anesthesiological visit) and in particular of the benefit/risk of the purpose tailored procedures must be provided before acquiring written consent for anesthesia. A specific risk such as difficult airway management, or cardiac, respiratory, neurological, and metabolic conditions, should be annotated on the anesthesiological chart and on the operatory list.

4.4 Premedication and Preoperative Fasting

At the end of the global evaluation (clinical history, physical examination, laboratory tests, imaging, cardiorespiratory tests), a pharmacological medication is considered. Sedative premedication is not always necessary, but when useful, midazolam 500 mcg/kg, orally, is currently the most frequently used drug. Midazolam can also be administered by nasal route (200 mcg/kg). Atropine in clinical practice is administered after vein placement only in the presence of clinical need. A local anesthetic emulsion (lidocaine 25 mg + prilocaine 25 mg) or medicated plaster (lidocaine 70 mg + tetracaine 70 mg, for children over 3 years) is applied on a detectable peripheral vein. Preoperative fasting is indicated for elective surgery and healthy patients, to avoid inhalation syndrome at anesthesia induction. Recent guidelines also consider the correct preoperative administration of drugs to decrease the risk for pulmonary aspiration in selected patients [6]. Parents are allowed to be present in the operating room at induction of anesthesia.

Table 4.1 Correlation between gastrointestinal/hepatic problems and potential anesthetic implications

Gastrointestinal/hepatic problems	Potential anesthetic implications
Vomiting, diarrhea	Electrolyte imbalance, dehydration, full stomach
Gastroesophageal reflux	Treat like a full stomach
Increased abdominal volume	Diaphragmatic cephalic displacement Decreased lung compliance Decreased systemic oxygenation
Ab ingestis inhalation	Aspiration pneumonia
Pulmonary infiltrates	Decreased lung compliance Increased V/Q mismatch Increased pulmonary shunt effect Decreased systemic oxygenation
Prolonged fasting	Dehydration, hypovolemia
Malabsorption	Anemia, malnutrition
Black stools	Anemia, hypovolemia
Jaundice	Drug metabolism/hypoglycemia
Liver dysfunction	Drug metabolism/toxicity

4.5 Anesthesiological Approach

Studies in the literature consider it very important in these patients to achieve a level of anesthesia which allows a safe execution of the surgical procedure. The entire staff, involving different professional figures, should be trained and educated in order to improve safety, ensure treatment of possible side effects, and guarantee the management of emergencies [7].

4.5.1 Monitoring

Standard intraoperative monitoring is both invasive and noninvasive and is well described in the guidelines for safety in the operating room.

Cardiovascular function is monitored by ECG (heart rate and rhythm), noninvasive systolic blood pressure (SBP), and diastolic blood pressure (DBP); if necessary, a radial arterial catheter is cannulated not only for invasive monitoring but also for intraoperative and postoperative blood gas analysis and laboratory tests. When clinical conditions and the fluid requirements are difficult to evaluate, a central venous catheter (CVC) is placed by a superior cava approach for invasive monitoring of central venous pressure (CVP).

The respiratory function is monitored by peripheral arterial oxygen saturation (SpO_2) and end-tidal CO_2 ($ETCO_2$). The mechanical ventilator permits the variation of all respiratory items including frequency, tidal volume (inspiratory and expiratory), minute volume, peak pressure, and mean airway pressure.

Monitoring also includes body temperature, urine output, and inspiratory and expiratory concentration of volatile anesthetics. In many patients, the neuromuscular blockade is monitored by stimulating the ulnar nerve using the train-of-four pattern of stimulation.

Temperature measurement is a must in pediatric abdominal surgery and in particular in neonates. The temperature is tested with the esophageal probe during major surgery. The use of pre-warmed fluids and active warming systems (mattress, convective warm air blanket, radiant heater) is necessary. Anesthesia interferes with the thermoregulatory response in all ages.

A new approach is oriented to measure cerebral oxygenation (using near-infrared spectroscopy technology) to reduce potential risks of neurolesive events caused by conventional intraoperative ventilation that influence intracranial pressure, cerebral blood flow, and cerebral perfusion pressure [8, 9].

4.5.2 Vascular Access

Vascular access is necessary in all types of surgery.

Adequate peripheral access is essential intraoperatively and also for fluid replacement in the postoperative period. One or two peripheral veins may be necessary.

Clinical conditions and the type of surgery indicate the placement of a single- or double-lumen central venous catheter, appropriate for the size of the patient. This vascular access is required both for monitoring and for rapid and safe infusions of fluid, plasma expanders, and blood derivatives. The upper cava vein approach is mandatory for the liver and oncologic abdominal surgery, particularly when it has been extended to or into the inferior cava vein (rarely until the right atrium), and surgery may foresee vein clamping. The use of ultrasonographic guidance during CVC placement has been demonstrated the better percutaneous procedure for decreasing the complications rate [10].

4.5.3 Intraoperative Fluids

Intra-surgical crystalloid infusion was 20 ml/kg during the first hour in patients under 3 years and 15 ml/kg for older patients; in the hours that followed, the infusion dosage was 8–10 ml/kg/h for all patients.

Extravascular or interstitial sequestration of fluid (the so-called "third-space" fluid loss) can occur during digestive surgery. Estimated third-space fluid deficits are replaced with isoosmotic fluids, at rates according to the type of surgery (approximately 4 ml/kg). The infusion used was 0.8–1 % dextrose in polyelectrolyte solution or in quarter-strength normal saline solution (0.2 % NaCl) and lactated Ringer's solution [11–13].

4.5.4 Anesthetic Techniques

General anesthesia is increasingly associated with regional anesthetic techniques, to optimize anesthesia and analgesia results throughout the perioperative period.

4.5.4.1 General Anesthesia (GA)

Anesthetic management can be performed by inhalation or intravenous hypnotics, associated with neuromuscular blocking agents, opioids, and adjuvant drugs, if necessary. Anesthesiological management, today, foresees combined general-regional anesthesia.

Balanced anesthesia is the most common GA applied, in which a mixture of small amounts of several drugs, administered by different routes (inhalation + intravenous), permits a correct anesthetic plan for the surgery. Recently, total intravenous anesthesia (TIVA) is chosen for pediatric patients. In all pediatric ages and in particular in neonates, many drugs cannot be legally used. The bispectral index is designed to observe the anesthetic plan and drug consumption although results do not differ from those of conventional clinical practice (Table 4.2) [14].

Inhalation Agents Sevoflurane is a halogenated general inhalation anesthetic drug and to date the most frequently drug employed in pediatric anesthesia. It is administered by vaporization vehicled by O_2/medical air at different FiO_2. The minimum alveolar concentration (MAC) in neonates (3.3 %) and children until 3 months (3.2 %) is similar, but older infants and children have a lower MAC of approximately 2.5 %. During mask induction, the incidence of agitation is near 14 %, but laryngospasm and bronchospasm are present in around 1 or 2 %. It is quite clear that the concomitant use of opioids requires a lower halogenated concentration. Inhalation anesthesia consents a rapid recovery, but agitation is frequently present and is considered an adverse effect [15–17].

Intravenous Agents Although in the past years sodium thiopentone, belonging to the pharmacological class of barbiturates, was considered the most commonly used intravenous agent for anesthesia induction, propofol is now the most frequently employed induction agent (1.5–3 mg/kg) in pediatric age. The current and recent literature contains many reports of good results in particular for anesthesia induction in procedural deep sedation [18–20]. In preterm neonates and in the first 10 days of life, there is a risk of propofol accumulation if given both for an intermittent bolus and infusion. It would seem sensible at present to limit its use to single-bolus administration [21–24].

Table 4.2 Drugs used during digestive general anesthesia in pediatric age

Drug	Induction doses	Maintaining doses
Anesthetic agents		
Sevoflurane*	1–8 %	2–3.5 %
Thiopental	3–6 mg/kg	
Propofol	2.5–3 mg/kg	9–12 mg/kg/h
Opioids		
Fentanyl	1–2 mcg/kg	1–3 mcg/kg/h
Alfentanil	7–15 mcg/kg	0.5–1.5 mcg/kg/min
Remifentanil	0.5–1 mcg/kg	0.3–1 mcg/kg/min
Neuromuscular blocking agents		
Atracurium besylate	0.3–0.5 mg/kg	0.2–0.4 mg/kg/h
Cisatracurium besylate	0.15–0.25 mg/kg	0.1–0.3 mg/kg/h
Vecuronium	0.08–0.1 mg/kg	0.06–0.08 mg/kg/h
Rocuronium	0.6 mg/kg	0.3–0.6 mg/kg/h

*Sevoflurane is a halogenated gas. Its administration is related to minimum alveolar concentration (MAC)

4.5.4.2 Regional Anesthesia (RA)

It is generally accepted that RA provides safe and effective pain relief, as it provides the block of sensory transmissions [25, 26]. Regional anesthetic techniques also in pediatric patients provide safe and effective pain relief during and after surgery with different techniques [27].

A recent study of the ADARPEF revealed a low incidence of complications related to regional anesthetic techniques and concludes that RA has a good efficacy and safety [28]. The application of pediatric regional anesthesia blocks has increased in recent years; neuraxial blocks are applied in all ages and peripheral blocks are rapidly expanding especially in children aged 5 years or older. In pediatrics RA is performed under GA or deep sedation to reduce potential damages from a loss of behavioral control during the procedure and to keep hypnosis during surgery. However, RA reduces intraoperative anesthetic requirements, supporting recovery and early ambulation and shortening the time to rehabilitation [29, 30]. A necessary condition to obtain the most benefits from RA is the knowledge and expertise of the specialist who chooses and applies the techniques and appropriate and adequate equipment and devices. Ultrasound guidance is the best clinical practice both for neuraxial and peripheral blocks. Ultrasonography could augment the success rate, since it allows anatomical structures and nerves to be visualized, permits the needle location to be identified, and reduces the amount of local anesthetic administered [31].

The drugs used are local anesthetics and opioids for both top-up boluses and continuous infusion. It should be noted that the binding of local anesthetics with plasmatic protein (albumin and α-glycoprotein) is reduced in both newborn and infants and can result in an accumulation of the drugs themselves, especially if a continuous infusion is planned, with potential toxic risks.

Currently, selected local anesthetics for pediatric techniques are left-handed enantiomers (levobupivacaine and ropivacaine), and this makes the technique safer. The association of local anesthetics with opioids allows the use of low doses of both. Morphine, which was once the most widely used opioid, owing to the increased incidence of respiratory depression, vomiting, and itching, is now often replaced by fentanyl.

Neuraxial Blocks Central neuraxial bock is suggested for patients undergoing major abdominal surgery. In the spinal approach, drugs are administered intrathecally into the cerebrospinal fluid, in epidural approach into the fatty tissues surrounding the dura [32]. Absolute contraindications are local infection at injection site, hypovolemia, shock, coagulopathy, high intracranial pressure, allergy to local anesthetics, and parent refusal. Relative contraindications include sepsis, neurological dysfunction, and anatomic abnormalities. Neurological injury, infection, ischemia, seizures, hypotension, and cardiac arrest are the risks of neuraxial anesthesia. It should be remembered that there are some anatomical differences between adults and children in the lumbosacral region [33].

Caudal Epidural Block Epidural block by caudal route, the most popular technique in pediatrics, is suggested in herniorrhaphy and other pathologies with surgical under umbilical approach. The caudal space is easy to find in patients less than 7 years of age, when block is commonly performed. The sacral hiatus is found by searching for a triangle with the base formed by a line joining the right and left sacral cornea and the apex at the lower IV sacral vertebrae. The sacral hiatus is situated higher in children than in adults. The dedicated needle passes, at a nearly 45° angle, through the sacrococcygeal ligament, and after loss of resistance, the local anesthetic is injected. This block is more frequently used as a "single shot." Adjuvants may be added to prolong the duration of analgesia. Over the past several years, caudal catheters were introduced upward even to thoracic level especially in neonates and infants, but this technique is no longer recommended, because of the risk of fecal soiling [34, 35].

Lumbar Epidural Block In contrast to the caudal block, lumbar epidural block is rarely used as a single injection, and usually a catheter is inserted. Catheter placement is based on surgical incision location corresponding to segmental levels to target analgesia. This technique should be performed by experienced anesthesiologists. In very small infants, epidural needles are inserted below L4 so, to achieve the desired segmental level, the catheters should be threaded for a long segment, monitoring the efficacy of the pain relief. Currently, the indication is to decrease the distance of insertion to as short as 3–4 cm inside the epidural space. Central blocks have a history of more than 100 years in adults, but in pediatrics RA was rarely applied/described [36, 37] and became an essential integrated, safe, and effective analgesic system producing excellent intraoperative analgesia, less than 20 years ago, when Anand published his work [38].

Peripheral Nerve Blocks Peripheral nerve blocks are a valid alternative to the neuraxial technique, with good sensory block and without the major complications of central block. Sympathetic block and hemodynamic changes are minimal as well as motor block and urinary retention. The use of neurostimulation and ultrasonography is recommended although, in the latter case, evidence is not strong. The length of block depends on the pharmacokinetics of the local anesthetic, long-acting anesthetics such as levobupivacaine or ropivacaine are preferred, while adjuvants such as clonidine may extend the duration.

Ilioinguinal-Iliohypogastric Nerve Block This block may be used for surgical procedures in the inguinal region such as herniorrhaphy. Using a landmark technique, the puncture site is about 1 cm medial to the anterior superior iliac spine, but this traditional technique is burdened with high failure rates. The point of injection by ultrasound is more lateral, and the transversus abdominis/internal oblique fascial plane needs to be identified, where the nerves could be found [39].

Rectus Sheath Block A rectus sheath block provides effective pain relief and muscle relaxation for laparoscopic surgery and other small midline incisions. It is performed bilaterally, between the rectus abdominis muscle and the posterior rectus sheath. The unpredictable depth of the posterior rectus sheath in children is a good argument for the use of ultrasound together with the advantage of allowing visualization of the bowel, which may decrease accidental puncture [40].

Transversus Abdominis Plane (TAP) Block TAP block is effective in laparoscopic procedures and open surgery. Its use is limited by the need for bilateral blocks when the incision crosses the midline. This, like the other abdominal wall blocks described above, is effective for somatic pain but not for visceral pain. TAP block may be useful when epidural analgesia is contraindicated. Local anesthetic should be placed between the internal oblique and transversus abdominis muscles; the triangle of Petit is used as landmark for injection; a relatively large volume of anesthetic is required [41].

Local Wound Infiltration Local wound infiltration is a component of multimodal postoperative analgesia. The single-shot infiltration of local anesthetics in laparoscopic working ports is more commonly performed than continuous wound infiltration for fear of complications. Also intraperitoneal instillation was rarely performed, although a systematic review and meta-analysis of its effectiveness in adults have given promising results [42].

4.5.5 Intraoperative Ventilation

The aim of intraoperative ventilation techniques is to maintain normal levels of oxygenation and normocapnia. The aim to facilitate the digestive intervention and the advice to avoid high pressure in the airway should be remembered.

Pulmonary mechanical ventilation for these patients reflects the traditional intraoperative ventilation techniques. Patients were mechanically ventilated using an oxygen/air mixture with oxygen inspired fraction (FiO_2) between 0.35 and 0.50; tidal volume was adjusted between 9 and 10 ml/kg, and respiratory rate (RR) was regulated on the basis of the patient's age. The ratio of inspiratory time to expiratory time was usually 1:2. Positive end-expiratory pressure (PEEP) was set at 3–4 cm H_2O.

4.6 Laparoscopy in Digestive Surgery

Laparoscopic videosurgery is becoming increasingly more important in pediatric abdominal surgery for both the diagnosis and surgical treatment. Several authors who have compared this technique to traditional surgery for the treatment of some pathologies have reported reduced surgical trauma, less postoperative pain, reduced perioperative morbidity, shorter period of postoperative ileus, earlier postoperative mobilization, shorter periods of disability, shorter hospital stays, and better cosmetic results in favor of laparoscopic videosurgery [43–45]. Other benefits, compared to traditional "open" operative techniques, include the avoidance of large incisions, less fluid loss, heat, and forced retraction of tissues.

An optimal approach to the planning of anesthesia for laparoscopy depends on a knowledge of the technical requirements and an understanding of the physiological alterations associated with the procedure.

Physiological changes during laparoscopic surgery are related to the changes associated with the increased abdominal pressure associated with insufflation of the abdomen, the patient's postural modifications (head-up or head-down), and the CO_2 absorption and its general effects [46].

The magnitude of the physiological perturbations associated with laparoscopy is influenced by the patient's age, the patient's underlying myocardial and respiratory function, and the administered anesthetic agents.

Tension pneumoperitoneum causes an elevation in intra-abdominal pressure (IAP) which produces important effects on cardiovascular, pulmonary, renal, and metabolic function.

4.6.1 Effects on Respiratory System

Pneumoperitoneum and increase in IAP cause cephalic displacement of the diaphragm, resulting in the reduction in lung volumes including vital capacity, total lung volume, and functional residual capacity (FRC). This phenomenon is exacerbated by cephalic shift of the abdominal contents in the head-down position. Pulmonary compliance is reduced and airway resistance is increased, producing a higher airway pressure for any given tidal volume with an increased risk of hemodynamic changes and barotrauma during intermittent positive pressure ventilation (IPPV). Restriction in diaphragmatic mobility promotes uneven distribution of ventilation to the nondependent part of the lung, resulting in ventilation-perfusion mismatch with hypercarbia and hypoxemia. This preferential ventilation is increased further by supine position, inhalational anesthetic agents, and neuromuscular blockade [47, 48].

Another important respiratory implication is represented by CO_2 insufflation. Insufflated CO_2 is rapidly absorbed across the peritoneum and can lead to an increase in the total body CO_2 content. If ventilation is controlled and not changed in response to this increase, then the arterial pCO_2 will rise.

4.6.2 Effects on Cardiocirculatory System

In recent years, important knowledge has been obtained about the cardiovascular changes induced by pneumoperitoneum in children. Routine clinical measurements, such as heart rate and blood pressure, have been used to assess the hemodynamic changes induced by laparoscopy. Studies so far have shown most effects on blood pressure, which often increases, while there are no or only slight effects on heart rate [47, 48]. Experimental studies on the intraperitoneal insufflation of young animals have also shown an increase in venous return, peripheral arterial resistance with impaired splanchnic circulation, cardiac output, and cardiac index [49]. In pigs weighing 3–8 kg, the presence of hypercarbia during peritoneal insufflation increased heart rate, left ventricular stroke work, and cardiac index, without changes in total peripheral resistance or central venous pressure [50]. A study concerning the hemodynamic effects of pneumoperitoneum in healthy infants, by continuous esophageal aortic blood flow echo Doppler, demonstrated that abdominal insufflation with a pressure of 10 mmHg resulted in a significant decrease in aortic blood flow and stroke volume and in a significant increase in systemic vascular resistance [51].

Another study examined cardiovascular changes associated with intra-abdominal insufflation (10 mmHg) using echocardiography with transthoracic approach. Systolic blood pressure and diastolic blood pressure increased during intra-abdominal insufflation. Heart rate remained regular. Pneumoperitoneum was associated with increases in left ventricular end-diastolic volume (EDV), left ventricular end-systolic volume (ESV), and left ventricular end-systolic meridional wall stress (LVESWS). Before, during, and after intra-abdominal insufflation, systolic function indexes, left ventricular fractional shortening (LVFS), and left ventricular ejection fraction (LVEF) underwent slight, insignificant changes. During the surgical procedure, LVFS and LVEF remained within a range above 25 % and 55 %, respectively. Furthermore, there were no variations in the LVESWS/LVFS ratio. In this study, pneumoperitoneum induction determined the increase in both EDV and ESV. The EDV is recognized as a good indicator of preload; the increase is mostly due to a drainage effect on the splanchnic circulation, with an increase in venous return to the right heart. The increase in ESV could be partly the result of slightly impaired contractility, probably affected negatively by anesthetic drugs, and partly of an acute increase in afterload, more correctly expressed as aortic impedance. The myocardial left ventricular performance remained stable in all patients of the study, as shown by the absence of any modification in the LVFS and LVEF. A parallel increase in ESV explains why LVFS and LVEF did not change significantly. These results could represent the balanced effect of the increase in both preload and afterload induced by elevated intra-abdominal pressure, through a combined action on venous return and aortic impedance [52].

Pneumoperitoneum in children has a major impact on cardiac volumes and function, mainly through the effect on ventricular load conditions. The acute increase in IAP affects both preload and afterload, while the systolic cardiac performance remains unchanged. The final advice of these studies was to remain prudent before subjecting a child with cardiopathy to laparoscopy. To date, the literature has reported many experiences of laparoscopy in children with cardiac disease, offering reassuring messages about this procedure and its outcome. Today, the culture and experience exist to improve or complete the mosaic of pediatric heart diseases, relating the cardiocirculatory changes of laparoscopy to the various pathophysiological and clinical profiles of homogeneous groups of children with similar heart lesions [53].

4.6.3 Management of Intra-abdominal Pressure

It is important not to exceed an intra-abdominal pressure of 6 mmHg in newborns, 8 mmHg in infants, and 12 mmHg in older children so as to minimize the negative effects on cardiocirculatory function and cardiac output. The IAP reading should be clearly visible to the anesthetist and documented on the record [46, 47].

After starting the pneumoperitoneum, the position of the tracheal tube needs to be checked again to exclude an endobronchial position which can result from the diaphragm and lungs being shifted upward relative to the tube.

4.7 Esophageal Atresia

4.7.1 Preoperative Management

Esophageal atresia (EA) and tracheoesophageal fistula (TEF) are congenital anomalies that commonly occur together with an incidence of 1:3000–4500 live births. Surgical repair should be performed within the first few days of life.

Careful preoperative management is mandatory for a good surgical result of this pathology. The essential components that need to be implemented after birth as early as possible are:

- Diagnosis
- Investigation of associated anomalies
- Suction of the upper pouch
- Prevention and treatment of gastric and bowel distension

Prenatally, esophageal atresia is often not identified and only suspected in the presence of polyhydramnios, cardiac malformation, or chromosomal abnormalities. In the absence of prenatal suspicion, the postnatal presentation typically includes respiratory distress with initial feedings associated with excessive drooling or salivation. An inability to pass a nasogastric or orogastric suction catheter is almost always diagnostic.

A preanesthetic plan included an evaluation of associated anomalies, present between 30 and 50 % of babies. The most common are the congenital heart diseases, particularly tetralogy of Fallot, pulmonary atresia, atrial or ventricular septal defects, patent ductus arteriosus, and aortic coarctation. Echocardiography is performed routinely on these babies preoperatively. Vascular anomalies and upper airway problems such as laryngo- or tracheomalacia may be present. Severe tracheomalacia is not unusual and may require prolonged intubation or even tracheostomy. Cleft lip and palate may be found in association with esophageal atresia, as may vertebral, renal, and anorectal defects.

The term VACTERL has been used to describe a syndromic complex with usual associated anomalies: *V* vertebral, *A* anorectal, *C* cardiac, *T* tracheoesophageal fistula, *E* esophageal atresia, *R* radial or renal, and *L* limb. The term CHARGE describes another syndrome represented by *C* coloboma, *H* heart disease, *A* atresia choanae or esophageal atresia, *R* retarded growth, *G* genital anomalies, and *E* ear anomalies.

To diagnose and manage this anomaly, it is imperative to carefully pass an orogastric tube into the proximal pouch, typically meeting resistance at 8–10 cm. Awake prudent aspiration of the proximal pouch is performed in the preoperative period.

To avoid inhalation in the respiratory tract, the neonate should be kept with the head of the bed elevated to 35–45°. A chest radiograph confirms the diagnosis, revealing the tip of the tube in a dilated, air-filled proximal atresic pouch. Distal bowel gas confirms the presence of a tracheoesophageal communication, most commonly a distal fistula.

A typical presentation of newborn with esophageal atresia is variable impairment in respiratory function. Often there is no respiratory distress, but it must be remembered that its presence may have different origins, sometimes associated: inhalation in the respiratory tract of saliva through the upper airway or gastric juice from the fistula, prematurity, failure in severe cardiac malformation, significant deformity of the rib cage, and excessive gastric distension.

In preoperative treatment it should not be underestimated that excessive crying can help increase the flow of air into the stomach through the distal fistula. A sedation with midazolam at low doses (0.5–0.8 mcg/kg/h) may be necessary. Similarly, aggressive abdominal palpation should be avoided, as this could lead to reflux of gastric content into the fistula and direct aspiration into the airway.

The onset of respiratory distress with the need of intubation and excessive gastric distension are clinical situations that can accelerate the surgical repair.

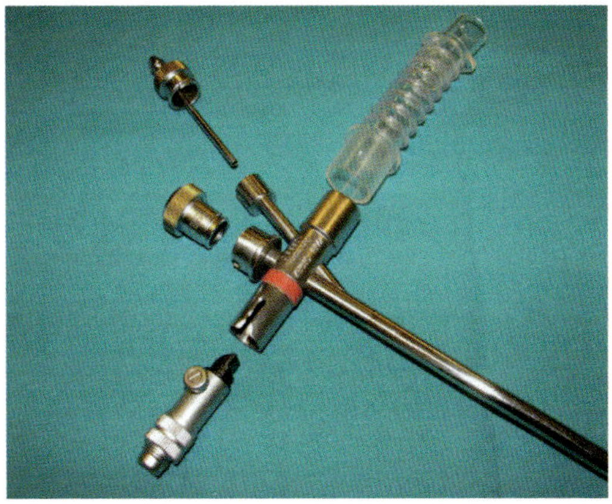

Fig. 4.1 The rigid bronchoscopy

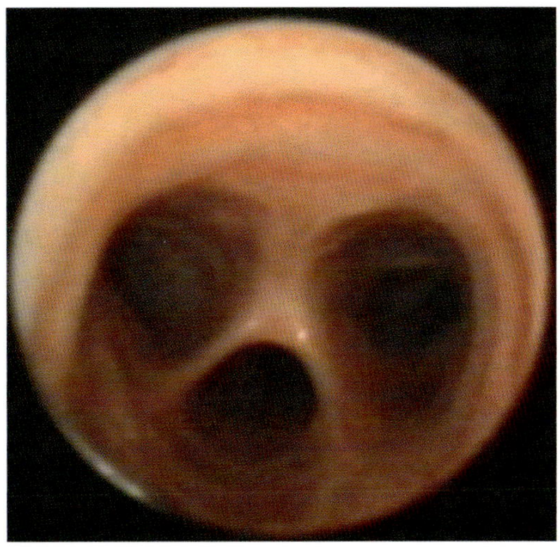

Fig. 4.2 Esophageal atresia type III. Tracheoesophageal fistula in the carina: trifurcation

4.7.2 Intraoperative Management

4.7.2.1 Anesthesia

The anesthesiological approach of esophageal atresia with tracheoesophageal fistula aims to avoid on the one hand an excessive gastric distension determined by positive pressure ventilation and, on the other hand, an acid reflux into the airway.

The literature suggests an induction of anesthesia maintaining spontaneous respiration, with topical administration of lidocaine (3–5 mg/kg), without application of a positive pressure via face mask. For this purpose, inhalation anesthesia is often indicated in several studies.

4.7.2.2 Airway Endoscopy

A preliminary procedure to surgery consists in the airway endoscopic evaluation, which is in fact the most reliable method for the recognition of tracheoesophageal fistula (TEF), and allows an exact classification of esophageal atresia.

The literature contains various descriptions of airway endoscopy used for the recognition of TEF, performed both with flexible and rigid instruments [54]. The use of the rigid endoscopy (Fig. 4.1) is reported in numerous studies and allows us to assure an open airway and assists operative management: in the presence of TEF, the airway endoscopic procedure was in fact diagnostic and operative at surgery [55, 56].

From a diagnostic standpoint, the endoscopy allows the identification of the EA type, the characteristics and size of the fistula, as well as the anatomic relationship with the esophageal pouches. From an operative point of view, the endoscopy allows the fistula themselves to be incannulated, which, in the case of distal TEF (Fig. 4.2), gives access to the stomach, which can then be drained, reducing the risks of aspiration pneumonia and improving the mechanical ventilation. The identification of the precise anatomic position of the TEF allows the tip of the endotracheal tube to be adjusted in order to achieve the optimal ventilation. Large or carinal fistula may bring about potential complications during anesthesia if the endotracheal tube happens to slip into them. The presence of the catheter or set of balloon catheters through the fistula (Figs. 4.3 and 4.4) prevents gastric insufflation, reducing the risk of pulmonary aspiration, and guides the surgical dissection during minimally invasive or open surgery [57].

The recognition of an upper fistula is particularly difficult because the fovea is smaller, or hardly visible, compared to lower TEF. This anatomical condition explains the need sometimes for a second endoscopy to better identify the presence of the upper fistula and plan correctly the therapeutic strategy: the presence of upper fistula led us to revise the diagnosis of two EAs at first considered of type III to EA of type IV (Fig. 4.5) and one EA of type I, without fistula, to EA of type II.

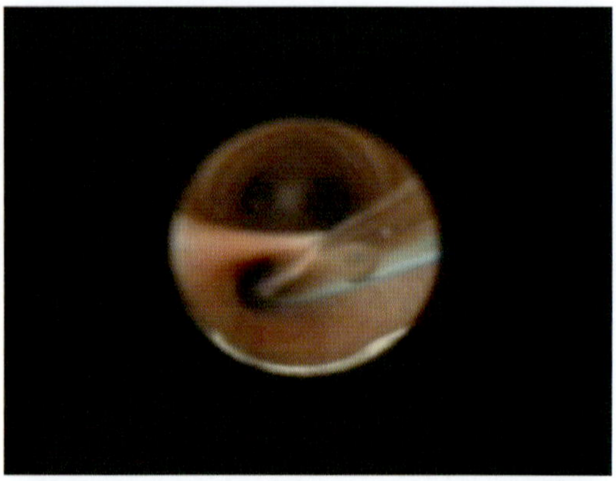

Fig. 4.3 Esophageal atresia type III: distal tracheoesophageal fistula with placement of catheter

The rigid ventilating tracheobronchoscopy, performed by experienced specialists, improves perioperative management of newborns affected by EA and appears to be a safe and effective procedure.

4.7.2.3 Thoracoscopic Implications

Esophageal atresia repair also foresees the thoracoscopic technique, which in newborns requires the lung to collapse, at least partially. There are two methods of achieving this. The first is lung exclusion which, using bronchial blocker with one-lung ventilation, allows the lung to collapse passively, and the second is lung compression by carbon dioxide insufflation. It should also be noted that the pathology and age of the patient often influence lung exclusion achievement. In neonatal age it is often impossible to perform lung exclusion.

Both methods are associated with serious respiratory and cardiocirculatory physiopathological problems that have been extensively studied in adult patients, but to a lesser extent in the neonatal and pediatric age.

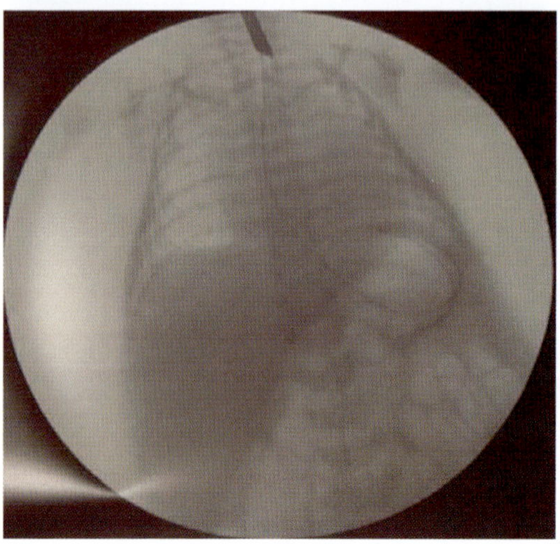

Fig. 4.4 Esophageal atresia type III: in rigid bronchoscopy the catheter, through the tracheoesophageal fistula, is placed in the stomach

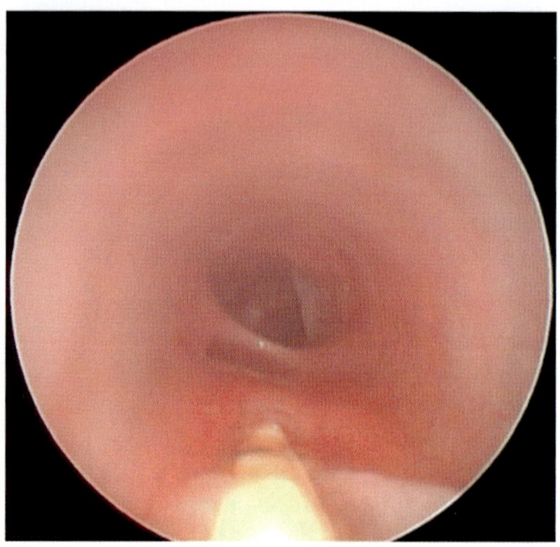

Fig. 4.5 Esophageal atresia type IV: double tracheoesophageal fistula, distal and upper with catheter

Lung exclusion presents extreme difficulties in newborns, although some cases are reported in literature [58, 59]. The difficulty in finding a suitable bronchial blocker for the newborn and the poor tolerance of prolonged lung ventilation are elements that favor the use of pleural insufflation. While during one-lung ventilation a marked decrease in oxygenation results from an increased intrapulmonary shunt due to the unventilated and collapsed lung, with pleural insufflation, the rise in pleural cavity pressure brings about notable hemodynamic effects that greatly decrease the preload, stroke volume, cardiac output, and mean arterial pressures. Cardiovascular function is penalized in direct proportion to the intrapleural insufflation values, while generally the respiratory parameters are only slightly compromised and hemogasanalytic changes are unremarkable. The pleural CO_2 insufflation always brings about a fall in cardiocirculatory performance, which is generally well tolerated in the euvolemic patient with normal cardiac function. An insufflating pressure limitation, a slow artificial pneumothorax, and a cardiovascular function optimization (by fluid administration or possible use of inotropic agents) can be useful to limit negative cardiocirculatory effects [60–62].

4.8 Abdominal Wall Defects

4.8.1 Preoperative Management

Abdominal wall defects are constituted by omphalocele and gastroschisis. The first is a herniation within the umbilical cord, and the second is a defect of the abdominal wall lateral to the umbilicus, usually on the right side. Omphalocele, with an incidence of 1 in 5000–10,000 live births, is more common than gastroschisis, which has an approximate incidence of 1 in 30,000 live births.

Surgical repair should be performed preferably within the first day of life; in gastroschisis the wait can be just a few hours. Timely and appropriate preoperative treatment is mandatory for a good surgical result of this disease.

These conditions are very readily diagnosed antenatally by ultrasonography, and often the birth of these children can be programmed. Many of these babies are of low birth weight, especially those with gastroschisis.

In the preoperative evaluation of the newborn, it is important to evaluate the common anomalies associated, more frequent with omphalocele. Other gastrointestinal malformations or genitourinary and craniofacial anomalies may be present, including harelip and cleft palate. Important syndromic abnormalities include Beckwith-Wiedemann syndrome (macrosomia, macroglossia, and hypoglycemia), imperforate anus, chromosomal anomalies (trisomies 13, 18, 21), as well as cardiac malformations including the pentalogy of Cantrell, characterized, in addition to omphalocele, by short sternum, anterior diaphragmatic hernia, left ventricular diverticulum, and deformity of the rib cage. Some patients have a very narrow "dog-type" chest with underlying hypoplastic lungs and may die early with respiratory failure or later with cor pulmonale.

The large surface area of exposed bowel out of the abdominal wall predisposes the patient to fluid and electrolyte disturbance due to gastroenteric loss and increased evaporation, heat losses, infections, and decreased mesenteric blood flow with risk of ischemia of the intestinal loops. The preoperative goals to appropriately resuscitate the newborn are:

- Predispose warming measures, including the increase of ambient room temperature, use of heating lamps and forced-air warming blankets, and infusion of heated fluids.
- Ensure an effective hydration, even with supplementation of blood and its derivatives, if necessary. Fluid resuscitation with isotonic solutions such as 1–2 % dextrose in polyelectrolyte solution, normal saline, or Ringer's lactate is recommended for the newborn with marked hypovolemia. Volume resuscitation is usually continued until the infant's urine output normalizes and/or blood gases indicate normal acid-base balance.
- Prevent infections by antibiotic therapy and placement of a plastic bag that encloses the entire infant below the nipples, including all externalized viscera.

- Ensure a good splanchnic perfusion by cardiovascular function optimization with fluid administration or possible use of inotropic agents. For this purpose, the position of the baby is important because it does not have to lead to a kinking or twisting of the bowel loops. Infants with gastroschisis should be positioned on their right side in a lateral decubitus position to enhance venous blood return from the gut.
- Predispose a gastroenteric decompression by naso-/orogastric tube, placed to intermittent suction. Decompression is important because it helps to prevent partial or total obstruction of blood flow and oxygenation to the bowel.

Stabilization and the decision about the most appropriate time for the surgical repair must take into consideration many factors, including thermoregulation, fluid volume status, gastric distension and intestinal compromise, infection, respiratory status, and preparation for surgery. Stability of the aforementioned factors is necessary before the impending surgical repair to optimize the infant's outcome [63].

4.8.2 Intraoperative Management

The treatment of choice for omphalocele and gastroschisis defects in newborn is primary repair, whenever possible. Primary closure carries the risk of placing the abdominal contents under excessive pressure and producing reduction of cardiac output, hypotension, bowel ischemia, anuria, and respiratory failure. Sometimes there is a chance that this clinical situation will develop into a full-blown abdominal compartment syndrome.

When primary closure cannot be achieved, either because of the large size of the defect or because it compromises respiratory and cardiovascular function, the alternative approach is a staged repair utilizing a pouch. This staged repair carries an increased risk of infection as well as the need of multiple anesthetic and surgical procedures.

The anesthetic technique must provide a good analgesia, obtained by opioids and a large use of muscle relaxants, to obtain the most effective help for the closing of the wall defect with replacement of the viscera in the abdomen. In addition to anesthetic support, surgical strategies to achieve primary repair include stretching of the abdominal wall, evacuating the contents of the stomach and small bowel, irrigating meconium from the intestines, and enlarging the defect by leaving a fascial hernia.

The determination of objective criteria that would predict safe, primary closure of abdominal wall defects is based mainly on intraoperative measurement of intra-abdominal pressures that should be kept less than 20 mmHg to prevent adverse hemodynamic consequences to other organs and tissues. However, during surgery, it is also necessary to consider changes of other intraoperative hemodynamic parameters such as central venous pressure, cardiac output, arterial blood pressure, and heart rate as well as of the urine output and of respiratory parameters such as oxygenation, $ETCO_2$, and airway pressure during mechanical ventilation [64].

References

1. Nasr VG, Davis JM (2015) Anesthetic use in newborn infants: the urgent need for rigorous evaluation. Pediatr Res 78(1):2–6
2. Sanders RD, Hassell J, Davidson AJ, Robertson NJ, Ma D (2013) Impact of anaesthetics and surgery on neurodevelopment: an update. Br J Anaesth 110(1):53–72
3. McCann ME, Soriano SG (2012) Perioperative central nervous system injury in neonates. Br J Anaesth 109(1):60–67
4. Serafini G, Ingelmo PM, Astuto M, Baroncini S, Borrometi F, Bortone L, Ceschin C, Gentili A, Lampugnani E et al (2013) Preoperative evaluation in infants and children: recommendations of the Italian Society of Pediatric and Neonatal Anaesthesia and Intensive Care (SARNePI). Minerva Anestesiol 80(4):461–469
5. Rajesh MC (2015) Anaesthesia for children with bronchial asthma and respiratory infections. Indian J Anaesth 59(9):584–588
6. ASA Committee on Standards and Practice Parameters (2011) Practice guidelines for preoperative fasting and the use of pharmacologic agents to reduce the Risk of pulmonary aspiration: application to healthy

patients undergoing elective procedures: an updated report by ASA Committee on Standards and Practice Parameters. Anesthesiology 114:495–511
7. Gregory GA (2012) Gregory's pediatric anaesthesia, 5th edn. Churchill-Livingstone, New York
8. Lerman J (2010) Perioperative respiratory complications in children. Lancet 376:745–746
9. Ing C, Chui I, Ohkawa S, Kakavouli A, Sun L (2013) Incidence and causes of perioperative endotracheal reintubation in children: a review of 28208 anesthetics. Paediatr Anaesth 23:621–626
10. Sang P, Yoon HK, Sang YS et al (2013) Ultrasound-guided subclavian catheterization in pediatric patients with a linear probe: a case series. Korean J Anesthesiol 64(6):541–544
11. Lindahal SG (1988) Energy expenditure and fluid and electrolyte requirements in anesthetized infants and children. Anesthesiology 69(3):377–382
12. Lönnqvist PA (2007) Inappropriate perioperative fluid management in children: time of solution. Paediatr Anaesth 17:203–205
13. Murat I, Dubois MC (2008) Perioperative fluid therapy in pediatrics. Paediatr Anaesth 18(5):363–370
14. Bresil P, Nielsson MS, Malver LP, Kraemer K, Schjørring O, Dethlefsen C, Lambert PH (2013) Impact of bispectral index for monitoring propofol remifentanil anaesthesia. A randomised clinical trial. Acta Anaesthesiol Scand 57(8):978–987
15. Keaney A, Diviney D, Harte S et al (2004) Postoperative behavioral changes following anaesthesia with sevoflurane. Paediatr Anaesth 14:866–870
16. Kuratani N, Oi Y (2008) Greater incidence of emergence agitation in children after sevoflurane anaesthesia as compared with halothane: a meta-analysis of randomized controlled trials. Anesthesiology 109:225–232
17. Faulk DJ, Twite MD, Zuk J, Pan Z, Wallen B, Fiesen RH (2010) Hypnotic depth and the incidence of emergence agitation and negative postoperative behavioral changes. Paediatr Anaesth 20(1):72–81
18. Ghanta S, Abdel-Latif ME, Lui K, Ravindranathan H, Awad J, Oei J (2007) Propofol compared with the morphine, atropine, and suxamethonium regimen as induction agents for neonatal endotracheal intubation: a randomized, controlled trial. Pediatrics 119(6):1248–1255
19. Papoff P, Mancuso M, Caresta E, Moretti C (2008) Effectiveness and safety of propofol in newborn infants. Pediatrics 121(2):448–449
20. Shah PS, Shah VS (2011) Propofol for procedural sedation/anaesthesia in neonates. Cochrane Database Syst Rev 3:CD007248
21. Allegaert K, de Hoon J, Verbesselt R, Naulaers G, Murat I (2007) Maturational pharmacokinetics of single intravenous bolus of propofol. Paediatr Anaesth 17(11):1028–1034
22. Allegaert K, Peeters MY, Verbesselt R et al (2007) Inter-individual variability in propofol pharmacokinetics in preterm and term neonates. Br J Anaesth 99(6):864–870
23. Allegaert K, De Hoon J, Naulaers G, Van De Velde M (2008) Neonatal clinical pharmacology: recent observations of relevance for anaesthesiologists. Acta Anaesthesiol Belg 59:283–288
24. Skinner AV (2010) Neonatal pharmacology. Anaesth Int Care 12(3):79–84
25. Tobias JD, Flannagan J, Brock J, Brin E (1993) Neonatal regional anaesthesia: alternative to general anaesthesia for urologic surgery. Urology 41(4):362–365
26. Bernstein S (1993) Regional anaesthesia for urological surgery. Int Anesthesiol Clin 31(1):57–66
27. Dalens B (2006) Some current controversies in pediatric regional anaesthesia. Curr Opin Anaesthesiol 19(3):301–308
28. Ecoffey C, Locroix F, Giaufre E (2010) Epidemiology and morbidity of regional anaesthesia in children: a follow up one-year survey prospective of the French-Language Society of Pediatric Anaesthesiologists (ADARPEF). Pediatr Anaesth 20:1061–1069
29. Bordet AEF, Duflo F, Lanais S, Combet S, Taylor P, Pouyau A, Paturel B, James R, Allaouchiche B, Chassard D (2003) Patient-controlled epidural analgesia versus continuous epidural infusion with ropivacaine for postoperative analgesia in children. Anesth Analg 97:1608–1611
30. Pavar D (2004) Regional anaesthesia in pediatric patients. Indian J Anaesth 48(5):394–399
31. Denny NM, Harrop-Griffiths W (2005) Location, location, location! Ultrasound imaging in regional anaesthesia. Br J Anaesth 94(1):1–3
32. Schug SA, Saunders D, Kurowski I, Paech MJ (2006) Neuraxial drug administration: a review of treatment options for anaesthesia and analgesia. CNS Drugs 20(11):917–933
33. Samol NB, Furstein JS, Moore DL (2012) Regional anaesthesia and pain management for the pediatric patient. Int Anesthesiol Clin 50(4):83–95
34. Spiegel P (1962) Caudal anaesthesia in pediatric surgery: a preliminary report. Anesth Analg 41:219–221
35. Fortuna A (1967) Caudal analgesia: a simple and safe technique in pediatric surgery. Br J Anaesth 39:165–170
36. Murrell D, Gibson PR, Cohen RC (1993) Continuous epidural analgesia in newborn infants undergoing major surgery. J Pediatr Surg 28:548–553
37. Ruston FG (1961) Epidural anaesthesia in pediatric surgery. Present status in the Hamilton General Hospital. Can Anaesth Soc J 11:12–34
38. Anand KJ, Sippell WG, Aynsley-Green A (1987) Randomized trial of fentanyl anaesthesia in preterm babies undergoing surgery: effects on the stress response. Lancet 1:62–66
39. Willschke H, Bösenberg A, Marhofer P, Johnston S, Kettner S, Eichenberger U et al (2006) Ultrasonographic-guided ilioinguinal/iliohypogastric nerve block in pediatric anaesthesia: what is the optimal volume? Anesth Analg 102(6):1680–1684
40. Willschke H, Bösenberg A, Marhofer P, Johnston S, Kettner SC, Wanzel O, Kapral S (2006)

Ultrasonography-guided rectus sheath block in pediatric anaesthesia – a new approach to an old technique. Br J Anaesth 97(2):244–249
41. Mai CL, Young MJ, Quraishi SA (2012) Clinical implications of the transversus abdominis plane block in pediatric anaesthesia. Paediatr Anaesth 22(9):831–840
42. Marks JL, Ata B, Tulandi T (2012) Systematic review and meta-analysis of intraperitoneal instillation of local anesthetics for reduction of pain after gynecologic laparoscopy. J Minim Invasive Gynecol 19(5):545–553
43. Bozkurt P, Kaya G, Altinas F, Yeker Y, Sarimurat N (2000) Systemic stress response during operations for acute abdominal pain performed via laparoscopy or laparotomy in children. Anaesthesia 55:5–9
44. Fujimoto T, Segawa O, Lane GJ, Esaki S, Miyano T (1999) Laparoscopic surgery in newborn infants. Surg Endosc 13:773–777
45. Georgeson KE, Cohen RD, Hebra A, Jona JD, Powell DM, Rothemberg SS et al (1999) Primary laparoscopic-assisted endorectal colon pull-through for Hirschsprung's disease. Ann Surg 5:678–683
46. Tobias JD (2002) Anaesthesia for minimally invasive surgery in children. Best Pract Res Clin Anaesthesiol 16(1):15–130
47. Petrat G, Weyandt D, Klein U (1999) Anesthetic considerations in pediatric laparoscopic and thoracoscopic surgery. Eur J Pediatr Surg 9:282–285
48. Tobias JD, Holcomb GW, Brock JW, Deshpande JK, Lowe S, Morgan WM (1995) Cardiorespiratory changes in children during laparoscopy. J Pediatr Surg 30:33–36
49. Masey SA, Koehler RC, Buck JR (1985) Effect of abdominal distension on central and regional hemodynamics in neonatal lambs. Pediatr Res 19:1244–1249
50. Rayman R, Girotti M, Armstrong K, Inman KJ, Lee R, Girvan D (1995) Assessing the safety of pediatric laparoscopic surgery. Surg Laparosc Endosc 5:437–443
51. Gueugniaud PY, Abiserror M, Moussa M, Godard J, Foussat C, Petit P et al (1998) The hemodynamic effects of pneumoperitoneum during laparoscopic surgery in healthy infants: assessment by continuous oesophageal aortic blood flow echo-doppler. Anesth Analg 86:290–293
52. Gentili A, Iannettone CM, Pigna A, Landuzzi V, Lima M, Baroncini S (2000) Cardiocirculatory changes during videolaparoscopy in children: echocardiographic study. Paediatr Anaesth 10:399–406
53. Gentili A, Landuzzi V, Pasini L, Lima M (2014) The laparoscopic approach in children with cardiopathy: a mosaic still awaiting completion. Paediatr Anaesth 24(3):351–352
54. Masciopinto F, Gentili A, Bianchini A, Baroncini S (2013) Airway endoscopy. In: Lima M (ed) Pediatric thoracic surgery. Springer, Milan, pp 181–192
55. Reed MF, Mathisen DJ (2003) Tracheoesophageal fistula. Chest Surg Clin N Am 13(2):271–289
56. Kane TD, Atri P, Potoka DA (2007) Triple fistula: management of a double tracheoesophageal fistula with a third H-type proximal fistula. J Pediatr Surg 42(6):E1–E3
57. Holcomb GW 3rd, Rothenberg SS, Bax KM, Martinez-Ferro M, Albanese CT, Ostlie DJ et al (2005) Thoracoscopic repair of esophageal atresia and tracheoesophageal fistula: a multi-institutional analysis. Ann Surg 242(3):422–428
58. Hammer GB (2004) Anaesthetic management for the children with a mediastinal mass. Paediatr Anaesth 14:95–97
59. Hammer GB, Harrison TK, Vricella LA, Black MD, Krane EJ (2002) Single lung ventilation in children using a new paediatric bronchial blocker. Paediatr Anaesth 12:69–72
60. Enk D, Rellensmann G, Brussel T, Van Aken H, Semik M, Schmidt C (2007) Ventilation management during neonatal thoracic surgery. Anesth Analg 104(1):218
61. Gentili A, Lima M, De Rose R, Pigna A, Codeluppi V, Baroncini S (2007) Thoracoscopy in children: anaesthesiological implications and case reports. Minerva Anestesiol 73(3):161–171
62. Mukhtar AM, Obayah GM, Elmasry A, Dessouky NM (2008) The therapeutic potential of intraoperative hypercapnia during video-assisted thoracoscopy in pediatric patients. Anesth Analg 106(1):84–88
63. de Buys Roessingh AS, Damphousse A, Ballabeni P, Dubois J, Bouchard S (2015) Predictive factors at birth of the severity of gastroschisis. World J Gastrointest Pathophysiol 6(4):228–234
64. Luo D, Wu L, Wu H, Huang W, Huang H (2015) Anesthetic management of a neonate receiving prenatal repair of gastroschisis. Int J Clin Exp Med 8(5):8234–8237

Intensive Care in Digestive Surgery

5

Andrea Gentili, Rosina De Rose, and Elisa Iannella

5.1 Introduction

Postoperative admission to the pediatric intensive care unit (PICU) is foreseen for all pediatric patients undergoing major digestive surgery and all children with a basic critical illness, often unrelated to the abdominal problem that leads to surgery, which requires monitoring and/or intensive treatment. Hospitalization in intensive care increases the security of critical patients in the delicate phase that follows the surgery, characterized by the need to maintain a proper respiratory, cardiovascular, and metabolic function and stabilization of these features, together with the need for analgesia and sedation, appropriate fluid therapy and electrolyte compensation, neurological monitoring, and prevention/treatment of infections.

It should also be pointed out that for some diseases, often typical of the neonatal age, such as esophageal atresia, abdominal wall defects, and necrotizing enterocolitis, the surgery is part of an intensive treatment, which begins at birth and which also involves an important phase of preoperative treatment and stabilization. For these clinical conditions, the more correct term is perioperative intensive care [1].

A. Gentili (✉) • R. De Rose • E. Iannella
Department of Pediatric Anaesthesia and Intensive Care, S. Orsola-Malpighi University Hospital, Via Massarenti 9, Bologna, Italy
e-mail: andrea_gentili@libero.it; rosina.derose@aosp.bo.it; elisa.iannella@aosp.bo.it

5.2 Intensive Monitoring

Monitoring is one of the main prerogatives of intensive perioperative hospitalization, which may involve pathologies with clinical controls and rapid autonomization or others requiring long and complex assistance.

Particular importance is given to respiratory monitoring, with attention to the type of mechanical ventilation, the respiratory weaning, and the techniques of noninvasive respiratory assistance, and to the cardiovascular, metabolic and electrolyte, temperature, and neurological monitoring carefully tailored to the level of consciousness and sedation of the patient.

The respiratory monitoring involves simple and noninvasive instrumentation ranging from pulse oximetry and capnography to the reading of volumes, pressures, and compliance curves present during mechanical ventilation. An important control is that of the arterial blood gases, which offers the opportunity to further monitor oxygenation parameters such as alveolar-arterial gradient oxygen (A-aDO_2), oxygenation index (OI), arterial-alveolar ratio (a/AO_2), and PaO_2/FiO_2 ratio, useful in the evaluation of the postoperative alveolar recruitment in many challenging diseases such as esophageal atresia, omphalocele, and gastroschisis. The traditional control of the chest with imaging through X-ray until the computed tomography is now usefully supplemented by the use of ultrasound lung, easily repeatable and usable in the control/treatment of conditions

M. Lima (ed.), *Pediatric Digestive Surgery*, DOI 10.1007/978-3-319-40525-4_5

such as pneumothorax, pleural effusion, and pulmonary atelectasis [2, 3].

Hemodynamic monitoring focuses on parameters of the conventional type such as ECG, invasive or noninvasive blood pressure, and central venous pressure as well as on parameters obtained through the method of pulse contour analysis and transpulmonary thermodilution, which allow the continuous evaluation of cardiac output, peripheral vascular resistance, and stroke volume, in addition to the measurement of preload in volumetric terms and the estimation of the intrathoracic blood volume (ITBV) and the amount of extravascular lung water (EVLW).

Furthermore, it is possible to obtain the evaluation of the perfusion of tissues such as the brain, renal, and splanchnic through the "near-infrared spectroscopy" (NIRS). Finally, again through ultrasound method, the monitoring of the filling fluid challenge can be obtained through the measurement of the size of the vena cava.

Monitoring in PICU includes control of the main laboratory tests and evaluation at regular intervals of daily input and output of fluid in order to accurately assess the volume status of the patient.

The children admitted require careful monitoring to prevent infectious complications. The monitoring follows a strict protocol of surveillance involving culture tests such as throat swabs, rectal samples, biological tracheobronchial secretions, gastric and urinary content, and material conducted by any drainage. The surveillance begins at the induction of anesthesia in the operating room or at the time of admission to the PICU. It should also examine all the types of principal invasive devices and drainage at the time of their removal. Blood cultures are programmed if the patient's clinical condition and the biohumoral markers suggest severe sepsis.

5.3 Respiratory Treatment

After major digestive surgery, often the main treatment in PICU is instrumental support of the respiratory function, which provides a gradation of interventions depending on the severity of the respiratory failure. Early respiratory weaning and extubation are safe and feasible in many patients, but in a significant minority, this might not be possible. A number of factors have been shown to contribute to delayed weaning from the ventilator. These include perioperative factors such as known chromosomal and neurological abnormalities, the age of the patients, the presence of airway problems and pulmonary disease, the complexity of the operation, postsurgical complications, and myocardial dysfunction.

The main objectives of such support are the insurance of an adequate alveolar ventilation, with CO_2 removal associated with a satisfactory oxygenation, improving the relationship of ventilation/perfusion (VA/Q), encouraging alveolar recruitment, and reducing the work of breathing (Table 5.1).

The first measures are constituted by methods of noninvasive ventilatory (NIV) assistance, combining oxygen therapy with the possible application of positive airway pressure and/or of a ventilatory support (high-flow nasal oxygen, NIV equipment), with the use of different interfaces depending on the age of the patient (nasal prong, masks, or helmets) (Figs. 5.1 and 5.2) [4].

If the newborn and children require intubation, the possibilities of ventilatory assistance can range from techniques of controlled ventilation (mainly controlled pressure) to assisted methods, used in the weaning of patients such as synchronized intermittent mandatory ventilation (SIMV), pressure support (PS), and continuous positive airway pressure (CPAP) [5, 6].

Table 5.1 Objectives of mechanical ventilation

Support or manipulate pulmonary gas exchange
Normalize alveolar ventilation (PaO_2, $PaCO_2$, and pH)
Achieve and maintain $PaO_2 > 90$ mmHg and peripheral Sat $O_2 > 95\ \%$
Increase lung volume and maintain adequate functional residual capacity (FRC)
Obtain lung expansion and prevent or treat atelectasis
Improve oxygenation and lung compliance
Reduce the work of breathing in the presence of high airway resistance and/or reduced compliance, when spontaneous breathing becomes ineffective

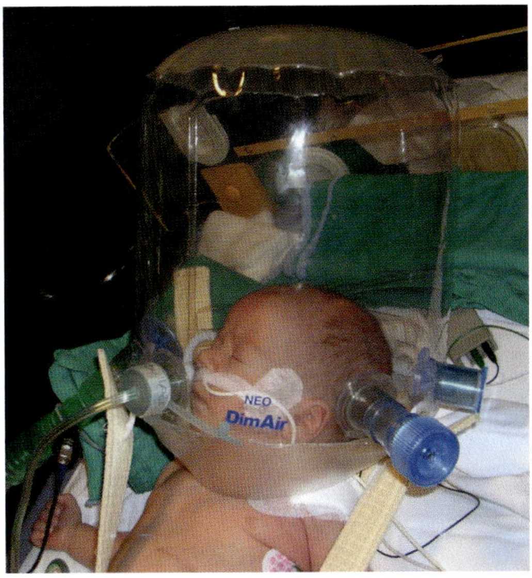

Fig. 5.1 Noninvasive ventilatory (NIV) assistance with helmet in neonatal age

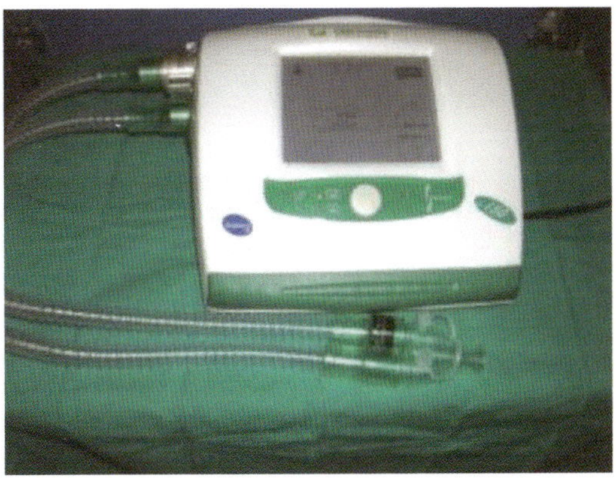

Fig. 5.2 Ventilator for noninvasive ventilatory (NIV) assistance

A particular method of ventilation is controlled high-frequency oscillatory ventilation (HFOV) characterized by very small volumes (less than the dead space) and extremely high respiratory rates between 5 and 15 Hz (300 and 900 breaths/min). Oscillatory ventilation produces a series of oscillations (positive and negative) in the airways, with an active expiratory phase, and during the entire respiratory cycle, lung volume is maintained almost constant (Fig. 5.3).

An interesting ventilatory approach, very useful for the weaning of patients, is the neurally

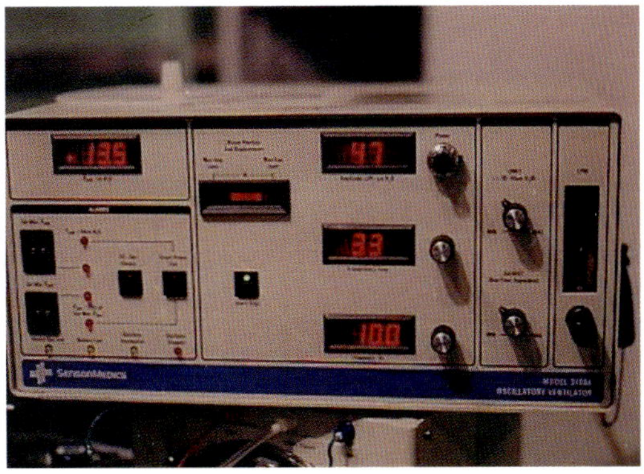

Fig. 5.3 Parameters of respiratory assistance with high-frequency oscillatory ventilation (HFOV)

adjusted ventilatory assistance (NAVA) based on neural respiratory control [7, 8]. By NAVA, the electrical activity of the diaphragm (Edi) is captured with an appropriate catheter, equipped with an array of nine miniaturized electrodes, which must interface in the lower esophagus at the level of the diaphragm, in order to obtain the best electrical signal from diaphragmatic fibers. The catheter sends the signals to the ventilator and is used to assist the patient's breathing [9, 10]. Since the mechanical ventilator and the diaphragm work with the same signal, the mechanical coupling between the diaphragm and the mechanical ventilation is virtually instantaneous (Fig. 5.4).

The ventilation in neonatal and pediatric age during the postoperative course after surgery requires a solid basic understanding of respiratory system mechanics (pressure-volume relationship of the respiratory system and the concept of its time constants) and cardiopulmonary physiology. Furthermore, careful attention has to be paid to avoid damaging the lungs by potentially injurious mechanical ventilation. Optimizing ventilator settings during controlled and assisted ventilation must lead to a progressive and gentle lung recruitment, avoiding the damage caused by strong and repetitive opening/collapse of distal airways and excessive alveolar hyperinflation.

Especially in neonatal age, in the presence of a still immature lung, and in association with problems such as pulmonary infections, sepsis, aspiration of saliva or gastric juice, and severe heart diseases, excessive mechanical ventilation

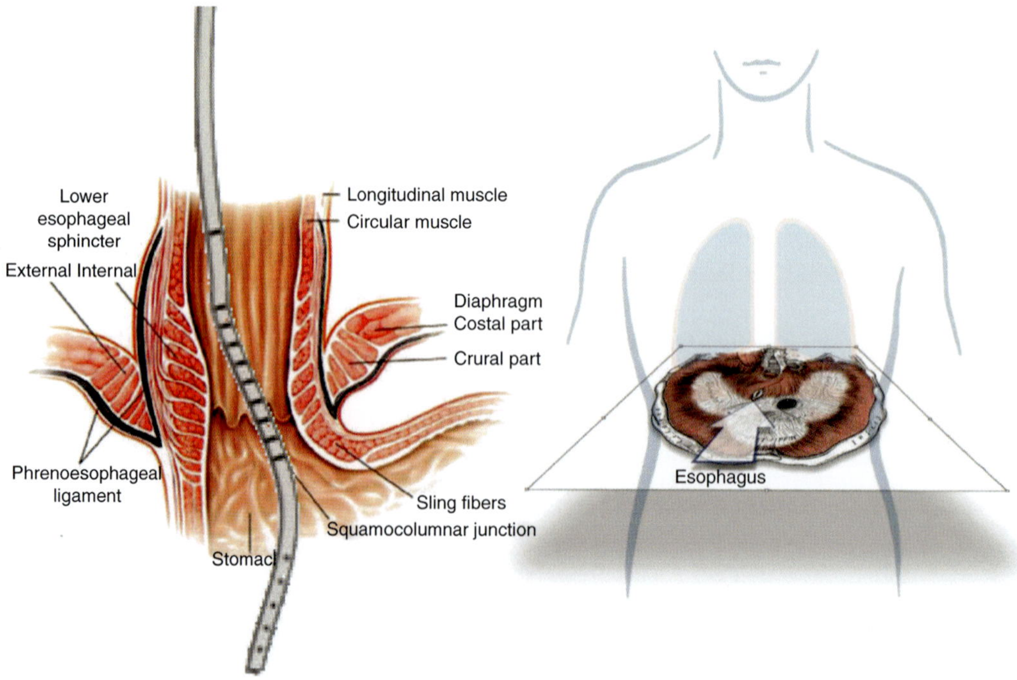

Fig. 5.4 The electrical discharge of the diaphragm captured through the introduction in the lower esophagus, at the level of the diaphragm, of a NAVA catheter equipped with an array of nine miniaturized electrodes

can lead to lung injury, emphasizing phenomena of volutrauma and barotrauma, which can result in a biotrauma, characterized by alveolar damage, with increased microvascular and epithelial permeability, fluid filtration, and pulmonary edema.

This clinical condition can approach an acute respiratory distress syndrome (ARDS), characterized by the absence of secretion or abnormalities in the action of surfactant, resulting in decreased lung compliance and significant hypoxemia. Administration of surfactant, associated with HFOV, may represent an effective method of lung recruitment and alveolar recovery in acute pulmonary injury and in ARDS. Bronchoscopic instillation offers the theoretical advantages that the surfactant may be distributed directly to the desired regions of the lung, with a more economical use of the drug and with the opportunity to lavage leaked serum proteins prior to instillation.

5.4 Cardiocirculatory Treatment

The cardiac output (CO) is the result of the heart rate multiplied by the stroke volume; it undergoes changes according to the variation of the two parameters.

Modifications of the heart rate are able to result in major reductions in cardiac output: bradycardia in children, especially at an early age, causes an important reduction of CO, as the systolic ejection volume does not increase in proportion to the decrease of the heart rate, because of poor ventricular compliance, due to the immaturity of the cardiac muscles.

Tachycardia, up to 200 beats/min, seems better tolerated, as it is accompanied by a proportional increase in CO.

Likewise, limitations in stroke volume also involve a significant lowering of cardiac output. Supporting cardiovascular disease in young patients with digestive surgery must include both principal actions for the overall improvement in stroke volume and specific interventions with antiarrhythmic therapy.

5.4.1 Increase of Stroke Volume

The increase of the CO is achieved, thanks to an increase in the volume of systolic ejection. It depends on and is influenced substantially by three mechanisms:

- Increase in the preload
- Increase in myocardial contractility
- Reduction of the afterload (vascular resistance against which the ventricle pumps the blood volume)

The volume expansion contributes to the increase in preload; it should benefit from the use of crystalloid, colloid, and blood and its derivatives. At first contributions of 10–20 ml/kg isotonic polyelectrolyte solutions are likely to improve the clinical condition with the recovery of peripheral perfusion, decreased heart rate, and the recovery of a viable diuresis. These quantities are usually well tolerated hemodynamically.

Secondly, volume resuscitation of a patient with hypovolemic or septic shock is an essential component of initial patient care. Massive amounts of intravenous fluid are usually administered to replace intravascular volume deficit and to minimize complications attributed to hypovolemia such as tachycardia, hypotension, acute kidney injury, and multiorgan failure. Goal-directed therapies focused on the restoration of normal blood pressure and organ perfusion have been advocated in the management of critically ill patients. Early goal-directed therapy, which is instituted in the initial phase of management of patients with severe sepsis or septic shock, has been shown to improve overall survival [11, 12].

In contrast to the notion of aggressive and liberal volume resuscitation, a growing body of evidence strongly suggests that fluid overload may be detrimental to critically ill patients. Relatively, little attention has been paid to the consequences of fluid overload such as respiratory failure, increased cardiac demand, and peripheral edema. Recent studies on patients with acute lung or kidney injury have reported that fluid overload has been associated with adverse outcomes [13, 14].

The treatment of choice for the optimization of myocardial contractility appears to be the correction of all unfavorable factors (hypoxia, acidosis, hypoglycemia, hypocalcemia, drugs, and toxic substances). Positive inotropic agents, pressor drugs, and vasodilators are indicated as appropriate [15]. Sympathomimetic amines are compounds used in optimizing hemodynamics.

Dopamine is a catecholamine most used in neonatal and pediatric age. Its action takes place on both beta and alpha receptors at a dose of 5–10 mcg/kg/min, respectively. The positive inotropic effect is still mainly due to the release of endogenous norepinephrine. Its positive inotropic effect is modest overall. In patients with renal impairment, it is the drug of choice because at a dose of 3–2 mcg/kg/min, in continuous administration, it ensures a vasodilatation of the splanchnic and renal vascular system. Such action however is discussed for renal and intestinal protection.

Dobutamine increases myocardial contractility, systolic ejection volume, and cardiac output; it decreases the systemic and pulmonary resistance when used in cardiac failure. Even at high doses, it has little effect on heart rate and does not cause an increase in peripheral resistance. It is therefore particularly indicated for patients with severe heart failure. Its action is predominantly beta-adrenergic. This drug is normally used in continuous infusion at a dose of 5–10 mcg/kg/min. It has no specific action on renal and mesenteric circulation and is therefore often used jointly with low-dose dopamine.

Epinephrine is the drug of choice in cardiopulmonary resuscitation (CPR). It possesses potent inotropic and chronotropic effects, associated with action on the alpha and beta receptors of the systemic vascular resistance. In moderate doses it proves to be a real inotropic support in critically ill patients, even when other medicines have not been fruitful; the risk of a response in generalized vasoconstriction is real only at high doses.

In other cases, it is necessary to resort to a reduction in the afterload; the decrease in systemic vascular resistance decreases afterload and increases the volume of systolic ejection, without being accompanied by increased myocardial oxygen demand.

Sodium nitroprusside is a vasodilator with effects on vascular resistance (arteries) and capacitance (veins). Arteriolar dilation produced by this drug reduces the afterload; increased vascular capacitance requires proper support of the preload. It is normally used at a dosage of 0.5–10 mcg/kg/min; its administration requires continuous monitoring of cyanide and thiocyanate metabolites [16].

Nitroglycerin dosage of 1–20 mcg/kg/min has an action prevailing on vascular capacitance with an effective reduction of the preload.

Amrinone is an inhibitor of phosphodiesterase, which has positive inotropic action and is a powerful vasodilator. It is administered slowly in boluses of 0.75–1 mg/kg, followed by continuous infusion of 5–10 mcg/kg/min.

5.4.2 Heart Rate and Rhythm Normalization

Tachyarrhythmias have recently been reported in childhood but can be related to the increased presence of circulating catecholamines, electrolyte abnormalities, metabolic acidosis, hypoxia, and hypercapnia. Pheochromocytoma and hyperthyroidism are the endocrine disorders that most frequently are associated with tachyarrhythmias. Often beta-blocker drugs, especially propranolol at a dose of 0.01–0.1 mg/kg/day, constitute the drugs mainly used, even only to reduce an excessive increase in heart rate.

Supraventricular tachycardia (SVT) is the most common rhythm disturbance in children. Adenosine is considered the drug of choice to correct the SVT. If administered quickly, at a dose of 0.1 mg/kg through a central venous catheter, it causes an immediate reduction in the frequency of the sinoatrial node and the conduction velocity of the atrioventricular node. The doses may be repeated and the dosage increased up to 0.2–0.3 mg/kg, with a maximum total dose of 12 mg.

Ventricular tachycardia, fortunately infrequent in children, requires immediate treatment. In the acute phase lidocaine (1 mg/kg), amiodarone (5 mg/kg) and procainamide (5–15 mg/kg) intravenous are recommended. Electrical cardioversion is indicated when the patient remains unstable despite drug treatment.

5.5 Fluid Management

Fluid management of the pediatric surgical patient represents an important aspect of clinical care, particularly for the initial treatment of the sick child. An understanding of the physiology of fluid requirements is essential for care of these children. Infants and children are sensitive to small degrees of dehydration, and commonly used protocols for pediatric fluid therapy do not consider the rapidly changing perioperative physiology in this patient population. Standard formulas for fluid therapy can be modified to account for these rapid changes in physiology (Table 5.2).

Control and distribution of body fluids in neonates, infants, and children are carried out in large part through the kidney and vary according to the different age groups: the total water of a premature infant represents approximately 85 % of body

Table 5.2 Postoperative fluid management

Patient weight	Daily fluid intake
<10 kg	85–100 ml/kg
10–20 kg	1000 ml + 50 ml every kg > 10 kg
>20 kg	1500 ml + 20 ml every kg > 20 kg

weight, with a redistribution percentage between the extracellular fluid volume (ECV) and intracellular fluid volume (ICV) of 55 % and 30 %, respectively; in term infant the total water constitutes 78 % with an ECV equals to 45% and an ICV to 33 %. Only at 1-year-old (total H_2O = 65 %) is the reversal of the percentages of the two compartments witnessed (ICV = 40 % and ECV = 25 %), which is the characteristic of adults (total H_2O 60 %, ICV 40 %, and ECV 20 %).

Two aspects are most relevant in designing a fluid therapy in all ages: fluid intake and volume replacement. Intravascular fluid guarantees tissue perfusion; therefore, paying attention to it must have the highest priority. Fluid replacement is necessary to maintain the hydroelectrolytic homeostasis and acid-base balance. Fluid distribution is regulated by osmotic pressure: hypothalamic nucleus is sensitive and responds to very low variations, and this condition causes a hormonal response, involving the secretion of ADH and aldosterone. The dehydrated patient produces more ADH to preserve the H_2O. It should be taken into account that during the intraoperative period, ADH secretions may increase due to factors other than the osmotic ones (pain, stress, drugs). For a correct fluid postoperative planning, consideration must be given to the metabolic requirements, intraoperative administration, "third-space" sequestration, blood loss related to surgery, and particular conditions such as the use of radiant lamps for neonates/preterms [17].

Fluid requirements depend on the metabolic expenditure, which is higher in neonatal age. Under normal conditions, 100 ml is required to metabolize 100 Kcal, according to the calculation of Holliday and Segar.

5.6 Analgosedation Management

Effective and adequate therapy to control pain and stress is essential in the management of children in perioperative digestive surgery treatment.

Analgosedation must meet different requirements: adequacy, appropriateness, effectiveness, and safety.

Much evidence confirms that pain and stress must be treated in order to prevent short- and long-term adverse outcomes [18–20].

Not rarely a correct analgosedation management is hard to achieve and overtreatment and undertreatment are both harmful. The complexity and the clinical difficulties due to the age of the patients sometimes induce therapeutic priorities to preserve cardiocirculatory stability or to ensure neurological evaluation, giving up analgesic and sedative drugs and underestimating the consequences of an inadequate pain control and prolonged stress.

Therapeutic necessities of a patient should be set up in advance on dedicated and shared internal protocols, integrated into local context and appropriate to the needs of specific situations, in order to prepare later and progressively an efficient and personalized analgosedation therapeutic plan, according to real needs of the patient.

5.6.1 Pain and Sedation Measurement

Analgesia must be regularly assessed and documented using validated age-related scales.

Self-report scales are preferred instruments for pain assessment in patients with adequate cognitive development. There are several proposals for different ages: the Faces Pain Scale (>3 years), the visual analog scale (VAS), and the numerical rating scale (NRS) (>7 years).

Observational scales must be applied in patients aged less than 3 years or unable to communicate and therefore are the most used in intensive care; some of them, multidimensional, also include the registration of physiological parameters such as heart rate, blood pressure, and SpO_2.

Observational scales recommended for neonatal age are the Premature Infant Pain Profile (PIPP) and the Crying, Requires increased oxygen administration, Increased vital signs, Expression, and Sleeplessness (CRIES) scale; for children the Face, Legs, Activity, Cry, and Consolability (FLACC) and the Children's

Hospital of Eastern Ontario Pain Scale (CHEOPS) are used.

Pain measurement must be carried out at regular intervals like other vital signs to monitor changes in pain intensity over time and the effectiveness of the treatment. Intervals of 4–6 h may be sufficient if pain control is adequate.

Sedation must be regularly assessed and documented using adequate monitoring scales. The COMFORT scale, validated also for the neonatal age, is the most utilized tool [21].

5.6.2 Drugs for Analgosedation

Measurement of pain and the identification of its underlying causes lead to the choice of analgesic drug, which must be of adequate power and targeted to causal mechanisms.

Acute pain is the form most frequently met in PICU, but complex patients with prolonged stay in intensive care may present with persistent, chronic forms of pain, for which a multimodality approach may be necessary (Table 5.3).

Acetaminophen in neonates and acetaminophen and nonsteroidal anti-inflammatory drugs in children above 3 months of age are recommended for treating mild pain (Table 5.4).

Opioids are the drugs recommended for treating moderate-to-severe pain (Table 5.5).

In some patients, adding nonsteroidal anti-inflammatory drugs or acetaminophen to opioids is useful.

Fentanyl is indicated in the presence of cardiocirculatory instability and in neonates with persistent pulmonary hypertension.

Table 5.3 Postoperative pain management. Multimodality approach

Acetaminophen
Nonsteroidal anti-inflammatory
Opioids
Regional anesthesia
Local infiltration of the trocar insertion in laparo- and thoracoscopy
Local wound infiltration
Nonpharmacological techniques

Regional techniques must always be considered in cases of localized pain such as procedures and surgery. Epidural analgesia is effective for acute pain after surgery or trauma to the chest, abdomen, pelvis, or lower limbs, although its safe management requires expertise and good skill level.

The aims of sedation are reduction of distress, fear, and agitation, improvement of patient-ventilator synchrony, and decrease in self-removing of invasive devices. Sedation cannot be pursued without an adequate analgesic treatment, since persistent not treated pain hampers the sedation strategy.

Midazolam is the most frequent benzodiazepine used for sedation in pediatric intensive care. Its administration by continuous intravenous infusion varies between 0.5 and 4 mcg/kg/min. Midazolam is not recommended in premature infants because of the high incidence of neurological adverse events related to continuous infusions.

Propofol is a sedative/amnestic agent with no analgesic properties. Although initially introduced into anesthesia practice, its rapid onset, rapid recovery time, and lack of active metabolites led to its evaluation as a drug for intensive care sedation. Its use for prolonged periods of time may cause adverse effects such as hyperlipidemia, hypercarbia, and the "propofol infusion syndrome," characterized by metabolic acidosis, rhabdomyolysis, arrhythmias, and cardiac failure [22].

5.6.3 Tolerance and Withdrawal Syndrome

Long-term treatments can be complicated by tolerance. Drugs and patient-related factors take part in developing tolerance, defined as the pharmacodynamic reduction of the secondary effects to long-term therapy.

Symptoms of withdrawal may develop during therapy discontinuation: hypersympathetic activity, neuroexcitability, and gastrointestinal impairment. Symptoms are not specific, and withdrawal syndrome may pass underdiagnosed

Table 5.4 Doses and method of postoperative administration of acetaminophen, main nonsteroidal anti-inflammatory drugs (NSAIDs), and tramadol used in children

Drugs	Administration	Dose (kg/day)	N° times (day)	Continuous
Acetaminophen	Oral, rectal	60–90 mg	4–6	
Acetaminophen	Intravenous	60–90 mg	4–6	
Ibuprofen	Oral, intravenous	20–40 mg	3–4	
Ketoprofen	Oral, intravenous	5–7.5 mg	3	
Ketorolac	Oral, intravenous	1–1.5 mg	3	
Naproxen	Oral, intravenous	10–20 mg	2	
Acetylsalicylic acid	Oral, intravenous	40–80 mg	4	
Tramadol	Oral, intravenous	2–3 mg	2–3	0.1–0.25 mg/kg/h

Table 5.5 Postoperative pain management. Drug doses, onset, duration, and potency of opioid narcotics

Drug	Potency	Doses (mcg/kg/h)	Onset (min)	Duration (h)	Respiratory depression
Morphine	1	10–50	20–30	3–4	+++
Fentanyl	100	0.5–4	3–5	0.5–1	+++
Alfentanil	20	3–15	1.5–3	0.2–0.3	+
Remifentanil	250	0.05–1 (mg/kg/min)	1–2	0.1–0.2	+

or not recognized, since such symptoms may be frequently ascribed to other pathologic conditions seen in PICU.

Risk factors have long been identified and must always be evaluated: length of the therapy (>5 days) and cumulative dose (fentanyl in neonates > 1.6 mg/kg, in infants > 2.5 mg/kg, midazolam > 60 mg/kg). Even if the incidence of the withdrawal syndrome is variable in different epidemiological studies, it seems clear that the syndrome develops mainly when analgosedation drugs are too rapidly reduced or abruptly withheld [23–25].

5.7 Nutritional Support

Clinical nutrition is a therapeutic act that helps meet the nutritional needs of patients unable to feed adequately in a natural way. Objectives of clinical nutrition are reduction of the damage produced by pain and surgical stress, preventing the onset of a condition of malnutrition, and/or the reduction of its implications if they were already present.

The quantitative and qualitative composition of the nutrition begins with the identification of needs in normal terms and assesses the changes related to the clinical status. Almost always it is good to take as a reference point the actual weight, considering the ideal weight only in cases that deviate significantly from normality.

Enteral and/or parenteral nutrition should aim at covering the nutritional needs of the patient in terms of basal metabolic rate and physical activity and correction of preexisting malnutrition, growth, and disease states.

Excessive nutritional intake can cause hyperglycemia, increased fat, fatty liver disease, disorders of the lipid, and protein metabolism. By contrast, a reduced intake can cause weight loss, malnutrition, impaired immune response, delayed tissue repair, and growth retardation.

The World Health Organization (WHO) indicates the adequate daily intake in pediatric age.

Tolerance of caloric intake is limited by the capacity to metabolize substrate calories, depending on the route of administration, the activity, the age, and the pathology of the patient.

A newborn subjected to parenteral nutrition (PN) requires a lower caloric intake compared to a similar neonate subjected to enteral nutrition (EN), since the consumption determined by the dynamic-specific action, related to intestinal absorption, is absent.

Early nutritional support is always necessary in newborns, especially in premature with reduced gestational age, such as very-low-birth-weight (VLBW) infants, whose birth weight is below 1500 g and that, because of their limited nutritional reserves, need a higher protein and calorie intake than a normal-weight newborn.

An important aspect of postoperative stress in pediatric surgery is that, after surgery, energy expenditure reaches a maximum value of 2–4 h after operation, returning to baseline within 24 h. The amount of energy expenditure is related to the severity of the surgery and remains higher in premature infants and in the first 48 h of life.

Pain, stress, and trauma surgery greatly influence a correct nutrition through hormonal imbalance initially characterized by reduced insulin secretion and increased release of the hormones with opposite action, such as catecholamines and glucagon. This early phase is characterized by a reduced utilization of metabolic nutrients. Subsequently, it develops into a tendency toward a hypermetabolic state, with an increased demand for protein and calories, which are drawn from the energy reserves of the organism, with a redistribution among deposit tissues, such as fat, toward organs with high metabolic needs such as the nervous tissue and viscera, including the liver and kidney. This altered nutritional, metabolic, and hormonal condition, if not supported by a gradual and controlled administration of nutrient intake, can lead to a state of catabolism and protein/caloric malnutrition, which in turn is responsible for:

- Increased susceptibility to infection
- Hypoprotidemia
- Slowing the healing of surgical wounds (gastrointestinal anastomosis)
- Increase of decubitus ulcers
- Increased presence of altered gastrointestinal bacteria
- Reduced intestinal absorption and nutrient loss with feces

After a major surgery, necessitating a state of starvation, it is mandatory to intervene through artificial feeding, of which there are two modes of administration: enteral and parenteral nutrition. On the basis of the age and the presence of endogenous reserves of nutrients, which are scarcer the lower the age of patients, it is necessary to program an artificial nutrition plan, which should not be delayed beyond 24 h in neonates and infants and beyond 48–72 h in later age bands. In the postoperative period following digestive surgery, parenteral nutrition is most frequently adopted.

The start and progressive increase of nutrients up to the desired values is called the induction phase of the parenteral nutrition (PN). Nutrients must be administered with well-calibrated increments, respecting a constant relationship between protein intake and energy intake (provided by nonprotein calories which are the sum between calories of carbohydrates and lipids). This ratio has to be carefully balanced (nitrogen grams/nonprotein calories = 1/150–250). In this phase the metabolic indexes should be checked frequently to test the tolerance of the patient to PN. In the following days, with the PN at a stability condition, if well tolerated by the patient, the biochemical controls may be weekly. With the achievement of the phase of stabilization, monitoring of the auxological parameters, such as nitrogen balance, visceral protein (retinol, prealbumin, transferrin), weight, height, and head circumference, is particularly useful [26].

As soon as bowel function is recovered, the PN can be suspended with a gradual reduction of the volume and amount of nutrients (weaning phase).

Table 5.6 shows the nutritional needs during total parenteral nutrition.

5.8 Abdominal Compartment Syndrome

5.8.1 Introduction

Abdominal compartment syndrome (ACS) is defined as the adverse physiologic consequences resulting from an increased intra-abdominal pressure (IAP). The organ systems most affected include the cardiovascular, renal, and pulmonary

Table 5.6 Nutritional needs during total parenteral nutrition

Age and weight	Protein (g/kg/day)	Carbohydrates (g/kg/day)	Lipids (g/kg/day)*
Premature	3–4	12–14–16	2–3
Neonate	3	18	2–3
3–10 kg	2.5–3	16–18	2
10–15 kg	2.5	12–14	2
15–20 kg	2	10–12	1.5
20–30 kg	1.5–2	<12	1.5
>30 kg	1.5	<10	1
Critically ill children	1.5–3	7.5	1–2

*Lipids in TPN
Lipid intake 25–35 % of nonprotein calories
Minimum 0.25 g/kg/day to prevent EFA deficiency
Maximum 2–3 g/kg/day in neonates and infants
Administration continuously over about 24 h

systems. If untreated, ACS can cause clinical deterioration and rapidly lead to crucial organ failure and death. On the other hand, abdominal decompression usually leads to a prompt reversal of the adverse pathophysiologic modifications.

5.8.2 Etiology and Pathophysiology

In pediatric age, ACS has been associated with several etiologies including abdominal injury with postoperative bleeding, abdominal hemangioma, trauma, bowel necrosis, mesenteric vein thrombosis, omphalocele, gastroschisis, intestinal graft-versus-host disease, intestinal perforation, peritonitis, necrotizing enterocolitis, hepatic veno-occlusive disease, shock, and burns requiring massive fluid resuscitation.

Intra-abdominal pressure under normal condition is usually 0 mmHg and is slightly positive in patients submitted to mechanical ventilation, because of transmission of intrathoracic pressure in the abdomen. Initially, IAP rises slowly as abdominal contents and girth increase. However, at a certain critical level, compliance of the abdominal wall reaches its limits, and any further distension results in a rapid rise in abdominal pressure, decreased organ perfusion, and development of clinical ACS.

As intestinal ischemia leads to bowel distension, bowel wall edema, and capillary leak, it can set up a vicious cycle by further increasing IAP and may eventually lead to both bowel necrosis and ACS [27].

5.8.3 Clinical Presentation

5.8.3.1 Cardiovascular

With advancing ACS, the patient presents a profound shock often unresponsive to fluid resuscitation and vasoactive drugs. Reduced cardiac output results primarily from decreased venous return because of compression of the inferior vena cava and the portal vein as well as from increased intrathoracic pressure, which markedly reduces cardiac preload.

Increased thoracic pressure, related to diaphragmatic elevation, was shown to decrease left ventricular compliance and a very high IAP to decrease myocardial contractility. Hemodynamic function is further impaired by increased systemic vascular resistances induced by increased IAP.

5.8.3.2 Respiratory

Respiratory failure is a major component of the ACS and is characterized by elevated peak ventilatory pressure, hypoxemia, and hypercarbia. The elevated IAP causes upward displacement of the diaphragm and compresses the lungs, resulting in progressively stiffer chest with extremely low compliance.

5.8.3.3 Renal

Oliguria progressing to anuria, both of which can be unresponsive to fluid therapy and diuretics, is the hallmark of the ACS. Elevated IAP results in markedly increased renal venous pressure and impaired renal venous drainage: this is thought to be the most important mechanism of renal dysfunction.

5.8.3.4 Gastrointestinal

Increased IAP was shown to significantly reduce splanchnic perfusion. At an IAP of 20 mmHg, significant decreases in blood flow to all segments of the bowel, the liver, the kidneys, and the spleen were demonstrated. Impaired intestinal perfusion results in anaerobic metabolism, lactic acidosis, and free radical production.

5.8.3.5 Cerebral

Increased intracranial pressure (ICP) is a recognized component of ACS. In recent years several case reports described prompt reductions in elevated ICP following abdominal decompression.

5.8.4 Intra-abdominal Pressure Determination

Intra-abdominal pressure can be determined by measuring intragastric pressure, inferior vena cava pressure through a long femoral venous catheter, or urinary bladder pressure. This last procedure is simple and practical in which an age-adjusted amount of saline is injected through a urinary catheter connected to a pressure transducer (Table 5.7).

5.8.5 Management

5.8.5.1 Medical Care

Critical care management of the patient with ACS consists of supporting the failing organ system until definitive therapy is instituted and the basic problem can be brought under control.

Volume resuscitation with repeated fluid challenges is the mainstay of cardiovascular support, aiming and improving the decreased preload that causes the reduced cardiac output. This should be increased by inotropic support (dopamine, dobutamine, epinephrine) if response is inadequate.

Most patients will require mechanical ventilation, and, as abdominal pressure rises, higher airway pressures and FiO_2 will be required to maintain gas exchange.

These measures, however, will at best result in temporary improvement, because they do not alleviate the underlying problem and may actually result in further deterioration as more fluids leak into the abdominal third space.

5.8.5.2 Surgical Care

The key to successful management of ACS is an early diagnosis and prompt surgical decompression of the abdomen.

In patients whose ACS is caused by intra-abdominal accumulation of fluid, such as ascites, peritoneal tap and continuous drainage may resolve the problem.

Following decompression, primary abdominal closure without excessive pressure is usually impossible, and the abdominal cavity is left open with the use of various temporary abdominal wall closure techniques.

Several techniques are described depending on the underlying disease, age, and severity of the clinical condition: the use of "only-skin" closure, the Dacron mesh, and the external sterile plastic pack (vacuum pack) or of sterile 2-L intravenous fluid bag ("Bogota" bag).

Table 5.7 Grading of abdominal compartment syndrome by intra-abdominal pressure and percentage of organ failures, with recommendation for treatment

Grade	Bladder pressure (mmHg)	Urine output <0.5 ml/kg/h	PIP >45 mmHg	SVR >1000 dyn/s/cm^{-5}	DO_2I >600 O_2/min/m^2	Recommendations
I	10–15	0 %	0 %	0 %	0 %	Maintain normovolemia
II	16–25	0 %	40 %	20 %	20 %	Hypervolemic resuscitation
III	26–35	65 %	78 %	65 %	57 %	Decompression
IV	>35	100 %	100 %	100 %	100 %	Decompression and re-exploration

PIP peak inspiratory pressure, *SVR* systemic vascular resistances, *DO_2I* oxygen delivery index

5.9 Necrotizing Enterocolitis

Necrotizing enterocolitis (NEC), which typically occurs in the second to third week of life in preterms, is characterized by variable damage to the intestinal tract, ranging from mucosal injury to full-thickness necrosis and perforation. NEC affects close to 10% of infants who weigh less than 1500 g, with mortality rates of 50%.

In surgical NEC, the anesthesia is carried out in a clinical condition characterized by a drastic and rapid deterioration, frequently involving complications such as acidosis, electrolyte imbalances, lethargy, abdominal compartment syndrome, acute renal failure, coagulopathy, RDS, and cardiocirculatory failure. Often the clinical picture is further complicated by the occurrence of toxic-septic shock with multiple organ dysfunction syndrome (MODS) which is triggered in an infant weighing <1000 g.

Often, especially in extremely low-birth-weight (ELBW) infants, the anesthesiological and intensive approach may become difficult [28–30].

Some points, almost always interdependent, need to be raised [31]:

- The choice of surgical option. This is between peritoneal drainage and laparotomy, depending on the clinical condition of the infant and the extent of the disease. However, the optimum choice remains controversial. Peritoneal drainage is a short procedure, requires a less risky anesthesia, but only offers a temporary decompression for the purposes of stabilizing the patient in expectancy of a more invasive surgical intervention. Laparotomy foresees an anesthesia with very high risk, its principal objective being the removal of gangrenous bowel in order to check sepsis while preserving as much bowel length as possible. The surgical options of laparotomy include enterostomy alone or intestinal resection with enterostomy.
- The decision about where to operate. This question is still open to debate, also considering that every hospital has its own logistic and organizational characteristics. The NICU may not be the optimal setting for a surgical procedure, but moving an infant weighing <1000 g in a serious and unstable condition to the operating theater entails very high risks. In a short space of time, various events may occur that could irreversibly precipitate their condition: the loss of body temperature, the discontinuation of the mechanical ventilation instituted, the modifications in posture during transfer, which could lead to serious cardiocirculatory complications such as bradycardia and hypotension.
- The decision as to whether, and for how long, it is possible to wait before undertaking the urgent intervention. The goal should be to obtain, in a brief space of time, the best possible clinical stabilization before undertaking surgery (optimization of the fluid resuscitation and inotropic and vasopressor drugs, correction of possible acidosis, anemia, or coagulopathy) without further compromising the general condition of the patient.
- The choice of which anesthetic drugs to use. Even though the pharmacokinetics is not fully understood, smaller doses of anesthetic are usually required, and their effects last longer due to low clearance and prolonged elimination half-lives. The literature is currently still discussing the neurotoxic effect of anesthetic drugs on the developing brain. It therefore remains unclear what role anesthesia exposure during infancy actually plays in determining neurobehavioral outcome. This could have very worrying implications in ELBW. Moreover, no important differences in neurodevelopmental outcomes were observed between the surgical and medical NEC.
- The choice of which intraoperative monitoring might constitute an additional aid in such small preterms in whom the scarce feasibility of monitoring is well known during high-risk interventions. Capillary blood-gas analysis could be useful. Other possibilities to be investigated in ELBW could be the reliability of central venous pressure in a peripherally inserted central catheter of extremely small caliber and the role of abdominal as well as cerebral near-infrared spectrometry (NIRS).

References

1. da Silva PS, de Aguiar VE, Fonseca MC (2013) Risk factors and outcomes of unplanned PICU postoperative admissions: a nested case-control study. Pediatr Crit Care Med 14(44):4420–4428
2. Gaspar HA, Morhy SS (2015) The role of focused echocardiography in pediatric intensive care: a critical appraisal. Biomed Res Int 2015:596451
3. Tan RN, Mulder E, Lopriore E, de Pas AB (2015) Monitoring oxygenation and gas exchange in neonatal intensive care units: current practice in the Netherlands. Front Pediatr 3:94
4. Milési C, Baleine J, le Bouhellec J, Pons-Odena M, Cambonie G (2015) High flow on the rise-pediatric perspectives on the FLORALI. J Thorac Dis 7(8):E230–E233
5. Nichols D, Haranath S (2007) Pressure control ventilation. Crit Care Clin 23:183–199
6. Nicolai T (2006) The physiological basis of respiratory support. Pediatric Resp Rev 7:97–102
7. Bengtsson JA, Edberg KE (2010) Neurally adjusted ventilatory assist in children: an observational study. Pediatr Crit Care Med 11(2):253–257
8. Biban P, Serra A, Polese G, Soffiati M, Santuz P (2010) Neurally adjusted ventilatory assist: a new approach to mechanically ventilated infants. J Matern Fetal Neonatal Med 23(3):38–40
9. Gentili A, Masciopinto F, Mondardini MC et al (2013) Neurally adjusted ventilatory assist in weaning of neonates affected by congenital diaphragmatic hernia. J Matern Fetal Neonatal Med 26(66):5598–5602
10. Verbrugghe W, Jorens PG (2011) Neurally adjusted ventilatory assist: a ventilation tool or a ventilation toy? Respir Care 56(3):327–335
11. Carcillo JA, Wheeler DS, Kooy NW et al. (2009) Shock: an overview. In: Wheeler DS et al (eds) Resuscitation and stabilization of the critically Ill child. Springer, London
12. Sinha R, Nadel S (2012) Understanding shock. Pediatr Child Health 23(5):187–193
13. Bouchard J, Soroko SB, Chertow GM et al (2009) Fluid accumulation, survival and recovery of kidney function in critically ill patients with acute kidney injury. Kidney Int 76:422–427
14. Payen D, de Pont AC, Sakr Y, Spies C, Reinhart K, Vincent JL (2008) A positive fluid balance is associated with a worse outcome in patients with acute renal failure. Crit Care 12:R74
15. Oishi PE, Teitel DF, Hoffman DF et al (2008) Cardiovascular physiology. In: Nichols DG (ed) Rogers' textbook of pediatric intensive care, 4th edn. Lippincott Williams & Wilkins, Philadelphia
16. Moffett BS, Price JF (2008) Evaluation of sodium nitroprusside toxicity in pediatric cardiac surgical patients. Ann Pharmacother 42:1600–1604
17. Murat I, Dubois MC (2008) Perioperative fluid therapy in pediatrics. Paediatr Anaesth 18(5):363–370
18. Anand KJ, Hickey PR (1987) Pain and its effects in the human neonate and fetus. N Engl J Med 317:1321–1329
19. Taddio A, Katz J, Ilersich AL et al (1997) Effect of neonatal circumcision on pain response during subsequent routine vaccination. Lancet 349:599–603
20. Anand KJ (2000) Pain, plasticity and premature birth: a prescription for permanent suffering? Nat Med 6:971–973
21. Playfor S, Jenkins I, Boyles C et al (2006) Consensus guidelines on sedation and analgesia in critically ill children. Intensive Care Med 32:1125–1136
22. van Dijk M, Tibboel D (2012) Update on pain assessment in sick neonates and infants. Pediatr Clin North Am 59(5):1167–1181
23. Cunliffe M, McArthur L, Dooley F, Hons BA (2004) Managing sedation withdrawal in children who undergo prolonged PICU admission after discharge to the ward. Pediatr Anesth 14(4):293–298
24. Ista E, van Dijk M, Gamel C, Tibboel D, de Hoog M (2007) Withdrawal symptoms in children after long-term administration of sedatives and/or analgesics: a literature review. "Assessment remains troublesome". Intensive Care Med 33(8):1396–1406
25. Birchley G (2009) Opioid and benzodiazepine withdrawal syndromes in the paediatric intensive care unit: a review of recent literature. Nurs Crit Care 14(1):26–37
26. Koletzko B, Goulet O, Hunt J, Krohn K, Shamir R, Parenteral Nutrition Guidelines Working Group (2005) Guidelines on Paediatric Parenteral Nutrition of the European Society of Paediatric Gastroenterology, Hepatology and Nutrition (ESPGHAN) and the European Society for Clinical Nutrition and Metabolism (ESPEN), Supported by the European Society of Paediatric Research (ESPR). J Pediatr Gastroenterol Nutr 41:S1–S4
27. Beck R, Halberthal M, Zonis Z et al (2001) Abdominal compartment syndrome in children. Pediatr Crit Care Med 2:51–56
28. Blakely ML, Tyson JE, Lally KP et al (2006) Laparotomy versus peritoneal drainage for necrotizing enterocolitis or isolated intestinal perforation in extremely low birth weight infants: outcomes through 18 months adjusted age. Pediatrics 117(4):680–687
29. Kinouchi K (2004) Anaesthetic considerations for the management of very low and extremely low birth weight infants. Best Pract Res Clin Anaesthesiol 18(2):273–290
30. Shah TA, Meinzen-Derr J, Gratton T et al (2012) Hospital and neurodevelopmental outcomes of extremely low-birth-weight infants with necrotizing enterocolitis and spontaneous intestinal perforation. J Perinatol 32(7):552–558
31. Gentili A, Landuzzi V, Lima M, Baroncini S (2013) Anesthesiological management in ELBW infants: like ductal ligation, does necrotizing enterocolitis similarly lie between 'simple anesthesia' and 'extreme art'? Paediatr Anaesth 23(2):200–201

Clinical Nutrition

6

Antonella Diamanti, Teresa Capriati, and Daniela Giorgio

6.1 Introduction

Pediatric patients are particularly vulnerable to the disease-related consequences of malnutrition that may be prevented by clinical nutrition [1]. The clinical nutrition applies in clinical practice the techniques of artificial nutrition (AN) that include enteral nutrition (EN) and parenteral nutrition (PN) [2]. EN consists in administration of complex nutrients into the gastrointestinal tract; PN delivers simple nutrients directly into the blood generally by central venous catheters or in some cases by peripheral veins [3, 4]. The most appropriate nutritional intervention will be determined by assessing patient's age, clinical condition, gastrointestinal function, attitude for oral intake, dietary habits, and costs [2]; however, decisional algorithm starts from the gut function. Following this assessment the patient may receive dietary advice, oral nutritional supplements, enteral nutrition (EN) regimens, or parenteral nutrition (PN) [2].

A. Diamanti, MD (✉)
Hepatology, Gastroenterology and Nutrition Unit, Bambino Gesù "Children Hospital", Piazza S. Onofrio 4, 00165 Rome, Italy
e-mail: antonella.diamanti@opbg.net

T. Capriati • D. Giorgio
Artificial Nutrition Unit, Bambino Gesù Children's Hospital, Piazza S. Onofrio 4, 00165 Rome, Italy

According to the ESPGHAN indications, EN support includes both delivery of liquid formulations via tube and provision of specialized oral nutritional supplements (ONSs) [2]. ONSs are suitable to completely replace intake by normal foods and they allow to avoid more invasive AN techniques. They have good taste and are available as liquids or creams. When oral intake is inadequate or intake of normal food is inappropriate to meet the patients' needs, EN by tubes should be approached. It is realized by the use of enteral formulations for the long-term use and subdivided as polymeric, based on cow's milk proteins (PFs); low molecular formulas, containing oligopeptides derived from protein hydrolysates and high amount of medium-chain triglycerides (MCTs) (HFs); and elemental feeds, based on free amino acids (AAs). EN support is the first choice in patients with maintained gut function. PFs are employed in about 50 % of the overall EN candidates; they are inadequate in some digestive diseases, in post-pyloric enteral feeding, and in cow's milk allergy [2, 5, 6].

When gut function is impaired, as in all forms of intestinal failure (IF), PN should be approached [2]. IF refers indeed to all states where the intestine has inadequate absorptive capacity to meet nutritional, fluid, and electrolyte needs to sustain life and growth requirements of a child [7].

The etiology of IF recognizes the short bowel syndrome (SBS) where congenital or acquired lesions have determined extensive loss of intestinal mass, as the most frequent underlying disease

M. Lima (ed.), *Pediatric Digestive Surgery*, DOI 10.1007/978-3-319-40525-4_6

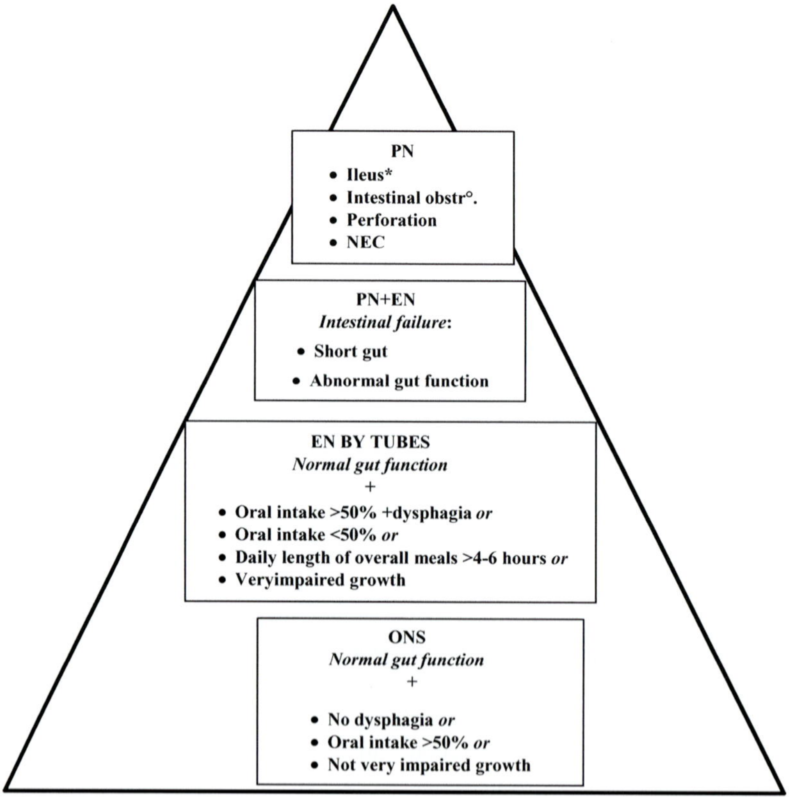

Fig. 6.1 Summary of clinical nutrition management in pediatric digestive diseases. *PN* parenteral nutrition, * paralytic or mechanical ileus, ° obstruction, *NEC* necrotizing enterocolitis, *EN* enteral nutrition, *ONS* oral nutritional supplements

[8]. Malabsorption due to ineffective mucosal surface (congenital enterocyte disorders, phenotypic diarrhea, and autoimmune enteropathy) and motility disorders with undamaged mucosal surface but wide motility dysfunctions (chronic intestinal pseudo-obstructions, gastroschisis not associated with small bowel resection, and Hirschsprung's diseases) are further categories of IF [7–10].

However, complete enteral starvation should be avoided whenever possible [2]. Therefore, although PN should be firstly considered in IF, EN should be also employed integrating the maximum tolerated amount of enteral intake with the ongoing support of PN. Even minimal quantities of nutrients in the gastrointestinal tract (so-called trophic feeding) may promote intestinal perfusion, initiate release of enteral hormones, and improve gut barrier function [11, 12]. Thus, few clinical conditions are now considered absolute contraindications to EN (see Fig. 6.1). We can ideally represent the nutritional approach to pediatric digestive surgery as a pyramid, in which, proceeding from the base to the tip, increasingly invasive techniques are encountered (see Fig. 6.1).

6.2 Clinical Nutrition and SBS

Nutritional management of SBS is of particular interest because it provides a model of combined PN/EN management. This model may be applied to several digestive diseases at neonatal onset. Following neonatal small bowel resection, IF occurs due to the residual reduced length of the

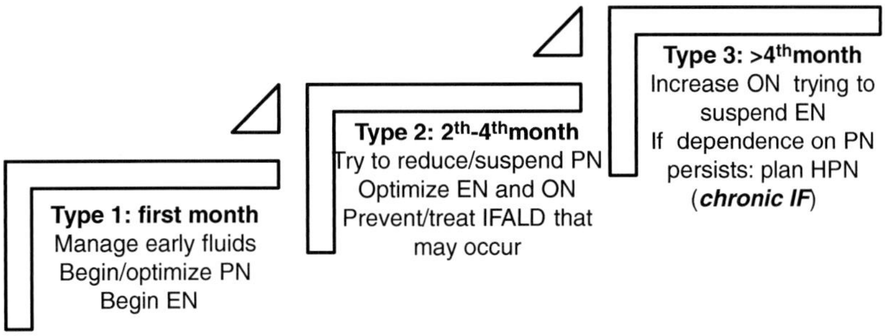

Fig. 6.2 Course of IF after neonatal small bowel resection. *IF* intestinal failure, *PN* parenteral nutrition, *EN* enteral nutrition, *ON* oral nutrition, *IFALD* intestinal failure-associated liver disease, *HPN* home parenteral nutrition

gut, responsible for SBS. The course of IF SBS related can be ideally subdivided into three phases, with distinct clinical characteristics and requiring different nutritional approaches. If long-term dependence on PN is expected (generally more than 3 months), IF can be defined as chronic, and it requires to plan home parenteral nutrition (HPN) programs (see Figs. 6.2 and 6.3) [13, 14].

Overall the nutritional care of neonatal SBS onset includes (1) early managing of fluid and electrolyte losses before starting PN and EN; (2) providing adequate PN, for growth and normal development; (3) promoting intestinal rehabilitation by optimizing EN; (4) discharging on home parenteral nutrition (HPN) the patients with protracted dependence on PN; and (5) preventing/treating complications related to the patients' underlying disease and their PN.

6.2.1 Early Managing of Fluid and Electrolyte Losses

SBS patients, at the early stages after bowel resection, have increased losses of fluids and electrolytes which can lead to significant electrolyte imbalance and dehydration. Early restoration of fluid and electrolyte homeostasis is therefore required, and it needs aggressive recovery with fluids [15]. Early fluid replacement is usually 1 mL for every mL of fluid loss. This phase is followed by PN beginning.

6.2.2 Providing Adequate PN

Before approaching each PN program, a reliable vascular access should be warranted. The choice of the access is dependent on the predicted length of the PN support. Peripherally inserted central lines are very effective means of providing PN over a short to medium term, while more definitive central venous access is required for prolonged PN. The expertise of a dedicated hospital-based nutritional team is required to tailor PN to the single patient and to manage central catheters; it is supported by official guidelines published by the pertinent societies [15–17].

SBS is at risk for developing intestinal failure-associated liver disease (IFALD) [18] due to IF-related factors, such as lack of enteral feeding, disturbed enterohepatic bile flow, presence of inflammation, oxidative stress, immaturity of the liver, and infections, but also PN-related factors [18]. Therefore, in patients who are predicted to require long-term treatments, PN should be tailored to reduce the risk of liver injury [9, 19]. To prevent/treat IFALD, some aspects of PN management can be modulated and in particular are the following:

A. Choosing lipid emulsions (LEs)
B. Optimizing non-lipid intake

6.2.2.1 Choosing LEs

Historically, a French study delineated IFALD in adult HPN patients as a value of at least 1.5-fold the upper limit of normal on two of three liver

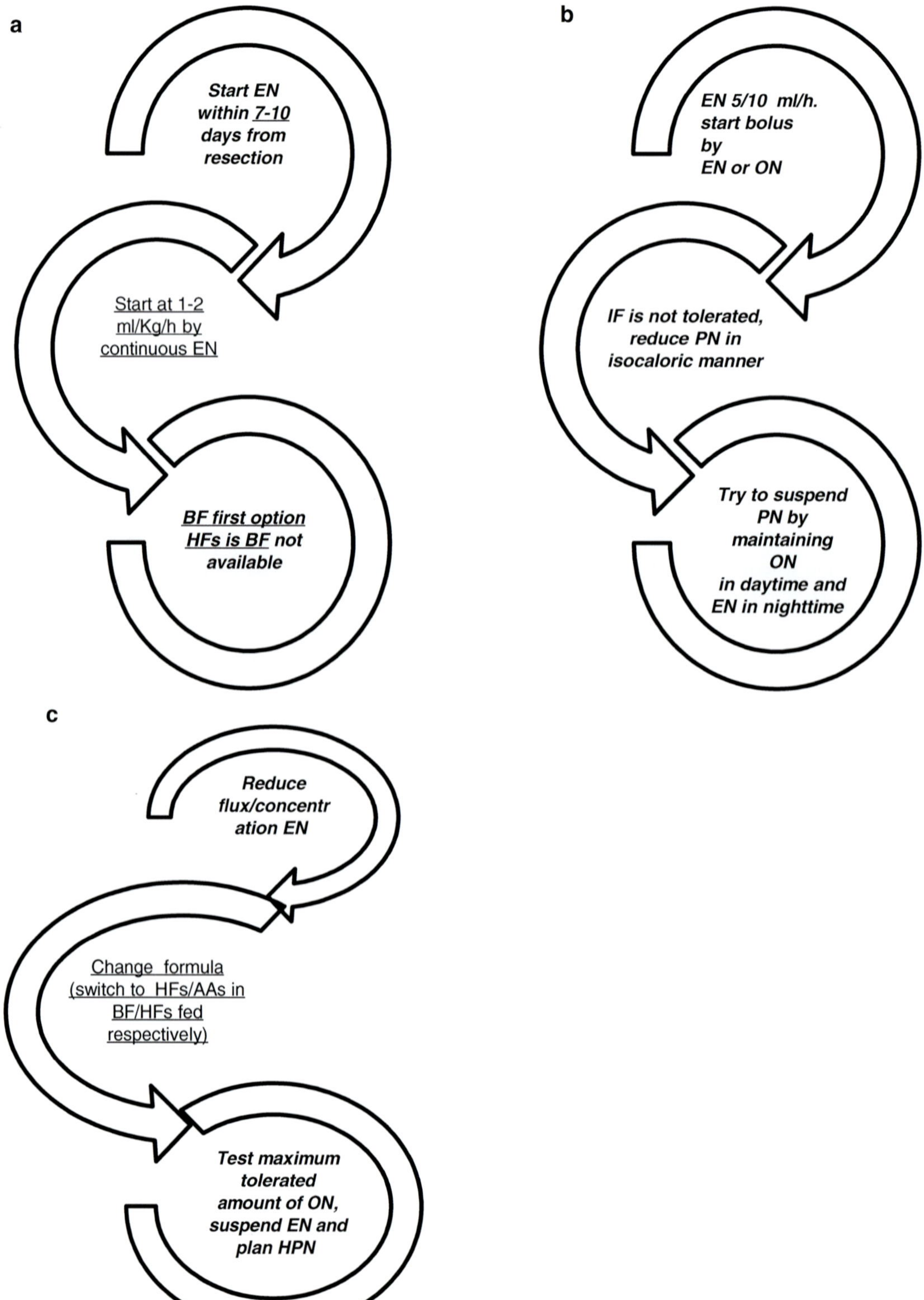

Fig. 6.3 Patterns of combined management of PN and EN after small bowel resection. *PN* parenteral nutrition, *EN* enteral nutrition. (**a**) Pattern of EN beginning. (**b**) Pattern of tolerance to advancing EN. (**c**) Pattern of intolerance to advancing EN. *BF* breastfeeding, *HFs* hydrolyzed formulas, *ON* oral nutrition, *AAs* amino acid-based formulas, *HPN* home parenteral nutrition

function measures for cholestasis that persists for more than 6 months [20]. This study also showed that chronic cholestasis predicts serious liver problems and is associated with the use of soybean oil-based lipids (SO) at doses >1 g/kg/day [20]. Several factors may explicate how LEs can impact on the development of IFALD:

(a) Activation of hepatic macrophages (Kupffer cells) by excess of ω–6 polyunsaturated fatty acids (PUFAs) in SO that leads to the production of proinflammatory cytokines derived from linoleic and arachidonic acids [21].
(b) High intake of phytosterols (e.g., stigmasterol and campesterol, equivalents of cholesterol in vegetable oils) derived from SO; they have structural similarity to bile acids and may act as antagonists to nuclear bile receptors that are protective against cholestasis [21].
(c) Overall content of vitamin E, especially of its most bioactive isoform α-tocopherol, which protects PUFAs from oxidative damage due to lipid peroxidation. The addition of this component to SO has been shown to reduce liver damage in a piglet model of IFALD [21].

Published surveys report that the use of a fish oil-based LEs (FO) is able to reverse IFALD [22, 23]. These surveys, nevertheless, are used at a markedly decreased dosage of FO (1 g/kg/d) if compared to that of SO in the control historic group (3 g/kg/day) [22]. That supports the hypothesis that the overall decreased fat intake rather than FO supplementation is important in reversing IFALD [21]. Interestingly a recently published paper reports two cases of reverted cholestasis by switching from SMOF lipid (Fresenius Kabi, Bad Homburg, Germany), an emulsion containing a mixture of 30 % of SO, 30 % of coconut oil, 25 % of olive oil, and 15 % of FO at 2.0–3.0 g/kg/day, to FO at 1 g/kg/day [24]. That supports the hypothesis that the reduced amount rather than the type of LEs may be hepatotoxic.

Anyway FO monotherapy has now been widely employed in clinical practice. FO alone may not be able to provide enough energy to sustain growth. A mixed LE containing soybean oil (SMOFlipid) compared with SO in a blinded randomized controlled trial in pediatric HPN patients resulted in mild changes in total bilirubin when administered four to five times per week at 2 g/kg/day and in normal growth pattern [25].

In North America, FO alone (Omegaven, Fresenius Kabi, Bad Homburg, Germany) is available on the market, whereas in Europe, it is possible to use LEs containing the mixture (SMOFlipid, Fresenius Kabi, Bad Homburg, Germany). That led to develop two different approaches to optimize LE use in the United States and Canada as compared with Europe.

Many institutions generally combine the use of novel lipid preparations and reduced rates of administration of SO to prevent the development of liver disease [21]; e.g., if bilirubin exceeds 34 μg/L, lipid intake is reduced at 1 g/k/day, while if it goes over 50 μg/L, the lipid source is changed to FO alone at 1 g/kg/day.

Table 6.1 summarizes the composition of available LEs employed in PN.

6.2.2.2 Optimizing Non-lipid Intake

Excessive glucose intake causes increased lipogenesis and fat tissue deposition together with subsequent liver steatosis and enhanced production of triglycerides by the liver [3]. The American Society for Parenteral and Enteral Nutrition (ASPEN) [26], the European Society for Pediatric Gastroenterology, Hepatology, and Nutrition [18], and the American Academy of Pediatrics guidelines (ESPGHAN) [27] recommend limiting the glucose infusion rate (GIR) at 12–14 mg/kg/min (18 g/kg per day) in infants and young children up to 2 years. Glucose intake should usually cover 60–75 % of nonprotein calories [3]. As reported above reduced LEs intake as strategy to prevent/treat IFALD may be required; in such cases increased glucose intake, to better satisfy the nutritional needs, resulted as well tolerated [28].

Furthermore, prophylactic cycling of PN may reduce the incidence of IFALD [21]. Cyclical PN is well tolerated and may be 3–6 months of age. In cyclical PN the maximal rate of glucose infu-

Table 6.1 Composition of lipid emulsions available for parenteral nutrition

Emulsion (% fat) (manufacturer)	Lipid source (%)	ω6:ω3 ratio	Phytosterols (mg/L)	α-Tocopherol (μmol/L)
Intralipid 20 % (Fresenius Kabi)	SO 100 %	7:1	348 ± 33	87
Lipofundin 20 % (B. Braun)	SO 50 % MCT 50 %	7:1	No data	502
ClinOleic-Clinolipid 20 % (Baxter)	SO 20 % OO 100 %	9:1	327 ± 8	75
Lipoplus 20 % (B. Braun)	SO 40 % MCT 50 % FO 10 %	2.7:1	No data	562
SMOF lipid 20 % (Fresenius Kabi)	SO 30 % MCT 30 % OO 25 % FO 15 %	2.5:1	47.6	500
Omegaven 10 % (Fresenius Kabi)	FO 100 %	1:8	0	505

SO soybean oil, *MCT* medium-chain triglycerides, *OO* olive oil, *FO* fish oil

sion may exceed the advised GIR. The maximal infusion rate should not exceed 1.2 g/kg per hour (20 mg/kg per min). A stepwise increase and decrease of glucose infusion rate at onset and at discontinuation of the infusion should be considered to avoid hyper- and hypoglycemia, respectively. A reliable method for tapering is to halve the rate for 30 minutes and then to halve this again for an additional 30 minutes. Glucose tolerance should be monitored during the first phases of the cycling PN [3].

With regard to the choice of amino acid solution, there is evidence that supplementation of TrophAmine may reduce the incidence of IFALD in certain high-risk populations such as those with NEC [19].

Furthermore, copper and manganese serum levels from PN solutions should be monitored closely in patients who have developed IFALD because they may exacerbate it [19].

6.2.3 Promoting EN

The provision of enteral nutrients is a critical component of the therapy of IF; in SBS patients it represents the fundamental driver of adaptation [15]. Early attempts of oral nutrition confer the critical window of opportunity for establishing normal suck and swallow patterns; if this is not attended, the child is at risk for oral aversion, which has many long-term negative consequences [29]. The most pragmatic way to address EN handling in IF should be to account that all patients regardless of the etiology of their IF may recover to a variable degree and that the strategies to promote EN should be reconsidered on a day-to-day basis. The overall care of IF is based on the judicious integration of two overlapped goals: progressive advancement of enteral calories and gradual weaning from the ongoing support of PN, maintaining a weight gain [15]. If tube feeding is used, the practice of inserting a gastrostomy early allows a more controlled method of delivering feed with an opportunity to preserve and promote voluntary feeding without the negative effects of the long-term presence of a nasal tube [29]. If patients with motility disorders but also with SBS show poor tolerance to gastric feeding, the post-pyloric EN approach should be tried [6]. Main aspects concerning EN management in SBS are:

A. Choosing the formula
B. Assessing methods of feeding
C. Assessing tolerance to EN
D. Using enteral supplements
E. Starting and handling complementary foods

6.2.3.1 Choosing the Formula

There is a paucity of evidence in favoring one type of feed over the other in this setting; however, breastfeeding (BF) should be used when tolerated as it helps and promotes adaptation [30]. The full advantages of BF include the optimal macronutrient composition for human infant growth, with a full complement of macro- and micronutrients [31, 32]. In addition, it contains trophic factors such as epidermal growth factor, which likely augment the adaptive process [7]. Furthermore, BF contains immunoglobulins and natural antimicrobial properties which both enhance mucosal barrier function and prevent dangerous overgrowth of bacteria within the intestinal lumen. Finally it promotes intestinal colonization by appropriate lactobacilli and related bacteria which are important elements of healthy microbiome [33, 34]. Bovine colostrum also seems to confer beneficial effects on IF [35].

Finally BF supports physiological and psychological relationship between infant and mother. If the mother's own milk is not available, banked breast milk, even with pasteurization, has nearly identical physiologic benefits [31]. Overall BF should be the first choice in SBS patients.

If BF is not available, formula selection should be based on:

(a) Low allergenicity, because SBS infants are at high risk for allergy [36]
(b) Fat profile based on a combination of medium-chain triglycerides (MCTs) and long-chain triglycerides (LCTs) (ratio of MCTs to LCTs of 30 %/70 %) that seems to favor fat absorption in patients with significant intestinal resection, with or without a colon in continuity [37]
(c) Pre-hydrolyzed protein content that may be more suitable than the whole proteins to give nitrogen source to an inefficient mucosal surface [32]
(d) Low osmolality (less than 310 mOsm/L) to minimize the risk for osmotic diarrhea [38, 39]]
(e) Glucose polymer as main carbohydrate source rather than lactose, due to the possible lactose intolerance, especially in SBS children [16]

Some HFs and AAs meet the above reported criteria. AAs have been shown effective in decreasing PN length in small and uncontrolled series of SBS patients [18, 40].

6.2.3.2 Methods of Feeding

EN should be started as soon as postoperative ileus resolves [16, 41, 42], by the most physiological mode. This ideally should be in the form of oral bolus feeding via the breast or bottle. In infants unable to tolerate oral feeds, nasogastric tube feeding is needed. Continuous tube feeding is associated with increased feed tolerance by improved mucosal contact and decreased transit time within the gut [16]. Bolus tube feeding helps gut motility and adaptation and provides periods of fasting, thus reducing persistent hyperinsulinemia. After establishing an appropriate base of enteral nutrients, the general pattern is to increase the provision of enteral nutrients by a slow but steady increment, beginning at 10–20 mL/kg/day (for the average newborn). After the infant can tolerate continuous feeds of 5 mL/h, it is extremely useful to begin transition to oral feeds, providing in small quantities, three to four bolus oral feedings a day (equal or less than the volume continuously tolerated per hour). After establishing a stable feeding pattern, feeds are steadily increased on a daily basis [16]. In order to maximize overall enteral intake, it is often helpful to have continuous drips overnight. To correctly switch from PN to EN, it needs to consider that the net caloric extraction from EN is not 100 % as from PN and that macronutrient absorption from EN is superior than that of electrolytes and fluids. Therefore, PN should be decreased according to the calories provided by EN and not volume for volume [41].

6.2.3.3 Assessing Tolerance to EN

In SBS infants, increasing stool output, vomiting, and irritability to the advancing EN may suggest poor tolerance to the current EN regimen. If stool output is between 30 and 40 mL/kg body weight, it needs to carefully increase EN. Doubled stool output or outputs >40 mL/kg/day are contraindications to increase enteral feeds and indications to deal with a short-term reduction in feeding volume that will be gradually reintroduced. Stool frequency greater than six times per day should induce to cautiously increase EN [16].

Carbohydrate intolerance, which determines frequent and liquid stools, is frequent in SBS

Table 6.2 Markers of impaired EN tolerance and of evolution toward chronic IF

		Reference (n°)
Anatomical markers	1. Residual small bowel length (≤40 cm) 2. Residual small bowel length assessed by GA (<10%) 3. Type of the remaining bowel (relevant loss of ileus) 4. ICV and colon loss (?)	[7, 8, 10, 17, 42]
Clinical markers	1. Frequency of stools (>6–8/day) 2. Impaired growth 3. Diaper rash due to liquid feces 4. Fecal or stoma output >30–40 ml/Kg	[17, 42, 43]
Biochemical markers	1. Plasma citrulline concentration (<12–15 μmol/L) 2. pH of feces (values <5 indicates acid and not absorbed stools) 3. Urine electrolytes (sodium <30 mEq/L and urine sodium-to-potassium ratio <1:1)	[7, 42, 43]

GA gestational age, *ICV* ileocecal valve

patients, and it can be suggested by the presence of reducing substances on the stools and by the stool pH <6.

The rise in plasma citrulline concentration frequently accompanies the successful achieving of enteral tolerance. Citrulline is a nonessential amino acid produced by the enterocytes of the small bowel; its serum level has been shown to reflect intestinal mass in various gastrointestinal diseases. Citrulline concentration of 12–15 μmol/L or greater following EN beginning seems to predict a successful PN withdrawal [41]. In Table 6.2 we report the markers of impaired EN tolerance useful in clinical practice. The combinations of several markers are associated with evolution toward chronic IF.

6.2.3.4 Use of Enteral Supplements

IF patients can loss bicarbonate and sodium in their stool or stoma which must be closely monitored and replaced, not only intravenously but also via enteral route [10]. It is important to monitor sodium balance, because sodium deficiency can limit growth in infants [7, 41]. The simple spot measurement of the urinary sodium and, in selected cases, the calculation of the fractional excretion of sodium are rapid and effective ways to monitor the sodium loss. If the spot urine sodium is <10 mEq/L, increased sodium intake, both in EN and in PN, is required. The sodium content in PN should be titrated to keep urine sodium >30 mEq/L and to maintain urine sodium-to-potassium ratio at least 1:1. Weekly monitoring of the urinary sodium is a preemptive way of assessing status, rather than waiting for the serum level to drop, and long-term monitoring of this parameter is suggested [7].

When increasing in feeds does not result in appropriate weight gain, it should consider supplementation with additional fat [15]. There is good rationale for using long-chain triglycerides (LCTs) as supplemental vegetable oils, or olive oil, or emulsified preparations. Additionally it may be reasonable to add MCTs because they are absorbed directly across the enterocyte membrane, without requiring lymphatic absorption. This occurs in the proximal small bowel and even the stomach; therefore, to add gradually increasing amounts of MCTs to the formula being used, especially if delivered by tube feeds, may favorably increase the overall caloric intake. MCTs are nevertheless less effective than LCTs in promoting intestinal adaptation [43].

6.2.3.5 Starting and Handling Complementary Foods

The introduction of complementary, age-appropriate foods between 4 and 6 months of age, as well as oral boluses of human milk/formula as soon as tolerated, is helpful to stimulate oral motor development and to prevent feeding aversion [10].

Early weaning (17 weeks) has the advantage of promoting feeding maturation with respect to solids and a reduction in milk fluid volume which may exacerbate a tendency to vomit or induce an increase in osmotically driven stomal losses [10]. Feeding therapy is usually required as these infants are likely to have some degree of oral aversion due to delayed introduction of oral feeds as a result of prematurity, prolonged intubation, and cardiovascular instability.

Patients without a colon tolerate better diets that are high in fat (30–40 % of caloric intake), whereas those with intact colons experience steatorrhea and magnesium and calcium loss with high-fat intake. With calcium loss, oxalate absorption is enhanced in the colon and kidneys, which can lead to the formation of oxalate renal stones [41, 44]. Hence, it is necessary to restrict oxalate intake in SBS patients with a colon to decrease the risk of oxalate renal stones. Oral calcium supplements can also reduce the formation of oxalate stones.

Soluble dietary fiber (pectin or guar gum) can slow gastrointestinal transit time allowing for improved absorption (see above). The soluble fiber in the colon is fermented to short-chain fatty acids, including butyrate which is an energy source for colonocytes. In addition, the butyrate regulates colonocyte proliferation and improves water and sodium absorption by upregulating the sodium-hydrogen exchangers [7]. However, excess pectin (>3 %) can lead to an osmotic diarrhea which can counteract its benefits.

In SBS children there is a potential for significant malabsorption of carbohydrates, especially lactose. Therefore, feed with a glucose polymer as a main carbohydrate source is likely to be better tolerated [16]. Solids rich in complex carbohydrates, such as cereals and soluble fibers, lean meat, and unsweetened fruits, are well tolerated in patients with little or intact colon. Patients without a colon or with a stoma tolerate foods at high lipid contents and poor of carbohydrates.

6.2.4 Discharging on HPN

HPN represents the best care option in infants who do not need hospitalization but are dependent on long-term PN. It is indicated if the transition from PN to full EN, although possible, is expected over a long period [45]. Patients eligible for HPN should be clinically stable. As soon as sufficient stability is reached, the child should be discharged under continued outpatient care with a team experienced in intestinal rehabilitation. A coordinated multidisciplinary approach is essential throughout, and the early training of parents in the complexity of HPN care is essential. A specialized nurse dedicated to the coordination of the HPN service is essential, and once the funding and provision of a HPN service are put in place, early discharge home benefits the child and family [10]. Transferring care of these children from hospital to home has a positive influence on CVC infections, social circumstances, as well as reducing the cost of treatment. At the same time, it also puts a significant burden on the family who has to spend a lot of time caring for the child and has difficulty in maintaining gainful employment [45].

6.2.5 Preventing/Treating Complications

The complications of IF SBS related [46–54] can be subdivided into two main categories:

A. CVC-related complications
B. IF-/PN-related complications

Main complications and suggested way of prevention are summarized in Fig. 6.4.

6.2.5.1 CVC-Related Complications

Administration of long-term PN requires placement of indwelling central venous catheter. The problems associated with central lines include infections, mechanical damage, blockages, and thrombosis. Infections are the commonest complication with incidence being around 1–6 per 1000 days of PN [17]. Prevention of infections is based on optimal catheter placement and strict hand hygiene. Taurolidine, a derivative of amino acid taurine, has been shown to have a role in reducing catheter-related sepsis [55]. With advances in the type of catheters used and insertion techniques, there has been a significant reduction in complications [17].

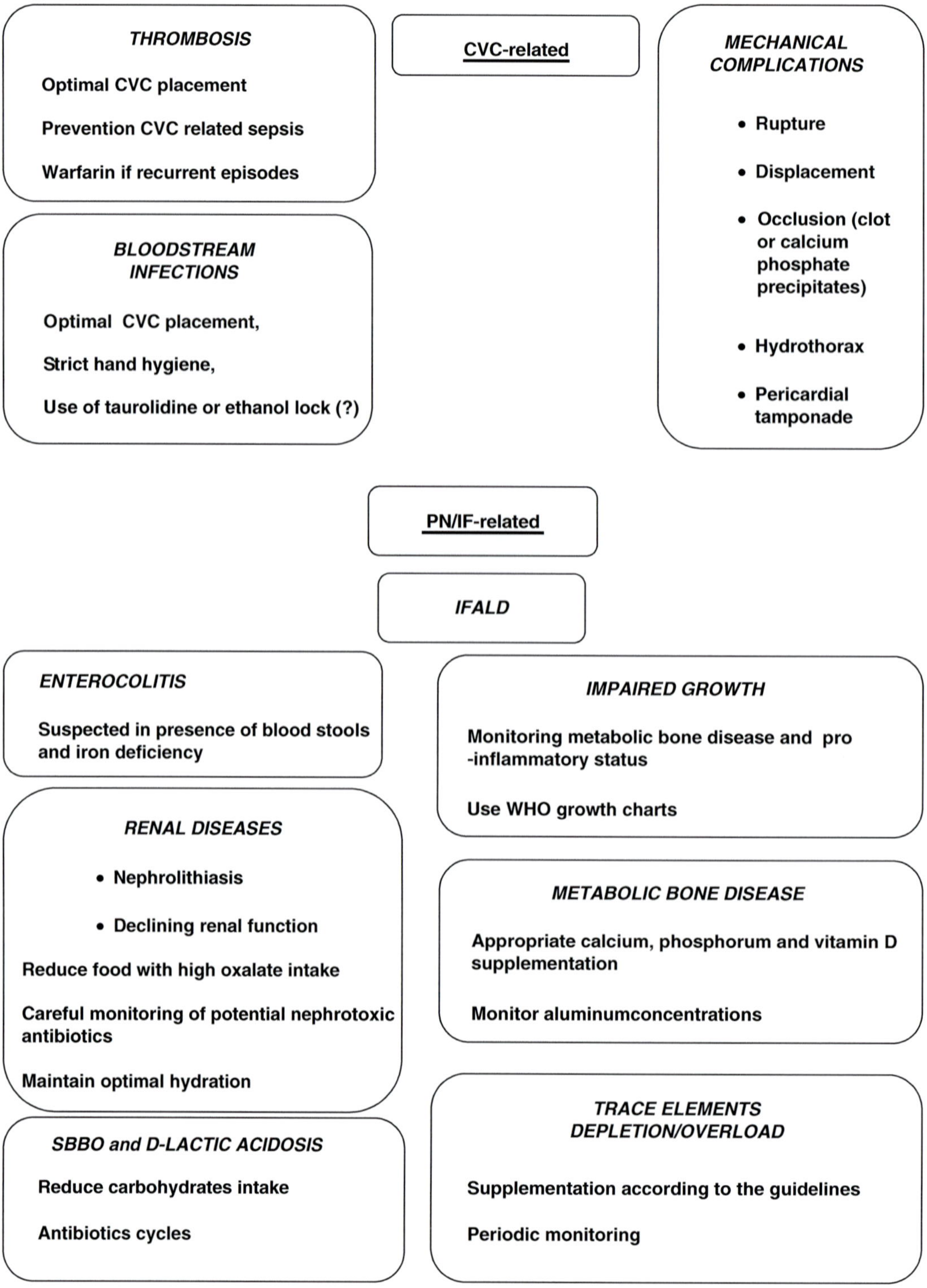

Fig. 6.4 Summary of short bowel syndrome complications. *CVC* central venous catheter, *PN* parenteral nutrition, *IF* intestinal failure, *IFALD* intestinal failure-associated liver disease, *WHO* World Health Organization, *SBBO* small bowel bacterial overgrowth

6.2.5.2 IF-/PN-Related Complications

Trace element depletion is very common among patients with surgical short bowel syndrome if parenteral administration is inadequate. Adequate parenteral zinc supplementation is particularly important; its deficiency is generally associated with high output from the stoma but also with congenital diarrhea. As zinc is a cofactor for alkaline phosphatase synthesis, an excellent surrogate marker for zinc deficiency is the serum alkaline phosphatase level, which is likely decreased in patients at risk for the clinical manifestations of zinc deficiency [7].

D-lactic acidosis occurs among patients whose gastrointestinal tract is colonized by D-lactate-synthesizing organisms. Humans have the ability to rapidly catabolize L-lactate, which is a product of human anaerobic metabolism, but D-lactate can be catabolized and cleared very slowly, and toxic blood levels can build up when the small intestine is overgrown with anaerobic bacteria. Signs and symptoms of D-lactic acidosis include confusion, somnolence, dementia, ataxia, or even seizures. This condition is characterized by acidosis associated with an anion gap but a normal blood L-lactate level. Lactobacilli and other bacteria, including *Clostridium perfringens* and *Streptococcus bovis*, when present, may ferment non-absorbed carbohydrate to D-lactic acid, which cannot be metabolized by L-lactate dehydrogenase [41]. These microorganisms may proliferate in the acidic environment of the colon that is the result of the metabolism of unabsorbed carbohydrate to SCFAs. D-lactic acidosis presents with encephalopathy (ataxia, blurred speech, decreased consciousness) and should be considered when there is a high anion gap metabolic acidosis with normal serum lactate and high gram+strains in the stools [41]. Preventive measures for D-lactic acidosis include the reduction of carbohydrate intake, followed by antibiotics (such as metronidazole or co-trimoxazole) when dietary changes fail [51].

Vitamin B12 absorption may be impaired among patients who have undergone distal small bowel resections. Serum levels of B12 are sometimes falsely elevated because of the production of biologically inactive B12 analogues among patients with bacterial overgrowth syndrome [43].

Provision of enteral water-soluble vitamins is unnecessary while patients are on parenteral vitamin supplements, but if adaptation occurs and patients are weaned off TPN, enteral provision of most water-soluble vitamins is advisable. Fat-soluble vitamin supplementation is delivered via parenteral vitamins and parenteral lipid generally preventing deficiency, but after weaning of TPN, enteral supplementation is advisable.

Iron deficiency can occur in patients with SBS, but it is frequently correctable with oral iron supplements because the efficiency of enteral iron absorption is maximal in the duodenum which is often maintained after neonatal surgical resections. For patients who cannot tolerate enteral iron or who remain deficient despite enteral supplementation, parenteral iron may be given. Iron deficiency can be also due to chronic gastrointestinal bleeding [41].

Another concern of the long-term PN is the potential exposure to toxic plasma aluminum concentrations. A recent Canadian survey found that in pediatric patients receiving long-term PN, aluminum intake is significantly greater than recommended by the US Food and Drug Administration to prevent aluminum toxicity [54]. In SBS patients on PN, aluminum is stored in the body because the protective gastrointestinal barrier is bypassed and renal function may be impaired. The long-term aluminum exposure can contribute to chronic bone disease (by inhibition of PTH) and to neurotoxicity of PN. In addition it is involved in IFALD (it accumulates in the liver) and in the development of hypochromic, microcytic anemia (binding to transferrin).

Colonic oxalate absorption is increased in patients with SBS, resulting in hyperoxaluria and in calcium oxalate nephrolithiasis. The risk of stone formation is reduced if the colon is partially or fully removed. Renal function can also be compromised by some antibiotics or by uncorrected control of fluids and electrolytes in the first phase of IF.

Growth is usually impaired in SBS at neonatal onset. These infants will be small and to push their weight gain to the 50th percentile or higher is not physiologic. It is more appropriate to examine the birth record and weight and to use these to guide the decision as to which percentile seems appropriate. There should be careful serial measures of length, head, and weight gain, with plotting of the appropriate normative or "Z" scores. It may be necessary to tolerate a modest growth in weight, so long as growth in height and especially head circumference are maintained. It is likely appropriate to follow the WHO growth curves.

Conclusions

The key concept of nutritional care in digestive pediatric surgery is to give the maximum tolerated EN to meet the nutritional needs for each patient. If the gut function is impaired, the maximum tolerated EN should be combined with the ongoing support of PN. The final objective is to achieve total or partial nutritional rehabilitation. Nutritional workup of neonatal onset SBS is usually complex and requires close attention. It should be tailored to the single case. The outcome is significantly improved if they are managed by a multidisciplinary team that allows for fully integrated care of inpatients and outpatients with IF by favoring coordination of surgical, medical, and nutritional management [7, 10, 15, 41, 56].

References

1. Agostoni C, Axelson I, Colomb V, Goulet O, Koletzko B, Michaelsen KF, Puntis JW, Rigo J, Shamir R, Szajewska H, Dl T (2005) The need for nutrition support teams in pediatric units: a commentary by the ESPGHAN Committee on Nutrition. J Pediatr Gastroenterol Nutr 41:8–11
2. Braegger C, Decsi T, Dias JA, Hartman C, Kolacˇek S, Koletzko B, Koletzko S, Mihatsch W, Moreno L, Puntis JW, Shamir R, Szajewska H, Turck D, van Goudoever J (2010) Practical approach to paediatric enteral nutrition: a comment by the ESPGHAN Committee on Nutrition ESPGHAN. JPGN 51:110–122
3. Koletzko B, Goulet O, Hunt J, Krohn K, Shamir R (2005) Guidelines on Paediatric Parenteral Nutrition of the European Society of Paediatric Gastroenterology, Hepatology and Nutrition (ESPGHAN) and the European Society for Clinical Nutrition and Metabolism (ESPEN), supported by the European Society of Paediatric Research (ESPR). J Pediatr Gastroenterol Nutr 41(Suppl 2):S1–S87
4. Gura KM (2009) Is there still a role for peripheral parenteral nutrition? Nutr Clin Pract 24:709–717
5. Axelrod D, Kazmerski K, Iyer K (2006) Pediatric enteral nutrition. J Parenter Enteral Nutr 30:S21–S26
6. Capriati T, Cardile S, Chiusolo F, Torroni F, Schingo P, Elia D, Diamanti A (2015) Clinical management of post-pyloric enteral feeding in children. Expert Rev Gastroenterol Hepatol 9:929–941
7. Kocoshis SA (2010) Medical management of pediatric intestinal failure. Semin Pediatr Surg 19:20–26. doi:10.1053/j.sempedsurg.2009.11.003
8. Barclay AR, Beattie LM, Weaver LT, Wilson DC (2011) Systematic review: medical and nutritional interventions for the management of intestinal failure and its resultant complications in children. Aliment Pharmacol Ther 33(2):175–184. doi:10.1111/j.1365-2036.2010.04514.x. Epub 2010 Nov 22
9. D'Antiga L, Goulet O (2013) Intestinal failure in children: the European view. JPGN 56:118–126. doi:10.1097/MPG.0b013e318268a9e3
10. Dalzell AM (2015) Management of intestinal failure in children. Arch Dis Child; Feb 20. pii: archdischild-2014-306101. doi:10.1136/archdischild-2014-306101. [Epub ahead of print]
11. Ohta K, Omura K, Hirano K, Kanehira E, Ishikawa N, Kato Y, Kawakami K, Watanabe G (2003) The effects of small amounts of a low residual diet against total parenteral nutrition. Am J Surg 185:79–85
12. Tyson JI, Kennedy KA (2005) Minimal enteral nutrition for promoting tolerance and preventing morbidity in parenterally fed infants. Cochrane Database Syst Rev 3:CD000504
13. Pironi L, Joly F, Forbes A, Colomb V, Lyszkowska M, Baxter J et al (2011) Long-term follow-up of patients on home parenteral nutrition in Europe: implications for intestinal transplantation. Gut 60(1):17–25
14. Petit LM, Girard D, Ganousse-Mazeron S, Talbotec C, Pigneur B, Elie C, Corriol O, Poisson C, Goulet O, Colomb V (2015) Weaning off prognosis factors of home parenteral nutrition for children with primary digestive disease. J Pediatr Gastroenterol Nutr 62(3):462–468
15. Goulet O, Olieman J, Ksiazyk J, Spolidoro J, Tibboe D, Köhler H et al (2013) Neonatal short bowel syndrome as a model of intestinal failure: physiological background for enteral feeding. Clin Nutr 32:162–171
16. Batra A, Beattie RM (2013) Management of short bowel syndrome in infancy. Early Hum Dev 89(11):899–904
17. Pittiruti M, Hamilton H, Biffi R, MacFie J, Pertkiewicz M et al (2009) ESPEN Guidelines on Parenteral Nutrition: central venous catheters (access, care,

diagnosis and therapy of complications). Clin Nutr 28:365–377
18. Tillman EM (2013) Review and clinical update on parenteral nutrition-associated liver disease. Nutr Clin Pract 28:30–39
19. Rangel SJ, Calkins CM, Cowles RA, Barnhart DC, Huang EY, Abdullah F et al (2012) Parenteral nutrition–associated cholestasis: an American Pediatric Surgical Association Outcomes and Clinical Trials Committee systematic review. J Pediatr Surg 47(1):225–240
20. Cavicchi M, Beau P, Crenn P, Degott C, Messing B (2000) Prevalence of liver disease and contributing factors in patients receiving home parenteral nutrition for permanent intestinal failure. Ann Intern Med 132:525–532
21. Wanten GJ (2015) Parenteral lipid tolerance and adverse effects: fat chance for trouble? J Parenter Enteral Nutr 2015(39):33S–38S
22. Gura KM, Lee S, Valim C, Zhou J, Kim S, Modi BP et al (2008) Safety and efficacy of a fish-oil–based fat emulsion in the treatment of parenteral nutrition–associated liver disease. Pediatrics 121:e678–e686
23. Diamond IR, Sterescu A, Pencharz PB, Kim JH, Wales PW (2009) Changing the paradigm: omegaven for the treatment of liver failure in pediatric short bowel syndrome. J Pediatr Gastroenterol Nutr 48(2):209–215
24. Lee S, Park HJ, Yoon J, Hong SH, Oh CY, Lee SK et al (2015) Reversal of intestinal failure–associated liver disease by switching from a combination lipid emulsion containing fish oil to fish oil monotherapy. J Parenter Enteral Nutr 40(3):437–440
25. Goulet O, Antebi H, Wolf C, Talbotec C, Alcindor LG, Corriol O et al (2010) A new intravenous fat emulsion containing soybean oil, medium-chain triglycerides, olive oil, and fish oil: a single-center, double-blind randomized study on efficacy and safety in pediatric patients receiving home parenteral nutrition. JPEN J Parenter Enteral Nutr 34:485–495
26. Forchielli ML, Miller SJ (2005) Nutritional goals and requirements. In: Merritt R (ed) The A.S.P.E.N. nutrition support practice manual, 2nd edn. A.S.P.E.N., Silver Spring,;pp 38–53
27. Kleinman RE (2009) Parenteral nutrition. In: Pediatric nutrition handbook, 6th edn. American Academy of Pediatrics, Elk Grove Village, pp 519–540
28. Jakobsen MS, Jørgensen MH, Husby S, Andersen L, Jeppesen PB (2015) Low-fat, high-carbohydrate parenteral nutrition (PN) may potentially reverse liver disease in long-term PN-dependent infants. Dig Dis Sci 60:252–2591
29. Byars KC, Burklow KA, Ferguson K, O'Flaherty T, Santoro K, Kaul A (2003) A multicomponent behavioral program for oral aversion in children dependent on gastrostomy feedings. J Pediatr Gastroenterol Nutr 37:473–480
30. Andorsky DJ, Lund DP, Lillehei CW, Jaksic T, Dicanzio J, Richardson DS et al (2001) Nutritional and other post operative management of neonates with short bowel syndrome correlates with clinical outcomes. J Pediatr 139:27–33
31. Lundqvist-Persson C, Lau G, Nordin P, Strandvik B, Sabel KG (2010) Early behaviour and development in breast-fed premature infants are influenced by omega-6 and omega-3 fatty acid status. Early Hum Dev 86:407–412
32. Underwood MA (2013) Human milk for the premature infant. Pediatr Clin North Am 60:189–207
33. Kau AL, Ahern PP, Griffin NW, Goodman AL, Gordon JI (2011) Human nutrition, the gut microbiome and the immune system. Nature 474(7351):327–336
34. Roger LC, McCartney AL (2010) Longitudinal investigation of the faecal microbiota of healthy full-term infants using fluorescence in situ hybridization and denaturing gradient gel electrophoresis. Microbiology 156:3317–3328
35. Sangild PT (2006) Gut responses to enteral nutrition in preterm infants and animals. Exp Biol Med (Maywood) 231:1695–1711
36. Diamanti A, Fiocchi AG, Capriati T, Panetta F, Pucci N, Bellucci F et al (2015) Cow's milk allergy and neonatal short bowel syndrome: comorbidity or true association? Eur J Clin Nutr 69(1):102–106
37. Jeppesen PB, Mortensen PB (1998) The influence of a preserved colon on the absorption of medium chain fat in patients with small bowel resection. Gut 43:478–483
38. Steele JR, Meskell RJ, Foy J, Garner AE (2013) Determining the osmolality of over concentrated and supplemented infant formulas. J Hum Nutr Diet 26:32–37
39. Di Lorenzo C, Youssef NN (2010) Diagnosis and management of intestinal motility disorders. Semin Pediatr Surg 19:50–58
40. Benjamin J, Singh N, Makharia GK (2010) Enteral nutrition for severe malnutrition in chronic intestinal pseudo-obstruction. Nutrition 26:502–505. doi:10.1016/j.nut.2009.07.012. Epub 2009 Dec 16
41. Kaufman SS, Matsumoto CS (2015) Management of pediatric intestinal failure. Minerva Pediatr 67(4):321–340
42. Cole CR, Kocoshis SA (2013) Nutrition management of infants with surgical short bowel syndrome and intestinal failure. Nutr Clin Pract 28(4): 421–428
43. Booth IW, Lander AD (1998) Short bowel syndrome. Baillieres Clin Gastroenterol 12(4):739–773
44. Nightingale JM, Lennard-Jones JE, Gertner DJ, Wood SR, Bartram CI (1992) Colonic preservation reduces need for parenteral therapy, increases incidence of renal stones, but does not change high prevalence of gall stones in patients with a short bowel. Gut 33:1493–1497
45. DiBaise JK, Young RJ, Vanderhoof JA (2004) Intestinal rehabilitation and the short bowel syndrome: part 1. Am J Gastroenterol 99:1386–1395

46. Colomb V, Ricour C (2003) Home parenteral nutrition in children. Clin Nutr 22(Suppl 2):S57–S59
47. Mermel LA, Alang N (2014) Adverse effects associated with ethanol catheter lock solutions: a systematic review. J Antimicrob Chemother 69(10): 2611–2619
48. Newall F, Barnes C, Savoia H, Campbell J, Monagle P (2003) Warfarin therapy in children who require long-term parenteral nutrition. Pediatrics 112(5):e386–e388
49. van Ommen CH, Tabbers MM (2010) Catheter-related thrombosis in children with intestinal failure and long-term parenteral nutrition: how to treat and to prevent? Thromb Res 126(6):465–470
50. Khan FA, Fisher JG, Bairdain S, Sparks EA, Zurakowski D, Modi BP et al (2015) Metabolic bone disease in pediatric intestinal failure patients: prevalence and risk factors. J Pediatr Surg 50(1):136–139
51. Uchida H, Yamamoto H, Kisaki Y, Fujino J, Ishimaru Y, Ikeda H (2004) D-lactic acidosis in short-bowel syndrome managed with antibiotics and probiotics. J Pediatr Surg 39(4):634–636
52. Hurwitz M, Garcia MG, Poole RL, Kerner JA (2004) Copper deficiency during parenteral nutrition: a report of four pediatric cases. Nutr Clin Pract 19(3):305–308
53. Erikson KM, Thompson K, Aschner J, Aschner M (2007) Manganese neurotoxicity: a special focus on neonates. Pharmacol Ther 113(2):369–377
54. Courtney-Martin G, Kosar C, Campbell A, Avitzur Y, Wales PW, Steinberg K et al (2015) Plasma aluminum concentrations in pediatric patients receiving long-term parenteral nutrition. J Parenter Enteral Nutr 39(5):578–585
55. Chu HP, Brind J, Tomar R, Hill S (2012) Significant reduction in central venous catheter-related bloodstream infections in children on HPN after starting treatment with taurolidine line lock. J Pediatr Gastroenterol Nutr 55(4):403–407
56. Torres C, Sudan D, Vanderhoof J, Grant W, Botha J, Raynor S, Langnas A (2007) Role of an intestinal rehabilitation program in the treatment of advanced intestinal failure. J Pediatr Gastroenterol Nutr 45(2):204–212

7 Vascular Rings and Pulmonary Sling

Gaetano Domenico Gargiulo, Francesco Petridis, Gabriele Egidy Assenza, and Emanuela Angeli

7.1 Introduction

Vascular rings are a group of congenital anomalies, in which the aortic arch and its branches form a complete or partial ring around the trachea, the bronchi, and the esophagus, with potential extrinsic compression leading to variable degrees of respiratory problems or feeding difficulties.

They constitute 1 % of all the congenital vascular abnormalities [1], and the term vascular rings was originally introduced for the first time in 1945 by Gross, when he performed the first surgical division of a double aortic arch [2].

Pulmonary sling describes a congenital vascular anomaly involving the development of the pulmonary arteries, more often the left one. Usually, the anomalous left pulmonary artery arises from the posterior aspect of the right pulmonary artery; it courses over the right bronchus and running from right to left, posterior to the trachea or carina and anterior to the esophagus; it reaches the hilum of the left lung, forming a sling around the trachea.

G.D. Gargiulo (✉) • F. Petridis • G. Egidy Assenza
E. Angeli
Department of Pediatric Cardiac Surgery and GUCH Unit, Azienda Ospedaliero-Universitaria S. Orsola-Malpighi, Via Massarenti, 9, Bologna 40138, Italy
e-mail: gaetano.gargiulo@unibo.it

The unifying characteristic of all these anomalies is the presence of a complete or incomplete vascular structure (in some cases with fibrous replacement) surrounding the tracheoesophageal unit.

The clinical picture can range from asymptomatic patients to patients presenting with breathing disorders and/or swallowing difficulties due to the bronchial and tracheal and/or esophageal constriction [3]. Vascular rings and pulmonary slings may be associated with genetic defects, such as 22q11.2 deletion (DiGeorge syndrome), or they may be combined with cardiac conotruncal anomalies, as tetralogy of Fallot (ToF), double outlet right ventricle (DORV), pulmonary atresia (PA), truncus arteriosus (TA), and interrupted aortic arch (IAA) [4].

7.2 Embryology

During fetal development, the brachial vascular system, which will give rise to the aortic arch and its branches, develops and completes within the second and seventh gestational week.

The complex and dynamic embryological development consists of six paired aortic arches (although never present at the same time during fetal life) connecting the dorsal and the ventral aorta, which will reorganize with differential growth and reabsorption during the fetal period by processes of apoptosis and remodeling (Fig. 7.1).

M. Lima (ed.), *Pediatric Digestive Surgery*, DOI 10.1007/978-3-319-40525-4_7

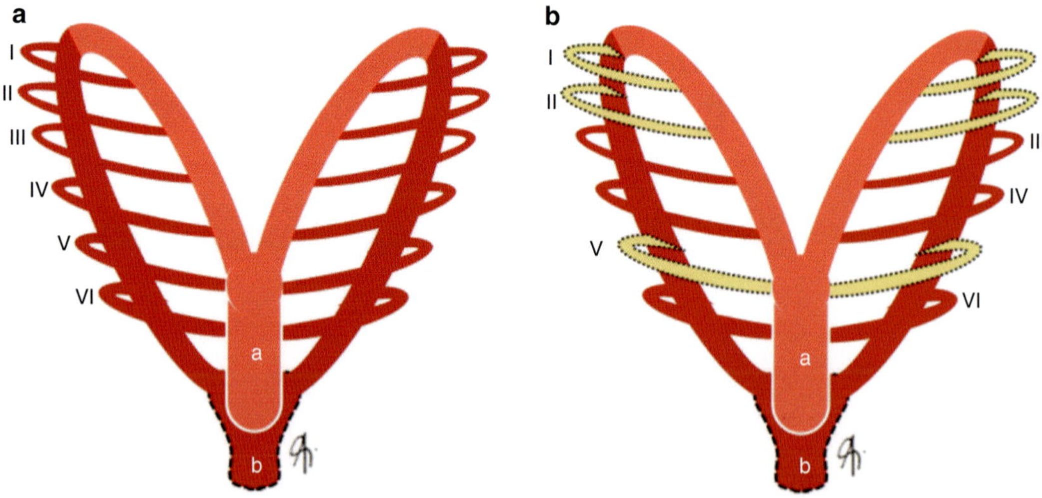

Fig. 7.1 The Rathke diagram: schematic representation of the six paired brachial arches (I–VI). (**a**) The brachial arches connect paired ventral aorta (*a*) and dorsal aorta (*b*). (**b**) Reabsorption of the first, second, and fifth arches

The first and second arches largely resorb and contribute to minor facial arteries; the fifth arches obliterate after the growth of the sixth ones; the third, along with the ventral aortic portion, will contribute to the development of the vessels arising from the mature aortic arch. The fourth will form the ultimate aortic arch, while the sixth will contribute to create the pulmonary arteries and the ductus arteriosus. On the right side, the segment of the dorsal aorta comprised between the fourth and sixth brachial arches will disappear; in the left side, it persists as the ductus arteriosus.

An unusual progression of obliterations and growth of this primitive vessel arrangement will result into a broad range of anatomical variations of vascular rings and slings [1].

A clear description of the possible anatomical variety is offered by Edward's scheme (Fig. 7.2); it condenses the conclusive phase of the brachial branches' embryogenesis, depicting the totipotent double (symmetrical) aortic arch, whose total or partial reabsorption or persistence may determine different anatomical variations.

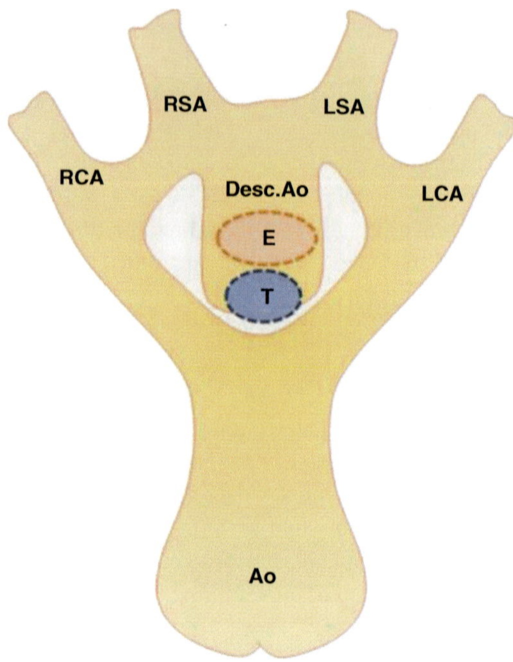

Fig. 7.2 Edward's diagram: totipotent double aortic arch system. Legend: *Ao* aorta; *Desc.Ao* descending aorta; *E* esophagus, *T* trachea, *RCA* right carotid artery, *RSA* right subclavian artery, *LCA* left carotid artery, *LSA* left subclavian artery

In case of persistence of both left and right fourth brachial branches, a double aortic arch will result; if an obliteration of the portion of the right aortic arch between the subclavian artery and dorsal aorta occurs, a normal formation of a left aortic arch will take place; instead, if the reabsorption involves the opposite fourth arch, a right-sided aortic arch with so-called "mirror image" arrangement of arch vessel will result. Obliterations affecting other segments will induce, in addition to the left or right location of the arch, the presence of an aberrant subclavian artery (Fig. 7.3).

7.3 Classification

There are different classifications of vascular rings, some of which take into account the morphology of the ring and some others considering the position and anatomy of the arch.

In relation to the *morphology*, vascular rings can be divided into two large groups [5]:

1. *Complete*: when fibrovascular elements create a complete ring around the trachea and esophagus
2. *Incomplete*: if the trachea and esophagus are not completely encircled by fibrovascular structures

The most common abnormalities in the complete form group are *double aortic arch, right-sided aortic arch with left aberrant subclavian artery and Kommerell diverticulum,* and *right-sided aortic arch "mirror image"* type with ligamentum arteriosum on the left side.

Among the incomplete forms, the most frequent are *left aortic arch with right aberrant subclavian artery* and *pulmonary sling.*

Regarding the *position* of the aortic arch and branching pattern of the great vessels, different *anatomical* types can be identified:

1. Left aortic arch
   (a) Normal branching
   (b) Aberrant right subclavian artery
2. Right aortic arch
   (a) Mirror image
   (b) Aberrant left subclavian artery
3. Double aortic arch
4. Pulmonary artery sling
5. Cervical aortic arch

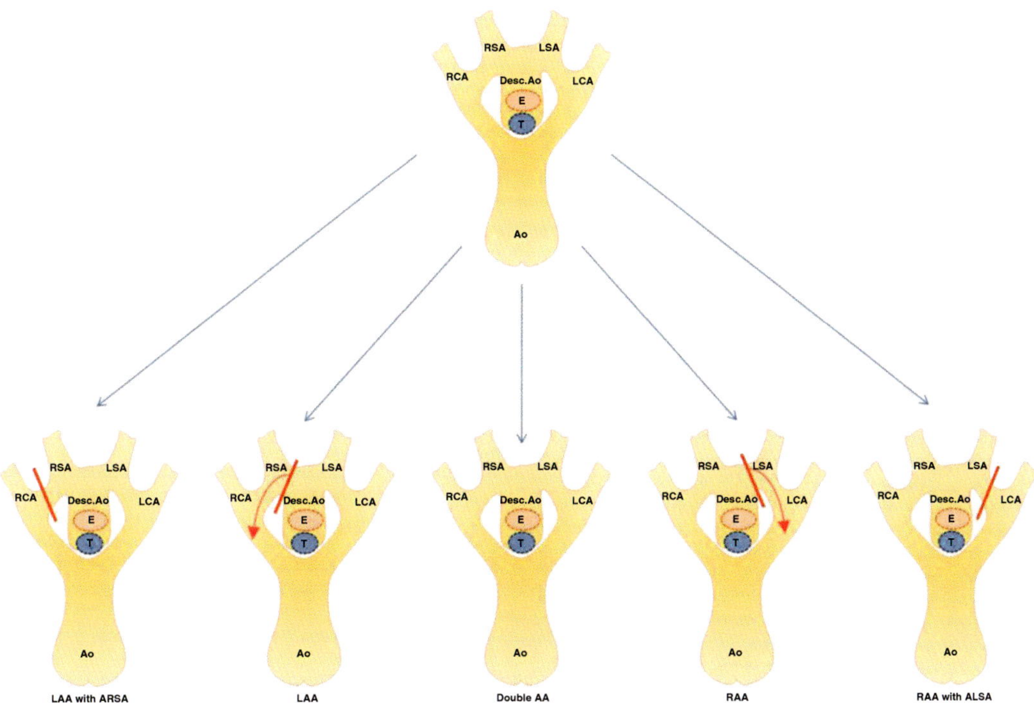

Fig. 7.3 Edward's diagram: hypothetical double arch system. Legend: *Ao* aorta, *Desc.Ao* descending aorta, *E* esophagus, *T* trachea, *RCA* right carotid artery, *RSA* right subclavian artery, *LCA* left carotid artery, *LSA* left subclavian artery, *LAA-ARSA* left aortic arch- aberrant right subclavian artery, *LAA* left aortic arch, *RAA* right aortic arch, *RAA-ALSA* right aortic arch-aberrant left subclavian artery, *Double AA* double aortic arch

Other anomalies exist, but they are either significantly less frequent or are usually asymptomatic.

7.4 Clinical Presentation and Diagnosis

Clinical presentation is heterogeneous (Table 7.1) and can vary from *asymptomatic* patients with incidental diagnosis during adulthood to *severe early symptoms* of either tracheal or esophageal compression, leading to early recognition of the more severe forms.

The breathing difficulty involves symptoms varying from wheezing, dry cough, and inspiratory dyspnea, with worsening during stress or meals. The wheezing can be misled as an asthmatic pathology.

Esophageal constriction is less frequent and characterized by increased risk of *ab-ingestis* events, gastroesophageal reflux, and progressive dysphagia, firstly at ingestion of solid food and only after for ingestion of liquids.

Eventually, recurrent infections of the respiratory tract can occur, in particular during the first year of patient life. Between 18 and 24 months, the symptoms tend to decline due to the physiological growth of body structures.

7.5 Imaging

Nowadays many possibilities exist to make a diagnosis in case of suspicion of vascular ring or pulmonary sling: *chest X-Ray (CXR), barium esophagram, echocardiography, computerized tomography scan (CT scan), magnetic resonance imaging (MRI), invasive angiography*, and *bronchoscopy.* All of these diagnostic techniques present advantages and disadvantages.

Table 7.1 Vascular ring and sling: clinical presentation

Asymptomatic	
Respiratory symptoms	Stridor, wheezing, chronic cough, recurrent respiratory infections, seal bark cough, tachypnea, intermittent cyanosis, asthma
Digestive symptoms	Feeding difficulty, dysphagia, recurrent emesis, gagging, choking, others

7.5.1 Chest X-Ray (CXR)

Chest radiography, with or without barium esophagography, can be considered the first-line imaging modality used in diagnosing tracheal or esophageal compression, particularly in children. CXR double projection (straight and leaning) can enlighten tracheal compression by nearby structures or tracheal displacement related to aortic arch location. In case of double aortic arch, the CXR image describes the trachea in axis, with two lateral compressions. The CXR with barium esophagography can display a posterior incision on the esophagus due to the presence of anomalous subclavian artery or Kommerell diverticulum, and in the presence of pulmonary sling, the cleft will be on the anterior wall of the esophagus. Moreover, there could be present signs of pulmonary atelectasis or lung hyperinflation in case of bronchial compression. Unfortunately, this technique does not allow direct images of vascular structures or vessels' anatomy, preventing from an accurate surgical planning.

7.5.2 Bronchoscopy

Bronchoscopy is nowadays an important tool to make a diagnosis when symptoms of respiratory distress are present. This procedure may demonstrate the presence of pulsatile compression and also the degree and precise location of such compression. In cases of pulmonary sling, bronchoscopy shows the length of hypoplastic tracheal segment, the diameter of this segment, and the presence of complete tracheal rings. Bronchoscopy is mandatory after surgical treatment to evaluate the results of surgery and in the postoperative period to follow the outcome of correction.

7.5.3 Echocardiography

The echocardiography can be considered the first tool to confirm the suspicion of vascular ring or sling. It is usually able to demonstrate the aortic side; the anomalies of vessels of the aortic arch, such as aberrant subclavian artery or aneurysm of the brachiocephalic trunk; the double aortic arch; and the anatomy of the pulmonary artery. However, echocardiography is a poor imaging tool to either establish or exclude the diagnosis of a vascular ring in case of poor acoustic windows such as in adult patients. In addition, it does not depict the ligamentous structures and hyperinflation of the lungs and the compression of the trachea or esophagus. Echocardiography is absolutely necessary for investigating associated cardiac defects.

7.5.4 Angiography

Angiography was the first procedure used to perform diagnosis in these patients until the last decade, but currently this imaging modality is rarely used, and it is useful only in selected cases. Angiography may be considered, if the anatomy of the patent vessels must be visualized, including the size of the two arches, in case of a double aortic arch, in order to make a proper selection of the arch that has to be cut. However, angiography is unreliable in demonstrating the tracheal or esophageal compression, and moreover it is an invasive procedure, requiring vascular access and the use of ionizing radiation and contrast agent.

7.5.5 Computed Tomography Scan (CT Scan)

Computed tomography angiography (CTA) allows for an accurate description of vascular and respiratory tract anatomy. Patent vascular channels are evident on CTA as contrast-enhancing segments and are well visualized on reconstructed 3D images. Conversely, atretic vascular segments and ligaments are not evident, but their presence can be inferred from traction on associated vascular structures or compression of the trachea [6]. Inspiratory and expiratory CTA studies allow the dynamic evaluation of tracheal caliber for narrowing or traction, which is particularly important in patients with associated tracheomalacia. CTA scanning times are shorter than magnetic resonance imaging (MRI), and therefore sedation is usually not necessary, which is a significant advantage in a young or respiratory distressed patient. The principal disadvantages of CTA are the need for intravenous contrast agents and the potential late consequences of radiation-dose exposure.

7.5.6 Magnetic Resonance Imaging (MRI)

MRI is currently the gold standard diagnostic modality, because of the anatomical definition of the anomaly with functional and dynamic study of the heart and vessels. Advantages of MRI over CTA include the freedom from exposure to both radiation and intravenous iodine contrast, as well as the ability to undertake functional studies in patients with intracardiac lesions. The limitations of MRI include longer scanning time than CTA and the need for sedation in pediatric patients.

7.6 Vascular Rings

7.6.1 Double Aortic Arch

The double aortic arch (Fig. 7.4) is the most frequent type of vascular ring and sums up about 40 % of the all anatomical varieties.

This vascular malformation consists of the presence of a double aortic arch, one left and one right, both completely patent; generally one of the two arches is larger than the other, and the descending aorta is generally left sided although it may be right sided or positioned in the midline.

In 75 % of the cases, the right arch is dominant, while in the remaining 25 %, the left is the dominant one or there is a balance between the two [7].

This malformation is often associated with other cardiac defects, such as tetralogy of Fallot, truncus arteriosus, or pulmonary atresia.

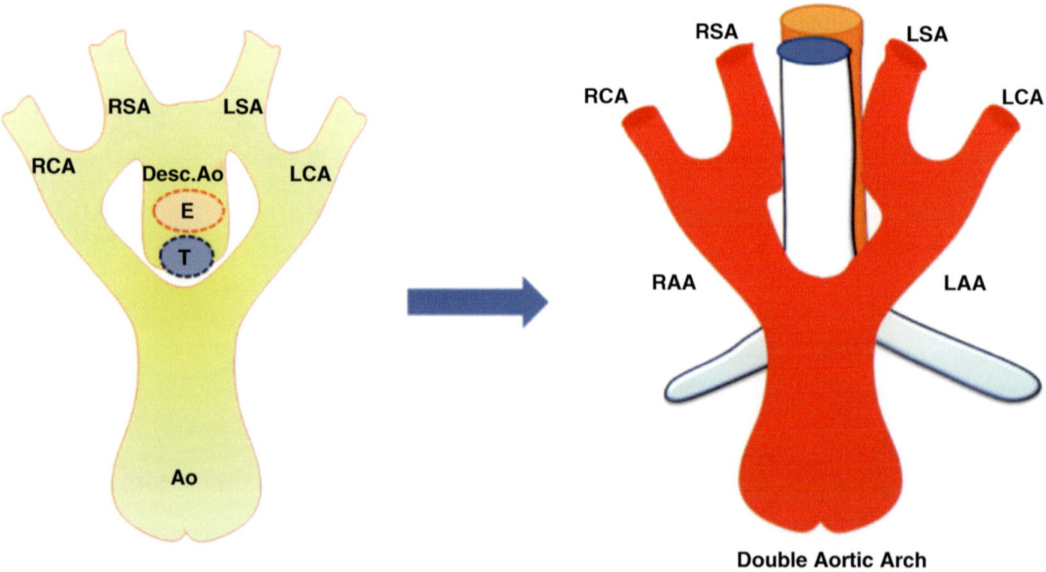

Fig. 7.4 Double aortic arch: persistence of the right and left aortic arch, both completely patent. Legend: *Ao* aorta, *Desc.Ao* descending aorta, *E* esophagus, *T* trachea, *RCA* right carotid artery, *RSA* right subclavian artery, *LCA* left carotid artery, *LSA* left subclavian artery

About 20 % of the cases are associated with chromosomal anomalies such as 22q11.2 deletion syndrome (CATCH 22) [7].

The clinical presentation can include respiratory and/or digestive symptoms, and the surgical correction includes the resection of the nondominant arch. In case of a balanced double aortic arch, it is preferred to maintain the right-sided arch. The surgical approach through a thoracotomy is usually performed on the opposite side of the dominant arch.

Surgical correction usually allows resolution of the symptoms, despite in some cases clinical improvement is not immediate but delayed in time, due to the persistence of the constriction previously established on the esophagus and trachea.

7.6.2 Right Aortic Arch, Aberrant Left Subclavian Artery, and Left Ligament (RAA-ALSA)

The presence of a right aortic arch with left subclavian artery arising from a Kommerell diverticulum is the second most common vascular ring and represents about 30 % of cases, and in 5–10 % of cases, it can be associated with other congenital cardiac abnormalities such as tetralogy of Fallot or ventricular septal defects (VSD).

The embryological development is related to a break occurring between the left common carotid artery and the left subclavian artery of the left-sided fourth brachial branch. The subsequent anatomy is a right aortic arch with aberrant left subclavian artery (ALSA) (Fig. 7.5). The ALSA usually takes origin from the Kommerell diverticulum, representing the remnant of the right dorsal aorta and, in some cases, can create a posterior compression of the esophagus.

This is the spot where the vestige of the ligamentum arteriosum connects the aortic arch to the ipsilateral pulmonary artery forming a complete vascular ring.

The existence, at once, of a bulky Kommerell diverticulum and the residual ligamentum arteriosum causes an important compression above the posterior esophageal wall, showing up with swallowing difficulty.

With the body growing, Kommerell diverticulum can evolve into an aneurysmatic formation, causing dysphagia in adulthood and could be the source of life-threatening collateral events, such as aortic dissection or wall rupture. The risks of rupture and aortic dissection are strictly related to the dimension of the diverticulum [8, 9].

The surgical repair is indicated in the presence of clinical symptoms and consists of the resection

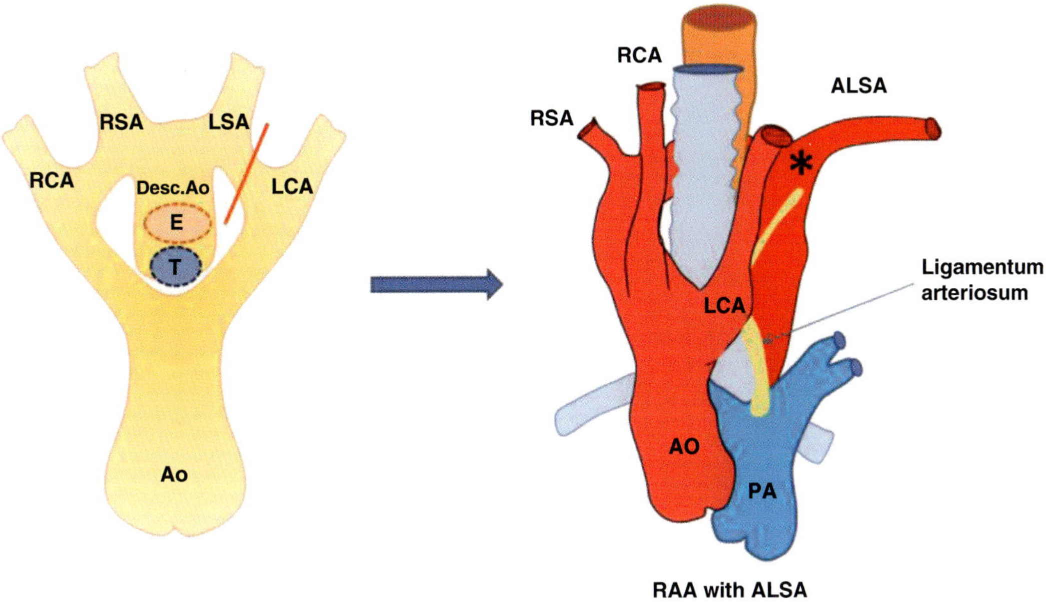

Fig. 7.5 Right aortic arch with aberrant left subclavian artery. Legend: *Ao* aorta, *PA* pulmonary artery, *RCA* right carotid artery, *RSA* right subclavian artery, *LCA* left carotid artery, *ALSA* aberrant left subclavian artery; * = Kommerell diverticulum

of the ligamentum arteriosum, resection of Kommerell diverticulum, and reimplantation of the left aberrant subclavian artery to the left common carotid artery. This surgery can be complex due to the extreme fragility of the diverticulum wall.

In adult patients when complete resection of the aneurysmatic segment of the thoracic aorta is required, the surgery must be performed with the aid of cardiopulmonary bypass with or without hypothermic circulatory arrest. In these cases, the surgery is very challenging and includes a significant risk of death (12 %) and paraplegia (4 %).

7.6.3 Right Aortic Arch with Mirror Image of the Arch Vessels and Retroesophageal Ligamentum (RAA)

This type of vascular ring named right aortic arch with *mirror image anatomy* results from the persistence of the fourth right aortic arch and obliteration of the left one. When reabsorption takes place in the posterior portion of left dorsal arch, behind the origin of the left subclavian artery, the consequent vascular anatomy will be characterized by a right aortic arch with the left brachiocephalic artery (BCA, Fig. 7.6).

Usually this anatomy is asymptomatic, and it does not form a vascular ring. However in rare cases, the presence of ligamentum arteriosum can pull back the BCA realizing an anterior tracheal compression. The RAA could be associated with conotruncal cardiac anomalies such as tetralogy of Fallot or double outlet right ventricle (DORV) and could be associated with genetic syndromes as CATCH 22.

Surgery is indicated only in cases when a tracheal compression is evident. In case of tracheal compression by the right ascending aorta or anomalous innominate artery, it may be performed as a simple aortopexy pulling the aorta toward the sternum, associated with the resection of ligamentum arteriosum.

7.6.4 Left Aortic Arch with Aberrant Right Subclavian Artery (LAA-ARSA)

The presence of a left aberrant subclavian artery is definitely the most common anomaly associated with the left aortic arch. This anomaly occurs

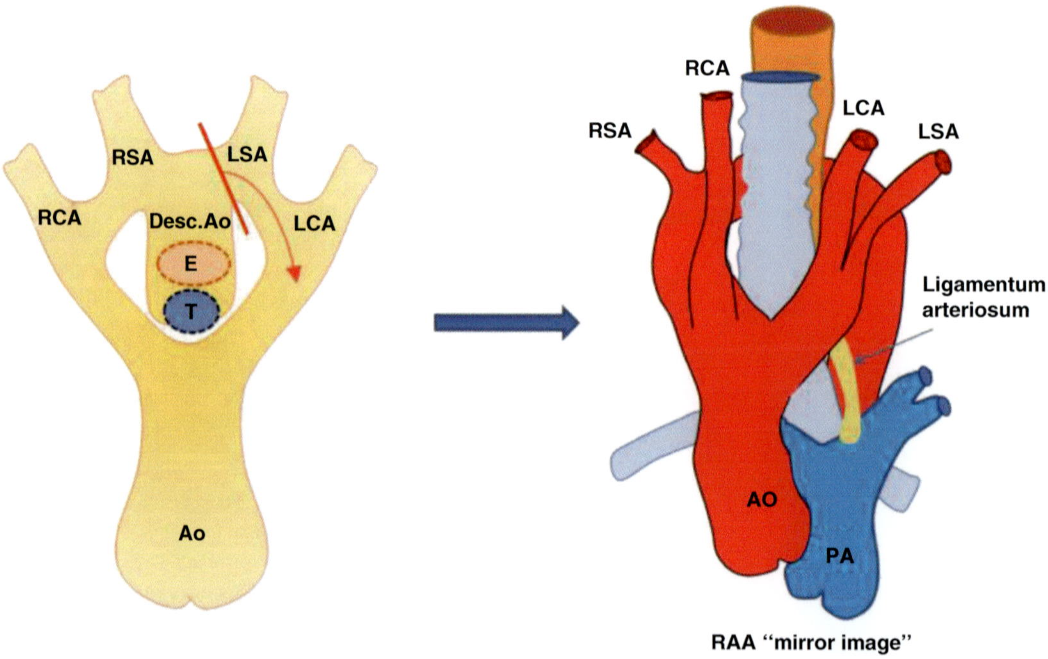

Fig. 7.6 Right Aortic Arch (RAA) "mirror image". Legend: *Ao* aorta, *PA* pulmonary artery, *RCA* right carotid artery, *RSA* right subclavian artery, *LCA* left carotid artery, *LSA* left subclavian artery

when the portion of the right arch, included between the origin of the right subclavian artery and the right common carotid artery, undergoes reabsorption; it usually is not associated with a vascular ring (Fig. **7.7**).

Sometimes the right aberrant subclavian artery arises from a Kommerell diverticulum, leading, in this case, to the formation of a vascular ring. This variant is rarely symptomatic, and symptoms usually depend on a voluminous diverticulum causing swelling discomfort or difficulty.

Occasionally, its presentation is associated with other cardiac defects, among which coarctation of aorta, hypoplastic left heart syndrome, tetralogy of Fallot, or a ventricular septal defect. Surgical repair is rarely indicated and consists of the resection of the ligamentum arteriosum and, if needed, resection of the Kommerell diverticulum. In many cases, the surgical treatment was found to be completely unsuccessful because the majority of these patients continued to have symptoms.

7.6.5 Pulmonary Sling

This anomaly is characterized by an unusual drift of the left pulmonary artery, climbing over the right bronchus, passing behind the trachea and in front of the esophagus, heading to the left hilum (Fig. 7.8).

The left pulmonary artery is often hypoplastic and smaller than the right artery, which can eventually be enlarged because of the volume overload; the small size of the left pulmonary artery may help to explain the high incidence of anastomotic problems that have been observed in the past with attempts to reimplant it.

Approximately 50 % of patients with a pulmonary artery sling have complete tracheal rings, that is, the posterior membranous component of the trachea is absent, and the tracheal cartilages, rather than being U shaped, are O shaped.

It usually presents as isolated malformation, but it can be associated with other congenital heart diseases like tetralogy of Fallot.

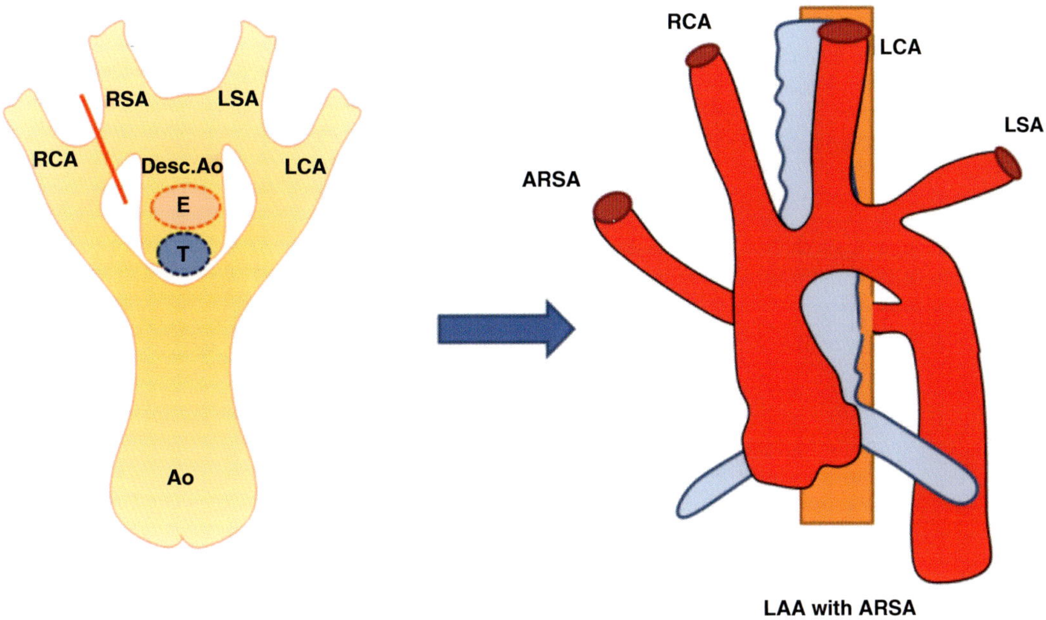

Fig. 7.7 Left aortic arch with aberrant right subclavian artery. Legend: *RCA* right carotid artery, *ARSA* aberrant right subclavian artery, *LCA* left carotid artery, *LSA* left subclavian artery

The clinical scenario is dominated by the compression of the distal part of the trachea associated with severe tracheal and/or bronchial hypoplasia and stenosis. Respiratory symptoms predominate because of the direct tracheal compression and are essentially the same respiratory symptoms as those described for vascular rings. In case of severe airway obstruction, it is necessary to establish a preoperative ventilator support or occasionally an extracorporeal membrane oxygenation (ECMO). Symptoms of esophageal compression are rarely present.

Surgical repair should be performed in those patients showing respiratory obstructive difficulty and consists of a relocation and reimplantation of the left pulmonary artery anterior to the trachea.

Additionally, surgery on the trachea can be required, because of the narrowing provoked by the compression around the portion surrounded by the sling; tracheal surgical repair can complicate the correction, increasing the risk of unsuccessful outcome. For the pulmonary artery relocation and tracheal repair, surgery is per-

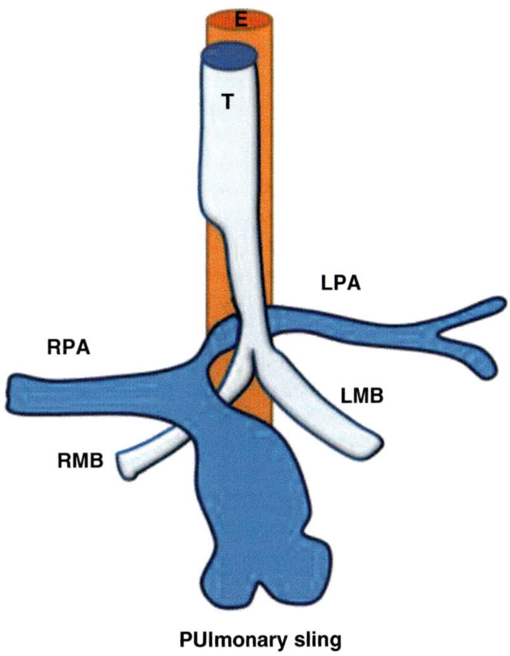

Fig. 7.8 Pulmonary artery sling. Legend: *T* trachea, *E* esophagus, *RPA* right pulmonary artery, *LPA* left pulmonary artery, *RMB* right main bronchus, *LMB* left main bronchus

formed by central sternotomy, and extracorporeal circulation may be required in order to maintain an adequate oxygenation of the patient.

The crucial point of this correction is represented by tracheal surgery. The experience in the treatment of tracheal stenosis remains limited, and the size criteria for tracheoplasty have not been clearly established. Many techniques have been proposed with related advantages and disadvantages.

Direct resection of the stenotic segment and direct anastomosis are ideal for locally limited stenosis. Tracheal reconstruction using pericardial patch is an option for more extended narrowing but currently is less used due to associated problems like patch collapse or excessive phenomenon of granulation in the midterm follow-up. Nowadays the technique of choice is considered the slide tracheoplasty. This technique, firstly introduced by Tsang [10] and popularized by Grillo [11], is used currently both for localized and diffuse stenosis. The main advantage of this technique is the possibility of avoiding the use of graft material with immediate stability of the trachea, reducing the ventilation time and consequently the excessive granulation process.

The trachea is divided transversely at the midpoint of the narrow segment. Subsequently, a longitudinal incision of the proximal and distal segment of the divided trachea is performed. Such incision is carried across opposite (facing) walls of the two segments, in order to complete a sliding oblique anastomosis to restore a final large working diameter.

In some cases with associated tracheobronchomalacia, it may be necessary, after repair, to stabilize the trachea by placing endotracheal stents.

7.7 Treatment and Results

7.7.1 Vascular Rings

Surgery is recommended in all symptomatic patients, especially those with severe respiratory distress. In those patients, the surgery is mandatory in order to avoid tracheobronchial damage or unexpected and graves events, like sudden death.

Asymptomatic patients do not require surgical repair, unless surgical treatment of an associated congenital heart defect is necessary.

The surgical approach depends on the type of vascular rings or sling, and it may be performed by sternotomy, thoracotomy, or in specific cases video-assisted thoracoscopic surgery (VATS).

Nowadays the surgical correction of vascular rings can be carried out with low mortality and morbidity, as described by Backer and coll [12]. In a cohort of 209 patients, who underwent surgery between 1949 and 2003; there was no operative mortality since 1959, and morbidity was mainly related to airway issues: four patients (2 %) required late aortopexy for recurrence of airway symptoms.

Recently Ruzmetov and coll. reviewed their experience in the treatment of vascular rings from 1970 to 2008 in 183 patients [13]. There was no intraoperative mortality, but three patients died within 30 days of surgery; mean follow-up was 9 ± 8.3 years, and overall survival was 96 % at 35 years [13]. Overall freedom from reoperation was 100 % at 35 years, and 75 % were free from compressive symptoms within 1 year of the operation; none of the patients showed any evidence of recurrent vascular ring anomalies at the last follow-up [13].

7.7.2 Pulmonary Sling

In cases of diagnosis of pulmonary sling, the repair is mandatory, in order to avoid the progressive damage of the trachea and lung and dangerous asphyctic spells. The results of pulmonary sling surgery without tracheal repair are excellent with low mortality and morbidity, and also the repair of associated anomalies can be performed with no added mortality. Yong and colleagues reported no mortality in nine patients who undergone pulmonary sling surgery alone and 25 % of mortality in patients with associated airways surgery [14].

The most important factor to achieve good results in surgery of pulmonary sling seems to be the diameter of the trachea. Huang and colleagues reviewed a small number of patients who underwent treatment of pulmonary sling showing no mortality in the cohort of patients with internal tracheal diameter larger than 3 mm and in which it was not associated a tracheal surgery [15].

Surgical treatment of tracheal stenosis has been reported having different results due to the complexity of the anatomy (length of the narrowing and diameter of stenotic segment), the presence of tracheomalacia, and the type of surgical techniques.

Backer and colleagues, in their series of 28 patients treated with pericardial patch tracheoplasty, reported 6 % of early mortality and 18 % of late deaths [16].

Similar results (11 % of mortality) are reported by Fanous and colleagues in their series of 26 patients who undergone patch tracheoplasty [17].

Recently, several reports demonstrated that slide tracheoplasty is the technique of choice because it is burdened by a lower mortality and postoperative airway complications. Manning and colleagues reported an operative mortality of 2.5 % after slide tracheoplasty in 80 patients operated between 2001 and 2009 [18].

References

1. Ganie IS, Amod K, Reddy D (2015) Vascular rings: a radiological review of anatomical variations. Cardiovasc J Afr 26:1–7
2. Gross RE (1945) Surgical relief for tracheal obstruction from a vascular ring. N Engl J Med 233: 586–590
3. Woods RK, Sharp RJ, Holcomb GW 3rd, Snyder CL, Lofland GK, Ashcraft KW, Holder TM (2001) Vascular anomalies and tracheoesophageal compression: a single institution's 25-year experience. Ann Thorac Surg 72(2):434–438; discussion 438–439
4. McElhinney DB, Clark BJ 3rd, Weinberg PM, Kenton ML, McDonald-McGinn D, Driscoll DA, Zackai EH, Goldmuntz E (2001) Association of chromosome 22q11 deletion with isolated anomalies of aortic arch laterality and branching. J Am Coll Cardiol 37(8):2114–2119
5. Backer CL, Mavroudis C (2000) Congenital Heart Surgery Nomenclature and Database Project: vascular rings, tracheal stenosis, pectus excavatum. Ann Thorac Surg 69(4 Suppl):S308–S318
6. Lowe GM, Donaldson JS, Backer CL (1991) Vascular rings: 10-year review of imaging. Radiographics 11(4):637–646
7. Stojanovska J, Cascade PN, Chong S, Quint LE, Sundaram B (2012) Embryology and imaging review of aortic arch anomalies. J Thorac Imaging 27(2):73–84
8. Austin EH, Wolfe WG (1985) Aneurysm of aberrant subclavian artery with a review of the literature. J Vasc Surg 2(4):571–577
9. Cinà CS, Althani H, Pasenau J, Abouzahr L (2004) Kommerell's diverticulum and right-sided aortic arch: a cohort study and review of the literature. J Vasc Surg 39(1):131–139
10. Tsang V, Murday A, Gillbe C, Goldstraw P (1989) Slide tracheoplasty for congenital funnel-shaped tracheal stenosis. Ann Thorac Surg 48(5):632–635
11. Grillo HC (1994) Slide tracheoplasty for long-segment congenital tracheal stenosis. Ann Thorac Surg 58:613–619
12. Backer CL, Mavroudis C, Rigsby CK, Holinger LD (2005) Trends in vascular ring surgery. J Thorac Cardiovasc Surg 129(6):1339–1347
13. Ruzmetov M, Vijay P, Rodefeld MD, Turrentine MW, Brown JW (2009) Follow-up of surgical correction of aortic arch anomalies causing tracheoesophageal compression: a 38-year single institution experience. J Pediatr Surg 44(7):1328–1332
14. Yong MS, d'Udekem Y, Brizard CP, Robertson T, Robertson CF, Weintraub R, Konstantinov IE (2013) Surgical management of pulmonary artery sling in children. J Thorac Cardiovasc Surg 145(4):1033–1039
15. Huang SC, Wu ET, Wang CC, Chen SJ, Chen YS, Chang CI, Chiu IS, Wang SS (2012) Surgical management of pulmonary artery sling: trachea diameter and outcomes with or without tracheoplasty. Pediatr Pulmonol 47(9):903–908
16. Backer CL, Mavroudis C, Gerber ME, Holinger LD (2001) Tracheal surgery in children: an 18-year review of four techniques. Eur J Cardiothorac Surg 19(6):777–784
17. Fanous N, Husain SA, Ruzmetov M, Rodefeld MD, Turrentine MW, Brown JW (2010) Anterior pericardial tracheoplasty for long-segment tracheal stenosis: long-term outcomes. J Thorac Cardiovasc Surg 139(1):18–23
18. Manning PB, Rutter MJ, Lisec A, Gupta R, Marino BS (2011) One slide fits all: the versatility of slide tracheoplasty with cardiopulmonary bypass support for airway reconstruction in children. J Thorac Cardiovasc Surg 141(1):155–161

8 Congenital Esophageal Stenosis

Michela Maffi and Mario Lima

8.1 Introduction

Congenital esophageal stenosis (CES) is a rare entity with an estimated incidence of 1:25,000–50,000 live births [1]. This anomaly was first reported in 1936 by Frey and Duschl who described the case of a dead 19-year-old girl with a suspected diagnosis of achalasia. The necropsy revealed cartilage in the cardia [2]. At the beginning of the past century, all the esophageal stenoses diagnosed in newborn were considered congenital so that Sir Arthur Keith in a report of 1910 did not differentiate between esophageal stenosis and atresia [3]. CES was also described as a further type of esophageal atresia (EA) and included in Gross classification as type F [4].

8.2 Classification

The most used classification of CES has been proposed by Nihoul-Fèkètè et al. in 1987 [5]. This classification delineates three forms of CES:

1. Tracheobronchial remnant
2. Segmental fibromuscular hypertrophy
3. Membranous web

M. Maffi (✉) • M. Lima
Pediatric Surgery, S. Orsola-Malpighi Hospital, Bologna University, Via Massarenti 11, 40138 Bologna, Italy
e-mail: michela.maffi@libero.it; mario.lima@unibo.it

8.2.1 Tracheobronchial Remnant

The embryological origin of the cartilaginous ring is to be found in the separation of the primitive esophagus and respiratory diverticulum, which is performed by the tracheoesophageal septum, formed by the proliferation of cells starting from the lateral crests of the primitive foregut. It may happen that, with the consequent cranial lengthening of the esophagus and the respiratory tree, mesenchymal cells belonging to the respiratory diverticulum can remain embedded in the esophageal wall. These ectopic tissue remnants are typically represented by seromucinous respiratory glands, respiratory epithelium, and cartilaginous tissue. Stenosis results from extrinsic compression by the ectopic tissue, as well as from inextensibility caused by the structure of the cartilaginous tissue. Heterotopic tissue of the tracheobronchial origin is most frequently seen in the distal esophagus, particularly in the lower third with a preference to the cardia level.

8.2.2 Segmental Fibromuscular Hypertrophy

This form is characterized by subepithelial proliferation of the smooth muscle and fibrosis. The embryologic origin of the esophageal stricture has to be found in developmental defects incurred within the first 10 weeks of gestation. The primitive gut separates from the trachea for the formation

M. Lima (ed.), *Pediatric Digestive Surgery*, DOI 10.1007/978-3-319-40525-4_8

of a tracheoesophageal septum to approximately the 36th day of development. After 4 weeks, the muscular and submucosal layers are well represented. Subsequently, between the seventh and the eighth week of gestational life, there is a process of rapid proliferation of epithelial cells that leads to an almost complete closure of the primitive esophagus lumen except for small vacuolated areas that remain in the context of obliterated lumen. These areas, at the end of the 10th week of gestational age, give rise to a process of channeling which leads to the reformation of a tubular cavity. The primitive fetal esophageal epithelium is composed of ciliated cells that are being replaced, at about the 4th month, by stratified squamous epithelium. The fibromuscular stenosis is mainly located in the middle third and in the proximal part of the lower third of the esophagus.

8.2.3 Mucosal Web

The development of this web is similar to that of the diaphragm which can be located in any other intestinal tract. These membranes are in fact strictly related to defects of recanalization of the previously obliterated lumen which occurred during the 10th week of gestation. Histologically these diaphragms are composed only by mucosa and submucosa.

8.3 Associated Anomalies

CES can be associated with other congenital anomalies in 17–33 % of cases [6]. The most reported association is with esophageal atresia and/or tracheobronchial fistula whose frequency ranges from 3 to 14 % [1]. Other anomalies include chromosomal anomalies, cardiac anomalies, intestinal atresia, anorectal malformation, and trisomy 21 [1, 3].

8.4 Symptoms

The clinical feature of the complete esophageal web appears at birth, and it is the same for esophageal atresia, characterized by drooling, coughing, and regurgitation. The inability to place a nasogastric tube in the stomach confirms the diagnosis. However if the diaphragm is incomplete or broken, or in case of fibromuscular stenosis or cartilaginous ectopic tissue, the clinical onset occurs later in life, usually when solid foods are introduced in the diet. In the literature, it is reported that the onset of symptoms can occur in a wide range of age, from 1 day old to 57 years of age, but it usually takes place during the first year of life, with dysphagia, vomiting during meals, regurgitation of undigested food, insufficient growth, and relapsing pneumonia due to aspiration.

8.5 Diagnosis

The diagnosis of esophageal stenosis is not particularly difficult and is done with a *barium esophagogram* performed on the indication of the clinical feature (Fig. 8.1). Less simple and certainly more important for a correct surgical therapy is the differential diagnosis that must be made between the various forms of esophageal stenosis; among these, achalasia and peptic strictures may also be included.

The radiologic appearance is morphologically similar in all cases of esophageal stenosis: an important esophageal dilation followed by a threadlike narrowing. The site of the stricture can be useful to reach a first differential diagnosis. It has been seen how the three different forms of congenital cause have different favorite localizations.

The ectopic cartilaginous tissue is found in more than 90 % of cases in the lower third of the esophagus and especially near the cardia; fibromuscular stenosis is more frequently found between the middle and the lower third with a predilection for the proximal part of the latter; in achalasia instead, by definition, the stenotic portion is always located in the cardia.

A first rough differentiation between the three types of CES can be made by examining the patient. Symptoms caused by tracheobronchial remnants and fibromuscular stenosis are typical in early infancy, while those caused by achalasia

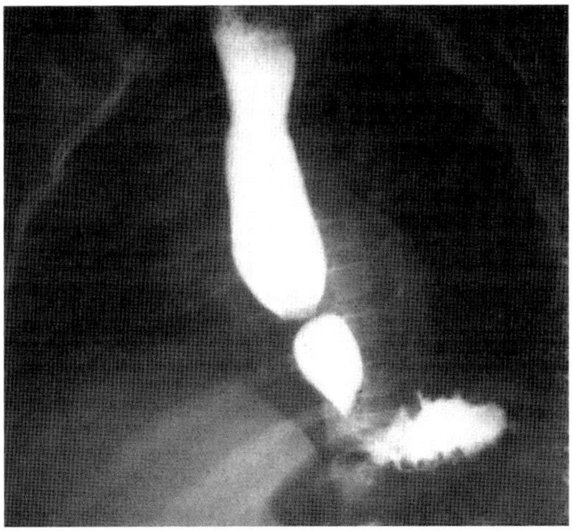

Fig. 8.1 Congenital stenosis of the distal third of the esophagus

usually occur later in school age; also peptic stricture typically affects older children. When radiographic examination is not able to identify the diagnosis, an *endoscopic study* can highlight the main characteristics of the lesion. The direct vision of the section affected by a peptic stricture will show an inflamed area also above the stenosis; the endoscopic images, associated with medical history and evaluation of symptoms, lead to the correct diagnosis. Regarding other types of stenosis, correct diagnosis can be made in the course of endoscopic examination, based on the ease or otherwise to overcome the restricted portion by the endoscope.

In case of achalasia, the cardia can be passed by the endoscope, forcing it kindly, and a mild dilation can be obtained, albeit only temporarily. In the presence of fibromuscular stenosis, the endoscope cannot exceed the stenotic tract that can be dilated with special probes. In ectopic cartilaginous ring, the direct vision does not allow the differential diagnosis, but the attempt to dilate the narrow tract is usually unsuccessful, and this causes the operator to desist. In case of cardia localization of fibromuscular stenosis, differential diagnosis with achalasia becomes more difficult and in some cases impossible even after endoscopy. Even if most of the patients' endoscopic examination can lead to diagnosis, further informations can be obtained with a manometric examination. Also the outcome of dilations can be used as a diagnostic criterion: in case of achalasia, improvement will only be transitional, while it will be present and often progressive in case of congenital stenosis sensitive to expansion.

Endoscopic ultrasonography (EUS) is a useful tool in differential diagnosis between the three types of congenital stenosis. In particular, EUS is able to evidence the presence of cartilage which is difficult to be seen with CT scan or MRI. EUS is available for pediatric patients from 2001, and recently, a 3D miniprobe has been used to obtain multiplanar and oblique views of the stenosis [7–9].

8.5.1 Therapy

The first-line treatment of CES is dilation. It can be performed with hydrostatic balloon probe or with Savary-Gilliard bougie. There is no strong evidence on which is the better technique, and the choice depends on the expertise of each center. Jones et al. reported advantages of balloon dilation because of radial and localized force applied by the baloon, rather than axial shearing force applied on stenosis by the bougie [10]. On the other hand, Romeo et al. reported a higher risk of perforation with balloon dilation affirming that bouginage seems safer [9]. An endoscopic check after dilation is mandatory, and in case of deep mucosal laceration, an esophagogram is recommended.

Whatever the technique chosen, the dilations are usually performed every 15 days until reaching a stable esophageal caliber. The subsequent dilations are established on the basis of clinics, age, and results obtained on each patient.

Some authors reported success in endoscopic electrocauterization or partial resection of mucosal web added to dilations [11, 12].

Fibromuscular stenosis and mucosal web usually respond successfully to dilations, while in case of cartilaginous remnant or dilation failure, it is necessary to undergo surgery (Fig. 8.2).

In these cases, the treatment of choice is the resection of the stenotic tract followed by end-to-end anastomosis (Fig. 8.3) and eventual fundoplication if the stenosis is closed to gastroesophageal

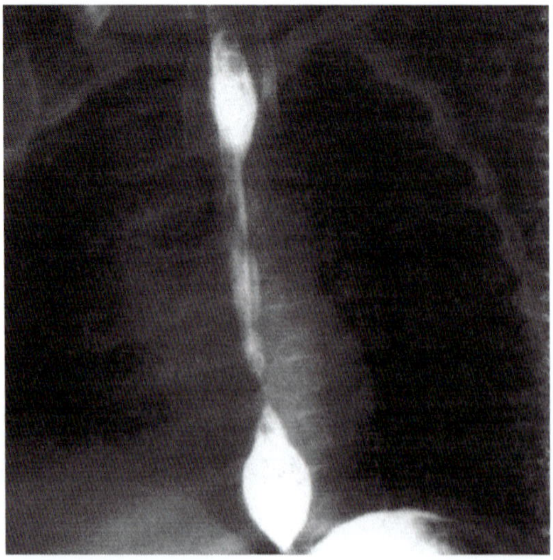

Fig. 8.2 Barium esophagogram after six dilations. The patient continued to complain of severe dysphagia

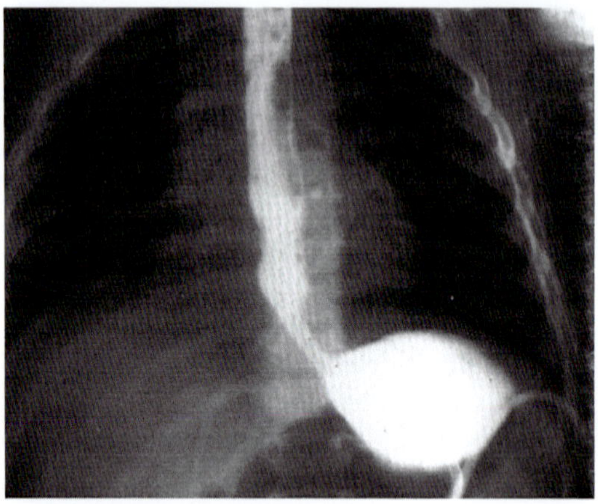

Fig. 8.3 The previous case after resection of the stenotic tract and end-to-end anastomosis

junction [2, 13]. The stricture can be identified externally by palpation or with the use of a catheter placed preoperatively. Maeda and Saito reported two patients affected by tracheobronchial remnant treated with circular extramucosal myectomy at the stenotic level followed by suture of the esophageal wall. This technique allows extirpation of the cartilage and muscular disarrangement avoiding lumen opening [14, 15].

8.6 Complications and Outcome

The most serious complication is surely the esophageal perforation whose reported incidence varies widely (from 10 to 44%) [9]. The treatment in these cases is initially conservative with fasting, nasogastric tube, and parenteral nutrition. In severe cases, segmental replacement of the esophagus may be necessary [13].

Despite various therapeutic options that could obtain a resolution of the stricture from a morphological point of view, a substantial proportion of patients (approximately 30–60%) continues to complain of dysphagia [7]. This suggests that these patients should be followed up for a long time.

References

1. McCann F, Michaud L, Aspirot A, Levesque D, Gottrand F, Faure C (2015) Congenital esophageal stenosis associated with esophageal atresia. Dis Esophagus 28(3):211–215
2. Rebelo PG, Ormonde JV, Ormonde Filho JB (2013) Congenital esophageal stenosis owing to tracheobronchial remnants. Rev Paul Pediatr 31(3):406–410
3. Appignani A (1993) Stenosi esofagee congenite. In: Dòmini R, Lima M (eds) Chirurgia delle malformazioni digestive. Piccin, Bologna
4. van Poll D, van der Zee DC (2012) Thoracoscopic treatment of congenital esophageal stenosis in combination with H-type tracheoesophageal fistula. J Pediatr Surg 47(8):1611–1613
5. Nihoul-Fèkètè C, De Backer A, Lortat-Jacob S et al (1987) Congenital esophageal stenosis: a review of 20 cases. Pediatr Surg Int 2:86–92
6. Vasudevan SA, Kerendi F, Lee H, Ricketts RR (2002) Management of congenital esophageal stenosis. J Pediatr Surg 37(7):1024–1026
7. Michaud L, Coutenier F, Podevin G et al (2013) Characteristics and management of congenital esophageal stenosis: findings from a multicenter study. Orphanet J Rare Dis 8:186
8. Bocus P, Realdon S, Eloubeidi MA, Diamantis G, Betalli P, Gamba P, Zanon GF, Battaglia G (2011) High-frequency miniprobes and 3-dimensional EUS for preoperative evaluation of the etiology of congenital esophageal stenosis in children (with video). Gastrointest Endosc 74(1):204–207
9. Romeo E, Foschia F, de Angelis P et al (2011) Endoscopic management of congenital esophageal stenosis. J Pediatr Surg 46(5):838–841

10. Jones DW, Kunisaki SM, Teitelbaum DH, Spigland NA, Coran AG (2010) Congenital esophageal stenosis: the differential diagnosis and management. Pediatr Surg Int 26(5):547–551
11. Chao HC, Chen SY, Kong MS (2008) Successful treatment of congenital esophageal web by endoscopic electrocauterization and balloon dilatation. J Pediatr Surg 43(1):e13–e15
12. Takamizawa S, Tsugawa C, Mouri N, Satoh S, Kanegawa K, Nishijima E, Muraji T (2002) Congenital esophageal stenosis: therapeutic strategy based on etiology. J Pediatr Surg 37(2):197–201
13. Amae S, Nio M, Kamiyama T, Ishii T, Yoshida S, Hayashi Y, Ohi R (2003) Clinical characteristics and management of congenital esophageal stenosis: a report on 14 cases. J Pediatr Surg 38(4):565–570
14. Maeda K, Hisamatsu C, Hasegawa T, Tanaka H, Okita Y (2004) Circular myectomy for the treatment of congenital esophageal stenosis owing to tracheobronchial remnant. J Pediatr Surg 39(12):1765–1768
15. Saito T, Ise K, Kawahara Y, Yamashita M, Shimizu H, Suzuki H, Gotoh M (2008) Congenital esophageal stenosis because of tracheobronchial remnant and treated by circular myectomy: a case report. J Pediatr Surg 43(3):583–585

9 Achalasia and Esophageal Motility Disorders

Olivier Reinberg

9.1 Etiology and Pathogenesis

Esophageal achalasia (EA) is a rare functional motility disorder of the esophagus of unknown origin, characterized by abnormal motility of the body of the esophagus associated with delayed or absent relaxation of the lower esophageal sphincter (LES), inducing stasis in the esophagus with subsequent dilatation.

Sir Thomas Willis described the disease in 1674 [1]. He did the first mechanical dilatation for achalasia, using an orally inserted cork-tipped whalebone. In 1881, Mikulicz described the disease as a cardiospasm, i.e., the symptoms were due to a functional problem rather than a mechanical one. Ernst Heller realized the first myotomy to release the symptoms in 1914 [2]. The procedure done by Heller was an anterior and a posterior myotomy. However it is still named after him, even if the procedure today differs. In 1929, Hurt and Rake realized that the disease was caused by a failure of LES to relax and coined the term achalasia (i.e., failure to relax).

The highest incidence in adults is between the fourth and seventh decades. Children count for 5 % of all cases of achalasia; thus it is an uncommon condition in pediatric population, appearing in 0.1–1/100,000 annually between 7 and 13 years of age. However today, progresses make diagnosis earlier than before. Our youngest patient was 1.1 year old [3–9].

The etiology is unknown. Achalasia is believed to be an acquired functional esophageal motility disorder. However its physiopathology remains unclear, and possibly there are several forms of the disease with different etiologies including primary disorder of the esophagus and "partial" achalasia. This could explain that the results of treatments are not as good as expected. Several studies have suggested that the genetic background may have a role in the pathogenesis [10]. It could be an autoimmune disease, genetically determined, then triggered by viral (*Herpes*), bacterial, or parasitic (Chagas' disease caused by *Trypanosoma cruzi*) infections resulting in a loss in inhibitory neurons of myenteric plexus [11, 12]. In some patients it could be malformative very similar to Hirschsprung's disease. The genetic theory is supported by the high frequency of congenital anomalies or associated syndromes such as the Down syndrome, the Allgrove syndrome (AAA syndrome, addisonianism-alacrima-achalasia), the congenital central hypoventilation syndrome, the Rozycki syndrome (deafness, vitiligo, esophageal achalasia), and the Hirschsprung disease [10, 13–16]. Achalasia is frequent in siblings or can be familial with an autosomal recessive mode [10, 17, 18]. It is frequently associated with an eosinophilic esophagitis.

O. Reinberg
Pediatric Surgery,
Rochettaz 24, CH – 1009 Pully, Switzerland
e-mail: olreinberg@gmail.com

M. Lima (ed.), *Pediatric Digestive Surgery*, DOI 10.1007/978-3-319-40525-4_9

However, this explains only partially the pathogenesis. Histology, electron microscopy, and immunohistochemistry provide answers. The Italian Camillo Golgi (1843–1926) invented the fixation and tissue stainings with methylene blue and silver impregnation. Thanks to this, the Spanish Santiago Ramon y Cajal (1852–1934) described the neuron and the organization of the central nervous system. They got together the Nobel Prize of Medicine for that in 1906. In 1911, Cajal, searching for a neural network to study, simpler than the brain, used the rabbit small intestine to find interstitial cells he believed to be the end cells of the sympathetic nervous system. His drawings of what we call after him the Interstitial Cells of Cajal (ICC) are still accurate. ICC can be studied due to electron microscopy and immunohistochemical staining for c-Kit [19].

The ICC are related to intestinal pacemaker activity [20]. However the esophagus has very few ICC associated with the myenteric plexus but has abundant intramuscular ICC (ICC-IM) dispersed throughout the circular and longitudinal muscle layers. ICC-IM are thought to be involved in pacemaking and slow-wave propagation in the stomach [20]. Three types of ICC have been described: the ICC-MY, ICC-IM, and ICC-SEP [20–23]. They are located, respectively, in the myenteric plexus between the circular and longitudinal muscle layers, within the muscle layers and within the septa between the circular muscle bundles. ICC are most frequent in the esophageal part of the LES but rare in the gastric part. The absence or reduction in the number of ICC causes abnormal electrical slow waves with a decreased contractility of smooth muscle cells, resulting in a diminished intestinal transit. Impaired production of nitric oxide (NO) and vasoactive intestinal peptide (VIP) affects both ICC and muscles thus inhibiting relaxation of the LES as it has already been suggested in intestinal pseudo-obstruction and Hirschsprung's disease [19, 24]. Anomalies of the ICC have been evocated in diseases such as idiopathic gastric perforation, hypertrophic pyloric stenosis, intestinal pseudo-obstruction, meconium ileus, and Hirschsprung's disease [21, 25]. Thus debated, ICC involvement in achalasia is highly probable [19, 21]. What is known today is that patients with achalasia have a loss of myenteric plexus and enteric neurons; a loss in number and modifications of the ultrastructure of the ICC, being replaced by fibrosis or inflammation ("plexitis"); and no immunoreactivity for VIP [19, 26, 27].

Because of the relatively low incidence of the disease in children, our knowledge is based on small series or extrapolated from adult studies. We ignore if achalasia in children differs from that in adults. For instance, esophageal manometry has allowed better description of esophageal primary disorders in children such as partial achalasia with various clinical conditions [28]. Unfortunately, no clinical or manometric features can differentiate the patients who present a favorable outcome under medication from those requiring surgery.

In addition, the environment could play a role that is not known yet. So achalasia appears to be a multifactorial and multimodal disease that remains partially understood.

9.2 Diagnosis and Pretreatment Work-Up

9.2.1 Symptoms

Achalasia can be difficult to recognize because there may be nonspecific symptoms that may include feeding aversion, failure to thrive, nonspecific regurgitation suggestive of gastroesophageal reflux (GER), and respiratory symptoms. The diagnosis is often delayed.

The most common complain is dysphagia. Children progressively refuse food intake, and then have special vomitings whose content is related to undigested previous meals. Dysphagia begins with solids but can reach the point where liquids cannot be absorbed (paroxysmal dysphagia). They complain retrosternal pains and pyrosis. Their relatives notice fetor. Secondary signs are dehydration, failure to thrive, and weight loss. Due to aspirations, respiratory symptoms (cough and repeated pneumonia) are often present [5, 7–9, 29].

9.2.2 Upper Gastrointestinal Contrast Study

The most common investigations performed in children are upper gastrointestinal contrast study (UGI) and manometry. The use of barium should be avoided in case of aspiration, and hydrosoluble contrasts should be preferred for the UGI. X-ray studies classically demonstrate a dilated esophagus that ends with "bird's beak" like tapering of the distal esophagus. The presence or the absence of esophageal contractions on serial views should be mentioned (Fig. 9.1).

Even if the esophagogram study alone with all the classical signs can be pathognomonic, as the disease is not clearly understood and as many variations may occur, it is wise to confirm the achalasia with an esophageal manometry [30].

9.2.3 Esophageal Manometry

Esophageal manometry should be performed following the recommendations of the North American Society for Pediatric Gastroenterology, Hepatology, and Nutrition (NASPGHAN) [31], the American Gastroenterological Association [32], and other experts [29, 33, 34]. However, the adult recommendation to use a continuously perfused low-compliance system should not be followed in infants as it may provide an unacceptable amount of water in the esophagus. Thus miniature strain-gauge pressure transducers mounted within thin pediatric catheters should be preferred. Manometries should not be done under sedation, but we place the catheter using inhaled equimolecular mixture of oxygen and nitrous oxide (EMONO, equivalent of MEOPA) [35, 36].

Elevated resting LES pressure (>22 ± 10 mmHg), absent or low-amplitude peri-

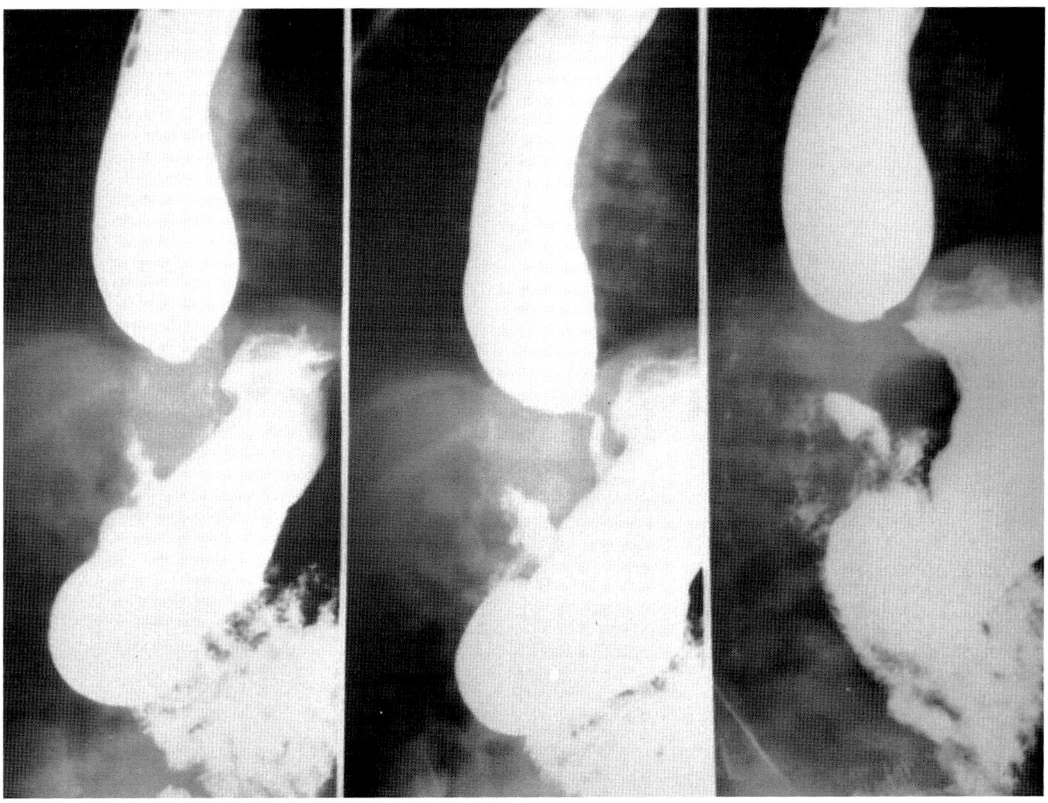

Fig. 9.1 Upper gastrointestinal contrast study showing a dilated esophagus that ends with "bird's beak" and the absence of esophageal contractions on serial views

stalsis, or non-relaxing LES upon swallowing (relaxation rate <90 %) are diagnostic findings on esophageal manometry in children [4, 6, 17, 37]. However, the absence of some of these findings does not rule out the diagnosis of achalasia as LES function in children is heterogeneous. Partial relaxations are common, and normal LES relaxations after wet swallows may also be present on manometries [29]. Only 4.2 % patients had all four common manometric features (elevated LES pressure, abnormal LES relaxation, aperistalsis, increased intraesophageal pressure) for achalasia in Agrawal's study (children and adults). Most of the 72 patients of his series had elevated increased intraesophageal pressure, elevated LES relaxation pressure, normal LES pressure, and low baseline impedance. The resting LES pressure can be normal in up to 40–70 % of achalasia patients [30].

9.2.4 Intraluminal Impedancemetry

Intraluminal impedancemetry (IIM) allows intraluminal measurements of electric impedance between several closely arranged electrodes during bolus passage. Impedance is inversely proportional to conductivity. When a highly conductive material is present inside the esophagus, the impedance decreases, i.e., with reflux, and increases with air. Combined multichannel IIM and esophageal manometry offers the ability to evaluate the relationship between esophageal contraction and bolus transit during the same swallow [30, 38]. Impaired bolus flow for liquid and viscous is found in most patients with achalasia as a translation of the aperistalsis of the esophagus. Thus, those combined investigations are useful to ensure achalasia and to understand the behavior of the esophagus.

9.2.5 High-Resolution Manometry (HRM)

The recently introduced high-resolution manometry (HRM) enlarges diagnostic investigations in esophageal dysmotility and may replace conventional manometry. However, the experience with using HRM in children is limited [39, 40]. HRM combines improvements in pressure-sensing technology with a greatly increased number of pressure sensors. In conventional manometry, the pressure sensors are spaced at 3–5 cm intervals. In HRM, 36 sensors are spaced at 1 cm and distributed longitudinally and radially along the probe. This allows simultaneous pressure recording in the esophagus. During swallow, the movements and pressure are recorded giving a topographic and cinematic view of the pressures in the esophagus from UES to LES. Pressure magnitude is encoded in color, conventionally in red for high pressures and blue for low [41].

This technique discriminates between different types of achalasia according to the LES but also to the intraesophageal pressure and movements. Thereby, achalasia has been classified into three types based on esophageal motility but helps to describe many other esophageal motility disorders as well (The Chicago Classification [42]). It provides an algorithmic scheme for diagnosis of esophageal motility disorders. Type I is characterized by the failed relaxation of the LES and 100 % failed peristalsis; Type II involves failed relaxation of the LES with no normal peristalsis and panesophageal pressurization with ≥20 % of swallows; Type III, or spastic achalasia, associates failed relaxation of the LES, with preserved fragments of distal peristalsis or premature (spastic) contractions with ≥20 % of swallows. Many other esophageal motility disorders are described such as distal esophageal spasm, hypercontractile esophagus, and absent peristalsis and statistically defined peristaltic abnormalities (weak peristalsis, frequent failed peristalsis, rapid contractions with normal latency, and hypertensive peristalsis). This Chicago classification has occasionally been used in children [39].

This technique contributes to better understand the variations of the outcomes after different treatments, as it appears that achalasia is not a unique pathology but that this term covers different diseases.

9.2.6 Endoscopy

Some authors use endoscopy only in case of unclear diagnosis. However, as others, we believe performing systematically an upper endoscopy is reasonable to rule out esophagitis, *Trypanosoma cruzi*, and other secondary causes of achalasia, eventually with biopsies [43]. In some cases we found food impactions filling the esophagus (like a fecaloma in the esophagus) that was not easy to empty. Once done, there was such an important underlying esophagitis that we postponed the surgery to give time to the inflammation to decrease and avoid perforation when doing the myotomy.

The Society of American Gastrointestinal and Endoscopic Surgeons (SAGES) provides guidelines on esophageal achalasia. The recommendations are that patients with suspected achalasia should undergo an UGI, an upper endoscopy, and an esophageal manometry to confirm the diagnosis, with strong evidences (level 3+) according to the GRADE system [44].

9.3 Treatments of Achalasia

As the pathogenesis of the disease remains unknown, no etiological therapy is available. Treatments focus on relief of symptoms by reducing the functional obstruction caused by a non-relaxing LES, in the hope that can restore esophageal emptying and peristalsis. They include medications, chemical paralysis of the LES, mechanical or pneumatic dilatations, and endoscopic or surgical esophagomyotomies with or without fundoplications. Because of the low incidence of the disease in children, treatments are based on small case series or extrapolated from adult studies. To date, there is no prospective randomized trial in the pediatric literature on achalasia, and a meta-analysis on seven retrospective reports is not conclusive due to the heterogeneity of the study designs and the various methods of treatment used both within and between studies [45]. Unfortunately adequate comparative data are lacking to determine the ideal treatment of pediatric achalasia.

9.3.1 Medications

Medications should be used sublingually because of the unpredictability of absorption if orally given. Nifedipine, a calcium channel blocker, inhibits the transmembrane calcium influx in cardiac and smooth muscle and has been primarily used to release the LES in adults, with efficiency between 13 and 19 % [46, 47]. It should be given 10–30 mg sublingually 30–45 min before meals in adults [44].

Other substances have been used in adults: long-acting nitrates (isosorbide dinitrate) and phosphodiesterase-5 inhibitors (sildenafil). There are few reports of short series on the use of nifedipine in children but with good results [48]. However the benefits are temporary, and the treatment cannot be used for long-lasting therapy due to secondary effects (orthostatic hypotension, headaches) occurring in 30 % of patients. However, it can be used as a bridge to relieve symptoms until another treatment is undertaken.

The SAGES recommendations are that medications play a very limited role in the treatment of achalasia and should be used in very early stages of the disease, temporarily before more definitive treatments, or for patients who fail or are not candidates for other treatment modalities with strong evidences (level 4+) according to the GRADE system [44].

9.3.2 Botulinum Toxin

Botulinum toxin is a potent neurotoxin that inhibits the release of acetylcholine at presynaptic terminals of motor neurons. It is endoscopically injected into the LES in the four quadrants [49]. Botulinum toxin has been used as diagnostic and therapeutic purposes. In children, the dose and the timing of injection frequency have not been well defined. Its effect is temporary, and the mean duration of symptom relief is 4 months in children, thus requiring repeated treatments [50]. In the 2014 Cochrane database, 80 % of patients experienced an immediate relief of their symptoms, but the recurrence rate was 60 % within a year [47, 51]. In the SAGES statements, 85 % of patients were initially improved, but the effect diminished over time (50 % at 6 months and 30 % at 1 year), and universal symptomatic relapse occurred at 2 years [44]. In case of failure, these patients need surgical treatments. They are the most difficult cases for the surgeons as the inflammation induced by the toxin evolves toward a fibrosis between the mucosa and the muscular layers with a subsequent increased risk of perforation [43, 44].

9.3.3 Dilatations

The aim of dilatations is to mechanically enlarge the LES. This can be done either using pneumatic dilatations or with bougies as the Savary-Gilliard bougies (M. Savary was our Chief of ENT in Lausanne, Switzerland) under general anesthesia in children. Both are endoscopically placed over a guidewire under fluoroscopic guidance. In both techniques, even under view control, passing the LES with the guidewire can be difficult in those cases where it is firmly tight. When using balloon dilatators, a radial pressure is performed on the LES that some authors thought to be better than a longitudinal direction of dilatations as done with the other method. When using balloon dilatations, it can be difficult to control the strength of expansion when the balloon inflates suddenly. For this reason, Savary's technique is softer and more progressive. Our belief is that all different techniques should be available and adapted to each case and dilatation. Multiple dilatations are often required [52]. The choice of dilator size is based on the size of the child. The sizes range from 12 to 35 mm [6, 45, 53, 54] The greater number of sessions per child varies from two to five [45].

Dilatations bear an immediate risk of perforation estimated at 2.4 % (0.5–5.6 %) [53, 55, 56], and 50 % or more of these patients with perforations required emergency surgery [57]. In addition, the release of the LES may induce a gastroesophageal reflux disease (GERD).

In the Cochrane database (children and adults), the initial release of symptoms was 70 %, and 40–50 % of patients remained asymptomatic after a year and several dilatations [47]. Hamza has reported a 90 % success rate in children treated with multiple pneumatic dilatations [54]. After dilatations, 61 % of patients were asymptomatic at 5 years of follow-up and 47 % at 10 years [55, 56]. These results are worse than those after surgery (see below). No long-term follow-up studies after dilatations are available for children. The advantages of dilatations are a shorter length of stay and decreased costs [53].

Many adult studies compare the effects of dilatation with laparoscopic Heller myotomy (LHM), with an advantage for the surgery on short- and long-term follow-up [57, 58]. The same results have been reported in pediatric series [6]. Some authors advocate for dilatations in older children suffering achalasia as safe and effective initial treatments thus avoiding surgery [53, 54, 59]. However, surgery after dilatations has an increased risk of perforation due to scarring adhesions between the mucosa and the muscle layers, not as high as after botulinum toxin but higher than if done as a first procedure.

The SAGES recommends dilatations as the most effective nonoperative treatment. However, it is associated with the highest risk of complications. It should be considered in selected patients who refuse surgery or are poor operative candidates with strong evidences (level 4+) according to the GRADE system [44].

9.3.4 Peroral Endoscopic Myotomy (POEM)

POEM is a new endoscopic technique for achalasia introduced by Inoue in 2008 [60]. It is one of the applications of the natural orifice transluminal endoscopic surgery (NOTES) concept. Under endoscopic vision, a mucosal incision is performed ≈ 15–20 cm above the LES. Then a submucosal tunnel is done downward to allow an endoscopic section of the muscular layers. At the end of the procedure, endoscopic clips are placed on the mucosal wound. To date, more than 3000 patients have been operated, and the number of publications is increasing. Some small pediatric and adolescent series have been reported, all but one including less than ten cases [61–64], the latest with 27 cases [65]. The youngest operated child was 3, suffering severe growth retardation, achalasia, and Down's syndrome [66]. Li gives a detailed description of the pediatric procedure with references for the equipments [63]. The selected cases had no previous treatment, and the reported problems are related to firm adhesions between the mucosa and the muscle. Caldaro has published a comparative study in children receiving nine LHM vs nine POEM with no conclusive results, but the series is very small [62].

In adults, there are 16 % reported minor complications and 3 % severe but nonfatal, as to mention: emphysema, pneumothorax (0.2 %), pneumoperitoneum (8.3 %), bleedings (1 %), leaks 0.2 %, and prolonged hospital stay >5 days (1 %) [67].

The results seem good with 82–100 % immediate relief of symptoms, but the longest follow-up published is 16–24 months [67–69]. The mean GERD rate is 35 % (limits 15–46 %). In the pediatric series by Chen, during the follow-up period of 24 months, 19.2 % patients develop a GERD [65]. A randomized study with a 6 months follow-up reports no difference between LHM and POEM [67]. However LHM has been shown to provide more durable symptom relief [70] and additionally could result in less post-intervention GER [71].

9.3.5 Surgeries

9.3.5.1 Heller Myotomy

The Heller myotomy is performed today doing an anterior incision of the muscular layers of the esophagus, approximately 5 cm above the esophagogastric junction and carried onto the gastric wall by 2–3 cm. Laparoscopic Heller myotomy (LHM) is the treatment of choice in adults and in children giving advantages of less pain, better cosmesis, shorter hospital stay, and faster return to normal activity [37, 43, 59, 72–74]. A survey concerning 64 pediatric centers worldwide done by Myers in 1994 could only conclude that "cardiomyotomy performed by the abdomen gives best results" [75]. The highly debated point is whether it is necessary or not to add a fundoplication to reduce the occurrence of iatrogenic GERD.

The HLM in children is performed under general anesthesia. We set the child supine at the foot end of the table, the legs being wrapped in the "frog position" for infants or extended on stirrups, with the knees slightly flexed by 20–30° in children and adolescents. The table is tilted to a 30° reverse Trendelenburg position. The surgeon stands at the foot of the table, facing the hiatus. A transumbilical port is inserted according to the Hasson technique for a 5 mm × 30° angulated telescope. We work with three ports (3 or 5 mm according to the age), the right upper one for an atraumatic liver retractor and the two remaining ones for the working instruments. The cardiophrenic membrane is opened anteriorly. The anterior face of the esophagus is freed by 5–8 cm according to the patient's size. The anterior vagus nerve is identified and mobilized so that the myotomy can be done high up on the esophagus beneath the nerve. We do not dissect the esophagus posteriorly, so we do not surround the esophagus with a traction loop. Traction is applied on the stomach below the esophagogastric junction using a Babcock clamp, to expose the anterior part of the distal esophagus. The myotomy is started on the esophagus just above the gastroesophageal junction with an incision in the anterior muscular wall down to the mucosa. Usually the mucosa separates easily from the muscular layers, if there have been no previous treatment with botulinum toxin or dilatations. The muscular section is done according to the surgeons' preference with scissors, with a monopolar hook, with a sealing-cutting device (LigaSure® LS 1500 Dolphin Tip or Maryland laparoscopic instrument by Covidien), or with a harmonic dissector (Ultracision® by Ethicon). A great care should be taken to lift up the muscle from the mucosa when using a monopolar hook or a harmonic dissector as those instruments heat and can perforate. The muscular incision must be undertaken down on the anterior face of the stomach by 2–2.5 cm. The transition from esophageal to gastric muscle fibers can be seen as they change from a horizontal circular orientation to an oblique one and are more adhered to the mucosa. This ensures having been enough downward. It is mandatory to check the integrity of the mucosa after the myotomy. This can be done using instilled water, air, or methylene blue in the esophagus at the level of the myotomy or better, as we do, performing a peroperative endoscopy for both perforation and adequacy of the myotomy. In case of a tear in the mucosa, an attempt of suture can be done, and we leave a suction probe at the level of the leak for a few days. Then according to the surgeon's preferences, an anti-reflux wrap can be built.

Antibiotics are not given routinely. Without perforation, the child is orally fed in the operative day or the next one. Some authors perform systematically an UGI to check the integrity of the esophagus before discharging the child [9, 37]. We do not.

The Cochrane review and other studies report good initial results after LHM, with 88–97 % relief of symptoms [44, 47, 51, 76]. This improvement appears to be long lasting. However, 79 % of patients remain asymptomatic after 5 years of follow-up and 76 % at 10 years [44, 55, 56].

Complications of surgery are related to perforations and GERD. Perforation rates occur from 0 to 15 % in large series [72, 77, 78]. Most of them heal spontaneously if recognized. In their comparative adult series, Weber and Chen have evidenced a higher risk of perforation with LHM (4.8 %) than with dilatations (2.4 %). However it should be noticed that the rate of reoperations was far smaller in the LHM group (0.6 %) than in the dilatation (2.4 %) as most of the perforations due to dilatations have been ignored whereas the one done under LHM are immediately identified and treated [55, 56].

The rate of perforation rises significantly during a redo procedure ranging from 4.7 to 30 % [58]. Several studies have suggested an increased risk of perforations during LHM up to 28 %, after previous endoscopic treatment (botulinum toxin or balloon dilatations). Reversely, other studies found no association between preoperative endoscopic treatment and perforations. The warning from the SAGES is that previous endoscopic treatment for achalasia may be associated with higher myotomy morbidity, but the literature is inconclusive. Then a careful approach by an experienced team is advisable [44].

9.3.5.2 Anti-reflux Procedures

A fundoplication can be added to prevent GERD following Heller myotomy. Whether it should be done, and with which wrap, is one of the most debated points among surgeons. Several authors don't believe it necessary, including in children [72, 79]. If done, several anti-reflux procedures can be used: a total fundoplication (loose 360° Nissen) [77, 80], a partial posterior 270° wrap (Toupet) [57, 81], or an anterior 180° wrap (Dor or Thal) [6, 37, 43, 74].

Several adult studies have compared the LHM with and without anti-GER procedure with an advantage for the combined procedure summarized by Tsuboi [57]. The 2012 guidelines of the SAGES also strongly recommended a combination of laparoscopic myotomy with anti-reflux surgery [44]. They did not precise which type of procedure is the best, as long as it is a partial one. The circular fundoplication (i.e., the Nissen) should be avoided because of the risk of persistence and/or recurrence of the disease.

The most efficient anti-GER is the Nissen. However, even a loose Nissen applies a pressure on an LES that we wanted to release [9, 72]. When doing a Toupet, the two rows of stitches of the 270° wrap are tied to the edges of the myotomy. Those who advocate for a Toupet believe that it helps to keep the myotomy open. On the other hand, a Toupet leaves the anterior mucosa exposed without coverage. Finally, both the Nissen and the Toupet require posterior dissections of the hiatus, which is not the case with an anterior wrap that preserves the periesophageal ligaments. In addition the anterior wrap protects the uncovered esophageal mucosa.

In a randomized controlled study on 144 adult patients followed up during 125 months, Rebecchi determined that laparoscopic Dor fundoplication after a LHM was superior to Nissen fundoplication because the recurrence rate of dysphagia was significantly higher in patients who received a Nissen fundoplication (15 %) than a Dor (2.8 %) [80]. However, as Franklin we wonder if recurrence of the dysphagia is a failure of the surgical treatment or is related to the nature of disease [37]. A pediatric multicenter prospective study, published by Rawlins and involving 85 children followed up for 36 months, compared LHM and Dor or Toupet showing no difference of the De Meester scores at pH-metries performed 6 and 12 months postoperatively. The conclusion was that "LHM provides significant improvement in dysphagia and regurgitation symptoms in achalasia patients regardless of the type of partial fundoplication" [82].

Laparoscopic surgery for esophageal achalasia provides symptomatic improvement, but some patients have a poor outcome. It can be related to the surgery (insufficient myotomy, too tight wrap, too lose wrap with subsequent esophagitis) thus requiring redo procedure. Esposito suggested that the experience contributes to decrease the rate of complications since their incidence of postoperative dysphagia dropped from 50 to 16 % with further experience [74]. Patients with severe preoperative dysphagia, aperistalsis, or esophageal dilatation have greater risks of a poor outcome [81]. Favorable factors in adults are the short duration of the symptoms without previous use of botulinum toxin [83]. An initial LES pressure >35 mmHg had more than 21 times the likelihood to achieve excellent dysphagia relief after myotomy as compared with those with an LES pressure ≤35 mmHg [84].

High-resolution manometry (HRM) has evidenced that there might be several types of achalasia and esophageal dysmotility including in children who may have primary dysmotility and "partial" achalasia [28, 32, 47]. To date, no investigation has a predictive value. However, several studies have evaluated the treatment outcome by type on HRM. The analysis found that Type II had the greatest therapeutic response (95.3 %), followed by Type I (85.4 %), and then Type III (69.4 %) [32, 85–87]. Thus, possibly Type III is another misunderstood form of the disease for which a new treatment should be developed. Very recently Sodikoff has reported a correlation between HMR types of achalasia and the immunohistological findings on surgical biopsies of the muscularis propria obtained from 46 patients during LHM [27].

9.4 Long-Term Follow-Up and Cancer

Chronic irritation of the esophageal mucosa increases the risk of squamous cell carcinoma and/or adenocarcinoma. Long-lasting achalasia increases 16 times the risk of developing a cancer. Due to residual GERD and poor peristalsis, the risk persists even after (surgical) treatment [88]. The risk of both squamous cell carcinoma and adenocarcinoma of the esophagus is believed to be significantly increased in patients with achalasia; however the absolute excess risk is small [89]. Leeuwenburgh has statistically evaluated the risk of cancer in non-treated achalasia vs treated by dilatations. The conclusion was that Barrett's esophagus is incidentally diagnosed in untreated achalasia patients despite high LES pressures but is more common after successful treatment, especially in the presence of hiatal hernia. Patients treated for achalasia should be considered for GERD treatment and surveillance of development of Barrett's esophagus, in particular, when they have low LES pressures and a hiatal hernia [90]. Thus, some authors recommend to perform repeated endoscopies since the second decade [76]. However, given limited data and conflicting opinions, it is unknown whether consensus regarding screening practices in achalasia among experts exists. Ravi created a worldwide survey distributed to 28 experts to assess screening practices in achalasia. While 82 % of experts endorsed long-term follow-up of patients, no consensus was found regarding its timing [91].

Conclusions

The pathogenesis of esophageal achalasia is not elucidated, and the pathogenic mechanism is not understood. Many questions remain unanswered. We don't know why we have a depletion of ICC and could this possibly be responsible for the lack of LES relaxation, because of missing inhibitory neurotransmission. Does achalasia in children differ from adults? Are biopsies with c-Kit staining of predictive value? The answers to these questions will help to promote optimal treatment in the future. At the moment, the LHM has become a good option for the treatment of achalasia. It gives symptomatic improvement to the majority of patients but not complete resolution of their disease.

References

1. Willis T (1674) The companation of madication and surgery of esophageal achalasia. In: Willis T (eds) Achalasia. Hgas-comitis, London, pp 18–19
2. Heller E (1914) Extramukose cardioplastik beim chronischen cardiospasmus mit dilatation des oesophagus. Mitt Grenzgeb Med Chir 27:141–145
3. Mattioli G, Cagnazzo A, Barabino A et al (1997) The surgical approach to oesophageal achalasia. Eur J Pediatr Surg 7(6):323–327
4. Walzer N, Hirano I (2008) Achalasia. Gastroenterol Clin North Am 37:807–825
5. Mayberry JF, Mayell MJ (1988) Epidemiological study of achalasia in children. Gut 29:90–93
6. Lee CW, Kays DW, Chen MK et al (2010) Outcomes of treatment of childhood achalasia. J Pediatr Surg 45:1173–1177
7. Hallal C, Kieling CO, Nunes DL et al (2012) Diagnosis, misdiagnosis, and associated diseases of achalasia in children and adolescents: a twelve-year single center experience. Pediatr Surg Int 28:1211–1217
8. Appignani A, Paico E, Lima M et al (1991) What is the role of achalasia in infancy? Presented at the OESO congress 1991. OESO Knowledge online, Volume: Primary Motility Disorders of the Esophagus Chapter: Infants and children https://www.hon.ch/OESO/books/Vol_4_Prim_Motility/Articles/ART345.HTML. Accessed 7 Jan 2016
9. Carlucci M, Mattioli G, Jasonni V (2013) Esophageal achalasia. In: Pediatric thoracic surgery. Mario LIMA Ed. Springer-Verlag, Italia
10. Gockel HR, Sehumacher J, Gockel I et al (2010) Achalasia: will genetic studies provide insights? Hum Genet 128:353–364
11. Boeckxstaens GE (2008) Achalasia: virus-induced euthanasia of neurons? Am J Gastroenterol 103: 1610–1612
12. Park W, Vaezi MF (2005) Etiology and pathogenesis of achalasia: The current understanding. Am J Gastroenterol 100:1404–1414
13. Ambrosino MM, Genieser NB, Bangaru BS et al (1986) The syndrome of achalasia of the esophagus, ACTH insensitivity and alacrima. Pediatr Radiol 16(4):328–329
14. Huebner A, Yoon SJ, Ozkinay F et al (2000) Triple A syndrome–clinical aspects and molecular genetics. Endocr Res 26(4):751–759
15. Prpic I, Huebner A, Persic M et al (2003) Triple A syndrome: genotype-phenotype assessment. Clin Genet 63(5):415–417
16. Zárate N, Mearin F, Hidalgo A et al (2001) Prospective evaluation of esophageal motor dysfunction in Down's syndrome. Am J Gastroenterol 96(6): 1718–1724
17. Zhang Y, Xu CD, Zaouche A, Cai W (2009) Diagnosis and management of esophageal achalasia in children: analysis of 13 cases. World J Pediatr 5(1):56–59
18. Chen CP, Lin SP, Lee CC et al (2006) Partial trisomy 1p (1p36.22→pter) and partial monosomy 9p (9p22.2→pter) associated with achalasia, flexion deformity of the fingers and epilepsy in a girl. Genet Couns 17(3):301–306
19. Gockel I, Bohl JRE, Eckardt VF et al (2007) Reduction of interstitial cells of Cajal (ICC) associated with neuronal nitric oxide synthase (n-NOS) in patients with achalasia. Am J Gastroenterol 102:1–9
20. Huizinga JD, Chen JH, Mikkelsen HB et al (2013) Interstitial cells of Cajal, from structure to function. Front Neurosci 7(43):1–3
21. Mostafa RM, Moustafa YM, Hamdy H (2010) Interstitial cells of Cajal, the Maestro in health and disease. World J Gastroenterol 16(26):3239–3248
22. Hirst GD (2001) An additional role for ICC in the control of gastrointestinal motility? J Physiol 537(1):1
23. Kraichely RE, Farrugia G (2006) Achalasia: physiology and etiopathogenesis. Dis Esophagus 19: 213–223
24. Hoshino M, Omura N, Yano F et al (2013) Immunohistochemical study of the muscularis externa of the esophagus in achalasia patients. Dis Esophagus 26(1):14–21
25. Streutker CJ, Huizinga JD, Driman DK et al (2007) Interstitial cells of Cajal in health and disease. Part I: normal ICC structure and function with associated motility disorders. Histopathology 50(2): 176–189
26. Villanacci V, Annese V, Cuttitta A et al (2010) An immunohistochemical study of the myenteric plexus in idiopathic achalasia. J Clin Gastroenterol 44(6):407–410
27. Sodikoff JB, Lo AA, Shetuni BB et al (2016) Histopathologic patterns among achalasia subtypes. Neurogastroenterol Motil 28(1):139–145
28. Devouge E, Michaud L, Lamblin MD et al (2002) Troubles moteurs primitifs de l'oesophage chez l'enfant, achalasie vraie exclue. Arch Pediatr 9(7):664–670
29. Morera C, Nurko S (2012) Heterogeneity of lower esophageal sphincter function in children with achalasia. J Pediatr Gastroenterol Nutr 54:34–40
30. Agrawal A, Hila A, Tutuian R et al (2008) Manometry and impedance characteristics of achalasia. Facts and myths. J Clin Gastroenterol 42:266–270
31. Di Lorenzo C, Hillemeier C, Hyman P et al (2002) Manometry studies in children: minimum standards for procedures. Neurogastroenterol Motil 14(4): 411–420
32. Pandolfino JE, Kahrilas PJ, American Gastroenterological Association (2005) AGA technical review on the clinical use of esophageal manometry. Gastroenterology 128:209–224

33. Murray JA, Clouse RE, Conklin JL (2003) Components of the standard oesophageal manometry. Neurogastroenterol Motil 15:591–606
34. Castell JA, Gideon RM (1999) Esophageal manometry. In: Castell DO, Richter J (eds) The esophagus. Lippincott Williams & Wilkins, Philadelphia, pp 101–117
35. Annequin D, Carbajal R, Chauvin P et al (2000) Fixed 50% nitrous oxide oxygen mixture for painful procedures: a French survey. Pediatrics 105(4):E47
36. Reinberg O, Augst MH (2014) Relief of painful procedures in children [Ces petits gestes qui font mal: stratégies de gestion ambulatoire de la douleur chez l'enfant]. Rev Med Suisse 415(10):222–226
37. Franklin AL, Petrosyan M, Kane TD (2014) Childhood achalasia: a comprehensive review of disease, diagnosis and therapeutic management. World J Gastrointest Endosc 6(4):105–111
38. Tutuian R, Castell DO (2004) Combined multichannel intraluminal impedance and manometry clarifies esophageal function abnormalities: study in 350 patients. Am J Gastroenterol 99:1011–1019
39. González-Rodríguez R, Ortiz-Olvera NX, González Martínez M et al (2015) Achalasia in pediatric population: use of high-resolution manometry in children. J Gastrointest Dig Syst 5(3):286–90
40. Singendonk MMJ, Smits MJ, Heijting IE et al (2015) Inter- and intrarater reliability of the Chicago Classification in pediatric high-resolution esophageal manometry recordings. Neurogastroenterol Mobil 27(2):269–276
41. Pandolfino JE, Kwiatek MA, Nealis T et al (2008) Achalasia: a new clinically relevant classification by high-resolution manometry. Gastroenterology 135:1526–1533
42. Bredenoord AJ, Fox M, Kahrilas PJ (2012) Chicago classification criteria of esophageal motility disorders defined in high resolution esophageal pressure topography. Neurogastroenterol Motil 1:57–65
43. Patti MG, Fisichella PM (2008) Laparoscopic Heller Myotomy and Dor Fundoplication for Esophageal Achalasia. How I do It. J Gastrointest Surg 12:764–766
44. Stefanidis D, Richardson W, Farrell TM et al (2012) SAGES guidelines for the surgical treatment of esophageal achalasia. Surg Endosc 26(2):296–311
45. Sharp NE, St Peter SD (2016) Treatment of idiopathic achalasia in the pediatric population: a systematic review. Eur J Pediatr Surg 26(2):143–149. [Epub ahead of print]
46. Chuah SK, Hsu PI, Wu KL et al (2012) 2011 update on esophageal achalasia. World J Gastroenterol 18:1573–1578
47. Leyden JE, Moss AC, MacMathuna P (2014) Endoscopic pneumatic dilation versus botulinum toxin injection in the management of primary achalasia. Cochrane Database Syst Rev 12:CD005046
48. Maksimak M, Perlmutter DH, Winter HS (1986) The use of nifedipine for the treatment of achalasia in children. J Pediatr Gastroenterol Nutr 5:883–886
49. Pasricha PJ, Ravich WJ, Hendrix TR et al (1995) Intrasphincteric botulinum toxin for the treatment of achalasia. N Engl J Med 332:774–778
50. Hurwitz M, Bahar RJ, Ament ME et al (2000) Evaluation of the use of botulinum toxin in children with achalasia. J Pediatr Gastroenterol Nutr 30:509–514
51. Wang L, Li YM, Li L (2009) Meta-analysis of randomized and controlled treatment trials for achalasia. Dig Dis Sci 54(11):2303–2311
52. Boyle JT, Cohen S, Watkins JB (1981) Successful treatment of achalasia in childhood by pneumatic dilatation. J Pediatr 99:35–40
53. Babu R, Grier D, Cusick E et al (2001) Pneumatic dilatation for childhood achalasia. Pediatr Surg Int 17:505–507
54. Hamza AF, Awad HA, Hussein O (1999) Cardiac achalasia in children. Dilatation or surgery? Eur J Pediatr Surg 9:299–302
55. Weber CE, Davis CS, Kramer HJ (2012) Medium and long-term outcomes after pneumatic dilation or laparoscopic Heller myotomy for achalasia: a meta-analysis. Surg Laparosc Endosc Percutan Tech 22(4): 289–296
56. Chen Z, Bessell JR, Chew A, Watson DI (2010) Laparoscopic cardiomyotomy for achalasia: clinical outcomes beyond 5 years. J Gastrointest Surg 14(4):594–600
57. Tsuboi K, Omura N, Yano F et al (2015) Data analyses and perspectives on laparoscopic surgery for esophageal achalasia. World J Gastroenterol 21(38): 10830–10839
58. Boeckxstaens GE, Annese V, des Varannes SB et al (2011) European Achalasia Trial: Pneumatic dilation versus laparoscopic Heller's myotomy for idiopathic achalasia. N Engl J Med 364:1807–1816
59. Hussain SZ, Thomas R, Tolia V (2002) A review of achalasia in 33 children. Dig Dis Sci 47:2538–2543
60. Inoue H, Minami H, Kobayashi Y et al (2010) Peroral endoscopic myotomy (POEM) for esophageal achalasia. Endoscopy 42:265–271
61. Familiari P, Marchese M, Gigante G et al (2013) Peroral endoscopic myotomy for the treatment of achalasia in children. J Pediatr Gastroenterol Nutr 57(6):794–797
62. Caldaro T, Familiari P, Romeo EF et al (2015) Treatment of esophageal achalasia in children: today and tomorrow. J Pediatr Surg 50(5):726–730
63. Li C, Tan Y, Wang X, Liu D (2015) Peroral endoscopic myotomy for treatment of achalasia in children and adolescents. J Pediatr Surg 50(1):201–215
64. Tang X, Gong W, Deng Z et al (2015) Usefulness of peroral endoscopic myotomy for treating achalasia in children: experience from a single center. Pediatr Surg Int 31(7):633–638
65. Chen WF, Li QL, Zhou PH et al (2015) Long-term outcomes of peroral endoscopic myotomy for achalasia in pediatric patients: a prospective, single-center study. Gastrointest Endosc 81(1):91–100

66. Maselli R, Inoue H, Misawa M et al (2012) Peroral endoscopic myotomy (POEM) in a 3-year-old girl with severe growth retardation, achalasia, and Down syndrome. Endoscopy 44(Suppl 2):E285–E287
67. NOSCAR POEM White Paper Committee, Stavropoulos SN, Desilets DJ, Fuchs KH et al (2014) Per-oral endoscopic myotomy white paper summary. Gastrointest Endosc 80:1–15
68. Teitelbaum EN, Soper NJ, Santos BF et al (2014) Symptomatic and physiologic outcomes one year after peroral esophageal myotomy (POEM) for treatment of achalasia. Surg Endosc 28(12):3359–3365
69. Bhayani NH, Kurian AA, Dunst CM et al (2014) A comparative study on comprehensive, objective outcomes of laparoscopic Heller myotomy with per-oral endoscopic myotomy (POEM) for achalasia. Ann Surg 259:1098–1103
70. Yaghoobi M, Mayrand S, Martel M et al (2013) Laparoscopic Heller's myotomy versus pneumatic dilation in the treatment of idiopathic achalasia: a meta-analysis of randomized, controlled trials. Gastrointest Endosc 78:468–475
71. Novais PA, Lemme EM (2010) 24-h pH monitoring patterns and clinical response after achalasia treatment with pneumatic dilation or laparoscopic Heller myotomy. Aliment Pharmacol Ther 32(10):1257–1265
72. Corda L, Pacilli M, Clarke S et al (2010) Laparoscopic oesophageal cardiomyotomy without fundoplication in children with achalasia: a 10-year experience: a retrospective review of the results of laparoscopic oesophageal cardiomyotomy without an anti-reflux procedure in children with achalasia. Surg Endosc 24:40–44
73. Salvador R, Costantini M, Cavallin F et al (2014) Laparoscopic Heller myotomy can be used as primary therapy for esophageal achalasia regardless of age. J Gastrointest Surg 18:106–111
74. Esposito C, Riccipetitoni G, Chiarenza SF et al (2013) Long-term results of laparoscopic treatment of esophageal achalasia in children: a multicentric survey. J Laparoendosc Adv Surg Tech A 23:955–959
75. Myers NA, Jolley SG, Taylor R (1994) Achalasia of the Cardia in children: a worldwide survey. J Pediatr Surg 29(10):1375–1379
76. Campos GM, Vittinghoff E, Rabl C et al (2009) Endoscopic and surgical treatments for achalasia: a systematic review and meta-analysis. Ann Surg 249(1):45–57
77. Pastor AC, Mills J, Marcon MA et al (2009) A single center 26-year experience with treatment of esophageal achalasia: is there an optimal method? J Pediatr Surg 44:1349–1354
78. Askegard-Giesmann JR, Grams JM, Hanna AM et al (2009) Minimally invasive Heller's myotomy in children: safe and effective. J Pediatr Surg 44: 909–911
79. Azizkhan RG, Tapper D, Eraklis A (1980) Achalasia in childhood: a 20-year experience. J Pediatr Surg 15(4):452–456
80. Rebecchi F, Giaccone C, Farinella E et al (2008) Randomized controlled trial of laparoscopic Heller myotomy plus Dor fundoplication versus Nissen fundoplication for achalasia: long-term results. Ann Surg 248:1023–1030
81. Khajanchee YS, Kanneganti S, Leatherwood AE (2005) Laparoscopic Heller Myotomy with Toupet Fundoplication. Arch Surg 140(9):827–833
82. Rawlings A, Soper NJ, Oelschlager B et al (2012) Laparoscopic Dor versus Toupet fundoplication following Heller myotomy for achalasia: results of a multicenter, prospective, randomized-controlled trial. Surg Endosc 26:18–26
83. Iqbal A, Tierney B, Haider M et al (2006) Laparoscopic re-operation for failed Heller myotomy. Dis Esophagus 19:193–199
84. Torquati A, Richards WO, Holzman MD et al (2006) Laparoscopic myotomy for achalasia: predictors of successful outcome after 200 cases. Ann Surg 243:587–591
85. Pratap N, Kalapala R, Darisetty S et al (2011) Achalasia cardia subtyping by high-resolution manometry predicts the therapeutic outcome of pneumatic balloon dilatation. J Neurogastroenterol Motil 17:48–53
86. Salvador R, Costantini M, Zaninotto G et al (2010) The preoperative manometric pattern predicts the outcome of surgical treatment for esophageal achalasia. J Gastrointest Surg 14:1635–1645
87. Zerbib F, Roman S (2015) Current therapeutic options for esophageal motor disorders as defined by the Chicago classification. J Clin Gastroenterol 49(6):451–460
88. Ríos-Galvez S, Meixueiro-Daza A, Remes-Troche JM (2015) Achalasia: a risk factor that must not be forgotten for esophageal squamous cell carcinoma. BMJ Case Rep 2015;2015. pii: bcr2014204418
89. O'Neill OM, Johnston BT, Coleman HG (2013) Achalasia: a review of clinical diagnosis, epidemiology, treatment and outcomes. World J Gastroenterol 19(35):5806–5812
90. Leeuwenburgh I, Scholten P, Caljé TJ et al (2013) Barrett's esophagus and esophageal adenocarcinoma are common after treatment for achalasia. Dig Dis Sci 58(1):244–252
91. Ravi K, Geno DM, Katzka DA (2015) Esophageal cancer screening in achalasia: is there a consensus? Dis Esophagus 28(3):299–304

Laryngotracheal Clefts 10

Lluís Nisa and Kishore Sandu

10.1 Introduction

Laryngotracheal clefts (LTC) constitute a rare cause of congenital upper airway malformation. First described in a doctoral dissertation on unavoidable causes of neonatal death in the eighteenth century by Richter, LTC incidence is estimated to be around 1 in 10,000–20,000 live births, accounting for 0.2–1.5 % of all congenital laryngeal anomalies [1, 2].

The presenting signs and symptoms as well as the age of diagnosis largely depend on the type of cleft (Table 10.1) as well as the eventual presence of associated malformations. Moreover, it has been previously pointed out that the actual incidence of LTC may be highly underestimated [3]. Potential reasons for this include asymptomatic or pauci-symptomatic disease especially in type I clefts, difficulties in endoscopic diagnosis mostly related to physician's unawareness, and immediate mortality in high-grade clefts without postmortem diagnosis. Furthermore, since LTC often occurs in a context of polymalformative disorders, endoscopic diagnosis may not be the priority in many cases [4, 5].

From an embryologic perspective, the larynx develops from endodermic tissues (which in turn derive from the primitive gut) as well as mesenchymal tissues derived from the IV–VI branchial arches. Toward the fourth week of development begins the midline fusion which is meant to lead to the separation of the digestive (esophageal) and respiratory (tracheal) axes. This fusion process takes place in the caudal to cranial direction [3]. The esophagus elongates and reaches its final relative length toward the seventh week. LTCs are pathological clefts thought to be the result of a closure failure between the tracheal and esophageal axes during embryogenesis, but despite the explanatory power of this theory, it is important to point out that it has been challenged as it does not allow explaining the origin of other pathological entities such as isolated tracheoesophageal fistulae.

10.2 Diagnostic Aspects

10.2.1 Grading

Several grading classifications for LTCs have been proposed, primarily based on the craniocaudal extent of the cleft. Such classifications are mainly descriptive, help in therapeutic choices, and have to some degree prognostic value. The

L. Nisa
Department of Clinical Research, University of Bern, 3010 Bern, Switzerland
e-mail: lluis.nisa@dkf.unibe.ch

K. Sandu (✉)
Department of Otorhinolaryngology – Head and Neck Surgery, Lausanne University Hospital, Lausanne, Switzerland
e-mail: kishore.sandu@chuv.ch

M. Lima (ed.), *Pediatric Digestive Surgery*, DOI 10.1007/978-3-319-40525-4_10

Table 10.1 Classification of laryngotracheal clefts

Benjamin and Inglis (1989)		Sandu and Monnier (2006)	
Type	Description	Type	Description
I	Supraglottic cleft	0	Submucosal cleft
		I	Interarytenoid cleft with the absence of the interarytenoid muscle
II	Cleft with partial cricoid involvement	II	Posterior cleft extending partially through the cricoid plate
III	Cleft beyond the cricoid cartilage with involvement of the cervical trachea	IIIa	Posterior cleft extending down to the inferior border of the cricoid plate
		IIIb	Posterior cleft extending into the cervical trachea, but not beyond the sternal notch
IV	Involvement of thoracic trachea	IVa	Laryngotracheal cleft extending into the intrathoracic trachea to the carina
		IVb	Intrathoracic extension of the cleft involving one main bronchus

most widely used classification is the one proposed by Benjamin and Inglis in 1989 [3]. Benjamin's classification was modified and updated by Sandu and Monnier [2] in 2006, in order to introduce parameters with therapeutic and prognostic implications previously overlooked (Table 10.1).

Unlike previous classifications, Sandu and Monnier introduce type 0 clefts ("occult" or more accurately submucosal), which appear as a consequence of a posteriorly defective cricoid cartilage accompanied by the absence of transverse interarytenoid muscles [6]. Type I clefts are manifest interarytenoid clefts with the absence of interarytenoid muscles which do not involve at all the cricoid cartilage. Type II clefts extend partially through the cricoid cartilage. By definition, type III and type IV clefts extend above and below the thoracic inlet, respectively. Sandu and Monnier's classification pays particular attention to two specific features in these severe forms of disease: (1) whether the cricoid plate is partially or completely involved by the LTC in type III clefts and (2) whether the cleft is supra- or infracarinal in type IV LTCs (Fig. 10.1).

10.2.2 Clinical Presentation

The classical diagnostic triad of LTC consists of husky cry, aspiration pneumonia, and swallowing disorders in a newborn child with associated congenital anomalies [7]. While such scenario should immediately prompt active search for LTC, disease spectrum can often complicate and delay LTC diagnosis. Indeed, LTCs are congenital laryngotracheal disorders which can present as submucosal closure defect in the mildest cases versus complete laryngotracheo-esophageal clefts (LTEC) in some other severe cases. Breathing difficulties are typically due to prolapsing of retroarytenoid mucosa caused by the absence of the aerodigestive party wall and obstruction of the posterior respiratory glottis (Fig. 10.2). Therefore, presenting signs and symptoms related to LTC may vary depending on disease severity [7, 8].

LTCs without involvement of the posterior cricoid plate (type 0 and I) may be asymptomatic or in the case of type I clefts present with mild occasional episodes of aspiration, hoarse cry, aspiration, cough, or in some cases dyspnea or cyanosis during feeding [8–10]. Due to their rarity, diagnosis of type 0 and I clefts requires a high-suspicion index.

Regarding clefts with cricoid (with or without tracheal involvement), the outstanding issue is severe aspiration and subsequent lower pulmonary tract infection, as well as respiratory problems in some cases [9, 11]. Finally, type IV LTCs have a dim prognosis due to respiratory distress, poor airway tone, and difficulties to maintain a patent airway even when using invasive procedures [11–13]. Table 10.2 summarizes the clinical presentation of LTCs [14].

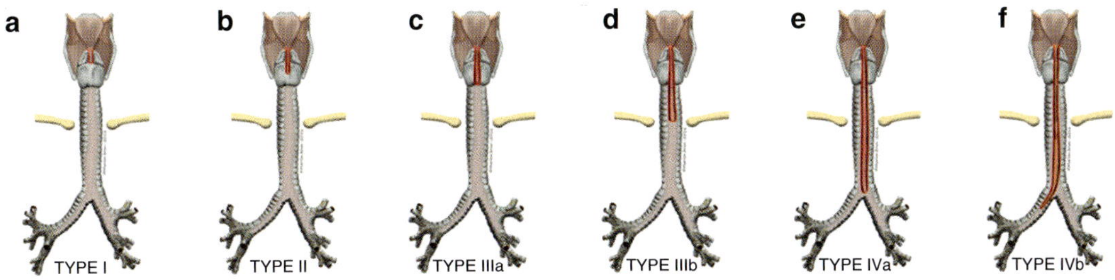

Fig. 10.1 LTC classification according to Sandu and Monnier

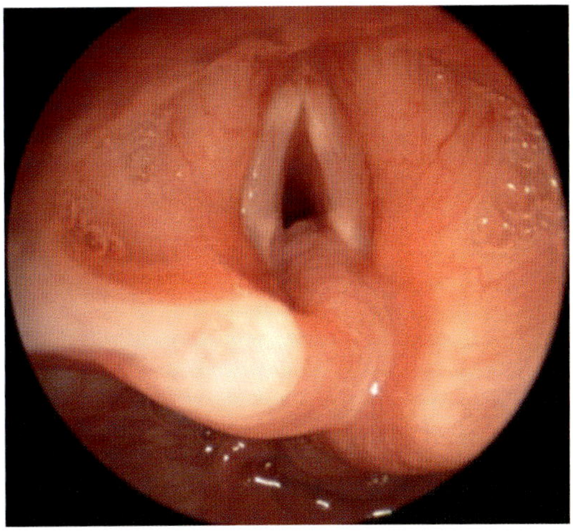

Fig. 10.2 Airway obstruction secondary to arytenoid prolapse and mucosal invagination into the trachea

Table 10.2 Clinical presentation of LTCs

Feature	Incidence (%)
Aspiration	53–80
Chronic cough	27–35
Stridor	10–60
Weak voice/cry	16
Salivary stasis in the pharynx	10–23
Aspiration pneumonia	16–54
Neonatal asphyxiation	33

10.2.3 Radiologic Studies

While the mainstay of LTC diagnosis is endoscopic (discussed below), some imaging exams may be contributive. Plain chest X-ray is often performed in children with persistent respiratory symptoms, whether or not such symptoms are secondary to an underlying LTC. Patients with LTC may present aspiration pneumonia or peribronchial cuffing, but chest X-ray is normal in up to 25% of type I and around 10% of type II LTCs [15].

Modified barium swallow (MBS) performed under the supervision of a speech and swallowing pathologist, testing diverse food consistencies, may help identifying patients with discoordinated swallow or aspiration. It has been previously pointed out that aspiration in an otherwise healthy child most often correlates with an underlying anatomic abnormality [16].

It is important to keep in mind that children with an undiagnosed LTC presenting with swallowing disorders may have undergone several MBSs in the past, and the cumulative radiation dose can be substantial.

10.2.4 Functional Endoscopic Evaluation of Swallowing (FEES)

FEES provides an extremely accurate dynamic assessment of the laryngeal function during swallowing. FEES is usually possible in children older than 1 year but is otherwise difficult to perform in younger children. During FEES, several food consistencies should be tested. Hypopharyngeal stasis and/or laryngeal penetration may be visualized in cases of early-stage LTCs [17].

Like MBS, FEES can be normal in children with grade I cleft with only intermittent aspiration.

10.2.5 Endoscopic Diagnosis

Definitive LTC diagnosis relies on endoscopic examination. Due to the high incidence of associated malformations, complete endoscopy of the upper aerodigestive tract is mandatory, and should include:

- Transnasal fiberoptic laryngoscopy, performed with the patient under spontaneous breathing. The entire airway is examined dynamically from the nostrils to the bronchi. The glottis ought to be sprayed with local anesthesia in order to examine the lower airway. In case the child bears a tracheotomy, the canula is removed intermittently during ventilation to facilitate comprehensive dynamic airway examination. Typically, LTC is associated with varying degrees of tracheobronchomalacia due to the absence of the trachealis muscle.
- Direct laryngoscopy and esophagoscopy:
  - Laryngoscopy must be performed using an anesthesia Macintosh spatula as well as 0°, 30°, and 70° telescopes, prior to airway intubation.
  - Suspension laryngoscopy in order to evaluate the morphology of the glottis and assess the posterior commissure using a Lindholm vocal fold retractor allows the diagnosis of a submucosal or small type I cleft. Palpation of the interarytenoid region using a blunt probe is the hallmark to the diagnosis of an LTC (Fig. 10.3). The probe dips down into the posterior commissure in the presence of a cleft. The lower limit of the probe and simultaneous visualization by a telescope gives an idea regarding the cleft depth and thus its type.
  - The esophagus and stomach are equally examined, paying particular attention to the presence of an eventual tracheoesophageal fistula [4, 18], GER, and microgastria (may be associated in type IV clefts).

Associated airway findings in LTC include:

- Narrowed interarytenoid distance with prolapsing retroarytenoid mucosa that blocks the posterior respiratory glottis

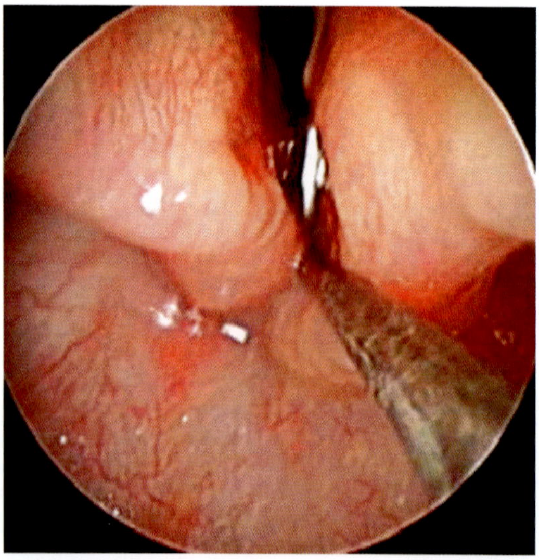

Fig. 10.3 The use of a blunt-angled probe to diagnose an LTC

- Paramedian position of the vocal folds
- Interarytenoid erythema
- Mucosal cobblestoning (secondary to gastroesophageal reflux)

10.3 Management

The therapeutic approach to the child with LTC largely depends on the extent of the cleft, severity of clinical manifestations, and associated or underlying disorders. All decisions should be taken in consultation with the parents and in the context of a multidisciplinary team, especially in children with severe comorbidities (such as cardiac, respiratory, etc.). In symptomatic patients, within the period between diagnosis and eventual surgical management, two issues stand out: respiratory and swallowing disorders.

Type 0 and I LTCs without respiratory symptoms may benefit of regular follow-up and eventually prophylactic-intermittent antibiotherapy in order to prevent pulmonary complications of recurrent pneumonia. Most of these patients are likely to require surgery at some point in their lives for chronic intractable aspiration. Type II clefts present with feeding difficulties and quasi-systematically require surgical management.

Type III and type IV LTCs may quickly degrade from a respiratory point of view, imposing oxygen therapy and pharyngeal aspiration tubes. The degree of invasiveness of oxygenotherapy may vary from nasal administration of oxygen to invasive ventilation (i.e., endotracheal tubes and even tracheostomy).

With respect to swallowing disorders, measures to avoid tracheobronchial aspiration and GERD must be considered a priority. Tracheobronchial aspiration in advanced-type LTCs represents a serious and immediate threat to the vital prognosis and consequently requires aggressive management approaches. More specifically, LTCs of type I and II require medical anti-GERD treatment and thickened food. More severe cases may impose suspension of oral feeding and enteral administration through a nasal or a gastrostomy tube, or even parenteral nutrition in case of longer clefts.

In summary, even though the management of LTCs is far from being consensual, there is some agreement that children with type I clefts may benefit from a trial of medical management and regular follow-up, while longer clefts (with cricoid involvement) require early surgical approaches to avoid the pulmonary complications of aspiration [7, 15, 17, 19]. Furthermore, a minimally invasive endoscopic approach has become standard for the management of types I, II, and IIIa (and even selected IIIb) LTCs, while major types IIIb and IV clefts most often require open approaches [2, 15, 20–22]. Open approaches are equally indicated as salvage for failed attempts of endoscopic repair.

10.3.1 Endoscopic Repair

Since the late 1970s, various endoscopic approaches have been successfully used primarily for types I and II clefts [25]. Injection laryngoplasty using different products (Gelfoam, bioplastic) has been reported [26, 27]. Endoscopic repair has progressively become the standard of care for types I and II clefts that remain symptomatic despite adequate medical treatment after an observation period of 4–6 months [14, 16, 17].

Sandu and Monnier reported a small series of patients with types IIIa and IIIb LTCs managed endoscopically [2]. In their reported experience carbon dioxide laser is used in ultrapulse mode to incise the cleft from caudal to cranial direction – cleft apex up to the cuneiform cartilages. The CO_2 laser is a precise cutting tool giving a bloodless field and causes no mucosal charring. Two layers of mucosae are created: laryngotracheal and pharyngoesophageal. Starting caudally, a set of inverted Vicryl 5.0 sutures are placed on the tracheal aspect of the cleft and the knots tied facing the pharyngoesophageal side. The second mucosal layer is sutured in similar fashion in distal to proximal direction with knots facing the esophagus while gradually withdrawing the suspension laryngoscope (Fig. 10.4). The procedure is performed under spontaneous respiration and without endotracheal intubation. At the end of the procedure, it is important to maintain an adequate posterior commissure and avoid posterior glottic stenosis (Fig. 10.5). Special endoscopic suturing instruments are a must and their role needs emphasis. The details of such instruments are described in related articles [2].

The advantages of the endoscopic repair are:

- The surgeon is axial to the larynx and gets the best view of the cleft. This is important so as to achieve a meticulous closure of the cleft and avoid excessive crowding of mucosa into the airway lumen and thus its obstruction.
- Maintains stability of the laryngotracheal framework.

10.3.2 Open Surgical Approaches

Several open surgical techniques for the repair of LTCs exist, depending on their extent. All approaches require a layer-by-layer closure of the cleft (esophageal and tracheal). The use of interposition material to reinforce the closure has been suggested by some authors (tibial periosteum, auricular cartilage, sternocleidomastoid muscle flap, fascia temporalis, or costal cartilage) [20, 22–24].

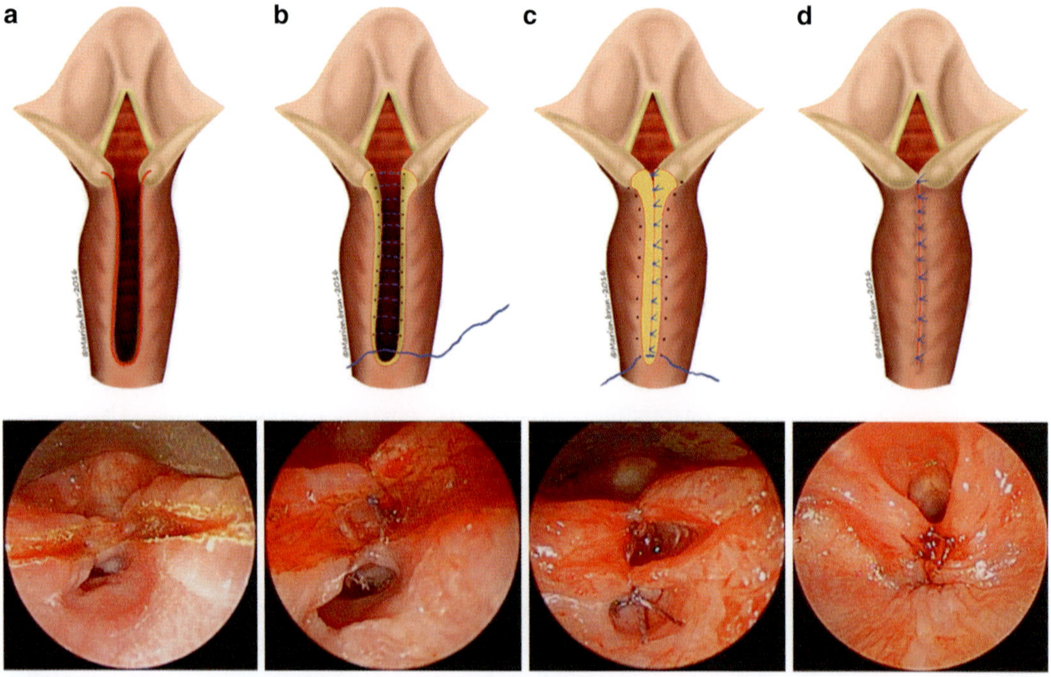

Fig. 10.4 Endoscopic closure of LTC: (**a**) Type IIIb LTC and the use of CO_2 laser to create two mucosal layers, laryngotracheal and pharyngoesophageal. (**b**) Vicryl 5.0 is used to suture the inner laryngotracheal layer from caudal to cranial, with the knots tied toward the esophageal side. (**c**) Caudo-cranial suturing of the pharyngoesophageal layer. (**d**) End of the two-layer LTC closure. Note that in the end, we should have an adequate posterior commissure and avoid a posterior glottic stenosis

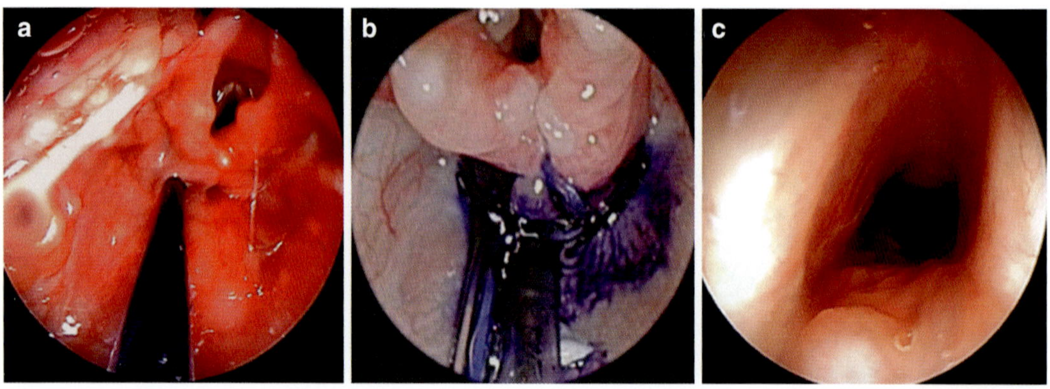

Fig. 10.5 Endoscopic closure of LTC – post-LTC repair endoscopy: (**a**) Placement of naso-esophageal suction catheter and injection of dilute methylene blue. (**b**) Avoid excessive spillage of the colored solution and airway soiling. (**c**) Simultaneous endoscopic visualization of the larynx and trachea shows complete healing of the LTC and no residual fistula

Cervical approaches differ in cases of extra- and intrathoracic LTCs and can be summarized as follows:

1. Extrathoracic LTEC

   The surgery begins with a nasotracheal intubation using a soft Portex blue line ET tube. Surgery begins with a horizontal neck incision and separating the pre-laryngeal strap muscles in the midline. The thyroid isthmus is divided and retracted. An extended laryngotracheofissure is performed dividing the anterior commissure exactly in the midline (Fig. 10.6a, b). The posteriorly placed laryngeal cleft is identified. The edges of the cleft are incised to create two layers: pharyngoesophageal and laryngotracheal depending on the cleft extension (Fig. 10.6c). These layers are then sutured independently in between tissue interpositions, using perichondrium, tibial periosteum, or rib cartilage graft that can be sutured to the splayed posterior cricoid plate similar to a posterior cartilage expansion graft (Fig. 10.6d). To calibrate the endolaryngeal reconstruction, Monnier's LT mold stent can be used temporarily.
2. Intrathoracic LTEC

   The repair is done under cardiopulmonary bypass or extracorporeal membrane oxygenation (ECMO) [7]. The long cleft is approached by a longitudinal incision along the right tracheoesophageal groove from the origin of the right main bronchus up to the level of the cricoid cartilage. A long laryngotracheofissure causes severe airway framework instability and is hence avoided. The right lateral esophageal wall is dissected in the groove, and the common tracheoesophageal space is entered. The objective of dissecting and mobilizing the right esophageal wall is to use this mucosa to reconstruct the

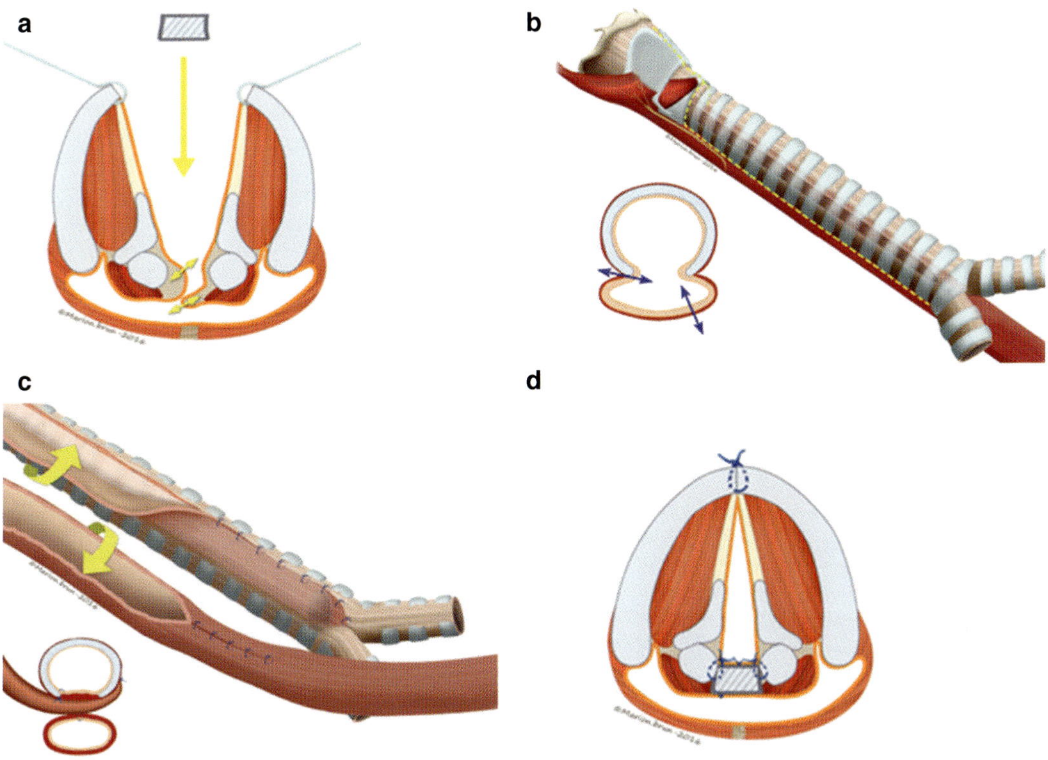

Fig. 10.6 Open repair of LTC. (**a**) Anterior extended laryngofissure. (**b**) Dissection in the right tracheoesophageal groove and (**c**) esophageal mucosa flipped over to the left that is used to reconstruct the posterior trachea. (**d**) A posterior costal cartilage graft is sutured into the cricoid defect. In addition, a small Monnier's LT mold is inserted for temporary airway calibration

posterior tracheal wall after identifying and incising the left tracheoesophageal cleft mucosa. The rest of the esophageal mucosa is rotated and sutured on to the left side. The trachea and esophagus are sutured longitudinally up to the cricoid. The laryngeal part of the cleft is then approached by laryngofissure. The posterior laryngeal cleft is identified and sutured as described above along with tissue interposition. A small LT mold (avoiding excess contact pressure on the suture line) is inserted to calibrate the airway and the laryngofissure closed. The LT mold is removed endoscopically at a later date.

Ideally and *if possible*, a tracheostomy is to be avoided in LTC management as it destabilizes the tracheal framework, erodes the posterior suture line of repair, and can potentially lead to severe tracheomalacia – albeit to say, it has to be done as per the patient requirements and for oxygenotherapy [19, 22]. In long LTC repairs, a well-fixed nasotracheal tube is preferred during the immediate postoperative period.

10.3.3 Transcervical Approach Using Cricotracheal Separation

Propst and Rutter [29] described a technique to repair a type IV LTC. The long cleft is approached transcervically, without sternum split and without deploying ECMO or a cardiopulmonary bypass (Fig. 10.7). The surgery is performed under spontaneous total intravenous anesthesia. An angioplasty balloon catheter is passed into the stomach and inflated, so as to avoid gastric insufflation by anesthesia gases and oxygen during the entire intervention. The surgery begins as described earlier up to exposing the laryngotracheal framework. The cricoid cartilage and the trachea are transected at the first tracheal ring. The dissection is continued posteriorly to identify the long LTC. Recurrent laryngeal nerves are not identified. The trachea is then peeled off from the esophagus up to the lower end of the cleft. A complete laryngofissure is performed, and the splayed cricoid is reconstructed using a rib cartilage. Proximal pharyngoesophageal and laryngotracheal mucosae are flipped across each other to close above the posterior cricoid and reaching the interarytenoid region. The front of the esophagus is sutured in the caudal to cranial direction. The excess of esophageal mucosa is used to reconstruct the posterior tracheal wall. The back of the trachea is then sutured in a similar fashion up to the cricoid cartilage. At this stage, the trachea is reconnected to the cricoid. The authors note the following advantages with this technique – improved visibility, access, airway stability, and coverage of the anastomosis with interpositional sternal periosteum – permitting a three-layer closure.

10.4 Associated Disorders

As previously mentioned, LTCs are often a manifestation of a larger spectrum of developmental disease and therefore are often embedded in a context of associated congenital malformations (Table 10.3). The most common comorbidities are esophageal atresia, considered to occur in 20–37 % of cases of LTCs, while various midline malformations including craniofacial and heart malformations would occur in around 10 % and 16–33 % of the cases, respectively [3, 19]. The co-occurrence of LTC and tracheoesophageal fistula is estimated to be between 10 and 15 % [28].

As mentioned above, complete digestive and respiratory examination is essential given the number of cases with associated malformations. LTCs can equally occur in a number of syndromic contexts, especially Opitz-Frias syndrome, Pallister-Hall syndrome, DiGeorge syndrome, CHARGE syndrome, and VACTERL association (Table 10.4).

Genetic counseling is a must in such cases.

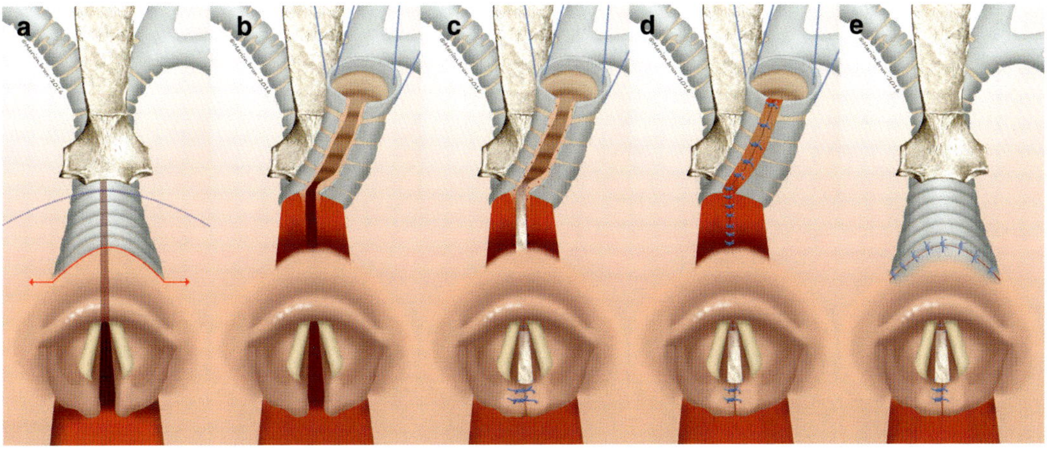

Fig. 10.7 Open repair (transcervical approach with cricotracheal separation): (**a**) Trachea transected from the cricoid at the first tracheal ring. (**b**) Trachea peeled off from the esophagus. (**c**) Complete laryngofissure and closure of the pharyngeal and laryngeal mucosae. An interpositional costal cartilage graft is used to reconstruct the splayed cricoid defect. (**d**) Repair of the back of the trachea and front of the esophagus. (**e**) Trachea is reconnected with the cricoid

Table 10.3 Most common associated malformations

System	Malformations
Head and face	Cleft lip and palate, micrognathia, glossoptosis, microtia, hypertelorism, and choanal atresia
Respiratory	Tracheoesophageal fistula, tracheomalacia, hyaline membrane disease, irregularities in size and shape of lower airways
Gastrointestinal	Esophageal atresia, duodenal atresia, imperforated anus, intestinal malrotation
Cardiac	Aortic coarctation, great vessel transposition, double outlet right ventricle, patent ductus arteriosus, and septal defects
Genitourinary	Renal malformations, hypospadias, and inguinal hernia

10.5 Prognosis

The outcome of LTCs depends on several factors, mainly cleft extent and associated comorbidities [22]. Early diagnosis and active prevention of lower airway infection and GER equally have an impact on disease progression. Longer clefts are associated with syndromic anomalies and comorbidities and carry a poor prognosis. The mortality rate of LTCs was around 50 % in the 1980s (43 % for types I and II, 42 % for type III, and 93 % for type IV) – but more recent series report rates of 6–25 % [19].

Table 10.4 Associated syndromes

Disease	OMIM ID	Chromosomal region	Inheritance mode	Incidence	Phenotypical manifestations
Opitz-Frias syndrome	145410	22q11.23	AD X linked	1:4000–1:10,000	Hypertelorism, telecanthus, cleft lip, palate, and uvula, hypospadias (male) and splayed labia majora (females), mental retardation, developmental delay, and congenital heart diseases
Pallister-Hall syndrome	146510	7p14.1	AD	Unknown	Extremity anomalies (polydactyly, syndactyly), hypothalamic hamartoma, bifid epiglottis, imperforated anus, and hydronephrosis/hydroureter
DiGeorge syndrome	188400	22q11.21	AD	1:2000–1:7000	Variable developmental delay, obesity, ear anomalies, eye anomalies, cleft palate/uvula, tetralogy of Fallot or multiple other heart malformations, endocrine and metabolic disorders *Mnemonic*: CATCH22 – *C*ardiac abnormality, *A*bnormal facies, *T*hymic aplasia, *C*left palate or VPI, *H*ypocalcemia/*h*ypoparathyroidism, 22q11.2
CHARGE syndrome[a]	214800	7q21.11 8q12.2	AD	1:8500–12,000	Variable phenotype Mnemonic: CHARGE – *C*oloboma, *H*eart defect, *A*tresia choanae, *R*etarded growth and development, *E*xtremity abnormalities
VACTERL association	192350			1.6 cases/10,000 live births	Variable phenotype Mnemonic: VACTERL – *V*ertebral anomalies, *A*nal atresia, *C*ardiovascular anomalies, *T*racheoesophageal fistula, *E*sophageal atresia, *R*enal anomalies, preaxial *L*imb anomalies

Source: Online Mendelian Inheritance in Man (www.omim.org)
Abbreviations: *AD* autosomal dominant
[a]Two different genetic lesions have been identified, and CHARGE syndrome overlaps with Kallmann syndrome

References

1. Richter RC (1972) Dissertation Medica de Infanticidio in Artis Obstetriciae Exercitio Non Semper Evitabili *Lipsiae ex oficina sommeria*. University of Leipzig, Leipzig
2. Sandu K, Monnier P (2006) Endoscopic laryngotracheal cleft repair without tracheotomy or intubation. Laryngoscope 116:630–634
3. Benjamin B, Inglis A (1989) Minor congenital laryngeal clefts: diagnosis and classification. Ann Otol Rhinol Laryngol 98:417–420
4. Parsons DS, Herr T (1997) Delayed diagnosis of a laryngotracheoesophageal cleft. Int J Pediatr Otorhinolaryngol 39:169–173
5. Wolfson PJ, Schloss MD, Guttman FM, Nguyen L (1984) Laryngotracheoesophageal cleft. An easily missed malformation. Arch Surg 119:228–230
6. Tucker GF Jr, Maddalozzo J (1987) "Occult" posterior laryngeal cleft. Laryngoscope 97:701–704
7. Pezzettigotta SM, Leboulanger N, Roger G, Denoyelle F, Garabedian EN (2008) Laryngeal cleft. Otolaryngol Clin North Am 41:913–933, ix
8. Schraff SA, Zur KB, Jacobs I, Darrow DH, Cotton RT, Rutter MJ (2007) The clinical relevance of the submucosal cricoid cleft. Int J Pediatr Otorhinolaryngol 71:1099–1104
9. Rahbar R, Rouillon I, Roger G et al (2006) The presentation and management of laryngeal cleft: a 10-year experience. Arch Otolaryngol Head Neck Surg 132:1335–1341
10. Parsons DS, Stivers FE, Giovanetto DR, Phillips SE (1998) Type I posterior laryngeal clefts. Laryngoscope 108:403–410
11. Koerte I, Nicolai T, Joppich I, von Schweinitz D, Dietz HG (2009) Type IV laryngotracheoesophageal cleft associated with microgastria and left lung hypoplasia: report of a long-term survivor. Eur J Pediatr Surg 19:120–121
12. Shehab ZP, Bailey CM (2001) Type IV laryngotracheoesophageal clefts – recent 5 year experience at Great Ormond Street Hospital for Children. Int J Pediatr Otorhinolaryngol 60:1–9
13. Iskit SH, Senyuz OF, Sander S (1998) Type IV laryngotracheoesophageal clefts: surgical management for long-term survival. J Pediatr Surg 33:1733
14. Garabédian ENLN (2011) Diastème. In: Denoyelle FCV, Froehlich P, Nicollas R (eds) *Le larynx de l'enfant*: Société Française d'Oto-Rhino-Laryngologie et de Chirurgie Cervico-Faciale. pp 279–302
15. Rahbar R, Chen JL, Rosen RL et al (2009) Endoscopic repair of laryngeal cleft type I and type II: when and why? Laryngoscope 119:1797–1802
16. Johnston DR, Watters K, Ferrari LR, Rahbar R (2014) Laryngeal cleft: evaluation and management. Int J Pediatr Otorhinolaryngol 78:905–911
17. Chien W, Ashland J, Haver K, Hardy SC, Curren P, Hartnick CJ (2006) Type 1 laryngeal cleft: establishing a functional diagnostic and management algorithm. Int J Pediatr Otorhinolaryngol 70:2073–2079
18. Triglia JM, Nicollas R, Ducroz V, Koltai PJ, Garabedian EN (1998) First branchial cleft anomalies: a study of 39 cases and a review of the literature. Arch Otolaryngol Head Neck Surg 124:291–295
19. Leboulanger N, Garabedian EN (2011) Laryngo-tracheo-oesophageal clefts. Orphanet J Rare Dis 6:81
20. Kubba H, Gibson D, Bailey M, Hartley B (2005) Techniques and outcomes of laryngeal cleft repair: an update to the Great Ormond Street Hospital series. Ann Otol Rhinol Laryngol 114:309–313
21. Eriksen C, Zwillenberg D, Robinson N (1990) Diagnosis and management of cleft larynx. Literature review and case report. Ann Otol Rhinol Laryngol 99:703–708
22. Myer CM 3rd, Cotton RT, Holmes DK, Jackson RK (1990) Laryngeal and laryngotracheoesophageal clefts: role of early surgical repair. Ann Otol Rhinol Laryngol 99:98–104
23. Garabedian EN, Ducroz V, Roger G, Denoyelle F (1998) Posterior laryngeal clefts: preliminary report of a new surgical procedure using tibial periosteum as an interposition graft. Laryngoscope 108:899–902
24. Donahoe PK, Gee PE (1984) Complete laryngotracheoesophageal cleft: management and repair. J Pediatr Surg 19:143–148
25. Yamashita M, Chinyanga HM, Steward DJ (1979) Posterior laryngeal cleft – anaesthetic experiences. Can Anaesth Soc J 26:502–505
26. Ahluwalia S, Pothier D, Philpott J, Sengupta P, Frosh A (2004) Laryngeal cleft type I: a novel method of repair using Bioplastique. J Laryngol Otol 118:648–650
27. Kennedy CA, Heimbach M, Rimell FL (2000) Diagnosis and determination of the clinical significance of type 1A laryngeal clefts by gelfoam injection. Ann Otol Rhinol Laryngol 109:991–995
28. Fraga JC, Adil EA, Kacprowicz A et al (2015) The association between laryngeal cleft and tracheoesophageal fistula: myth or reality? Laryngoscope 125:469–474
29. Propst EJ, Ida JB, Rutter MJ (2013) Repair of long type IV posterior laryngeal cleft through a cervical approach using cricotracheal separation. Laryngoscope 123:801–804

11 Esophageal Atresia and Tracheoesophageal Fistula

Arnold G. Coran, Steven W. Bruch, and
Shaun M. Kunisaki

Esophageal atresia (EA) with or without tracheoesophageal fistula (TEF), a defect occurring in about 1 in 3000 live births, remains a challenging problem for pediatric surgeons [1]. Since Cameron Haight performed the first successful primary anastomosis in 1941 [2], survival rates have improved due to refinements in surgical technique and advances in neonatal care. In 1994, Spitz predicted survival based on birth weight (greater or less than 1500 g) and associated complex anomalies usually cardiac in nature [3]. Spitz reexamined this in 2006 and found that survival for babies without cardiac anomalies and weighing more than 1500 g was 98.5 %, similar to that in 1994. However, survival rates improved from 59 to 82 % in babies born less than 1500 g or had a major cardiac anomaly over this time. And during this same period, survival rates improved from 22 to 50 % in babies who were born less than 1500 g and had a major cardiac anomaly [4]. Using the Kids' Inpatient Database (KID) in 2014, Brindle calculated the odds ratio for significant predictors of inhospital mortality in babies born with EA and TEF. Table 11.1 describes the risk factors with their associated scores, and Table 11.2 shows the mortality stratified by risk factor scores [5].

A.G. Coran (✉)
C.S. Mott Children's Hospital, University of Michigan Hospital and Health Systems, Ann Arbor, MI, USA
e-mail: acoran@umich.edu

S.W. Bruch, MD • S.M. Kunisaki, MD
C.S. Mott Children's Hospital, University of Michigan, Ann Arbor, MI, USA

11.1 Anatomy

An understanding of the anatomy involved with each case of EA and TEF is important when devising a treatment strategy. There have been several classification systems, but a description of each type is the easiest and most practical way to classify the five different types of EA and TEF as shown in Fig. 11.1. The most common configuration is EA with a distal TEF. This configuration occurs in 86 % of cases [6]. The proximal esophagus ends blindly in the upper mediastinum. The distal esophagus is connected to the tracheobronchial tree usually just above or at the carina. The second most common type is the isolated EA without a TEF. This configuration occurs in 8 % of cases [6]. The proximal esophagus ends blindly in the upper mediastinum, and the distal esophagus is also blind ending and protrudes a varying distance above the diaphragm. The distance between the two ends is often too far to bring together shortly after birth. The third most common configuration, occurring in 4 % of cases [6], is a TEF without EA. The esophagus extends in continuity to the stomach, but there is a fistula between the esophagus and the trachea. The fistula is usually located in the upper mediastinum running from a proximal orifice in the trachea to

M. Lima (ed.), *Pediatric Digestive Surgery*, DOI 10.1007/978-3-319-40525-4_11

Table 11.1 Odds ratio for significant predictions for mortality

Risk factor	Odds ratio	Risk points
Birth weight <1500 g	9.05	9
Chromosomal abnormality	5.80	6
Major cardiac anomaly[a]	2.68	3
Renal anomaly	1.89	2

CNS and GI abnormalities did not contribute to mortality
[a]Major cardiac anomaly defined as all other than PDA or ASD

Table 11.2 Mortality stratified by risk factor scores

Risk score	% of EA TEF population	% mortality
Low risk (0–6)	86.3	4.4
Intermediate risk (7–14)	12.0	33.8
High risk (15–20)	1.7	67.5

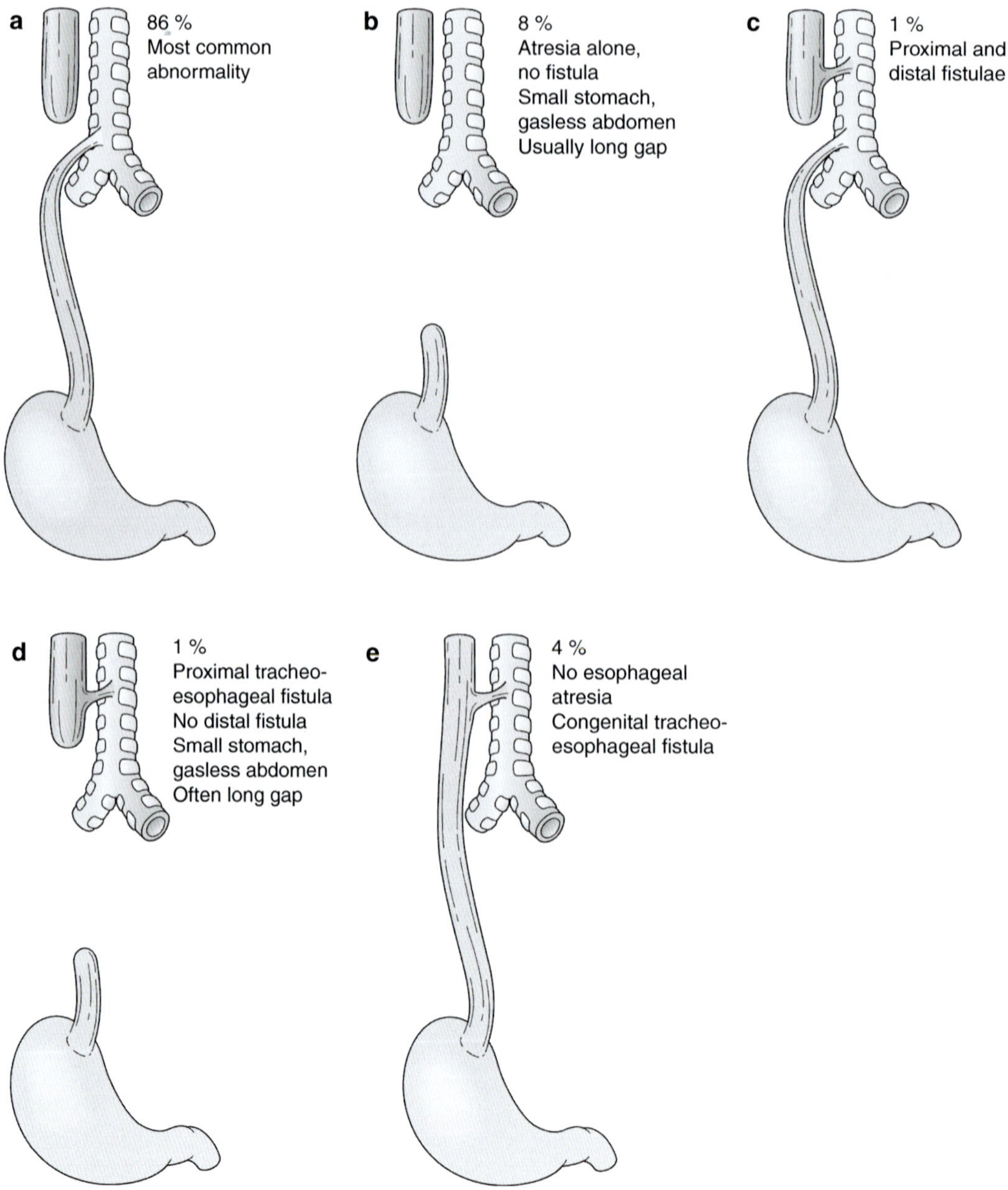

Fig. 11.1 Types of esophageal atresia and tracheoesophageal fistula with rates of occurrence. (**a**) Esophageal atresia with distal tracheoesophageal fistula. (**b**) Isolated esophageal atresia. (**c**) Esophageal atresia with proximal and distal tracheoesophageal fistulas. (**d**) Esophageal atresia with proximal tracheoesophageal fistula. (**e**) H-type tracheoesophageal fistula

a more distal orifice in the esophagus. This is also known as an "H"-type or "N"-type TEF. Two more forms of EA and TEF exist, both of which occur about 1 % of cases [6]. These are EA with both proximal and distal TEF and EA with a proximal TEF. These two forms correspond to the first two forms described with the addition of a proximal fistula between the upper pouch and the trachea. A proximal fistula is often difficult to diagnose preoperatively even when bronchoscopy is performed, resulting in the real incidence being higher than previously reported [7]. Again the EA with proximal TEF, similar to its counterpart without the proximal fistula, will have a long gap between the two ends of the esophagus, making it difficult to repair shortly after birth.

11.2 Associated Anomalies

As noted earlier, prematurity and associated cardiac and chromosomal anomalies often determine the outcome of a baby with EA and TEF. Babies with EA and TEF are often born prematurely due in part to the polyhydramnios resulting from fetal esophageal obstruction [8]. Recent series revealed a mean gestation age of 36.5 weeks with 3.5 % being born between 24 and 29 weeks estimated gestation age (EGA), and 38.3 % between 30 and 36 weeks EGA [9], and a birth weight of 2500 g [10]. Up to two thirds of EA and TEF babies have one or more associated anomalies that are usually chromosomal or related to the VACTERL association [9, 11]. The VACTERL association includes abnormalities in the following areas: *v*ertebral, *a*norectal, *c*ardiac, *t*racheal, *e*sophageal, *r*enal, and *l*imb. A breakdown of the individual incidences of the anomalies in babies with EA and TEF is presented in Table 11.3 [9]. The VACTERL syndrome requires three or more of these abnormalities and occurs in up to 33 % of babies with EA and TEF [9]. Chromosomal abnormalities occur in 5 % and include trisomies 13, 18, and 21 [12]. Other syndromes associated with EA and TEF include the Feingold syndrome, CHARGE syndrome, anophthalmia-esophageal-genital (AEG) syndrome, Pallister-Hall syndrome, Opitz syndrome, and Fanconi's anemia [13]. Infants with EA and TEF also have a higher incidence of pyloric stenosis compared to the normal population [14].

Table 11.3 Incidence of associated anomalies with EA and TEF

Associated anomalies	Occurrence (%)
Vertebral	25.4
Atresia, anorectal, and duodenal	16.3
Cardiac	59.1
Renal	21.8
Skeletal	6.4

11.3 Clinical Presentation and Diagnosis

Prenatal diagnosis of EA remains difficult with only 16–32 % of babies born with EA and TEF having the diagnosis before delivery [15, 16]. The use of fetal ultrasound to screen for polyhydramnios and a small or absent stomach followed by MRI looking for a dilated upper esophageal pouch for confirmation can lead to a correct diagnosis of EA and TEF in 66.7 % of those suspected [17]. The majority of babies diagnosed prior to delivery will have pure EA as it is more difficult to diagnose EA with a distal TEF [16, 18]. The vast majority of cases of EA and TEF are initially diagnosed shortly after birth with inability to handle saliva and episodes of coughing, choking, and cyanosis, especially with the first attempt to feed. This usually leads to the placement of a tube in the esophagus, which meets resistance. Plain films of the chest and abdomen will show the tube coiled in the upper mediastinum. This confirms the presence of esophageal atresia. If there is gas in the distal bowel, a distal TEF is present, while a pure EA will present with a gasless abdomen. The remainder of the preoperative evaluation targets the associated anomalies and looks to determine the presence of a proximal fistula between the trachea and the esophagus. The VACTERL anomalies can be identified using physical exam (limb and anorectal), plain films (tracheal, esophageal, vertebral, and limb), abdominal ultrasound (renal and a tethered spinal cord), and an echocardiogram (cardiac). The position of the aortic arch needs to be identified during the echocardiogram. If a right-sided arch is present, which occurs in 2–6% of series [19], evaluation with a CT scan or an MR angiogram will find a complete vascular ring 37% of the time [20]. A chromosome analysis should also be considered. A proximal pouch fistula can be interrogated in two ways. A pouchogram, or contrast evaluation of the proximal esophageal pouch, will often reveal a proximal fistula if present. An experienced radiologist should perform this exam with 1 or 2 ml of contrast material to decrease the risk of aspiration. Rigid bronchoscopy looking for a proximal fistula just prior to surgical repair is often used in conjunction with the pouchogram. During the dissection of the proximal pouch, the surgeon should always look carefully for a proximal fistula. If the proximal pouch is not thick walled and dilated, there may be a proximal fistula that has relieved the usual distending pressure in the proximal pouch. A TEF without EA (H-type fistula) may not present in the initial neonatal period and is more difficult to diagnose. The tube will go into the stomach when originally passed, but persistent coughing and choking with feeds by mouth should prompt a search for an isolated fistula. A prone pullback esophagram and bronchoscopy with esophagoscopy are used to identify the isolated fistula.

11.4 Treatment

After the diagnosis is confirmed, plans for operative repair should be made. In healthy newborns, the operation can take place within the first 24 h of life to minimize the risk of aspiration and resulting pneumonitis. Before the operation, the baby should be kept supine with the head elevated 30–45°. A tube should be in the proximal pouch to constantly suction saliva and prevent aspiration. Intravenous access should be established and fluids instilled along with perioperative antibiotics and vitamin K.

The goal of operative therapy for EA and TEF is to establish continuity of the native esophagus and repair the fistula in one setting. Most of the time, primary repair can be achieved. There are special situations where this may not be possible or advisable. These situations will be described later. In the usual scenario, the baby, who is stable both hemodynamically and from a pulmonary standpoint, is brought to the operating room and placed under a general anesthetic. Rigid bronchoscopy may be performed to locate the distal fistula, usually at or near the carina, look for a proximal fistula or cleft, and assess for tracheomalacia. The baby is then placed in the left lateral decubitus position in preparation for a right posterolateral thoracotomy. If the preoperative echocardiogram reveals a right-sided aortic arch, which occurs in 2–6% of cases, the repair should be approached from the left chest [19, 21]. Attempting to bring the ends of the esophagus together over a right-sided aortic arch results in a high anastomotic leak rate in the range of 40% due to increased tension [22]. The preoperative echocardiogram identifies a right-sided aortic arch correctly in 20–62% of the cases [20, 22]. A right-sided arch discovered intraoperatively should prompt an attempt at repair of the esophagus through the right chest. If this cannot be completed due to tension, divide the fistula, close the right chest, and complete the anastomosis through a left-sided thoracotomy.

In the typical case, a right-sided posterolateral thoracotomy using a muscle-sparing, retropleural approach gives access to the mediastinal structures. An extrapleural axillary approach provides another option to gain exposure. The azygos vein is divided, revealing the tracheoesophageal connection. The distal esophagus is divided, and the tracheal connection is closed with 5-0 monofilament suture. Manipulation of the distal esophagus is minimized to protect the segmental blood supply to this portion of the esophagus. The proximal esophagus has a rich blood supply coming from the thyrocervical trunk and may be extensively dissected as depicted in Fig. 11.2. The dissection of the upper esophageal pouch proceeds on the thickened wall of the esophagus to prevent tracheal injury. Dissection is carried as high as possible to gain length for a tension-free anastomosis and to look for a proximal fistula, which occurs rarely. A single-layered end-to-end anastomosis is performed as depicted in Fig. 11.3. A tube placed through the anastomosis into the stomach allows decompression of the stomach and eventual enteral feeding. A chest tube placed in the retropleural space next to the anastomosis controls any subsequent leak. Some surgeons prefer not to use a chest tube if the pleura remains intact. The advantage of a retropleural approach is that if the anastomosis leaks, the baby will not soil the entire hemithorax and develop an empyema.

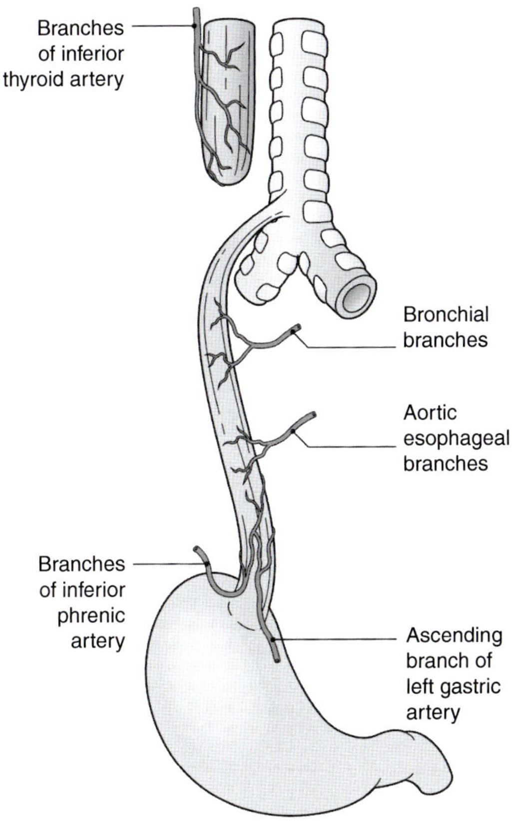

Fig. 11.2 The vascular supply of the esophagus in esophageal atresia and tracheoesophageal fistula

A leak into the retropleural space will result in a controlled esophagocutaneous fistula that will almost always close spontaneously.

Since the first thoracoscopic repair of EA by Lobe in 1999, this approach has become increasingly popular [23]. Visualization of the posterior mediastinum depends on patient position and creation of a pneumothorax. The baby is placed in a semi-prone position elevating the right chest about 30°. The camera trocar avoids competing with the working ports by being placed just posterior to the scapula tip in the fifth intercostal space. The two working ports are then placed two interspaces above the midaxillary line and one to two interspaces below and slightly posterior to the camera port. This allows the instruments to meet at a 90° angle at the site of the anastomosis [24]. Insufflation of CO_2 gas at a flow of 1 L/min and a pressure of 4 mmHg provides an adequate working space. The improved visualization allows for a precise division of the fistula at the membranous portion of the trachea and an extensive mobilization of the proximal fistula up into the neck while preserving the recurrent laryngeal nerves. Suture placement proves to be the biggest challenge especially when the ends of the esophagus are brought together under tension. Advantages of the thoracoscopic approach include better cosmetic results, improved musculoskeletal function of the thorax, and improved visualization. Disadvantages include a steep learning curve even for those with excellent thoracoscopic skills,

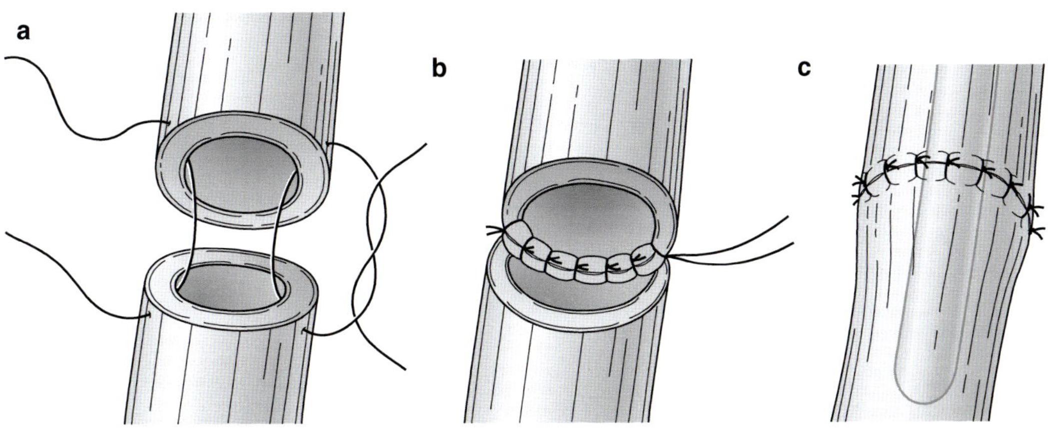

Fig. 11.3 Single-layer end-to-end esophageal anastomosis. (**a**) Corner sutures are placed. (**b**) Posterior row sutures are placed. A tube is then passed through the anastomosis into the stomach. (**c**) Anterior row sutures complete the anastomosis

difficulty in small (<2,000 g) infants or in neonates with significant cardiac or pulmonary disease, and the potential impact of elevated pCO_2, acidosis, and cerebral hypoperfusion from prolonged carbon dioxide pneumothorax [25]. A meta-analysis comparing thoracoscopic and open repair of EA with or without TEF found no difference in leakage rate or anastomotic strictures [26].

Postoperatively, the baby is returned to the intensive care unit and continued on intravenous nutrition and antibiotics. Special care should be directed toward preventing aspiration with frequent oropharyngeal suctioning and elevation of the head of the bed 30–45°. Feedings may be started through the transanastomotic tube into the stomach 2–3 days after the operation. Acid-suppressive therapy should be instituted to prevent acid irritation of the anastomosis and subsequent stricture. On postoperative day 5–7, an esophagram is obtained to check the integrity of the anastomosis. Feeds are initiated orally, and if there is no leak clinically or radiographically, the chest tube is removed. If a leak is present, it is treated conservatively with intravenous antibiotics, nutrition, and chest tube drainage. Another esophagram is ordered in a week. These leaks will invariably close without further operative intervention [27]. Only a complete disruption of the anastomosis requires further operative procedures. In that case the proximal esophagus should be brought out of the left neck as a cervical esophagostomy, the distal esophagus should be tied off, and the mediastinum and chest should be adequately drained.

11.5 Special Situations

Three unique situations require different tactics: babies with EA and TEF with concomitant respiratory insufficiency where the fistula contributes to the ventilator compromise, long-gap EA, and H-type TEFs. Babies with respiratory insufficiency and a TEF are usually premature neonates with lung immaturity requiring significant ventilatory support. The connection between the trachea and the distal esophagus may be the preferred path for air provided by the ventilator. The stiff lungs have a higher resistance than the fistulous tract, allowing a significant portion of each inspiratory volume to go into the distal esophagus and then the stomach, resulting in abdominal distention and elevation of the hemidiaphragms, further impeding ventilation. Various strategies have been developed to deal with this situation. A change to high-frequency ventilation decreases the portion of tidal volume lost to the fistula [28]. A number of techniques designed to prevent ventilation through the fistula have been proposed: advancing the endotracheal tube past the fistula opening [29], bronchoscopically placing and inflating Fogarty catheters for temporary occlusion [30], and temporarily occluding the esophagus at the gastroesophageal junction [31]. If a gastrostomy tube is present, the tube can be placed to underwater seal to increase the resistance of the tract and reduce airflow through the fistula [6]. However, to prevent further respiratory decompensation, and to ameliorate the risk of gastric perforation, these babies often require an urgent thoracotomy and control of the TEF. If the baby stabilizes, the remainder of the repair can proceed at that time, which is the usual case [32]. However, if the baby remains unstable, the esophagus is secured to the prevertebral fascia, the chest is closed, a gastrostomy tube is placed, and the definitive repair is completed when the baby is stabilized. In very low birth weight infants, less than 1500 g, a staged repair should be considered. Compared to a primary repair in these very low birth weight infants, staged repair resulted in fewer anastomotic leaks and strictures [33].

The second special situation occurs when there is a long gap between the two ends of the esophagus. This often occurs with pure EA or EA with a proximal TEF. On occasion, a baby with EA and distal TEF may fit into this special group. If the baby presents with a gasless abdomen, a long gap should be suspected. The baby is brought to the operating room for a gastrostomy tube placement to allow enteral feedings while waiting for the two ends of the esophagus to grow spontaneously, so a primary anastomosis can be attempted. The stomach is quite small in these babies because it was unused during fetal life and has not yet stretched to its full capacity. Care must be taken to avoid injury to the small stomach and its blood supply while placing the gastrostomy tube. Careful placement will not compromise the use of the stomach for an esophageal replacement if necessary. During gastrostomy tube placement, an estimate of the distance between the two ends of the esophagus is made using a neonatal endoscope in the distal esophagus and fluoroscopy. If the two ends of the esophagus are more than three vertebral bodies apart, they will not be easily connected. The baby is then nursed with a tube in the proximal pouch to remove the saliva and is fed via the gastrostomy tube. During the first several months of life, the gap between the two ends of the esophagus shortens because of differential growth of the atretic esophagus [34]. The upper pouch may undergo serial dilation attempting to stretch the pouch [35]. The gap distance is measured every 2–4 weeks, and, if the two ends are within two to three vertebral bodies, a thoracotomy and attempt at anastomosis are performed. Waiting longer than 4 months rarely provides extra growth of the esophageal ends. The gap will close to within two to three vertebral bodies in close to 70 % of these babies [36]. Intraoperatively, several techniques help gain length on the esophageal ends if needed. These include complete dissection of the upper pouch to the thoracic inlet. A circular myotomy of livaditis performed on the upper pouch produces about 1 cm of length for each myotomy as depicted in Fig. 11.4 [37]. A tubularized graft of the upper pouch can be created and connected to the distal esophagus [38]. If these techniques do not allow an adequate anastomosis, the distal esophagus is mobilized, despite its segmental blood supply, to gain length [6]. If these maneuvers do not allow an adequate anastomosis, then one of three options must be chosen. The first

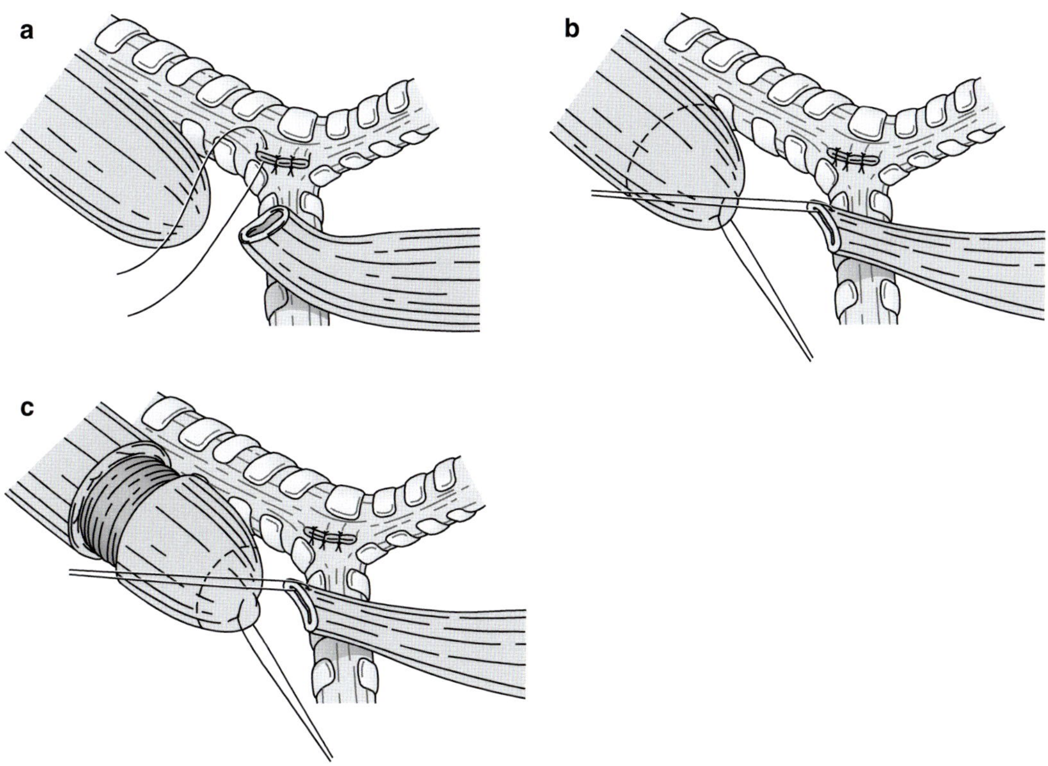

Fig. 11.4 Repair of esophageal atresia and distal tracheoesophageal fistula using a circular myotomy to provide adequate length. (**a**) The tracheoesophageal fistula is closed with 5-0 monofilament suture. (**b**) The feasibility of primary anastomosis between the two esophageal segments is assessed. (**c**) A proximal esophagomyotomy provides extra length to allow for a primary anastomosis

option is a two-stage procedure in which a cervical esophagostomy is initially created in the left neck followed by an esophageal substitution at a later time. The esophagostomy will allow the baby to take sham feeds to prevent oral aversion without the risk of aspiration while awaiting esophageal replacement. The replacement operation usually takes place between 9 and 12 months of age. The second option is a one-stage esophageal-substitution procedure using a gastric transposition, a gastric tube, or a colon interposition to replace the native esophagus. Currently, a gastric transposition is our preferred approach and has been shown to be a reliable and reproducible procedure at other centers worldwide [39]. A third option for esophageal reconstruction in long-gap esophageal atresia involves the placement of traction sutures on both ends of the esophagus and either attaching them under tension to the prevertebral fascia if the gap is moderate length or bringing them out through the back and increase the tension on them sequentially over the ensuing 2 weeks (Foker technique). A delayed primary anastomosis is carried out after the two ends of the esophagus are in close proximity [40]. Although the Foker technique allows for a primary repair, it requires multiple thoracotomy incisions, is associated with a very high stricture rate, and invariably requires a gastric fundoplication procedure to control gastroesophageal reflux [41]. Thoracoscopic techniques have been introduced for both the gastric transposition [42] and the Foker technique [43].

The third special situation is the H-type tracheoesophageal fistula without esophageal atresia. An H-type fistula will often escape the discovery in the neonatal period but will be found later during evaluation of coughing and choking episodes with feeds. Often the fistula is identified by contrast studies, usually a prone pullback esophagram as shown in Fig. 11.5. However, it is not unusual to also require bronchoscopy and esophagoscopy to make the diagnosis. To repair this fistula, rigid bronchoscopy and esophagoscopy are used to find the fistula, place a glidewire through it, and bring the two ends out of the mouth to aid in its identification during the exploration. The right neck is then explored through an incision just above the clavicle. The fistula is identified and divided. If possible, the muscle or other available vascularized tissue is placed between the two suture lines to help prevent a recurrence.

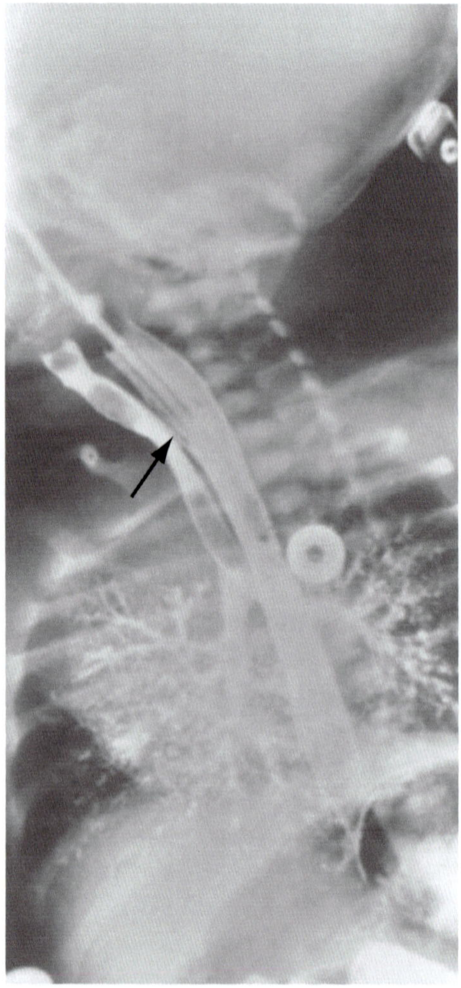

Fig. 11.5 An H-type tracheoesophageal fistula is demonstrated as contrast is injected through a nasoesophageal tube. Contrast is noted passing from the esophagus, through the fistula, and filling the upper trachea and larynx

11.6 Postoperative Complications

Complications following repair of EA and TEF relate to the anastomosis and to the underlying disease. The anastomotic problems include anastomotic leaks, anastomotic strictures, and recurrent TEFs. The issues related to the underlying disease include gastroesophageal reflux and tracheomalacia.

The number of anastomotic problems that occur after repair is directly dependent on the amount of tension that is used to create the anastomosis. The incidence of leak at the anastomosis varies from 5 to 20 % [44] and has remained stable over the years [45, 46]. The majority of these leaks seal within 1–2 weeks with conservative management. Complete disruption of the anastomosis, a rare complication occurring in less than 2 % of cases, presents with a pneumothorax and significant salivary drainage from the chest tube. This scenario may require early thoracotomy and revision of the anastomosis or a cervical esophagostomy and gastrostomy for feeding with subsequent esophageal replacement.

Anastomotic strictures occur in one third to one half of repairs, a rate that has remained stable over the past 25 years [47]. All repairs will show some degree of narrowing at the anastomosis, but dilations are not instituted unless the stricture is symptomatic, causing dysphagia, associated respiratory difficulties, or foreign body obstruction. Most strictures respond to repeated dilations. These are carried out every 3–6 weeks over a 3–6-month period. Strictures that are recalcitrant to dilations are often related to gastroesophageal reflux disease and will not resolve until the reflux is controlled. The perforation rates for uncomplicated esophageal strictures for balloon dilation and bougienage are 0–2 % and 8–9 %, respectively [48]. Esophageal stenting may be useful to temporize an esophageal stricture but has not yet been successful as a definitive treatment [49].

The incidence of recurrent TEF formation ranges from 5 to 10 % in recent series [50]. These children present with coughing, choking, and occasional cyanotic episodes with feeding and with recurrent pulmonary infections. Recurrent fistulas are often associated with anastomotic leaks, but the possibility of a missed proximal fistula must also be entertained. A prone, pullback esophagram and bronchoscopy with esophagoscopy are useful to diagnose recurrent fistulas. A repeat right thoracotomy with closure of the fistula is a difficult operation. Identification of the fistula tract is improved with placement of a glidewire or ureteral catheter through the fistula at bronchoscopy just before opening the chest. After the fistula is identified and divided, a viable piece of tissue, usually a vascularized muscle flap or a portion of pleura or pericardium, should be placed between the suture lines to prevent recurrence of the fistula, which occurs in up to 20 % of these repairs [51]. Endoscopic techniques may be attempted prior to surgical closure of a small recurrent TEF. It appears that the combination of de-epithelialization of the fistula tract with an energy source (diathermy or laser) combined with tissue adhesives (Histoacryl or fibrin glue) works better than either techniques alone to close the fistula tract with a reported short-term success rate of 75 % [50].

Gastroesophageal reflux is commonly associated with EA and TEF. This stems from a number of issues including the abnormal clearance of the distal esophagus due to poor motility and the altered angle of His that occurs as a result of tension on the distal esophagus and proximal stomach to allow for an adequate anastomosis. Using videomanometry with topographic analysis, Kawahara et al. found two subgroups of patients with repaired EA and TEF. Neither group had esophageal contractions at the anastomosis. One group had distal esophageal contractions and did not develop reflux, whereas the other group lacked distal contractions, and 15 of 17 developed symptomatic reflux [52]. In multiple series over the past 30 years, the incidence of significant gastroesophageal reflux following EA and TEF repair has remained stable with an average incidence of 43 % [53]. The reflux is treated medically with acid-reducing medication. Close to half of those who develop reflux will require a fundoplication, especially if an anastomotic stricture develops that remains resistant to dilation, or repeated pulmonary aspiration secondary to reflux complicates the postoperative course [53]. Careful consideration should be given to a partial fundoplication in these children, but a loose Nissen fundoplication remains the preferred method following EA and TEF repair [54, 55]. A

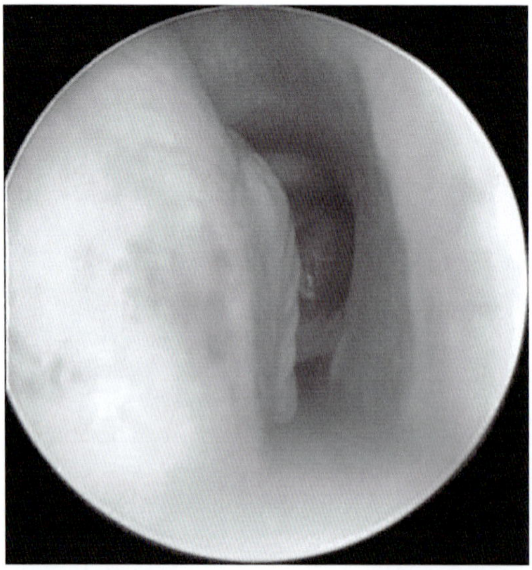

Fig. 11.6 Tracheomalacia after repair of esophageal atresia and tracheoesophageal fistula. Bronchoscopic view of the tracheal lumen during spontaneous respirations shows almost complete collapse or the trachea during expiration (please rotate figure counterclockwise 90° for final view)

comparison of fundoplications done in babies with and without EA and TEF revealed that those with EA had more intra- and postoperative complications and more problems with recurrent reflux, dysphagia, and dumping after the fundoplication [56].

Symptomatic tracheomalacia occurs in 10–20 % children after repair of EA and TEF [44, 57]. Tracheomalacia refers to collapse of the trachea on expiration leading to expiratory stridor and episodes of desaturations, apnea, cyanosis, and bradycardia that are often associated with feeds. This is thought to originate from weakening of the tracheal cartilage due to pressure exerted during fetal life from the fluid-filled dilated upper esophageal pouch. The tracheomalacia may be severe enough to prevent extubation after the original repair. Determining the etiology of this symptom complex can sometimes be difficult because tracheomalacia and gastroesophageal reflux both occur frequently in this population and produce similar symptoms. Tracheomalacia is diagnosed with rigid bronchoscopy in the spontaneously breathing patient. The trachea will flatten anteroposteriorly, or "fishmouth" on expiration, as depicted in Fig. 11.6. Recently, the use of dynamic airway multidetector CT scanning in the diagnosis of tracheomalacia has been described [58]. Tracheomalacia is often self-limiting but may require intervention in children with severe life-threatening symptoms. If treatment with continuous positive airway pressure is not effective, then aortopexy [59] or tracheal stenting may be required [60]. Intervention for tracheomalacia is required in up to 5 % of children with EA [61].

11.7 Outcome

The outcome for babies with EA and TEF has improved over time to the point where now, unless major cardiac anomalies, significant chromosomal abnormalities, severe pulmonary complications, or birth weight less than 1500 g exist, almost all will survive. The long-term problems in children after repair of their EA and TEF include pulmonary issues, especially reactive airway disease, bronchitis, and pneumonias and upper gastrointestinal complaints of dysphagia and gastroesophageal reflux. Pulmonary symptoms severe enough to require hospitalization occur in close to half of children after repair of EA and TEF [62] Both obstructive defects with airway hyperresponsiveness resulting in asthma-like symptoms and restrictive defects often related to thoracotomy-induced rib fusions and gastroesophageal reflux disease occur [63, 64]. A recent meta-analysis of outcomes at least 10 years after EA and TEF repair revealed a pooled prevalence of recurrent respiratory tract infections of 24 %, persistent cough of 15 %, doctor-diagnosed asthma of 22 %, and persistent wheezing of 35 % [65]. Although the pulmonary symptoms tend to persist into adulthood [66], they tend to be mild and not affect activities of daily living [12].

The dysphagia and gastroesophageal reflux commonly seen in these children stem from the altered innervation of the distal portion of the esophagus be it intrinsic or secondary to operative dissection of the esophageal pouches. This dysmotility persists into adulthood. In manometric studies of adolescents and adults with repaired EA, the main long-term motility deficits are uncoordinated peristaltic activity and low-amplitude contraction of the distal esophagus. Interestingly, the swallow-induced relaxation of the lower esophageal sphincter occurs normally [67]. This abnormal esophageal motility sets the stage for dysphagia and gastroesophageal reflux. Using 24-h pH probe and esophageal biopsy data, the incidence of gastroesophageal reflux has been documented in infants (41 %), in children up to the age of 10 (45–50 %), and in adults (40 %) after EA repair. No new cases of histologic esophagitis or abnormal pH probes occurred in children after age 5. The gastroesophageal reflux appears to develop early and persist in patients after EA repair [68]. Esophageal strictures are uncommon as a late complication. If a stricture occurs late in the course, it is usually associated with gastroesophageal reflux. Symptoms do not appear to predict abnormal endoscopic findings in patients with EA suggesting that routine endoscopy may be useful [69]. Chronic reflux may lead to Barrett's esophagus, a precursor to adenocarcinoma of the esophagus. Risk factors for Barrett's following EA repair include early stricture requiring resection, recurrent TEF, age over 30, long-gap EA, and an esophageal stricture as an adult. To date, eight cases of esophageal cancer have been reported in patients who had their EA repaired at birth. All but one presented in the mid-esophagus or at the anastomosis, five were squamous cell, and three were adenocarcinomas, and they presented at a mean age of 38 years with the earliest at age 20 [70]. The meta-analysis referenced above revealed a pooled prevalence of dysphagia (50.3 %); gastroesophageal reflux symptoms (40.2 %), of those 56.5 % had esophagitis on biopsy; Barrett's esophagus (6.4 %); and esophageal cancer (1.4 %) [65]

Several quality-of-life (QOL) measures have been used to assess the long-term outcomes after EA repair as an infant. The health-related QOL in children with EA was decreased related to healthy controls but higher when compared to children with chronic diseases like asthma and diabetes [71]. The decrease in health-related QOL in children appears to be due to ongoing morbidity and associated anomalies resulting in lower physical functioning and general health perception. Following EA repair, adults have a comparable QOL to the general population in most domains [72]. A Dutch study of QOL in adults following repair of EA compared to healthy subjects found no difference in overall physical and mental health between the two groups. However, former EA patients reported worse "general health" and less "vitality" than the healthy subjects because of continued gastrointestinal difficulties reported in up to a quarter of the EA group. Marital and family status did not differ from that of the general Dutch population [73]. The QOL of adults after a colonic interposition as an infant is not as good as it is for adults who had a primary repair [74]. A recent review of QOL following repair of EA at birth concluded that the overall health-related QOL was reduced compared to healthy controls but that the associated effect of EA repair on overall QOL seems less than expected [75].

References

1. Prato AP, Carlucci M, Bagolan P et al (2015) A cross-sectional nationwide survey on esophageal atresia and tracheoesophageal fistula. J Pediatr Surg 50:1441–1456, http://dx.doi.org/10.1016/j.jpedsurg.2015.01.004
2. Haight C, Towsley H (1943) Congenital atresia of the esophagus with tracheoesophageal fistula: extrapleural ligation of the fistula and end-to-end anastomosis of esophageal segments. Surg Gynecol Obstet 76:672
3. Spitz L, Kiely EM, Morecroft JA et al (1994) Oesophageal atresia: at-risk groups for the 1990's. J Pediatr Surg 29:723–725
4. Spitz L (2007) Oesophageal atresia. Orphanet J Rare Dis 2:24
5. Turner B, Dasgupta R, Brindle ME (2014) A contemporary prediction rule for esophageal atresia (EA) and trachea-esophageal fistula (TEF). J Pediatr Surg 49:1758–1761
6. Harmon CM, Coran AG (2006) Congenital anomalies of the esophagus. In: O'Neill Jr JA. Rowe MI, Grosfeld JL et al (eds) Pediatric surgery, 6th edn. Mosby, St Louis, pp 1051–1081
7. Bax KMA, Roskott AMC, van der Zee DC (2008) Esophageal atresia without distal tracheoesophageal fistula: high incidence of proximal fistula. J Pediatr Surg 43:522–525
8. Losty PD, Baillie CT (2003) Esophageal atresia and

tracheo-esophageal fistula. In: Puri P (ed) Newborn surgery, 2nd edn. Oxford University Press, New York, pp 337–352
9. Lautz TB, Mandelia A, Radhakrishnan J (2015) VACTERL associations in children undergoing surgery for esophageal atresia and anorectal malformations: implications for pediatric surgeons. J Pediatr Surg 50:1245–1250
10. Sfeir R, Bonnard A, Dhen-Dunlop N et al (2013) Esophageal atresia: data from a national cohort. J Pediatr Surg 48:1664–1669
11. Brosens E, Ploeg M, van Bever Y et al (2014) Clinical and etiological heterogeneity in patients with tracheo-esophageal malformations and associated anomalies. Eur J Med Genet 57:440–452
12. Lilja HE, Wester T (2008) Outcome in neonates with esophageal atresia treated over the last 20 years. Pediatr Surg Int 24:531–537
13. Bednarczyk D, Sasiadek MM, Smigiel R (2013) Chromosome aberrations and gene mutations in patients with esophageal atresia. JPGN 57:688–693
14. Spitz L, Hitchcock RJ (1994) Oesophageal atresia and tracheo-oesophageal fistula. In: Freeman NV (ed) Surgery of the newborn, 1st edn. Churchill Livingstone, New York, pp 353–373
15. Fallon SC, Ethun CG, Olutoye OO et al (2014) Comparing characteristics and outcomes in infants with prenatal and postnatal diagnosis of esophageal atresia. J Surg Res 190:242–245
16. Spaggiari E, Faure G, Rousseau V et al (2015) Performance of prenatal diagnosis in esophageal atresia. Prenat Diagn 35:1–6
17. Garabedian C, Verpillat P, Czerkiewicz I et al (2014) Does a combination of ultrasound, MRI, and biochemical amniotic fluid analysis improve prenatal diagnosis of esophageal atresia? Prenat Diagn 34:839–842
18. Kunisaki SM, Bruch SW, Hirschl RB et al (2014) The diagnosis of fetal esophageal atresia and its implications on perinatal outcome. Pediatr Surg Int 30:971–977
19. Berthet S, Tenisch E, Miron MC et al (2015) Vascular anomalies associated with esophageal atresia and tracheoesophageal fistula. J Pediatr 166:1140–1144
20. Allen SR, Ignatio R, Falcone RA et al (2006) The effect of a right-sided aortic arch on outcome in children with esophageal atresia and tracheoesophageal fistula. J Pediatr Surg 41:479–483
21. Bonkett B, Beasly SW, Myers NA (1999) The frequency, significance, and management of a right aortic arch in association with esophageal atresia. Pediatr Surg Int 15:28–31
22. Babu R, Pierro A, Spitz L et al (2000) The management of oesophageal atresia in neonates with right-sided aortic arch. J Pediatr Surg 35:56–58
23. Lobe TE, Rothenberg S, Waldschmidt T et al (1999) Thoracoscopic repair of esophageal atresia in an infant: a surgical first. Ped Endosurg Innov Tech 3:141–148
24. Rothenberg S (2014) Thoracoscopic repair of esophageal atresia and trachea-esophageal fistula in neonates: the current state of the art. Pediatr Surg Int 30:979–985
25. Dingemann C, Ure BM (2013) Minimally invasive repair of esophageal atresia: an update. Eur J Pediatr Surg 23:198–203
26. Borruto FA, Impellizzeri P, Montalto AS et al (2012) Thoracoscopy versus thoracotomy for esophageal atresia and tracheoesophageal fistula repair: review of the literature and meta-analysis. Eur J Pediatr Surg 22:415–419
27. Nambirajan L, Rintala RJ, Losty PD et al (1998) The value of early postoperative oesophagography following repair of oesophageal atresia. Pediatr Surg Int 13:76–78
28. Ho AMH, Dion JM, Wong JCP (2015) Airway and ventilator management options in congenital tracheo-esophageal fistula repair. J Cardiothorac Vasc Anesth 30(2):515–520 [epub ahead of print 2015]
29. Salem MR, Wong AY, Lin YH et al (1973) Prevention of gastric distension during anesthesia for newborns with tracheoesophageal fistulas. Anesthesiology 38:82–83
30. Filston HC, Chitwood WR Jr, Schkolne B et al (1982) The Fogarty balloon catheter as an aid to management of the infant with esophageal atresia and tracheo-esophageal fistula complicated by severe RDS or pneumonia. J Pediatr Surg 17:149–151
31. Margain L, Perez-Etchepare E, Varlet F et al (2015) Lower esophageal banding in extremely low birth weight infants with esophageal atresia and tracheo-esophageal fistula is a life saving practice followed by successful delayed primary thoracoscopy reconstruction. J Pediatr Surg 50:489–492
32. Conforti A, Morini F, Bagolan P (2014) Difficult esophageal atresia: trick or treat. Sem Pediatr Surg 23:261–269
33. Petrosyan M, Estrada J, Hunter C et al (2009) Esophageal atresia/tracheoesophageal fistula in very low-birth-weight neonates: improved outcomes with staged repair. J Pediatr Surg 44:2278–2281
34. Ein SH, Shandling B, Heiss K (1993) Pure esophageal atresia: outlook in the 1990's. J Pediatr Surg 28:1147–1150
35. Mahour GH, Woolley MM, Gwinn JL (1974) Elongation of the upper pouch and delayed anastomotic reconstruction in esophageal atresia. J Pediatr Surg 9:373–383
36. Nakayama DK (2003) Congenital abnormalities of the esophagus. In: O'Neill Jr JA, Grosfeld JL, Fonkalsrud EW et al (eds) Principles of pediatric surgery, 2nd edn. Mosby, St Louis, pp 385–394
37. Livaditis A, Radburg L, Odensjo G (1972) Esophageal end-to-end anastomosis, reduction of anastomotic tension by circular myotomy. Scand J Thorac Cardiovasc Surg 6:206–214
38. Gough MH (1980) Esophageal atresia – use of an anterior flap in the difficult anastomosis. J Pediatr Surg 15:310–311
39. Holland AJA, Ron O, Pierro A et al (2009) Surgical outcomes of esophageal atresia without fistula for 24 years at a single institution. J Pediatr Surg 44:1928–1932

40. Foker JE, Kendall Krosch TC, Cotton K et al (2009) Long-gap esophageal atresia treated by growth induction: the biological potential and early follow-up results. Semin Pediatr Surg 18:23–29
41. Bairdain S, Hamilton TE, Smithers CJ et al (2015) Foker process for the correction of long gap esophageal atresia: primary treatment versus secondary treatment after prior esophageal surgery. J Pediatr Surg 50:933–937
42. Ng J, Loukogeorgakis SP, Pierro A et al (2014) Comparison of minimally invasive and open gastric transposition in children. J Laparoendosc Adv Surg Tech 24:742–749
43. Van der Zee DC, Gallo G (2015) Thoracoscopic traction technique in long gap esophageal atresia: entering a new era. Surg Endosc 29:3324–3330
44. Engum SA, Grosfeld JL, West KW et al (1995) Analysis of morbidity and mortality in 227 cases of esophageal atresia and/or tracheoesophageal fistula over two decades. Arch Surg 130:502–508
45. Dingemann C, Dietrich J, Zeidler J et al (2015) Early complications after esophageal atresia repair: analysis of a German health insurance database covering a population of 8 million. Dis Esophagus doi: 10.1111/dote12369 [Epub ahead of print]
46. Koivusalo AI, Pakarinen MP, Lindahl HG et al (2015) Revisional surgery for recurrent tracheoesophageal fistula and anastomotic complications after repair of esophageal atresia in 258 infants. J Pediatr Surg 50:250–254
47. Baird R, Laberge J-M, Levesque D (2013) Anastomotic strictures after esophageal atresia repair: a critical review of recent literature. Eur J Pediatr Surg 23:204–213
48. Serhal L, Goffrand F, Steir R et al (2010) Anastomotic stricture after surgical repair of esophageal atresia: frequency, risk factors, and efficacy of esophageal bougie dilations. J Pediatr Surg 45:1459–1462
49. Manfredi MA, Jennings RW, Anjum MW et al (2014) Externally removable stents in the treatment of benign recalcitrant strictures and esophageal perforations in pediatric patients with esophageal atresia. Gastrointest Endosc 80:246–252
50. Lal DR, Oldham KT (2013) Recurrent tracheoesophageal fistula. Eur J Pediatr Surg 23:214–218
51. Bruch SW, Hirschl RB, Coran AG (2010) The diagnosis and management of recurrent tracheoesophageal fistulas. J Pediatr Surg 45:337–340
52. Kawahara H, Kubota A, Hasegawa T et al (2007) Lack of distal esophageal contractions is a key determinant of gastroesophageal reflux disease after repair of esophageal atresia. J Pediatr Surg 42:2017–2021
53. Tovar JA, Fragoso AC (2013) Gastroesophageal reflux after repair of esophageal atresia. Eur J Pediatr Surg 23:175–181
54. Wheatley MJ, Coran AG, Wesley JR (1993) Efficacy of the Nissen fundoplication in the management of gastroesophageal reflux following esophageal atresia repair. J Pediatr Surg 28:53–55
55. Esposito C, Langer JC, Schaarschmidt K et al (2005) Laparoscopic anti-reflux procedures in the management of gastroesophageal reflux following esophageal atresia repair. J Pediatr Gastroenterol Nutr 40:349–351
56. Holschneider P, Dubbers M, Engelskirchen R et al (2007) Results of the operative treatment of gastroesophageal reflux in children with particular focus on patients with esophageal atresia. Eur J Pediatr Surg 17:163–175
57. Filler RM, Rossello PJ, Lebowitz RL (1976) Life threatening anoxic spells caused by tracheal compression after repair of esophageal atresia: correction by surgery. J Pediatr Surg 11:739–748
58. Ngerncham M, Lee EY, Zurakowski D et al (2015) Tracheobronchomalacia in pediatric patients with esophageal atresia: comparison of diagnostic laryngoscopy/bronchoscopy and dynamic airway multidetector computed tomography. J Pediatr Surg 50:402–407
59. Schwartz MZ, Filler RM (1980) Tracheal compression as a cause of apnea following repair of tracheoesophageal fistula: treatment by aortopexy. J Pediatr Surg 15:842–848
60. Filler RM, Forte V, Fraga JC et al (1995) The use of expandable metallic airway stents for tracheobronchial obstruction in children. J Pediatr Surg 30: 1050–1056
61. Mortell AE, Azizkhan RG (2009) Esophageal atresia repair with thoracotomy: the Cincinnati contemporary experience. Semin Pediatr Surg 18:12–19
62. Chetcuti P, Phelan PD (1993) Respiratory morbidity after repair of oesophageal atresia and tracheo-oesophageal fistula. Arch Dis Child 68:167–170
63. Delacourt C, deBlic J (2011) Pulmonary outcome of esophageal atresia. JPGN 52:S31–S32
64. Sistonen S, Malmberg P, Malmstromk K et al (2010) Repaired oesophageal atresia: respiratory morbidity and pulmonary function in adults. Eur Respir J 36:1106–1112
65. Connor MJ, Springford LR, Kapetanakis VV et al (2015) Esophageal atresia and transitional care – step 1: a systematic review and meta-analysis of the literature to define the prevalence of chronic long-term problems. Am J Surg 209:747–759
66. Gatzinsky V, Wennergren G, Jonsson L et al (2014) Impaired peripheral airway function in adults following repair of esophageal atresia. J Pediatr Surg 49:1347–1352
67. Pedersen RN, Markow S, Kruse-Anderson S et al (2013) Esophageal atresia: gastroesophageal functional follow-up in 5–15 year old children. J Pediatr Surg 48:2487–2495
68. Rintala RJ, Sistonen S, Pakarinen MP (2009) Outcome of esophageal atresia beyond childhood. Semin Pediatr Surg 18:50–56
69. Castilloux J, Bouron-DalSoglio D, Faure C (2010) Endoscopic assessment of children with esophageal atresia: lack of relationship of esophagitis and esophageal metaplasia to symptomatology. Can J Gastroenterol 24:312–316

70. Rintala RJ, Pakarinen MP (2013) Long-term outcome of esophageal anastomosis. Eur J Pediatr Surg 23:219–225
71. Legrand C, Michaud L, Salleron J et al (2012) Long-term outcome of children with oesophageal atresia type III. Arch Dis Childhood 97:808–811
72. Glinianaia SV, Embleton ND, Rankin J (2012) A systematic review of studies of quality of life in children and adults with selected congenital anomalies. Birth Defects Res 94:511–520
73. Deurloo JA, Ekkelkamp S, Hartman EE et al (2005) Quality of life in adult survivors of correction of esophageal atresia. Arch Surg 140:976–980
74. Bouman NH, Koot HM, Hazebrock FWJ (1999) Long term physical, psychological, and social functioning of children with esophageal atresia. J Pediatr Surg 34:399–404
75. Dellenmark-Blom M, Chaplin JE, Gatzinsky V et al (2015) Health-related quality of life among children, young people and adults with esophageal atresia: a review of the literature and recommendations for future research. Qual Life Res 10:2433–2445

Hiatal Hernia and Gastroesophageal Reflux

12

Philippe Montupet and Reva Matta

12.1 Introduction

A hiatal hernia is a partial gastric pull-up across the hiatal orifice. Gastroesophageal reflux (GER) is frequently associated. On the contrary, a GER disease can exist without anatomical hiatal hernia. In many instances, a small hiatal hernia and slight or transient GER are asymptomatic or well tolerated.

There is a broad spectrum of symptoms related to hiatal hernia and GER. Postprandial regurgitations and failure are suggestive, although upper respiratory or pulmonary symptoms can prevail. In addition, ENT and allergic manifestations, or a failure to thrive, can be the main consequences in terms of symptomatology. Diagnostic techniques are required to confirm GER and associated hiatal hernia and also to assess its repercussions. Although the X-ray barium meal suffers from numerous limitations, it remains a useful tool. The pHmetry has gained popularity, performed over a 24-h period in ambulatory conditions. The endoscopy allows a simple and fast evaluation of the possible repercussions of reflux on the esophageal mucosa and may show a cardial gaping openness or a hiatal malposition. The manometry goes further since it is also a mean to investigate possible motor troubles and abnormalities of the lower esophageal sphincter (LES) pressure. Newly the impedancemetry [1–3] combines 24-h records of pH, motility, and pressures – an alkaline GER may be detected as well.

Many children who suffer from a GER disease remain under-investigated. When a GER induces severe complications or escapes a prolonged medical treatment, surgical indications have to be considered. That is always the case for a large hiatal hernia. Surgery could also be more frequently indicated since advanced laparoscopic techniques and skill have improved dramatically surgical results [4].

All the techniques performed prior to the era of minimally invasive surgery (MIS) are reproducible under laparoscopy. However, the surgeon's skill is related to a solid training, and as a matter of fact any surgeon is faithful to a favored technique. Thus, this chapter describes various approaches and also current trends.

12.2 Pathophysiology

The esophagogastric junction is an anatomical functional system anchored by anatomical elements which create an antireflux barrier. The fac-

P. Montupet (✉)
Hôpitaux Universitaires Paris-Sud, Bicêtre Hospital, Université Paris XI, 78 avenue du Général Leclerc, 94275, Le Kremlin-Bicêtre Cedex, France
e-mail: philippe.montupet@wanadoo.fr

R. Matta
Assistant Professor of Clinical Surgery, University of Balamand, El-Koura, Lebanon

Division of Pediatric Surgery, Department of Surgery, Saint George Hospital University Medical Center, Beirut, Lebanon
e-mail: mattareva@gmail.com

M. Lima (ed.), *Pediatric Digestive Surgery*, DOI 10.1007/978-3-319-40525-4_12

tors of anchorage are intrinsic (sphincter and His angle) and extrinsic (crura, membrane of Laimer, gastrophrenic ligament).

The LES extends for about 1–2 cm above the diaphragm to reach the cardia. Its function partly depends on the vagus nerve. The LES pressure ranges in children from 10 to 20 mmHg, influenced by sympathetic and parasympathetic innervation.

The anatomical or physiological incompetence of the crural sphincter may be responsible for reflux during LES relaxation. Inadequate responses of the LES to an increase of intragastric pressure – due to a physiologic event or to a delayed gastric emptying – are also causes of GER.

Esophageal clearance and peristalsis consist in expelling material coming from the stomach. Their failure induces alteration of the esophageal mucosa. Ultimately, the columnar metaplasia of Barrett's esophagus may appear.

These anatomo-physiologic features have to be reminded to emphasize some details of the surgical repair, such as vagus nerve preservation, careful knotting on crural muscles, and right positioning of the LES.

12.3 Surgical Indications

Best results with drugs are achieved by an effective initial therapy. However, the effects of long-term treatment are little known. Moreover, a long-lasting medical treatment implies regular controls [5].

As such, it might be not cost-effective because the duration of this treatment is unpredictable; otherwise, when it is not totally successful, the chronic evolution of the disease consists in a great challenge for both parents and children. In addition, numerous families are concerned by several GER among their members, and this should be correlated with a genetic factor; some of those children need an operation, and some others do not.

In terms of surgical indications regarding a GER, especially because the parents' expectation and their anxiety about complications or failure are great, surgeons are strongly required to be cautious and advised. Since there are four categories of possible investigations – endoscopy, pHmetry, manometry, and barium meal – at least two of them must clearly establish abnormal results. Eventually, a form of gentlemen agreement should impose a postoperative checking [14] and a long-term follow-up after the surgery.

As for associated pathologies, they can induce more surgical indications, despite the suitable choice of investigation and time for decision doesn't make a consensus. If huge hiatal hernias are operated sooner, on the contrary, in case of beforehand operated esophageal atresia or diaphragmatic hernia, the time for surgical indication is unclear. The correction of the GER represents a second operation, and the success is more difficult to warrant due to the age and fragility of the patients. The question is somewhat similar regarding neurologically impaired patients (NIP).

Finally, various arguments make the surgeon trends to increase or on the contrary to reduce his own indications: center's ability to investigate GER, devotion to associated abnormalities, and own skill are the main factors.

12.4 Initial Treatments and Preoperative Preparation

Initial therapy has to be prolonged to a minimum of 6–8 months prior to discussing the surgery. This period of time is under the control of the pediatrician, who usually several drugs are prescribed; among them are a prokinetic and a proton-pump inhibitor. The choice of therapy for a GER disease depends on the severity of signs and the degree of esophagitis. After a break off, if there is a clear relapse of symptoms, investigations are required again – at least a barium meal and a manometry [5] – which will be used also as preoperative workup.

The preoperative workup has several goals:

- To confirm the surgical indication
- To precise the anatomical condition, i.e., hiatal hernia
- To make a checkup regarding associated pathologies or anesthetic risk

A thorough history of troubles and physical exam are the essential initial stage of any workup for gastroesophageal disease, including compliance with treatments, familial status, and growth landmarks. Complementary investigations appear to be objective arguments. Nevertheless, all are neither available in a single center nor suitable in a single patient. In fact, it seems correct to discuss a surgical indication only if two of them show a continuous and severe GER.

When a child and his parents are referred to the surgeon's consultation, most of them spent a long time of treatment, underwent several more or less invasive investigations, and are anxious to obtain a better result. Their pediatrician briefly informed them about surgical procedures and possible side effects, while they could also get information from internet. The surgeon has to take these informations into account, in order to provide detailed and precise surgical ones. A draft of the planned procedure helps the understanding, also the reasons of its choice, the right description of the postoperative period, and eventually the long-term follow-up. Information should be given concerning the risk of recurrences and the way to treat them. Anesthetic consultation has to be planned separately, to allow parents asking new questions as well.

12.5 Surgical Procedures

The aim of the surgery is to create an efficient sphincter process at the bottom of the esophagus [5]: principles are repositioning of the abdominal part of the esophagus, calibration of the hiatal orifice, and creation of an antireflux mechanism.

Children fast for an average of 6 h before surgery (4 under 12 ms). A general anesthesia is required, while vecuronium is given for muscle relaxation only if necessary. Monitoring is standardized. A nasogastric tube is inserted.

As for laparoscopic surgery, a locoregional anesthesia is added by injection of marcaine laterally to the umbilicus along the right muscles. The gas insufflation is controlled at an 8–12 mmHg level but varies during the different steps of the procedure in order to preserve a suitable ventilation and to prevent hypercarbia.

12.5.1 Positioning and Setup

In case of laparoscopic approach, the patient is supine in the reverse Trendelenburg position. If the child is under 6–8 years of age, the legs are folded at the bottom of the table in a frog position. If he is older, they are placed in the lithotomy position, and the surgeon sits between the legs. The video equipment is placed at the right side of the patient's head. All the cables are fixed at the level of the right leg. The assistants and the instrument's table are on the right hand of the surgeon, facing the video screen.

As for open approach, the incision can be on the medial supraumbilical line or more often transversal on the right side. A rigid retractor lifts up the parietal wall. The left liver lobe is carried up and to the right by a smooth retractor held by an assistant. There is no special instrumentation devoted to the open approach.

Laparoscopic instrumentation depends more on the patient size than on the chosen technique. For infants and children less than 10 kg, 3-mm instruments of 18–20 cm are suitable. A 30°-angled endoscope is preferentially used. The choice of energy source is related to the instruments used, scissors or hook, sealing devices which continuously are improved. Limitations are also their relative cost.

12.5.2 Laparoscopic Antireflux Surgery

Laparoscopic antireflux surgery (LARS) has more and more replaced the open approach worldwide [4], thanks to an excellent clinical outcome and success rates. It was first reported in children in 1993 [6]. This evolution in terms of MIS is especially to be considered for children with neurological impairments who represent a large part of the surgical indications.

At the beginning of LARS, it was advocated to reply the same procedures as made by an open approach. Then, the tendency has been to compare the results of the three main used procedures [4], and reports regarding the others became scarce. In spite of their progressive abandon, we will briefly describe them as well.

Nissen, Toupet, and Thal techniques are equally important to know, because even if a pediatric surgeon is more trained with one, the two others can be useful and applied to peculiar cases, for instance, the redo cases. They are total fundoplication and partial – posterior or anterior – fundoplication. In addition to differences concerning the type of the wrap which is created around the esophagus, these techniques can differ by some techniques of dissection; the latter will be emphasized within the discussion.

12.5.2.1 Laparoscopic Nissen

First described in 1959, it has been one of the standards for antireflux surgery (ARS) for the last 50 years, because a 360° wrap was considered as the most effective antireflux valve.

Laparoscopy is started with a 30° endoscope placed through the umbilical site. The left lobe of the liver is retracted. The procedure is started by dividing the gastro-hepatic ligament; it is advised to respect an aberrant left hepatic artery, present in about 25 % of cases. Both diaphragm crura are cleared to allow adequate mobilization of the intra-abdominal esophagus. Then the stomach is retracted medially, and the upper short gastric vessels are divided in order to free a large part of the gastric fundus. As such, a large retroesophageal window is safely made (and the wrap will be tension-free). The retroesophageal window is enlarged, taking care not to injure the posterior vagus nerve. Mobilization of a good length of intra-abdominal esophagus is critical to ensure the formation of an adequate wrap. Once this has been completed, time is to reparation.

Even if the hiatus looks to be of normal size, one or several crural stitches are placed using a strong nonabsorbable suture; this routine closure will help to prevent the development of a hiatal hernia, one of the most common complications following a Nissen. A 360° wrap is formed with the fundus brought around behind the esophagus with a stent inside. The wrap is made 2–3 cm in length and consists in three to four sutures going from the stomach to the anterior wall of the esophagus and to the wrapped portion of the stomach; the inclusion of the esophagus in each suture should prevent a slipped Nissen. The top stitch may also include the anterior diaphragmatic rim with the same goal. Additional stitches may be placed between the wrap and the right crus to help secure the wrap in the abdomen [6–11].

12.5.2.2 Laparoscopic Nissen Rossetti

Rossetti worked close to Nissen and finally described his own modification of the technique. His principle is to use the anterior wall of the stomach as a short and floppy wrap around the esophagus. Moreover, the anterior wall of the esophagus is not concerned by the wrap sutures.

Dissection does not differ from a Nissen. Short gastric vessels are divided as far as it is considered useful to free the wrap. However, there is a minimal hiatal dissection; the posterior vagal nerve is always identified first but never dissected and always left close to the esophagus. The esophagus is pushed downward, but there is a minimal hiatal dissection. Division of short gastric vessels is not always necessary.

The sutures include only the stomach and no other structures (Fig. 12.1).

The risk of tension and stricture after Nissen Rossetti or Nissen is the same, depending on the surgeon's training.

12.5.2.3 Laparoscopic Toupet

Toupet described a partial wrap some years after the complete one described by Nissen. A partial wrap seemed to him to be more physiological than a complete one.

Dissection approaches the hiatal area on its right side, thanks to a liver retractor. A small nasogastric tube is on place. The lesser omentum is widely opened, and the right crus is easily identified. Then the posterior vagal nerve should be the main landmark to find the relief of the left crus. When the fascia of the left crus has been found, a large window toward the splenic area is opened. In fact, because the short gastrosplenic vessels will never been divided in this technique, this step is only focused on the enlargement of a retrocardial window, which will allow the wrap to be not twisted or stretched.

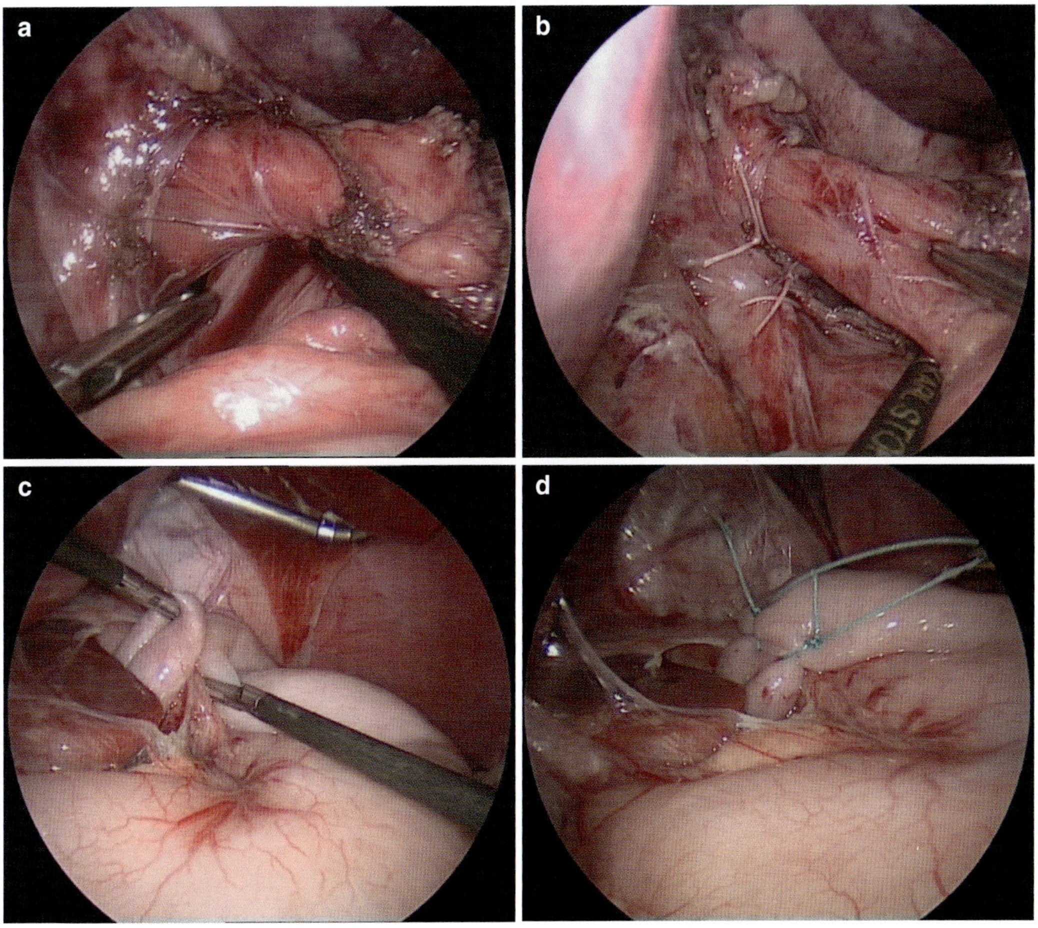

Fig. 12.1 Laparoscopic Nissen Rossetti fundoplication. Creation of the retroesophageal window (**a**), suture of the diaphragmatic crura (**b**), the fundus is brought around behind the esophagus to create a wrap (**c**), suture of the wrap including only the stomach (**d**)

The main feature of the wrap is to be only a translation of the gastric fundus behind and around the esophagus. Then this wrap is fixed onto the right crus by three stitches. Two other rows of three stitches make the wrap encircling the esophagus only on three-fourth of its girth. The final aspect shows an anterior esophagus wall kept free [12–14] (Fig. 12.2).

12.5.2.4 Laparoscopic Thal

This partial fundoplication according to Thal was described in the 1970s by an open approach. Then, laparoscopic series were provided, especially by the team of Utrecht. Hiatal dissection allows a mobilization of the distal esophagus until a sufficient part has reached an intra-abdominal position. The hiatus is calibrated by one or two sutures, while a stent is temporarily introduced into the esophagus.

The fundoplication consists in two rows of three stitches between the anterior wall of the fundus and the anterior wall of the esophagus, in two layers. The last one fixes the wrap to the anterior rim of the hiatus and to the right crus.

12.5.2.5 Other Techniques of LARS

Many procedures have been described. All are feasible under laparoscopy; all were invented to obviate some pitfalls or imperfect results of the main techniques. Here are summarized some of them which knew popularity.

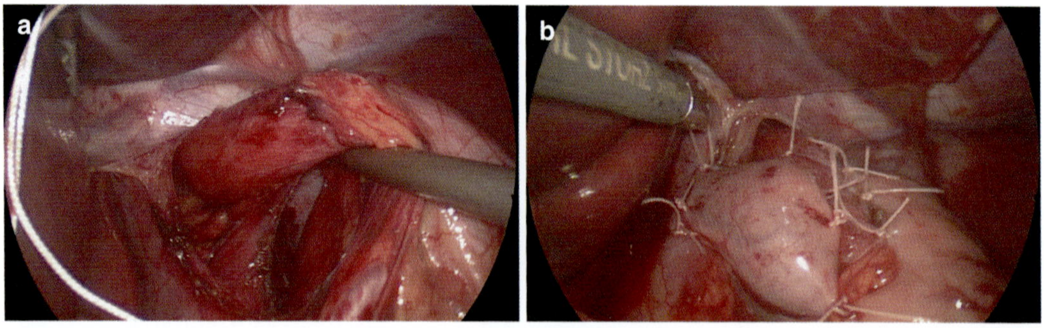

Fig. 12.2 Laparoscopic Toupet fundoplication. Creation of retroesophageal window (**a**), suture of the wrap to the esophagus (**b**)

Jaubert de Beaujeu procedure's combines a reconstruction of the His angle according to the Lortat-Jacob principle, an anterior fundoplication as described by Thal and Dor, pulling the esophagus down as far as possible and also anchoring it to the crus and diaphragm. There is no need to divide short gastric vessels. Intra-abdominal fixation of the esophagus around the hiatus is the main step of the procedure. Both edges of the pulled down esophagus are sutured to the adjacent crus and the anterior part of the esophagus to the diaphragm. Then, when recreating the Hiss angle, sutures include also the fascia of the left crus. Anterior fundoplication ends the procedure.

Boix-Ochoa procedure gained popularity in the 1980s. Again, the fundamental aim of this procedure was to restore and maintain the length of the infradiaphragmatic segment of the esophagus. After dissection, several stitches are put between the esophagus and the hiatal orifice. The latter is calibrated by one or several stitches. Then the greater curvature of the stomach is mobilized and fixed to the undersurface of the diaphragm, and an anterior fundoplication is performed.

Other techniques were developed by gastroenterologists for adult patients; however, either they need sized devices which are not adapted to children like endoluminal plication or Stretta procedure or their follow-up is too short in order to apply them to young patients, like injectable fluids.

12.6 How to Choose an Antireflux Procedure

Any pediatric surgeon today received a training for LARS, with a favorite technique which is depending on his/her team of learning. However, trends and scientific studies moved, so that we must be interested to learn different possible procedures. Nissen and Toupet are first; Thal is also mandatory, for instance, in case to end a Heller intervention.

Having said that, our most frequent practice guaranties our best results. Another consideration is a professional trend to be adapted to a new scientific evidence, such as repeated conclusions from large series and among them RCT (randomized controlled trials). Nowadays, these studies are available [14–19] to prove that postoperative dysphagia is reduced after a partial wrap without impair of efficacy regarding the ARS.

Then, the result of LARS in children is supposed to be maintained life lasting, while a redo [20, 21] is acceptable in case of failure and has also to be explained properly before any parent's decision is made. Thanks to MIS, this possibility is acceptable and rates of failures as well.

There are some advices in order to propose suitable details in case of specific indications which are not depending on the selected procedure.

Huge hiatal hernia makes more cautious and complicated the step of dissection. In addition, more stitches are needed to close the orifice prior to the ARS.

Because a large amount of cases concern NIP, who often have to undergo heavy cares and possibly other surgeries, LARS has to be successfully performed before pulmonary reflux complications make it at risk. First, the hiatus must be reinforced by several stitches. Second, a very large wrap, without possibility of tension or twist, anchored to the right crus, taking in account the gastrostomy implantation, is recommended. The same advice can be applied to children with a previous diaphragmatic hernia.

Many patients are not investigated regarding the esophageal motility because manometric studies are not available everywhere. Even if a Nissen floppy wrap is performed, dysphagia is more often a complication, as proved by multicentric RCTs. This is especially the case for patients cured from an esophageal atresia, and moreover the stomach size makes a difficult total wrap. A posterior partial wrap obviates this problem.

Statistically, a beating vasculonervous pedicle going to the left liver is visible in 15 % of cases. Even if it makes the procedure more demanding, it must be respected.

12.7 Complications of Antireflux Surgery

At the beginning of experience, a bleeding, a perforation, and an abnormal duration of the procedure can induce a conversion to an open approach in order to control it. Although later, these are possible complications to better manage laparoscopically.

Bleeding can occur during the dissection for different reasons. Younger is the child, more fragile is the liver. A suitable choice of the liver retractor, a regular checking of its position must avoid a tear of the liver. Other causes of bleeding are injuries of retrocardial vessels or splenic parenchyma when creating the retrocardial window. The last one is an injury of the inferior diaphragmatic vessels, more often the left one when we release the superior part of the fundus.

Perforations may mainly concern the esophagus or the stomach, when the proper plan of dissection is missed. We have to keep in mind that the posterior vagus nerve is the main landmark to identify in order to follow a good direction close to the left crus.

Perforation can also concern the pleura, and it is immediately recognized by the anesthesiologist. More often it is a small tear, and the solution is to leave this area for a while, without attempt to close it.

Any injury of the posterior vagus nerve will have consequences, mainly a prolonged diarrhea and then a dumping syndrome. We observed four cases, but symptoms disappeared spontaneously in 4–8 months.

Because LARS is a repairing surgery, its success depends on a lot of details and careful attention. Some of them merit a special mention. Knotting has to be minutely controlled, thanks to the video magnification, so that cutting knots, disruption of knots, and transmural stitches can be avoided. The size of the wrap is a main factor of its efficacy. Dividing or not dividing the short gastric vessels is frequently advocated. In fact, if the anterior wall of the fundus is used, there will be no tension and no twist; in addition, the translation can be enlarged on request, even if there is a small stomach. The calibration of the hiatus is mandatory in two cases: NIP who have spastic crisis and for them several stitches, never too tight, are used and large hiatal hernia, for obvious reasons. In our practice, one-third of normal-sized orifice requires a stitch calibration. But when we calibrate the hiatal orifice, be very careful.

The goal of LARS is to create a wrap, partial or total, to reinforce the pressure around the LES pulled down in right position. Main causes of failures are disruption, migration, or being a too loose or too tight wrap. According to these requests, a partial wrap cannot be too tight because the anterior esophagus wall is maintained free.

12.8 Redo Surgery

According to literature review, it appears that redo surgery in GERD was challenging in the times of open approaches. This has completely moved since LARS [20, 21]. The reasons can be fewer adhesions and also a magnification which allow a more precise dissection. Also the rate of redo decreased, as a confirmation of a progress due to MIS.

As for the dissection, it is easier to separate the liver from the wrap and to avoid a large bleeding at this step. New coagulating devices help to do it.

Moreover, a total reconstruction of the wrap is rarely requested. Either it is pulled up or slipped behind the cardia. After a gentle dissection, the wrap has to enlarge below or on the right side of the hiatus. Then, some stitches will ensure the stability of the montage.

Thanks to this evolution, the redo could become a part of the initial information to the parents, with an acceptable rate of 5 %.

Conclusions

Hiatal hernia and GERD are associated and much more frequent than diagnosed in pediatric population. Pediatricians keep a fair memory of the open surgery and also trend toward prolonged medical treatments, which are not without side effects.

Children and families confronted with this disease are suffering more than it is generally thought. Useful investigations are delayed or repeated without a proper surgical advice.

The success of LARS is underestimated. Since the pioneer period, numerous progress and scientific reviews proved that it is an efficient and cost-effective treatment of severe GERD.

This is a demanding surgery [26], in terms of training rather than skills. All pediatric surgery centers are able to teach a suitable technique for the majority of those children. Some of them need to obtain new investigation devices within their pediatrician teams.

Up to now, LARS for children is awarded by excellent results; even if several techniques are in competition, the best one must remain the choice of the expert surgeon.

References

1. Ayazi S, Hagen JA, Zehetner J et al (2009) The value of high- resolution manometry in the assessment of the resting characteristics of the lower esophageal sphincter. J Gastrointest Surg 13:2113–2120
2. Bredenoord AJ, Fox M, Kahrilas PJ, Pandolfino JE, Schwizer W, Smout AJ (2012) International High Resolution Manometry Working Group Chicago classification criteria of esophageal motility disorders defined in high resolution esophageal pressure topography. Neurogastroenterol Motil 24(Suppl 1):57–65
3. Hoshino M, Srinivasan A, Mittal SK (2012) High-resolution manometry patterns of lower esophageal sphincter complex in symptomatic post-fundoplication patients. J Gastrointest Surg 16(4):705–714
4. Esposito C, Montupet P, van Der Zee D, Settimi A, Paye-Jaouen A, Centonze A et al (2006) Long-term outcome of laparoscopic Nissen, Toupet, and Thal antireflux procedures for neurologically normal children with gastroesophageal reflux disease. Surg Endosc 20(6):855–858
5. Lind JF, Burns CM, MacDougall JT (1965) 'Physiological' repair for hiatus hernia manometric study. Arch Surg 91:233–237
6. Lobe TE, Schrop KP, Lunsford K (1993) Laparoscopic Nissen fundoplication in childhood. J Pediatr Surg 28:358–361
7. Nissen R (1961) Gastropexy and fundoplication in surgical treatment of hiatal hernia. Am J Dig Dis 6:954–961
8. Rothenberg SS (2005) The first decade's experience with laparoscopic Nissen fundoplication in infants and children. J Pediatr Surg 40:142–147
9. Rothenberg SS (2006) Laparoscopic redo Nissen fundoplication in infants and children. Surg Endosc 20:1518–1520
10. Rothenberg SS (2012) The effect of laparoscopic Nissen fundoplication on patients with severe GERD and steroid-dependant asthma. J Pediatr Surg 47(6):1101–1104
11. Nissen R (1956) A simple operation for control of reflux esophagitis. Schweiz Med Wochenschr 86(Suppl 20):590–592
12. Kathouda N, Khalil M, Manhas S, Grant S, Velmahos G, Umbach T, Kaiser A (2002) "Andre Toupet" surgeon technician by excellence. Ann Surg 235(4):591–599
13. Mickevicius A, Endzinas Z, Kiudelis M, Jonaitis L, Kupcinskas L, Maleckas A et al (2008) Influence of wrap length on the effectiveness of Nissen and Toupet fundoplication: a prospective randomized study. Surg Endosc 22:2269–2276
14. Memon MA, Subramanya MS, Belal Hossain M, Yunus RM, Khan S, Memon B (2015) Laparoscopic anterior versus posterior fundoplication for gastroesophageal reflux disease: a meta-analysis and systematic review. World J Surg 39:981–996

15. Mauritz FA, van Herwaarden-Lindeboom MY, Stomp W, Zwaveling S, Fischer K, Houwen RH et al (2011) The effects and efficacy of antireflux surgery in children with gastroesophageal reflux disease: a systematic review. J Gastrointest Surg 15:1872–1878
16. Kubiak R, Andrews J, Grant HW (2011) Long-term outcome of laparoscopic Nissen fundoplication compared with laparoscopic Thal fundoplication in children: a prospective, randomized study. Ann Surg 253:44–49
17. Broeders JA, Roks DJ, Jamieson GG et al (2012) Five-year outcome after laparoscopic anterior partial versus Nissen fundoplication: four randomized trials. Ann Surg 255:637–642
18. Peters MJ, Mukhtar A, Yunus RM, Khan S, Pappalardo J, Memon B, Memon MA (2009) Meta-analysis of randomized clinical trials comparing open and laparoscopic antireflux surgery. Am J Gastroenterol 104(6):1548–1561
19. Mardani J, Lundell L, Engstrom C (2011) Total or posterior partial fundoplication in the treatment of GERD. Results of a randomized trial after 2 decades of follow-up. Ann Surg 253:875–878
20. Ostlie DJ, Holcomb GW (2007) Reiterative laparoscopic surgery for recurrent gastroesophageal reflux. Semin Pediatr Surg 4(16):252–258
21. Lopez M, Kalfa N, Forgues D et al (2008) Laparoscopic redo fundoplication in children: failure causes and feasibility. J Pediatr Surg 43:1885–1890

Esophageal Replacements in Children

13

Olivier Reinberg

13.1 Introduction

For historical reasons, our University Hospital has been involved for a long time in esophageal replacements: in 1907, Cesar Roux performed successfully the first total esophageal replacement on a 12-year-old child in Lausanne, Switzerland. The child suffered from caustic stenosis. It was a presternal jejunoplasty, so-called *esophago-jejuno-gastrostomose, a new procedure for untreatable esophageal stenosis* [1]. His patient died at 53. His pupil, Henri Vulliet, was the first one to use the colon in 1911. Since then, many surgical procedures have been used to replace the injured or abnormal esophagus. From 1966 to 1989, our Master Noël Genton did 46 esophageal replacements in children, and that was a large series at that time [1–5].

13.2 Indications for Esophageal Replacements

From 1989 to 2014, we have done 285 esophageal replacements in children aged 9 months–18 years (mean age 5.9) as first attempts. They were a majority of boys (62 %) as 95 % of our replacements were for caustic burns.

The indications for esophageal replacements differ according to the children's native countries. Both in low- and high-income countries, ingestion of corrosive substances, alkalis or acids, is the most common cause for esophageal replacement, to minimize the hazards of household products and laws for containers with child-resistant closures. The majority of ingestions occurs in children younger than 5 years and could be preventable [6–9]. Ingestion in children older than 5 years is suspect, and, in adolescents, mainly in girls, is usually intentional with larger volumes swallowed [7]. In addition, there might be an unknown number of cases of abuse. The true prevalence of these injuries is unknown. According to the report on pediatric trauma done by the World Health Organization and the UNICEF, more than 120,000 children under 6 years old suffered caustic injuries in the United States in 2004 [6, 10]. In the pediatric group, 90 % of esophageal burns are caused by alkali substances and 10 % by acids [11]. (For more details see Chap. 16.)

Other indications for esophageal replacements are uncommon. As other authors, we got involved in the treatment of isolated cases of postinfectious strictures, fungal (*Candida*) or viral (*Herpes*) [12], malformations (long congenital strictures, long duplications of the esophagus), tumors (giant leiomyoma [13]), stenosis post-radiotherapy, or related to epidermolysis bullosa. We do not believe dilatations can release strictures in epidermolysis bullosa as the injury on the

O. Reinberg
Pediatric Surgery, Rochettaz 24, CH – 1009 Pully, Switzerland
e-mail: olreinberg@gmail.com

M. Lima (ed.), *Pediatric Digestive Surgery*, DOI 10.1007/978-3-319-40525-4_13

mucosa produces the recurrence [14]. However, they are the most difficult surgeries that we had to deal with. Other authors have also reported unusual cases such as postinfectious strictures after *Pseudomonas* infections [15] and ingested tablets of salicylic acid [16] (Table 13.1).

On the opposite, since 1989, we have never performed an esophageal replacement, neither for a peptic stricture nor for an esophageal atresia born in our hospital. In our team peptic strictures are released with dilatations following anti-reflux procedures. The definition of a "long-gap esophageal atresia" as the "inability to achieve primary end-to-end anastomosis" is surgeon dependent. Most anastomosis of "long-gap esophageal atresia" can be done as delayed procedures, waiting sometimes for several months with a gastrostomy, as long as no cervicostomy has been done impeding from spontaneous lengthening. There is a strong correlation between too early procedures and complications including graft necrosis, anastomotic leaks, and sepsis [17–19].

Lee has compared delayed primary anastomosis with esophageal replacement with gastric tubes in a series of 44 patients with "long-gap esophageal atresia." There was no difference in perioperative complications, but replacements had more long-term complications (86 %) compared to delayed primary anastomosis (30 %). Almost all patients experienced gastroesophageal reflux (GER) [20]. Pierro and coworkers, who has a large experience in esophageal replacements for long-gap atresia, very recently published a series of ten esophageal atresias without fistula with primary delayed anastomosis without replacement [21]. He concluded that the management of pure EA continues to be challenging, but the preservation of native esophagus is possible with significant morbidity, and the long-term outcomes are favorable.

Table 13.1 Indications for esophageal replacements ($n=285$)

Acquired	Congenital
273 Caustic stenosis	Four malformations Two long congenital stenosis One long esophageal duplication One achalasia
Two stenosis post-radiotherapies	One giant esophageal leiomyoma
Two stenosis post-viral infections (*Herpes*)	Two sequelae of epidermolysis bullosa
Two stenosis post-fungal infections (*Candida*)	

13.3 Pathogenesis

(For more details, please refer to Chap. 16.)

Acids and bases can be defined as caustics, which cause significant tissue damages upon contact with the esophagus. Most acids produce a coagulation necrosis by denaturing proteins, inducing a coating coagulum that protects the underlayers from deeper penetration. Bases induce more severe injuries known as liquefaction necrosis, i.e., the denaturation of proteins together with a saponification of fats, which penetrate deep through the esophageal wall and can perforate.

The severity of the damages is related to several factors, including the pH, the concentration, and the volume of the agent. The contact time is of little interest as a lesion occurs within a few seconds. The physical form of the agent plays a significant role: the ingestion of solid pellets results in prolonged local contact time with the esophagus, thus deeper localized burns, while liquids generate superficial but more extensive lesions. For this reason, it is of major importance to refrain from drinking after pellet ingestion as it may induce both types of lesions.

Due to stagnation, lesions are more frequent and more serious at the level of anatomic narrowings of the esophagus (superior esophageal sphincter, aortic arch and left main bronchus at the level of T4–T5, and above the esophagogastric junction).

Like skin, the long-term effect of caustic esophageal burns is a hypertrophic scarring process, which can result in stricture formation. In addition, with the disappearance of the mucosa, the facing surfaces adhere to each other worsening the stenosis of the esophagus or occluding its lumen moving toward a fistula. Mucosal reepithelization is a slow process, usually not complete before 4–6 weeks. Not until a complete reepithelization, the inflammation continues, and granulation tissue comes to maturity. Thus, a stricture formation is detectable after 2 weeks and is definite by the fourth week. This is the best time to start dilatations.

If the muscular layers of the esophagus have been destroyed, they will not regenerate and be replaced by fibrous tissue. Even if the lumen has been kept open, the contraction waves will never overpass that point.

The caustic burn induces a shortening of esophagus and a motility disorder resulting in reflux and poor esophageal clearance, which adds a peptic stenosis to a caustic one evidenced by histology (O. Reinberg, unpublished). For this reason, all our patients under conservative treatment with dilatations receive proton-pump inhibitors (PPIs) as early as possible, even if their efficiency has not been proven [6, 9, 19].

13.4 Initial Treatment and Preoperative Preparation

(For more details, please refer to Chap. 16.)

The rate of stricture formation reported in literature varies from 2 to 63 % (!). About a month after caustic ingestion, the diagnosis of stenosis can be assessed by an esophagogram and an endoscopy, once the edema has gone. Then, according to the severity of the stenosis, a dilatation program can be started. The optimal frequency of dilatation is not well established in the literature, and our practice was to use a symptom-based approach, but an interval of 3 weeks seems appropriate in most cases.

Isolated short stenosis of the esophagus, i.e., 1–2 cm, can be treated by dilatations with good results. Long ones (more than 3 cm), multiple stenosis (more than 2), or those with a tracheo-esophageal fistula cannot be solved by dilatations and require an esophageal replacement [5, 17]. However, the decision should not be precipitated as spontaneous improvement can occur within a few months until the lesions are stabilized. We have seen children with long narrow stenosis at 6 months that would have been candidates for esophageal replacement, who have been "forgotten" in their native countries. When they "reappeared" a year later, they only required dilatations of short narrow strictures. Subsequently, indications for esophageal replacements and their timing vary widely. As a result, children are often subjected to prolonged courses of dilatations prior to esophageal replacement or, conversely, may be exposed to unnecessary surgery [17]. A strong predictor of poor outcome was the delay from ingestion to the beginning of dilatations [17, 18]. Without improvement after 12 months of repeated dilatations, we consider doing an esophageal replacement as other authors [5, 22].

Esophageal replacements are major surgeries that require the child to be in a good nutritional condition. Esophageal strictures usually produce dysphagia for solids, liquids, or both, with slow and insidious progression of weight loss and malnutrition. If the stenosis is important with subsequent dysphagia lasting for more than a month, a gastrostomy should have been done. Most patients referred to us, even those with a previously done gastrostomy, were in poor nutritional conditions and must be placed under refeeding program before surgery.

The way the gastrostomy was done on the anterior stomachal wall is a major concern for the surgeon. When intending to replace an esophagus, the surgeon never knows which transplant he can use: if the gastrostomy has been placed too close from the greater curvature, he may face an interruption of the gastroepiploic artery, and the vascularization of the stomach can be compromised. When performing a gastrostomy for caustic stenosis, it is wise to place it far away from the greater curvature. In some cases, we used an interesting artifice suggested in 1974 by Papahagi and Popovici: when performing the gastrostomy, these authors ligated the middle colonic artery and sometimes the right one to stimulate the development of the left one, anticipating a possible transverse isoperistaltic colonic replacement [23].

A preoperative evaluation of the oropharynx and larynx has to be done preoperatively as associated lesions are not unusual: 15 % in our experience [5]. This initial evaluation should include vocal cord movements before surgery in the neck as paralysis can occur at the time of the caustic injury. We recommend the use of the consensual classification of benign laryngotracheal stenosis done by the European Laryngological Society [24]. The level of a preexisting tracheo-esophageal fistula has to be defined by tracheoscopy. The length of the intact proximal esophagus above the first stenosis should be carefully measured to anticipate swallowing problems.

As other authors, we have abandoned mechanical preparation (enemas) [25, 26]. The day before surgery, we give an oral preparation of polyethylene glycol (= macrogol, 4 l/1.73 m^2) through the gastrostomy (similar to those used before a colonoscopy), independently of the planned procedure, as we never know which transplant will be used.

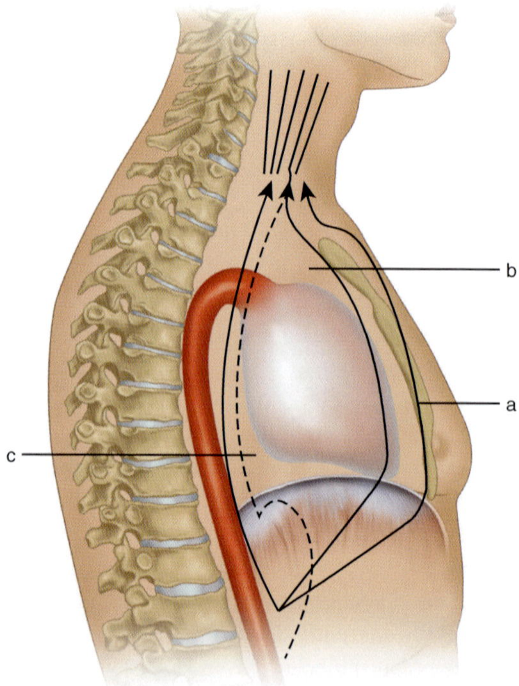

Fig. 13.1 The routes for substitute placement [2]: (*a*) historic presternal, (*b*) retrosternal, (*c*) orthotopic mediastinal posterior

13.5 Surgical Managements

13.5.1 Where Should the Esophageal Substitute Be Placed?

Choosing the appropriate route for esophageal replacement is an important decision.

The historic route was presternal (Fig. 13.1a) as the thorax could not be open at that time. Then the transplants were placed in the retrosternal position in a first procedure, and the native esophagus was removed in a second stage (Fig. 13.1b). We introduced the one-stage procedure in 1989, placing the transplant in the orthotopic position, i.e., in the posterior mediastinum, following a closed-chest esophagectomy (Fig. 13.1c) [27]. The path for an orthotopic plasty is straighter and shorter than that of the retrosternal route but requires removal of the native esophagus [28]. It avoids the two kinks at the upper thoracic inlet and at the reentry into the abdomen. It is our favorite procedure as it seems that the periesophagitis limits dilatation and redundancy of the transplant [2, 5, 27–29].

However, in some circumstances, the retrosternal route had to be used when it appears impossible to dissect safely the esophagus or a previous transplant from the mediastinum. This is most often the case in the multiple redo procedures. In his series of redo procedures, Tovar had also to use the retrosternal route and even to go back to the old presternal path for one patient [30, 31]. It is easy to build a path behind the sternum in a space with very few adhesions. But with time, any transplant placed in this space will widen, especially if there is a narrowing at the distal end where it reintegrates the abdomen. This is more frequent in colonic transplants than in gastric tubes. Colonic transplants placed retrosternally have a strong tendency to become redundant, and we have had to tailor some of them. A gastric tube is more appropriate if the transplant is placed in the retrosternum.

13.5.2 Should We Remove the Native Esophagus and How?

There are two reasons to remove the native esophagus before an esophageal replacement: (i) to place the transplant in the orthotopic position, as mentioned above and (ii) because of the oncologic risk induced by the burned esophagus. The prevalence of malignancies, mostly carcinoma, is unknown but has been shown in several reports to range from 1.8 to 16 %, and the malignancies are known to take decades to develop. They were believed to be related to the abrasion of food intake on the burned esophagus. Subsequently, it was said that a disconnected burn esophagus did not bear that risk. Actually, no one knows the fate of a disconnected burned esophagus, and cases have been reported of carcinoma appearing on disconnected unused native esophagus after replacements [22, 32, 33]. For this reason, we remove as much as possible a native burned esophagus before replacement. However, a demucosed short segment of an abandoned disconnected esophagus is an acceptable risk.

In 1978, Orringer was the first to describe a blind esophagectomy without thoracotomy [34]. Since 1989, we introduced the one-stage orthotopic esophageal replacement following a closed-chest esophagectomy [27, 35]. The esophagus was removed through a left cervical incision after its transhiatal dissection by laparotomy without thoracotomy. A blind dissection by digitoclasy was performed in the middle part of the esophagus. At this level, adhesions to the major vascular structures and to the bronchi are the most severe and can lead to serious life-threatening injuries [35]. Some anatomical considerations on the vascularization of the esophagus are particularly useful when doing the hemostasis from the cervical opening and from the hiatus [36]. The greater danger remains at the level of the aortic arch and left bronchus where the most important adhesions are and which is the farthest point from skin incisions during the blind dissection. When total esophagectomy became too dangerous, we have abandoned some esophageal remnants at the level of the aortic arch after removal of the mucosa without subsequent narrowing of the esophageal substitute. Even after the experience in more than 200 cases, we considered this step as the most dangerous part of the procedure, showing 18 % of various complications. It allowed the esophagus to be totally removed in 45 % of cases and partially in 40 % [37] (Table 13.2).

In addition, several complications related to anesthesia can occur during blind esophagectomy. The most frequent were (i) endotracheal tube displacement during the dissection of the esophagus which requires tractions on it and through it and (ii) obstructions of the endotracheal tube or of the bronchi (mainly the left one) because of the mobilization of mucous plugs from the lungs during the esophagectomy.

For these reasons, we have tried to achieve esophagectomy under visual control without opening the thorax. Since 2006, we have used a standardized procedure through a laparoscopic transhiatal approach [38, 39]. This technique has been used by other surgeons since then [40]. Some cases of esophageal dissection using a thoracoscopy [41] or a combination of thoracoscopy and laparoscopy in children have also been reported [42–44]. The problem of the thoracoscopic approach is that it gives a lateral view of the esophagus that is hidden in the scarring process. It is safer to start the dissection from below by a transhiatal approach and to follow the intact esophagus up into the adhesions.

During the laparoscopic procedure, the child lays supine at the foot end of the table. The legs are wrapped in a "frog position" as for an antireflux procedure, and the table is tilted to a 30° anti-Trendelenburg position. In order to allow a good access to the esophagus, the right-hand port is placed in relation to the position of the gastrostomy, i.e., slightly inward and inferior to it. This will not only help the dissection of the esophagus, especially during dissection in the mediastinum, but also allow easier insertion of instruments by giving the appropriate direction to the mediastinum through the open hiatus. The esophageal diaphragmatic hiatus is enlarged by a 2–3 cm incision at 10 o'clock. Two large (0 or 2) trans-parietal monofilament threads are passed through the two crura from both sides of the patient and taken out through the skin. They allow a wide opening of the crura similar to the raising of a stage curtain. The transhiatal dissection of the esophagus is pursued under direct vision in close contact with the esophageal wall using a sealing device (Ligasure® LS 1500 Dolphin Tip or Maryland laparoscopic instrument by Covidien). The use of the harmonic dissector (Ultracision® by Ethicon) can be more dangerous as it heats in a very narrow field. Once the distal third of the esophagus has been freed, the liver retractor can be introduced into the mediastinum below the heart to allow a wider view of its major anatomical structures. A rotation of the 30° angulated camera helps to have a better view of both sides of the esophagus. This approach provides a clear view of the vagus nerves and facilitates their preservation. Should a pleural tear occur, a drainage tube is inserted under direct vision. The anatomical structures which run the greatest danger of being damaged during dissection are the left bronchus, whose soft posterior membrane usually adheres firmly to the esophagus, and the left brachiocephalic vein (innominate vein). The esophagus can be freed as far up as possible, usually one or two centimeters below the clavicle. With this technique of and more than 40 cases, no vascular or bronchial wound occurred, and the rate of the total removal of the esophagus raised up to 83 % without complication [38, 39] (Table 13.2). Moreover, it appeared that the delay to extubation and the length of stay in the pediatric intensive care unit (PICU) were shorter after laparoscopic transhiatal esophagectomy [38, 39].

The cervical dissection of the esophagus requires the greatest care to avoid a tracheal tear or a lesion to the left recurrent laryngeal nerve. Preserving the most proximal centimeters of the native esophagus is crucial to avoid swallowing disorders.

A preexistent or preoperative tracheoesophageal fistula must be identified and occluded. The healing of such a suture requires coverage with a well-vascularized tissue because of the firm scarry processes in the mediastinum. For this purpose, several flaps can be used, such as pericardial flap, muscular flap taken from the intercostal muscles, or a flap from the latissimus dorsi in the most severe cases. However in some cases, we have left a part of the native esophagus after the removal of its mucosa and used it as a tracheal or bronchial coverage with success.

Table 13.2 Esophagectomies: comparison according to the techniques used

Techniques	Blind dissection (1989–2006)		Laparoscopic transhiatal (2006–2014)	
N	244		41	
Mean ages	5.9		6.0	
Total esophagectomies	111	45 %	34	83 %
Partial esophagectomies	97	40 %	5	12 %
Failure	36	15 %	2	5 %
Major accidents	44	18 %	0	0 %

13.5.3 Which Transplant?

The esophagus can be replaced by a segment of the colon, the entire stomach, a gastric tube, or a part of the small bowel. However, none is perfect and can operate as a normal esophagus.

Gallo has performed a meta-analysis on 15 studies to compare three techniques for esophageal replacement of long-gap atresia in children: jejunal interposition, colon interposition, and gastric pull-up. The gastric pull-ups and colon interpositions appeared comparable regarding postoperative mortality, anastomotic complications, and graft loss. On long-term follow-up, the gastric pull-ups seem to be associated with a higher respiratory morbidity but fewer gastrointestinal complications than the colon interpositions. They were only two studies with jejunum and none with gastric tubes [45]. Loukogeorgakis and Pierro have published an extensive comparison of recent literature published over the last 5 years on the four main types of esophageal substitution that must be carefully read [46].

We are frequently asked which is our favorite transplant. We cannot answer this question and

Table 13.3 Choice and place of 285 transplants

Transplant	*N*	Direction	*N*	Position	*N*
Transverse colon	234	Isoperistaltic	224	Posterior mediastinum	221
		Antiperistaltic	10	Retrosternal	3
				Posterior mediastinum	10
Right colon	8	Isoperistaltic	5	Posterior mediastinum	8
		Antiperistaltic	3		
Colon mixt	3	Isoperistaltic	3	Posterior mediastinum	3
Gastric tube	36	Antiperistaltic	36	Posterior mediastinum	26
				Retrosternal	10
Jejunum	4	Isoperistaltic	2	Cervico-mediastinal	4
		Antiperistaltic	2		

we used several of them [5] (Table 13.3). When intending to replace an esophagus, the surgeon never knows which transplant can be used: if the gastrostomy has been placed too close from the greater curvature, he may face an interruption of the gastroepiploic artery, and a gastric tube cannot be achieved. Should he plan a colonic transplant, a missing artery could make it impossible. Therefore, he must be able to adapt his technique to the patient's condition and so must be aware of several techniques.

13.5.3.1 Colonic Transplants

The colon is the most frequently used conduit to replace the esophagus; the transverse, ascending, or descending colon has been used, either in an antiperistaltic or isoperistaltic fashion. It offers the advantage of a segment of bowel with several possible vascular supplies that is long enough to be mobilized. Its width is approximately the same as the esophagus. Its length can be adjusted to the requirement [18, 22, 29]. This operation requires meticulous attention to technical details for a successful outcome. The use of the colon provides a good length of transplant and allows a tube of an appropriate diameter.

The operation is carried out through a midline incision from the xyphoid process to the umbilicus. The best transplant is taken on the transverse colon, vascularized by the left colonic artery and placed isoperistaltically (Fig. 13.2). Before ligating the unused vascular bundles, it is wise to generously mobilize the colon from the right to the left severing the gastrocolic ligament and to explore carefully its arteries. An efficient left colonic artery is missing in about 10 % of patients, and the anastomotic transverse colonic arcade can be absent. We check the quality of the chosen arterial supply by clamping the unused arteries during 10–15 min with atraumatic vascular bulldogs clamps. The superficial arteries must remain pulsating, especially those at the farthest end from vascular supply and the peristaltism be present. Once appropriate length is chosen, the transplant is prepared by severing the unused vessels while preserving long arcades. We use conventional ligatures and never coagulate them to prevent from vascular spasms. Once freed the transplant is cleaned and preserved in warm cloths avoiding any tension on its vascular supply.

The colonic transplant has no efficient propulsive contraction and empties by gravity. However, in 1971, Jones first demonstrated on animals [47] and since then in humans [48] that an acid reflux in the transplant can induce a contraction that protects the colonic mucosa against acid aggression. When a reflux occurs, this intrinsic contraction, which can be reproduced with the amplitude of 15–20 mmHg for 45–50 s, rapidly clears the colon. For this reason, we believe that colonic transplants should be placed as far as possible in an isoperistaltic position to benefit from this self-protection.

If the right colon is used, it can be placed in an isoperistaltic fashion using a vascular supply from the middle colonic artery or antiperistaltically on the ileocolic artery. As the right colon is shorter than the transverse, the distal ileum is used with sacrifice of the valve to gain some extra length.

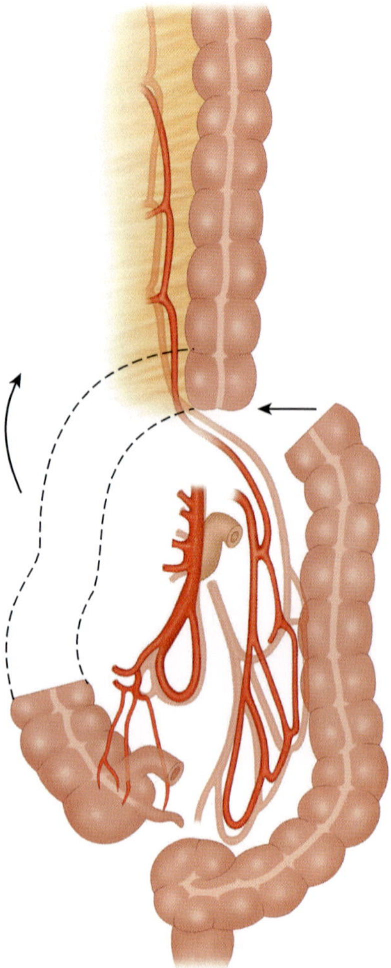

Fig. 13.2 Isoperistaltic transverse colon vascularized by the left colonic artery

In some cases, we used an interesting artifice suggested in 1974 by Papahagi and Popovici: when performing the gastrostomy, these authors ligated the middle colonic artery and sometimes the right one to stimulate the development of the left one, anticipating a transverse isoperistaltic colonic replacement [23].

To bring the transplant to the neck, we use a large (40 mm) Penrose drain, the proximal end of the transplant being placed inside and sutured to it. This avoids any friction to its proximal edge when pulling it up. Before and after this maneuver, we check the arterial pulse with Doppler ultrasounds and the venous return as well. We handle the colon to find the best position for an optimal venous return. Some studies have been dedicated to the arterial supply of transplants but none about the venous return. However, it seems obvious that it is of great importance. Should compression or kinking occur on the drainage vein, the transplant could have a venous engorgement that may induce an ischemia with subsequent leak or stenosis [5].

We always perform the proximal end-to-end anastomosis using a single layer of full thickness interrupted resorbable sutures, with a V-shape incision of the proximal esophagus to make the colon width fit to its diameter if needed. In some cases if a short stenosis is present in the upper part of the native esophagus, we widen it using a Mikulicz procedure to avoid the anastomosis too close from the upper esophageal sphincter.

The distal cologastric anastomosis is performed on the anterior wall of the stomach by the upper third of the small curvature. The suture is done using two layers of resorbable stitches, with disrupted stitches on the seromuscular suture and a running one on the mucosa. A decompression tube is placed into the transplant though the gastrostomy together with a gastrostomy tube and a jejunal feeding tube.

As we placed the colons in an orthotopic position, we experienced frequent reflux and/or stasis in the transplants. Thus, we felt for the need of a new anti-reflux procedure as the standard ones (Nissen, Toupet) were too efficient on the weak wall of the colon. We described in 1993 a new anti-reflux procedure for colonic transplants using an anterior wrap similar to the one described by Dor that was made out of the fundus but fixed to the right crus [5, 49] (Fig. 13.3). It covers 3 cm of the distal transplant. The wrap must be loose enough not to compress the vascular pedicle located behind the transplant. The opening of the hiatus behind the transplant is never closed. This loose anterior wrap is efficient enough on a colonic transplant to prevent reflux as shown on esophagograms performed on day 10. It reduces the reflux at day 10 from 48 to 7,5 % using the anti-reflux wrap and from 40 to 21 % on later

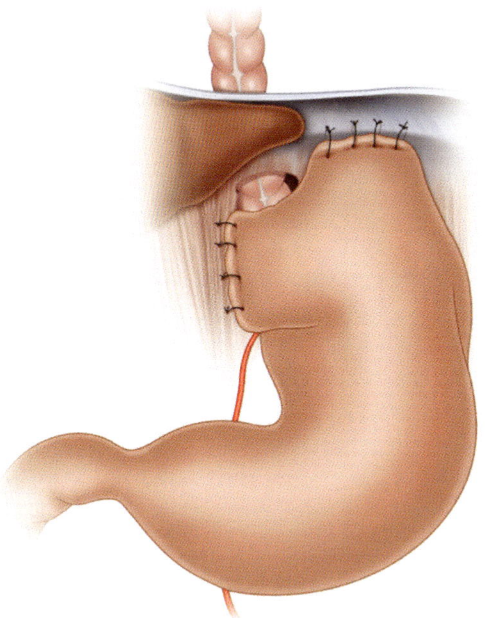

Fig. 13.3 The anti-reflux wrap for colonic transplant [49]

esophagograms. The 20 % long-term rate of stasis in the transplant is not increased with this valve [49].

We never performed a gastric drainage procedure or a Mikulicz pyloroplasty even if damage to the vagus nerves was suspected. We observed some stasis in the stomach and in the transplant, but they all resolved spontaneously within a few days or weeks. Some children had delayed gastric emptying before surgery, so we believe that vagus nerves have suffered from trans-parietal burns as they were in the scar of the periesophagitis.

Gastric Tubes

The concept of a gastric tube comes from the experiments on gastrostomies undertaken during the second half of the nineteenth century. The use of a gastric tube as an esophageal substitute was first done by Dan Gavriliu from Romania in 1951. Heimlich claimed he did it first, but in 1957 after visiting him, he paid tribute to Gavriliu. The first gastric tube performed in North America was by James Fallis from Canada. Dan Gavriliu built two different tubes using the greater curvature vascularized by the gastroepiploic artery. The first one was a reversed gastric tube, the prepyloric antrum being brought to the neck and vascularized by the left gastroepiploic artery; the second one was isoperistaltic supplied by the right gastroepiploic artery. Both required a splenectomy at that time [2, 3]. Today most gastric tubes are reversed, built from the greater curvature of the stomach with blood supply from the left gastroepiploic artery without splenectomy (Fig. 13.4). It brings the antrum to the neck, this part of the stomach producing less acid than the fundus. However, some teams keep doing isoperistaltic tubes [51].

The procedure involves at first the division of the gastrocolic ligament preserving the gastroepiploic artery from the pyloroduodenal artery to the splenic one. Usually the short gastric vessels can be preserved. The free edge of the tube should be taken at about 3 cm from the pylorus. The gastric curvature is molded around a 24-Fr tube, using two to three shots of a 75-mm-long GIA stapler or is hand sewn. It is brought to the neck in the same manner as for a colonic transplant. Care must be taken to the hinge between the tube and the stomach, and some reinforcement stitches can be useful. The upper anastomosis is done the same way as for the colon. A gastrostomy is performed on the anterior wall of the stomach. A decompression tube into the transplant, a gastrostomy tube, and a jejunal feeding tube are placed through it [5].

The gastric tube is an excellent substitute to the esophagus with a reliable blood supply, better than the colon. We never encounter the complication described of a leak along the long suture line. Possibly, this was true at the era of hand sewing, but not anymore with careful stapling. However, a major problem is related to the position of a previously done gastrostomy along the greater curvature, interrupting the gastroepiploic artery. We had to deal with several redo esophageal replacements for severe stenosis of the upper part of gastric tubes because the surgeons had closed gastrostomies along the curvature to build their tubes. When performing a gastrostomy for caustic stenosis, it is wise to place it far away from the greater curvature, just in case a tube could be done. Even with an apparently intact gastroepiploic artery, defects in its continuity

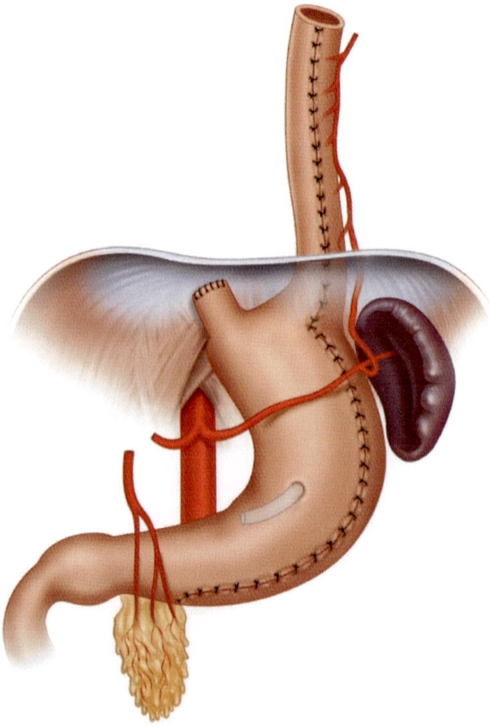

Fig. 13.4 Reversed gastric tube vascularized by the left gastroepiploic artery [50]

have been shown on cadaver studies by Koskas and Ndoye [52, 53].

Because a part of the stomach has been used, an anti-reflux wrap is not possible. Thus, the gastric tube has the disadvantage of an associated gastroesophageal reflux with subsequent possible ulcer. The long suture carries the risk of progressive dysfunctional propulsion. It appears to act purely as a passive conduit. The volume of the stomach, reduced at the beginning, grows with time. The gastric tube keeps its tubular shape without developing dilatation as the colon does.

Gastric Pull-Ups

In the last two decades, the gastric pull-up became predominant after the works of Sweet (1948) in adult patients with esophageal cancer [54] and Spitz in children (1984) [55]. Discouraged by the long-term results of colonic transplants at his institution, Spitz reintroduced it for esophageal atresia at first.

The gastric pull-up involves mobilization of the entire stomach, creating a space in the mediastinum and achieving only one anastomosis in the neck with the cervical esophagus. However, they are three additional sutures to close the gastrostomy, to close the esogastric junction, and to perform a pyloroplasty. The patient is positioned supine with the neck, chest, and abdomen prepared and draped. A midline laparotomy is done, and the gastrostomy is taken down and closed. The stomach should be totally freed from adhesions: the gastrocolic ligament with the short gastric vessels should be carefully divided as well as the gastro-hepatic omentum. The right gastroepiploic artery is preserved and the left one is divided. This may imply the removal of the spleen. The gastroesophageal junction is closed with two layers of sutures. The stomach has to be completely freed, preserving the blood supply via the right gastric artery and the right gastroepiploic vessels. The stomach is brought to the neck through the mediastinum. Extra length can be obtained by the addition of a Kocher maneuver or by some other improvements of the technique such as an additional Collis procedure [56]. The esophagus is sutured to the fundus of the stomach using a single layer of full-thickness interrupted sutures. This gives the longest possible conduit [57].

The vagus nerves are divided bilaterally during the gastric pull-up, so most authors recommend a Mikulicz pyloroplasty. However, Cowles advocates for an extramucosal pyloromyotomy considering that a formal Mikulicz pyloroplasty is placed under tension when the conduit is pulled into the neck and a pyloromyotomy is suitably efficient. A feeding jejunostomy should be done for the postoperative period [57].

The gastric pull-up requires a single cervical anastomosis, and the conduit has an excellent blood supply. However, the closures of the gastrostomy, of the esogastric junction, and of the pyloric procedure are at risk of leak in case of gastric distension [18].

Hirschl found no deaths in 41 patients operated on between 1985 and 2002, but a high incidence of leaks (36 %) and strictures (49 %) was noted [58]. In a large, single-center updated series of 192 gastric pull-ups over a 25-year period, Spitz reported no transplant failure but 5.2 % deaths. Morbidity is not unusual and includes cervical fistula (12 %), anastomotic strictures (19.6 %), swallowing dysfunctions (30.6 %), and delayed gastric emptyings (8.7 %) [59]. Even an intrathoracic volvulus has been reported [60]. In his most recent review, Spitz reports on 236 gastric transpositions with a mortality rate of 2.5 %, leak rate of 12 %, and stricture of 20 % [61].

For the sake of comparison, from 1989 to 2014, we performed 280 esophageal replacements (included redo procedures for referred patients) using either the colon or a gastric tube (but no gastric pull-up): no deaths were observed and no transplant was lost. The complications were cervical leaks in 6 % (all of which resolved spontaneously within a few days), proximal stenosis requiring 1–12 dilatations (and two enlargement surgeries, see below) in 24 %, and 16 % refluxes in the transplants [5]. In 2009, Tovar reviewed his series of 33-year median follow-up of 65 patients with colonic interpositions, reporting 9 % deaths. Patients experienced mild symptoms of reflux (43 %), scoliosis, (22 %), and some other complications [22].

Gastroesophageal reflux is a major problem encountered by 25–30 % of patients with gastric transplants with acid and/or biliary reflux even if pyloroplasty is not carried out. The prevalence of reflux esophagitis in the upper native esophagus when the stomach is used as a substitute ranges from 30 to 78 %. It should be pointed out that the gastric conduit is aperistaltic and surgically denervated even if studies have shown mass contractions of the body of the stomach without any obvious rhythmic peristaltic contractions [62].

Another major problem is related to the volume of the stomach in the chest of small children that compromises the lung function and the venous return. We were involved in undoing 12 gastric pull-ups for life-threatening events, and possibly some of the reported deaths were related to that. According to Newman, reports suggest that several patients undergoing gastric pull-up in the 1960s required colon transposition in the 1980s because of lung problems associated with chronic acid reflux, aspiration pneumonia, and compression by the dilated intrathoracic stomach [50].

Parilli has described a modification of the gastric pull-up (TEGPUL), performed by transhiatal laparoscopy, without pyloroplasty or pyloromyotomy, bringing the transplant through the distal esophagus. It has been successfully done on ten children for esophageal atresia and seems promising, but studies with a larger number of patients and longer follow-up are needed [40].

Small Bowel Interpositions

Several techniques have been tried using either jejunum or ileum on their pedicles [63–66]. Bax reports a series of 19 cases done between 1988 and 2005 for esophageal atresia at a mean age of 76 days with no necrosis [66].

The vessels of the jejunum are built in short arcades with no long unique artery. As to get a segment of jejunum with a long pedicle, the first jejunal branches of the mesenteric vessels are divided close to the upper mesenteric artery. The jejunum is transected between the first and the second loop to allow for reanastomose. After careful measurement of the transplant length, a pedicle is created by withdrawing a segment of jejunum distal to the transplant. The resection has to be very close to the removed segment as to avoid any damage to the vascular arcade. Then the transplant is brought to the upper esophagus and sutured. In most studies, jejunal transplants are anastomosed directly to the stomach [64–66].

Jejunal interpositions are scarcely used in children as blood vessels are thin and frequently compromised. According to its vascular disposition, the jejunal transplant requires the withdrawal or a greater length than needed to divide the vascular arcades and to allow curves in the jejunum to be straightened [2, 63, 67] (Fig. 13.5). Furthermore, the jejunum is fragile to the erosion of acid, so the jejunum should not be the first choice. However, we have used the jejunum as a rescue transplant for referred patients after the failure of colonic or gastric transplant as did Simms [65].

The use of jejunal transplant in children is one of the most difficult procedures for esophageal replacements. It is a demanding surgery with considerable morbidity that requires a great expertise to achieve acceptable results.

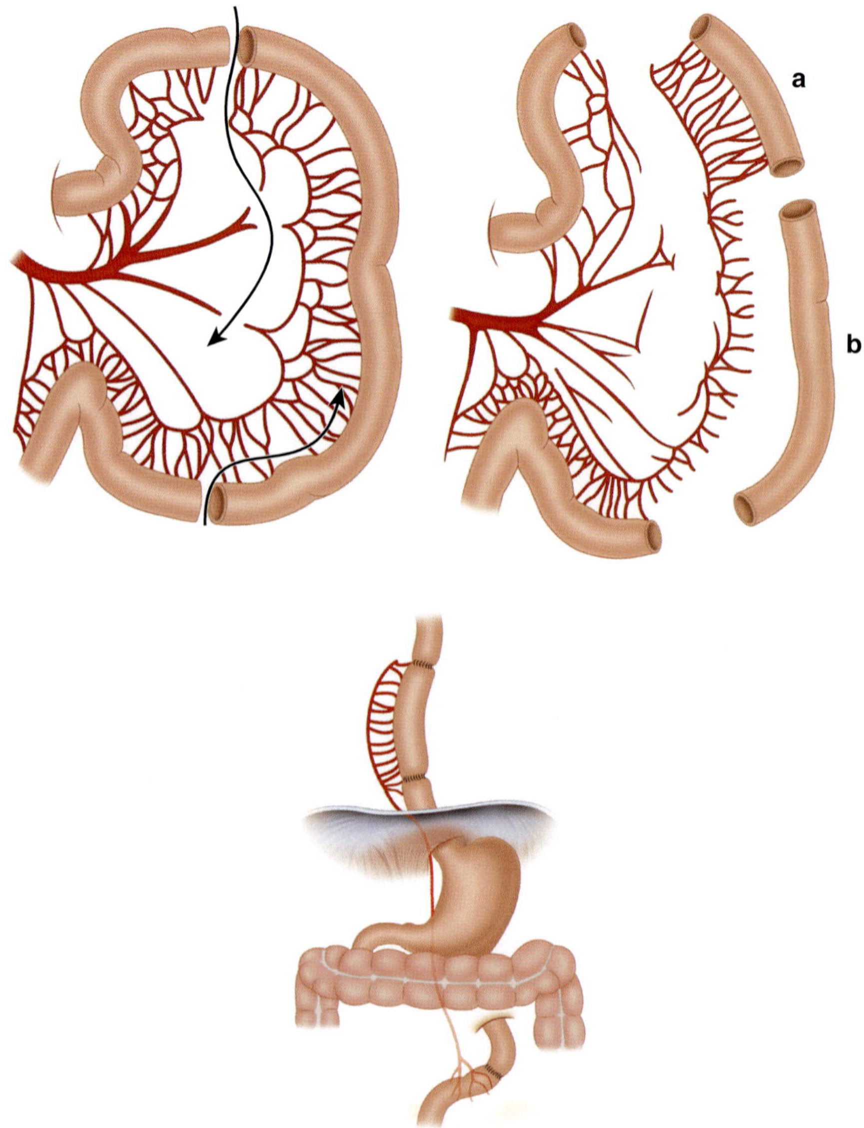

Fig. 13.5 Jejunal transplant: (*a*) pediculated jejunal transplant; note the unused segment with a greater length than that of the transplant (*b*) [66]

Free Grafts and Patches

In some circumstances, it can be interesting not to replace the whole esophagus or to widen a short segment as adults are used to do for cervical cancers. For instance, after ischemic stenosis of a segment of transplant, when the rest of the transplant remains usable, it could be wise to replace only the stenotic segment [5, 65, 67, 68].

In those cases, a free graft of jejunum (or of ileum or colon) can be used in the neck or the upper thorax with microvascular anastomosis on the facial or superior thyroid arteries. The vascularized segment can be used as a circular interponed graft or as a patch. In the latter, after a careful identification of the level of the stenosis by endoscopy, the stricture is open longitudinally. Then the vascularized graft is tailored as a diamond-shaped patch and sutured to the margins of the open esophagus. A soft suction tube is left for a week at the level of the patch to prevent a leak. We used successfully four free jejunal grafts with microanastomosis, measuring from 2 to 4 cm, for short stenosis of the cervical esophagus or after recurrent stenosis of the proximal anastomosis of transplants [5].

13.5.4 Pharyngeal-Associated Burns

Burns from ingestion of caustic agents may include the oral, pharynx, and larynx as well. Combined lesions of the esophagus and the pharynx represent a challenging problem. Among 285 replacements performed for caustic burns since 1989, 25 children had associated pharyngeal burns with partial or total destruction of the epiglottis, pharyngo-laryngeal stenosis, and/or obstruction of one or both pyriform sinuses with variable severity including total closure of the airways in four cases. In spite of severe narrowing of the airways related to subglottic diaphragm with respiratory impairment, only three had tracheostomies when referred. However, they all had intact vocal cords. This is the most important point. The closure reflex of laryngeal vestibule during accidental ingestion of caustic materials acts as a protective measure at the level of the larynx [5, 69]. For those unusual very difficult cases, we proceed in a one-stage reconstruction of the larynx and of the esophagus. At the beginning of the procedure, the ENT surgeons (Prof. Ph. Monnier) resect totally the pharyngo-epiglottic stenosis and the scarring bands with C02 laser under suspension micropharyngoscopy. This allows the resection of the two pyriform sinuses with excellent homeostasis and locates exactly the place where the transplant should be brought.

Then a one-stage esophagoplasty is done using an isoperistaltic colonic interposition or a gastric tube associated with an endoscopic pharyngoplasty, the proximal anastomosis being done at the level of the arytenoids on the larynx and somewhat higher in the oropharynx posteriorly. Thus, the proximal end of the transplant is 3–5 mm from the vocal cords. A long stay in the pediatric intensive care unit (PICU) is needed after surgery because of possible pharyngeal and pulmonary complications, in spite of tracheostomies.

All but one child were able to recover normal swallowing within 2–6 months. After this time, they did not present with aspiration during the day once the tracheostomy was closed. It took 3–12 months until they stopped coughing at night. During this period, pulmonary aspirations were frequent, and a high rate of pneumonias (from 1 to 5 per child) was noted. With a follow-up ranging from 1 to 10.6 years, all children are healthy eating and breathing normally.

We believe that very proximal pharyngeal anastomosis of esophageal replacements can be attempted as long as children have no impairment of vocal cord mobility by glottic scars or lesion to the laryngeal recurrent nerve. However, the rehabilitation is very long until they learn how to occlude their larynx and swallow with their vocal cords. During this time, aspirations and subsequent pneumonia are frequent. Regardless to the used transplant, there is an important difference in those where the proximal anastomosis is done a few centimeters below the upper esophageal sphincter or if it has been destroyed.

13.6 Postoperative Period, Complications, and Follow-Up

13.6.1 Postoperative Period

The patients leave the operating theater with several equipments:

We place a low-pressure suction tube into the transplants to avoid their postoperative distension. We believe that most vascular problems are not related to the arterial supply but due to venous stasis. Deflating the transplants improves venous return.

The children cannot eat postoperatively, sometimes for an extended period, so we avoid total parenteral nutrition placing gastrostomies in all cases. It is used to deflate the stomach while the gastric sutures heal and a transpyloric jejunal tube is placed through it to feed the child promptly.

Intraoperatively, we always place a non-resorbable never-ending thread through the nose, the throat, and the transplant and exteriorized through the gastrostomy. This never-ending thread is left in place for months. It can be used to replace a probe in the transplant if needed, without the risk of perforation related to blind introduction in a tortuous conduit. Furthermore, it gives the advantage of safe dilatations, using the Tucker-Rehbein bougies for the same reasons.

Postoperative care demands a stay in the PICU because of pharyngeal and pulmonary respiratory possible complications. For these reasons, we keep our patients intubated for a period of 2–5 days as the dissection in the neck can create an important edema of the upper airways. We ask the intensivists to administer adequate fluids and sometimes amines during the first 24 h, to maintain a mean arterial pressure as high as possible, thereby avoiding a poor perfusion in the transplant.

An esophagogram is performed between day 7 and day 14 related to the difficulty of the procedure. This is done per os but also through the tube left in place in the transplant to fill it completely, as children do not have a sufficient oral intake at that time. If no leak appears, the tube is removed and the child is allowed to eat soft food. Should a leak occur, the tube is left in place under soft suction for another week.

13.6.2 Complications

The most frequent short- and long-term complications of esophageal replacements are stenosis and leaks of the proximal anastomosis. We have had, respectively, 33 % and 8 % of them (Table 13.4). Leaks at the proximal anastomosis occur even when the transplant is well vascularized and the suture line free of tension on an intact proximal esophagus. We believe they are related to ischemia of the farthest end of the transplant. A slight ischemia seems to be related to venous stasis rather than poor arterial supply, as evidenced by the fact that a straighter transplant would give better results with less leak and stenosis than a tortuous one.

The same explanation can be ascribed to stenosis of the proximal anastomosis but may follow persistent ischemia. We noticed that all patients with a leak of the proximal anastomosis required dilatations.

Table 13.4 Complications

Complications	Nb	%
Stenosis (upper anastomosis)	67	24
Stasis in transplant	45	16
GER	41	14
Leak-fistula	17	6
Pyloric spasm-delayed gastric emptying	12	4
Occlusion	6	2
Redundant transplant	4	1
Septicemia	4	1
Severe bronchospasms	3	1
Transplant too long – kinking	3	1
Chylothorax	2	1
Tamponade	2	1
Tracheomalacia	2	1
Transient left phrenic nerve palsy	1	<1
Ulcer in transplant (gastric tube)	1	<1
Cervical abscess	1	<1
Transplant necrosis	0	0
Death	0	0

Two children developed cervical stenosis 3 months after the replacements, and two others developed cervical stenosis 3 years and 5 years after the surgery even though the radiological, endoscopic, and surgical aspects were normal and they were already eating. They were probably related to a recurrent hypertrophic healing process, induced by the surgical procedure and/or by subsequent oral feeding. These recurrences raise the question how long these children should be kept under observation.

Other complications are summarized in Table 13.4.

13.6.3 Long-Term Follow-Up

We have a long-term follow-up for 69 % of our patients with a mean long-term follow-up of 8.6 years. All patients are eating normally, with no failure to thrive and no growth retardation. Most children or their parents have no complaints. Those who are now adult lead a normal life. Nevertheless, many children experience noisy breathing and coughing refluxes and have acquired strange eating habits, for instance, drinking between each bite.

Lima has published a long follow-up review of 72 patients having had a colonic esophageal replacement, regarding their general conditions, functional outcomes, and quality of life. The mean follow-up was 345 months (range 180–552 months). The working activity for those who were concerned was good: 64 patients (89 %) did not feel that surgery influenced their daily work activity, and four patients (6 %) had minor difficulties. Regarding daily life activity, 60 patients (83 %) had no limitations, and seven patients (10 %) had minor difficulties. Thirty-six patients (50 %) complained of clinical symptoms. This can be related to the 71 % suffering from gastroesophageal reflux and 35 % using daily pharmacological therapies. About 30 % complain aesthetic result of the surgery. He concludes that esophageal replacements are major procedures associated with a low mortality rate and have an acceptable benefit-to-risk ratio. The long-term results show that quality of life is acceptable even if adolescents are unsatisfied with aesthetic results [70].

Conclusions

According to Cowles and Coran, the "ideal" esophageal replacement conduit for children should (a) be long lasting, (b) be associated with minimal reflux, (c) be technically feasible, (d) not affect cardiac or pulmonary function, and (e) allow oral consumption of nutrition [33]. With a personal experience of more than 280 esophageal replacements during 24 years, I still don't know which is the best procedure, and my perplexity increases when I read studies such as the one by Pierro [46].

Our belief remains that a successful replaced esophagus does not behave as a normal one. The best esophagus for a child is his own one. Everything has to be done to preserve it and esophageal replacement should be last resort.

References

1. Roux C (1907) L'oesophago-jéjuno-gastrostomose, nouvelle opération pour rétrécissement infranchissable de l'oesophage. Sem Méd 27:37–40
2. Reinberg O (1989) Les oesophagoplasties chez l'enfant. Thèse, Faculté de Médecine de l'Université de Lausanne. p 166
3. Danielou T (2012) Histoire de l'oesophagoplastie chez l'enfant, Master under supervision of O. Reinberg, Faculty of Biology and medicine, University of Lausanne, Switzerland, p 47
4. Reinberg O (1993) A propos de l'oesophago-jéjuno-gastrostomose de César Roux. Rev Med Suisse Romande 113(2):162–163
5. Reinberg O (2014) Les oesophagoplasties chez l'enfant. E-Mem Acad Natl Chir 13(2):011–022
6. Peden M, Oyegbite K, Ozanne-Smith J et al (2008) World report on child injury prevention. World Health Organization/UNICEF, Geneva
7. Millar AJ, Cox SG (2015) Caustic injury of the oesophagus. Pediatr Surg Int 31:111–121
8. Rossi A (2015) Acute caustic ingestion: state of art and new trends. J Gastroenterol Hepatol Res 4(3):1501–1506
9. Riffat F, Cheng A (2009) Pediatric caustic ingestion: 50 consecutive cases and a review of the literature. Dis Esophagus 22:89–94
10. Watson W et al (2005) Annual report of the American Association of Poison Control Centers Toxic Exposure Surveillance System. Am J Emerg Med 23:589–666
11. Janousek P, Kabelka Z, Rygl M, Lesny P, Grabec P, Fajstavr J, Jurovcík M, Snajdauf J (2006) Corrosive injury of the esophagus in children. Int J Pediatr Otorhinolaryngol 70(6):1103–1107
12. Diaz M, Leal N, Olivares P, Larrauri J, Tovar JA (2001) Infectious strictures requiring esophageal replacement in children. J Pediatr Gastroenterol Nutr 32(5):611–613
13. Cheng BC, Chang S, Mao S et al (2005) Surgical treatment of giant esophageal leiomyoma. World J Gastroenterol 11(27):4258–4260
14. Ksia A, Mosbahi S, Ben Brahim M et al (2012) Sténoses œsophagiennes de l'épidermolyse bulleuse (Esophageal strictures in children with epidermolysis bullosa). Arch Pediatr 19(12):1325–1329
15. Shih SL, Huang FY, Sheu JC et al (2005) Esophageal stenosis in infants: unusual complication after Pseudomonas aeruginosa sepsis. J Pediatr Surg 40:e11–e13
16. Waasdorp Hurtado CE, Kramer RE (2010) Salicylic acid ingestion leading to esophageal stricture. Pediatr Emerg Care 26(2):146–148
17. Panieri E, Rode H, Millar AJW, Cywes S (1998) Esophageal replacement in the management of corrosive strictures: when is surgery indicated? Pediatr Surg Int 13:336–340
18. Arul GS, Parikh D (2008) Esophageal replacement in children. Ann R Coll Surg Engl 90(1):7–12
19. de Jong AL, Macdonald R, Ein S et al (2001) Corrosive esophagitis in children: a 30-year review. Int J Pediatr Otorhinolaryngol 57:203–211
20. Lee HQ, Hawley A, Doak J et al (2014) Long-gap oesophageal atresia: comparison of delayed primary anastomosis and oesophageal replacement with gastric tube. J Pediatr Surg 49(12):1762–1766

21. Zani A, Cobellis G, Wolinska J, Chiu PP, Pierro A (2016) Preservation of native esophagus in infants with pure esophageal atresia has good long-term outcomes despite significant postoperative morbidity. Pediatr Surg Int 32:113–117, Epub ahead of print
22. Burgos L, Barrena S, Andrés AM, Martínez L, Hernández F, Olivares P, Lassaletta L, Tovar J (2010) Colonic interposition for esophageal replacement in children remains a good choice: 33-year median follow-up of 65 patients. J Pediatr Surg 45:341–345
23. Papahagi E, Popovici Z (1974) Procédé pour améliorer l'irrigation de la plastie dans l'oesophagoplastie par le côlon transverse et le côlon ascendant isopéristaltique. J Chir (Paris) 108:229–240
24. Monnier P, Dikkers FG, Eckel H et al (2015) Preoperative assessment and classification of benign laryngotracheal stenosis: a consensus paper of the European Laryngological Society. Eur Arch Othorhinolaryngol 272(10):2885–2896
25. Leal AJ, Tannuri AC, Tannuri U (2013) Mechanical bowel preparation for esophagocoloplasty in children: is it really necessary? Dis Esophagus 26(5):475–478
26. Chattopadhyay A, Prakash B, Vepakomma D et al (2004) A prospective comparison of two regimes of bowel preparation for pediatric colorectal procedures: normal saline with added potassium vs. polyethylene glycol. Pediatr Surg Int 20(2):127–129
27. Reinberg O, Genton N (1997) Esophageal replacement in children: evaluation of the one-stage procedure with colic transplants. Eur J Pediatr Surg 4(7):216–220
28. Ngan SY, Wong J (1986) Lengths of different routes for esophageal replacement. J Thorac Cardiovasc Surg 91(5):790–792
29. Hamza AF, Abdelhay S, Sherif H et al (2003) Caustic esophageal strictures in children: 30 years' experience. J Pediatr Surg 38(6):828–833
30. Andres AM, Burgos AL, Encinas JL et al (2007) What can we do when a esophagocoloplasty fails? Cir Pediatr 20(1):39–43
31. Ortiz R, Galan AS, Martinez L et al (2015) Tertiary surgery for complicated repair of esophageal atresia. Eur J Pediatr Surg 25(1):20–26
32. Kochhar R, Sethy PK, Kochhar S et al (2006) Corrosive induced carcinoma of esophagus: report of three patients and review of literature. J Gastroenterol Hepatol 21:777–780
33. Fékété F, Rongère C, Assens P (1987) Cancérisation d'un œsophage restant exclu après œsophagoplastie pour sténose caustique. [Cancerous degeneration of an excluded esophagus after esophagoplasty for caustic stenosis]. Ann Chir 41(5):341–343
34. Orringer MB, Sloan H (1978) Esophagectomy without thoracotomy. J Thorac Cardiovasc Surg 76:643–654
35. Reinberg O (1990) Les oesophagoplasties chez l'enfant. Med Hyg 48:2553–2565
36. Caix M, Descottes B, Rousseau D (1981) La vascularisation artérielle de l'oesophage thoracique moyen et inférieur. Anat Clin 3:95–106
37. Reinberg O, Lutz N, Joseph JM et al (2001) Video-assisted repair or major vascular and bronchial tears occurring during esophageal replacements in children. Eur J Coeliosurg 37(3):81–84
38. Reinberg O (2008) Laparoscopic esophagectomy in esophageal replacements in children. J Laparoendosc Adv Surg Tech 18(3):503
39. Vasseur Maurer S, de Buys Roessingh A, Reinberg O (2013) Comparison of transhiatal laparoscopy versus blind closed-chest cervicotomy and laparotomy for esophagectomy in children. J Pediatr Surg 48:887–892
40. Parilli A, García W, Mejías JG et al (2013) Laparoscopic transhiatal esophagectomy and gastric pull-up in long-gap esophageal atresia: description of the technique in our first 10 cases. J Laparoendosc Adv Surg Tech A 23(11):949–954
41. Cury EK, Schraibman V, De Vasconcelos Macedo AL et al (2001) Thoracoscopic esophagectomy in children. J Pediatr Surg 36(9):e17
42. Kane TD, Nwomeh BC, Nadler EP (2007) Thoracoscopic-assisted esophagectomy and laparoscopic gastric pull-up for lye injury. JSLS 11:474–480
43. Chokshi NK, Guner YS, Ndiforchu F et al (2009) Combined laparoscopic and thoracoscopic esophagectomy and gastric pull-up in a child. J Laparoendosc Adv Surg Tech 19(Suppl 1):197–200
44. Nwomeh BC, Luketich JD, Kane TD (2004) Minimally invasive esophagectomy for caustic esophageal stricture in children. J Pediatr Surg 39:1–6
45. Gallo G, Zwaveling S, Groen H, Van der Zee D et al (2012) Long-gap esophageal atresia: a meta-analysis of jejunal interposition, colon interposition, and gastric pull-up. Eur J Pediatr Surg 22(6):420–425
46. Loukogeorgakis SP, Pierro A (2013) Replacement surgery for esophageal atresia. Eur J Pediatr Surg 23(3):182–190
47. Jones EL, Booth DJ, Cameron JL (1971) Functional evaluation of esophageal reconstructions. Ann Thorac Surg 12:331–346
48. Stein HJ, DeMeester TR, Hinder RA (1992) Outpatient physiologic testing and surgical management of foregut motility disorders. Curr Probl Surg 29:415–550
49. Vasseur Maurer S, Estremadoyro V, Reinberg O (2011) Evaluation of an anti-reflux procedure for colonic interposition in pediatric esophageal replacements. J Pediatr Surg 46(3):594–600
50. Newman KD, Anderson KD (1998) Esophageal replacement. In: Stringer MD, Mouriquand PDE, Oldham KT, Howard ER (eds) Pediatric surgery and urology: long term outcomes. W.B. Saunders, London, pp 214–219
51. Borgnon J, Tounian P, Auber F et al (2004) Esophageal replacement in children by an isoperistaltic gastric tube: a 12-year experience. Pediatr Surg Int 20(11–12):829–833
52. Koskas F, Gayet B (1985) Anatomical study of retrosternal gastric esophagoplasties. Anat Clin 7:237–256

53. Ndoye JM, Dia A, Ndiaye A, Fall B et al (2006) Arteriography of three models of gastric esophagoplasty: the whole stomach, a wide gastric tube and a narrow gastric tube. Surg Radiol Anat 28:429–437
54. Sweet RH (1948) A new method of restoring continuity of the alimentary canal in cases of congenital atresia of the esophagus with tracheoesophageal fistula not treated by immediate primary anastomosis. Ann Surg 127(4):757–768
55. Spitz L (1984) Gastric transposition via the mediastinal route for infants and children with long-gap esophageal atresia. J Pediatr Surg 19(2):149–154
56. Schneider A, Ferreira CG, Kauffmann I, Lacreuse I, Becmeur F (2011) Modified Spitz procedure using a Collis gastroplasty for the repair of long-gap esophageal atresia. Eur J Pediatr Surg 21(3):178–182
57. Cowles RA, Coran AG (2010) Gastric transposition in infants and children. Pediatr Surg Int 26:1129–1134
58. Hirschl RB, Yardeni D, Oldham K et al (2002) Gastric transposition for esophageal replacement in children: experience with 41 consecutive cases with special emphasis on esophageal atresia. Ann Surg 236:531–539
59. Spitz L (2009) Gastric transposition in children. Semin Pediatr Surg 18(1):30–33
60. Greenspon J, Yu J, Warner BW (2012) Late volvulus of an intrathoracic gastric pull-up. J Pediatr Surg 47(4):792–794
61. Spitz L (2014) Esophageal replacement: overcoming the need. J Pediatr Surg 49(6):849–852
62. Gupta DK, Charles AR, Srinivas M (2004) Manometric evaluation of the intrathoracic stomach after gastric transposition in children. Pediatr Surg Int 20:415–418
63. Ring WS, Varco RL, L'Heureux PR, Foker JE (1982) Esophageal replacement with jejunum in children: an 18 to 33 year follow-up. J Thorac Cardiovasc Surg 83:918–927
64. Saeki M, Tsuchida Y, Ogata T, Nakano M, Akiyama H (1988) Long-term results of jejunal replacement of the esophagus. J Pediatr Surg 23:483–489
65. Simms MH, Brearley S, Watson D, Roberts KD (1989) Reconstruction of the esophagus using a free jejunal graft in complicated esophageal atresia. Pediatr Surg Int 4(3):159–161
66. Bax KM (2009) Jejunum for bridging long gap esophageal atresia. Semin Pediatr Surg 18(1):34–39
67. Cusick EL, Batchelor AA, Spicer RD (1993) Development of a technique for jejunal interposition in long-gap esophageal atresia. J Pediatr Surg 28:990–994
68. Shirakawa Y, Naomoto Y, Noma K et al (2004) Free jejunal graft for hypopharyngeal and esophageal reconstruction. Langenbecks Arch Surg 389(5):387–390
69. Saetti R, Silvestrini M et al (2003) Endoscopic treatment of upper airway and digestive tract lesions caused by caustic agents. Ann Otol Rhinol Laryngol 112(1):29–36
70. Lima M, Destro F, Cantone N et al (2015) Long-term follow-up after esophageal replacement in children: 45-year single-center experience. J Pediatr Surg 50(9):1457–1461

14 Pyloric Stenosis

Olivier Reinberg

14.1 Introduction

Infantile hypertrophic pyloric stenosis (IHPS) is a mechanical obstruction of the gastric outlet, due to a simple benign hypertrophy and hyperplasia of the smooth muscle fibers of the pylorus. The result is a narrowing and elongation of the pyloric channel. The origin remains unknown more than a century after the first treatments.

Gastric outlet obstructions in infants have been described several times (Fabricius Hildanus, 1627 [1]; Patrick Blair, 1717 [2–4]; Christopher Weber, 1758 [5]; George Armstrong, 1777 [6, 7]; H. Beardsley, 1788 [7, 8], Williamson, 1841 [9], Siemon-Dawoski, 1842 [10]) before the first unequivocal modern description of IHPS in 1887 by the Danish Harald Hirschsprung who gave complete clinical details and accurate pathological findings [9, 11, 12] and then by Sir William Osler, from Ontario, Canada, in 1903 [13]. Probably the first successful surgical attempt to solve the problem was by Pietro Loreta from Bologna in 1887 [14]. He described an antral opening to dilate the pylorus from the stomach. Then several procedures were performed, such as a gastroenterostomy by Lobker in 1898 on a 10 weeks old infant. The surgical treatment still in use today is an extramucosal pyloromyotomy (EMP) which bears the names of Fredet-Weber-Ramstedt, referring to those who were supposed to have done it first. However, the procedure performed in 1907 by Pierre Fredet was an extramucosal pyloroplasty [15, 16]. In 1910 Weber did an extramucosal splitting of the muscle followed by a transverse suturing [17], and on August 23, 1911, Conrad Ramstedt (also written Rammstedt, due to a misspelling of his name) performed an EMP leaving the two muscular margins free, but covered the myotomy with an omentoplasty [18]. So the first true EMP was done in Edinborough on February 7, 1910 by Sir Harold Stiles as attested by his original operating report (thanks to Gordon McKinley). However, he did not report it at that time, and the date and records of his operation were published by Mason Brown only in 1956 [19].

14.2 Epidemiology

Infantile hypertrophic pyloric stenosis (IHPS) is the most common cause of vomiting in the postnatal period, occurring with a prevalence rate of ≈2 per 1000 live births in Europe and North America, predominantly in boys compared to girls (4:1 up to 5:1). IHPS is less frequent in children of African or Asian origin [20–23]. In 1927, Still already noticed that it is more frequent in the firstborn [4, 24], but this point is debated by epidemiologists [25]. A decline in the incidence of IHPS has been reported over the past two decades

O. Reinberg
Pediatric Surgery, Rochettaz 24, CH – 1009 Pully, Switzerland
e-mail: olreinberg@gmail.com

M. Lima (ed.), *Pediatric Digestive Surgery*, DOI 10.1007/978-3-319-40525-4_14

in Northern European countries and the United States [20, 25–28]. Decreases in rates of IHPS were observed among foreign-born Hispanics and foreign-born Asians, but not among their US-born counterparts, suggesting an environmental origin [22].

In a case-control study, Svenningsson reports cesarean section, prematurity, primiparity, young maternal age as significant risk factors for IHPS [28].

IHPS affects infants between 3 and 8 weeks. The mean age at diagnosis is about 40 days; 95 % of the cases being diagnosed between age 2 and 11 weeks [25]. However, delayed cases up to 4 years of age have been reported [29].

On the other hand, prematurity is associated with a higher rate of IHPS than term babies [25]. Premature infants develop IHPS at a later chronological age, than term infants [30] and have a higher female preponderance [31], the sex-ratio in preterm being nearly 1:1 [25]. Small weight for gestational age babies have also a significantly higher rate of pyloric stenosis compared with heavier infants [25].

14.3 Etiology

More than a century after its first description, IHPS remains a disease of unclear origin. IHPS can occur as an isolated disease, but it is also well established that it can be associated with chromosomal abnormalities, congenital malformations, and clinical syndromes, which indicate a genetic involvement associated with environmental factors. However, no causal gene or sequence variant has been identified to date and the pathophysiology at a molecular level remains unclear [32].

14.3.1 Genetic Factors

The cases of IHPS reported by Armstrong in 1777 were three siblings [6]. Recurrence risk in families and twin studies [33, 34] provide a high suspicion of a genetic origin, even if debated [32]. Yang recommends that the asymptomatic co-twin should be investigated when one of the twins presents with IHPS [33]. Carter first demonstrated non-syndromic pyloric stenosis as a complex, multifactorial, sex-modified threshold trait [35, 36]. A reanalysis by Mitchell of data from several studies concluded that IHPS is determined by two or three loci of moderate effect conferring individual genotype relative risks of up to 5 [37]. To date five genetic loci (IHPS1 to IHPS5) have been identified. IHPS1, which encodes the enzyme neuronal nitric oxide synthase (NOS1), was considered as a possible evidence that a defect in nitric oxide production may play a role in the etiology of IHPS. However, the evidence for linkage and association is weak and has not been confirmed. Two other loci, IHPS2 (16p13-p12) and IHPS5 (16q24.3), have been identified, suggesting autosomal dominant inheritance [38, 39]. A genome-wide single nucleotide polymorphism (SNP) identified IHPS3 on chromosome 11q14–q22 and IHPS4 on Xq23 [40]. Further analysis provided suggestive evidence for a third locus on chromosome 3q12–q25 [41].

Seven percent of children with IHPS had a major malformation compared with 3.7 % of the general population [20]. IHPS is associated with many clinical syndromes that have known causative mutations, such as Cornelia de Lange and Smith-Lemli-Opitz syndromes, chromosomal abnormalities, including translocation of chromosome 8 and 17, and partial trisomy of chromosome 9. An extensive detailed up-to-date review of what we know in the genetics, the molecular studies, and the metabolic studies in IHPS has been published by Peeters et al. [42].

14.3.2 Environmental Factors

A variety of environmental and mechanical factors have been implicated in the occurrence of IHPS. Sleeping position, maternal smoking, and postnatal erythromycin administration are the most commonly evocated factors [21, 32].

In several studies, the rate of IHPS is higher in infants of smoking mothers than among infants of nonsmoking mothers [25, 28].

Sharp decline in the incidence of IHPS in Denmark and Sweden, during the 1990s, coincides with successful campaigns to discourage the prone sleeping position as a prevention of sudden infant death syndrome. This led to the hypothesis that sleeping prone may be a risk factor for IHPS [21, 32]. This could be related to the place where the milk accumulates in the stomach according to the position. However, a similar German study concluded that a common cause was unlikely [27].

Several studies have suggested an increased risk of IHPS following child exposure to erythromycin in the postnatal period, but not through the mother pre- or post birth. Erythromycin is known for its prokinetic effects mediated by its action as a motilin receptor agonist, which could affect gastric motility and/or pyloric contraction [43–45].

The diet itself could play a role as it seems that formula feeding is associated with significantly increased risk of IHPS compared to breastfed children [46]. The development of a delayed pyloric stenosis during transpyloric feedings has also been reported [47, 48].

14.4 Physiopathology

IHPS results in an important thickening of the muscular lays of the pylorus. The enlarged pylorus becomes longer and thicker. This enlargement impairs the normal release of the pyloric sphincter thus occluding the lumen and realizing a gastric outlet obstruction with subsequent vomiting failure to thrive and dehydration.

The pyloric sphincter function involves intrinsic myogenic activity of the smooth muscle, the interstitial cells of Cajal (ICC) which play a role of intestinal pacemaker, gut hormones, and the autonomic and enteric nervous systems. Associated to IHPS, abnormalities have been observed in gastrin levels, enteric nerve terminals, nerve supporting cells, ICC, smooth muscle cells, growth factor synthesis and receptors, and extracellular matrix [49]. But the major hypothesis is that a primary defect in production of nitric oxide (NO) by nitrergic nerves of the enteric nervous system leads to failure of relaxation of the pyloric smooth muscle [50, 51]. Abel brought evidence that nitric oxide synthase (NOS) has been implicated in the pathogenesis of IHPS, since NOS expression is diminished in both circular and longitudinal muscles, as well as in the myenteric plexus [52]. Looking for the ontogeny of the peptide innervation of the pylorus, Abel reports that NOS and vasoactive intestinal polypeptide (VIP) are colocalized to the same nerves in the circular muscle and in the myenteric plexus; they are diminished by the same proportion in IHPS; so he concluded that the initial lesion occurs by 12 weeks of gestation and could be the increment in vasoactive intestinal polypeptide (VIP) in pyloric myenteric ganglia [50, 52].

14.5 Clinical Presentation and Diagnosis

Non-syndromic IHPS affects normally fed healthy children. The story begins with gradually increasing non-bilious vomiting becoming projectile. The vomiting and the inability to be fed lead to dehydration with associated physical signs: loss of weight, skin fold, depressed fontanel, dry mucosa, oliguria, and constipation. Children are hungry and are eager for more to eat without nausea. Given a test meal, visible gastric peristalsis may be seen when the child lays supine.

The palpation of the pylorus is often possible for an experienced examiner. The pylorus must be searched for on the midline just below the edge of the liver. It can be felt as an olive, hence the world "pyloric olive." It was described in 1923 by Sir G. Frederic Still (1868–1941), who is considered to be the "Father of British pediatrics" [24], as "a small barrel-shaped hard tumor (…) varying in size from the thickness of an ordinary lead pencil up to that of a hazelnut" or "as hard as a calcareous gland" [3, 24]. The term "olive" was given by Ladd in 1946 [53]. The palpation of an olive has a 99 % positive predictive value [54].

The patient history, the clinical conditions, and the abdominal palpation of a pyloric olive allowed for a diagnosis of IHPS. Historically, the diagnosis of IHPS was only made by clinical history and physical examination. By the years 1930s, as radiology improved, the upper gastrointestinal (UGI) came to support diagnosis of IHPS. Today ultrasounds (USs) have replaced UGI. However, UGI can still be used in some unusual circumstances or places where US is not available. Then an isotonic hydrosoluble contrast media should be preferred to the old barium meal, in case of aspiration in a vomiting child [55]. The radiological signs of IHPS are gastric retention, parenthesis shape of the antrum ("shoulder sign") ending with a "beak sign" (the narrowed gastric antrum entering the pylorus), and lengthening of the pylorus with the typical "double-track" sign, or even triple (small trickle of contrast in the thickened and elongated pylorus).

The first diagnostic use of ultrasounds (USs) for IHPS was done by Teele and Smith in 1977 [12, 56]. Today in almost all pediatric medical centers, the high-resolution, real-time US is the modality of first choice to confirm the diagnosis of IHPS [12]. It is a noninvasive technique not using ionizing radiations. It is commonly available with relatively low cost. Ultrasounds have accuracy and sensitivity approaching 100 % [57]. False-positives are rare. However, the distended stomach filled with gas can rotate the pylorus dorsally, thus resulting in its difficult localization and measurements. Thus it requires appropriate equipment, expertise, and clinical experience to produce best results [12].

The positive US diagnosis is based on precise measurements of canal length and muscle thickness. A pylorus is considered hypertrophic when the single hypoechoic muscle layer measured transversely exceeds 3 mm [57–63]. There is some variability for pyloric channel length criteria ranging from 14 to 17 mm in literature, as the pyloric canal lengthens with age [58–63].

US diagnosis can be difficult in infants below 3 weeks or preterms because of the thin pyloric muscle thickness [57]. However, it seems that the normal values are not affected by weight, corrected gestational age, or duration of symptoms [31]. When in doubt, repeated US within 1 or 2 days can be an issue.

14.6 Preoperative Management

IHPS is a medical emergency. The vomiting associated with IHPS leads to depletion of sodium, and hydrochloric acid, thus resulting in hypochloremic metabolic alkalosis that can be partially compensated by a respiratory acidosis. Anesthesia and surgery on an infant in poor metabolic condition can be harmful. Because IHPS is not a surgical emergency, the hypochloremic metabolic alkalosis should be corrected before surgical intervention with adequate fluid and electrolyte IV replacement. This can require a few days. As the potassium is mostly intracellular, its loss may not appear immediately in the kalemia. However, it must be anticipated [64].

14.7 Surgical Treatment

The surgical procedure used to relieve the pyloric obstruction remains the extramucosal pyloromyotomy (EMP) as described more than a century ago. The pyloric serosa is open longitudinally with a blade on its avascular part. Then the thick muscle is split using a smooth grasper or a pyloric spreader, until the mucosa is exposed and bulges out between the muscular edges. It is essential to ensure total opening of the pylorus. Most of the "recurrences" are incomplete myotomies. The splitting of the muscle has to run from the gastric antrum to the pyloroduodenal junction. This is the most dangerous point. At this very place, the mucosa comes up as the muscular wall becomes suddenly thinner, bearing a risk of mucosal perforation (Fig. 14.1). For this reason the surgical procedure must end with a search for potential perforation, using gas insufflation in the stomach via a gastric tube. Bubbles appearing on the pyloric mucosa evidence a leak. A perforation per se is not a major problem as long as it is immediately recognized and sutured. It will only differ the first postoperative meals.

14.7.1 Open Surgery

If EMP has not evolved over time, the surgical access has changed substantially. The initial

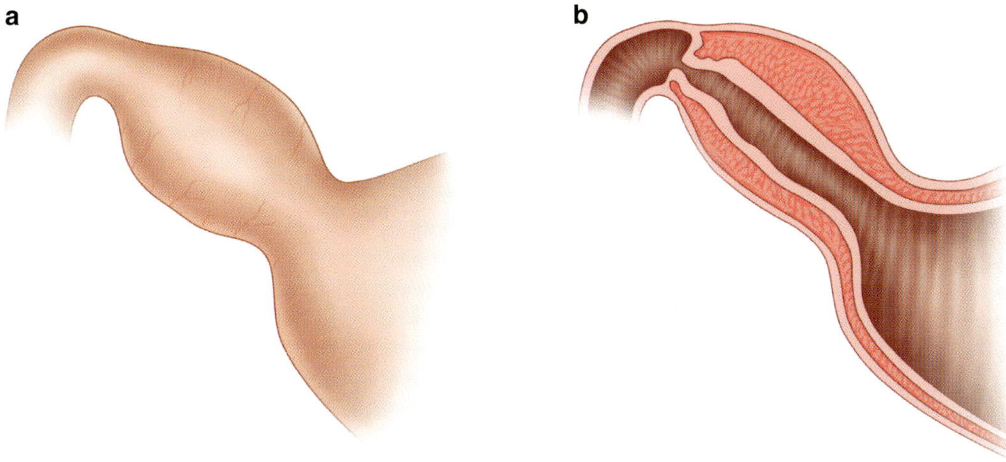

Fig. 14.1 Drawing of the hypertrophic pylorus showing the dangerous place where the mucosa comes up as the muscular wall becomes suddenly thinner

open approach was a midline laparotomy, which has moved toward a transverse laparotomy and then a smaller transrectal (from the rectus abdominis) approach in the right upper quadrant. A first major change toward minimal invasive surgery was suggested by Bianchi, with a circumumbilical approach, which rapidly spreads among pediatric surgeons [65]. Tan and Bianchi described in 1986 a semicircular supraumbilical skinfold incision leaving an almost invisible scar. Through this minimal incision, the pylorus is palpated, seized with a Babcock clamp, and delivered through the umbilicus to perform the EMP out of the abdomen. Somehow it can be difficult to bring out a big firm pylorus. Then the aponeurotic fascia must be open longitudinally on the midline as far as needed, to allow easy extraction. Once the EMP is done, the fascia is sutured. The transumbilical incision for EMP allows excellent access to the pylorus, while leaving an almost undetectable scar.

Modifications of the Bianchi's umbilical approach were suggested by some authors. As there are some obvious technical difficulties in delivering a large pyloric tumor through the umbilicus even after opening the midline fascia, instead of bringing the pylorus out through the umbilicus with subsequent traction, the pylorus is kept in situ and the EMP is performed intracorporeally [66–69]. To stabilize the pylorus and draw it up just under the umbilical wound, suspension threads are placed in the hypertrophic muscle [67, 69].

14.7.2 Laparoscopic Pyloromyotomy

One of the first laparoscopic procedures even done in children were pyloromyotomies performed by Dominique Grousseau and Jean-Luc Alain from Limoges, France, in 1989, and published first in French in 1990 [70] then in English with ten cases in 1991 [71]. The technique was long to gain popularity but by some pediatric surgeons involved in pediatric minimal invasive surgery.

Initially three ports were used: a 5 mm in the umbilicus for the telescope, using the Hasson's open technique, and two 3 mm for instruments, one on the midline, the second on the right midclavicular line just below the liver. The pylorus was caught in a Babcock grasper. The pyloric serosa was opened longitudinally on its anterior face using a 3-mm retractable knife. Then the pyloric muscle was split with a laparoscopic pyloric spreader.

The laparoscopic EMP has evolved toward simpler technique. Nowadays, only one 5-mm port is placed in the umbilicus and none for the instruments. As the left hand is used only to seize the pylorus, the instrument is left in place from beginning to end and do not require a port. As it appeared difficult to grab the big firm pylorus with a small Babcock grasper, today we use a smooth Johann grasper placed transversally on the duodenum just below the pyloroduodenal junction. This allows to lift up or to rotate the pylorus with a good exposure of the pyloroduodenal junction. A small 2–3-mm disposable knife (designed for ophthalmology or for arthrotomies) is inserted through the skin on the midline just in front of the pylorus. The blade is not pushed down to the pylorus, but the pylorus is lifted up toward the blade. Then the wound site is used to insert a smooth 2 or 3-mm grasper (Johann, Maryland) to split the muscle. The use of one of the specially designed pyloric spreaders is helpful but not mandatory.

There are no contraindications to laparoscopic IHPS. However, prematures bear a risk of cerebral bleeding due to the elevation of pressure in the superior vena cava related to insufflation, even done at a low pressure (5–6 mmHg). Children with cardiac defect shunting from left to right could embolize in their brain and therefore should be recused for laparoscopy as those with lung anomalies (Figs. 14.2 and 14.3).

14.7.3 Which Is Better: Lap or Open?

We have had to wait for more than a decade until data were available to compare open with laparoscopic EMP (lap).

The French team of Nantes has performed a randomized prospective study of respectively 50 EMPs done by laparoscopy with 52 open. The

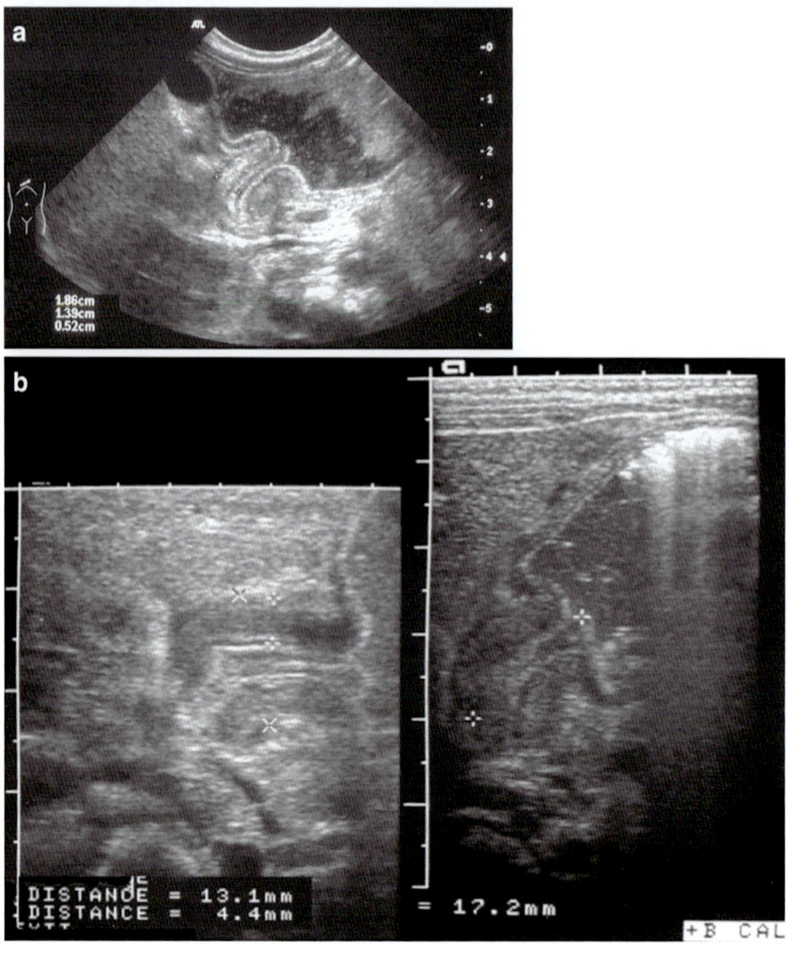

Fig. 14.2 (a, b) Ultrasounds of IHPS. Measures are taken between calipers + and X. The lamina muscularis mucosae appear as a white stripe in the thick muscle. Note the dilated stomach filled with echoes

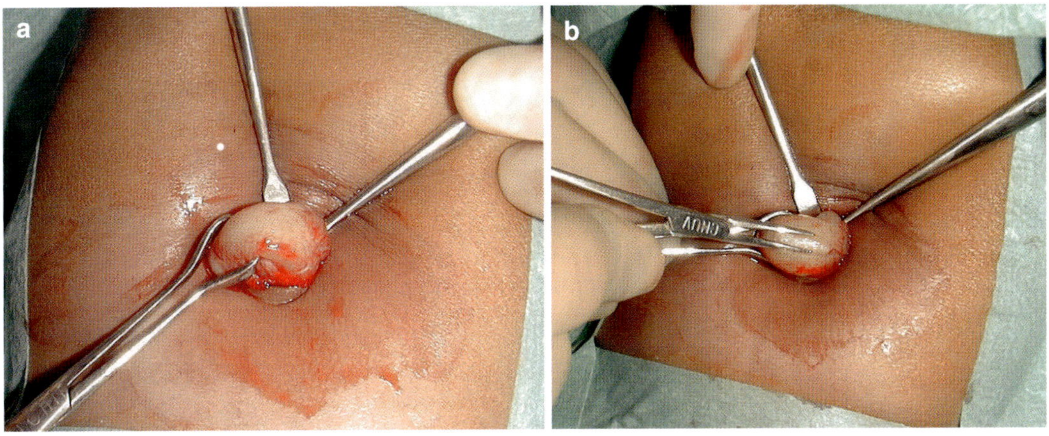

Fig. 14.3 Extramucosal plyloromytotomy through the umbilical approach. (**a**) The pylorus has been delivered through the umbilicus. (**b**) The pyloric muscle is split using a mosquito and the mucosa is exposed between the muscular edges

durations of surgery and anesthesia were longer in the lap group. There was no difference in the incidence of postoperative vomiting, and the complications were similar (1 perforation each ie 1 %; 2 wound complications open versus 1 lap ie 3 %; 3 incomplete myotomies after lap ie 3 %) but significantly with less pain in the lap group ($p < .0001$) [72].

A multicenter international double-blind controlled trial across six tertiary pediatric surgical centers has been published with 180 infants randomly assigned to open ($n = 93$) or laparoscopic EMP ($n = 87$) [73]. Complications were similar (17 vs 15). All perforations (1 vs 2) and the 3 incomplete myotomies by laparoscopy were done by nontrainees. Full oral feeding was achieved faster in the lap group ($p = .002$); there were less pain in the lap group ($p = .011$); and the postoperative hospital stay was shorter in the lap group ($p = .027$). The postoperative vomiting and complications were similar. The parental satisfaction was higher for the lap group ($p = 0.011$). The design of the study was to recruit 200 infants (100 per group). However, the data monitoring and ethics committee recommended halting the trial before full recruitment because of significant treatment benefit in the laparoscopy group at interim analysis. Their conclusions were: "Both open and laparoscopic pyloromyotomy are safe procedures for the management of pyloric stenosis. However, laparoscopy has advantages over open pyloromyotomy, and we recommend its use in centers with suitable laparoscopic experience."

Keith Georgeson and his team from Birmingham, AL, have compared the incidence and type of technical complications seen in a retrospective series of pyloromyotomies done by open (225) and by laparoscopic (232) EMP in similar groups performed by multiple surgeons. The overall incidences of complications were similar in the two groups (open 4.4 %; lap 5.6 %). There was a greater rate of perforation with the open technique (3.6 % vs 0.4 %) and a higher rate of postoperative problems including incomplete myotomy in the laparoscopic group (0 vs 2.2 %). They conclude that: "This lower rate of perforation could be attributed to improved visualization because of the magnification provided by laparoscopy. Alternatively, the lower perforation rate could be owing to a less "aggressive" pyloromyotomy" [74].

Sola published a meta-analysis upon six prospective studies of level 1 (5) or 2 (1) in which it appeared that laparoscopic EMP had a lower total complication rate ($p = .04$) due to a lower wound complication rate ($p = .03$). The laparoscopic EMP had shorter time to full feedings ($p < .00001$) and shorter postoperative hospital stay ($p = .0005$) with no statistically significant differences in mucosal perforation (0.9 % vs 1.3 %), wound infections, and postoperative vomiting. There were six incomplete myotomies (4 lap vs 2 open).

The conclusion was: "This systematic review and meta-analysis favors the laparoscopic approach with significantly reduced rate of total complications, which is mostly due to a lower wound complication rate" [75].

Finally, Carrington and the British team from Great Ormond Street Hospital for children, London, have compared the costs of the laparoscopic EMP with the open approach in a multicenter randomized double-blind controlled trial, for which the primary outcomes were time to full feeds and time to discharge. Operation costs were similar between the two groups. A shorter time to full feeds and shorter hospital stay in lap versus open patients resulted in a highly significant difference in ward costs ($ 2,650 ± 126 lap versus $ 3,398 ± 126 open; $p = .001$) and a small difference in other costs. Overall, laparoscopic patients were $ 1,263 less expensive to treat than open patients [76].

To summarize, the quoted advantages of laparoscopic pyloromyotomy compared to the open approach are reduced postoperative pain, shorter hospital stay, earlier return to normal activity, and cosmetic benefits [77, 78].

14.7.4 Postoperative Period

Postanesthetic apnea in the premature <60 WGA is well known and specific recommendations have been made to prevent them. However, postanesthetic apnea can occur in full-term babies without perinatal problem after some surgical procedures including cures of IHPS [79]. Some recommendations have been made but a strict postoperative monitoring and supervision in a specialized environment is wise [80, 81].

The nasogastric tube is suctioned at the end of the procedure before its removal, except in case of sutured perforation. Wounds are infiltrated with 0.25 % bupivacaine 2 mg/kg for postoperative pain relief. Antibiotics are given only in case of mucosal tear. Oral feeding may be resumed on return to the ward and increased as tolerated.

Isolated vomiting can endure for a few hours/days (≤2 days) after surgery in 10–15 % of cases. They are related to the gastric irritation associated with preoperative vomiting and to the traction on the pylorus during the procedure [82]. Subsequently, they are less frequent after laparoscopic or transumbilical intracorporeal EMP than after exteriorized one. However, they must not be minimized as they can reveal a perforation.

The more electrolyte abnormalities children have at the time of diagnosis, the longer they stay in the hospital [64].

14.7.5 Complications

Complications are between 1 and 3 % in the hands of pediatric surgeons and mostly related to incomplete myotomies or perforations [72, 82]. Infections of the umbilical wounds have been described (1–7 %). However, with the increment of laparoscopy in neonates and infants, pediatric surgeons have learned how to clean the umbilicus, and the rate of umbilical infections is decreasing.

Complications per surgeon drop with experience. This has been evidenced in laparoscopic EMP. Mucosal perforation was experienced by 8.3 % of the patients in the initial series, as compared with 0.7 % in the later series reported by Van der Bilt [78]. Insufficient pyloromyotomy occurred in 8.3 % of the initial series, as compared with 2.7 % of the later series. He suggested that the learning curve could be 15 laparoscopic IHPS [78] (Fig. 14.4).

14.8 Nonsurgical Conservative Treatment for IHPS

Before the era of the EMP and until the years 1960s, IHPS were treated conservatively using atropine or equivalents (belladonna, atropine methylnitrate (eumydrin)). Although pyloromyotomy became the first choice of treatment in Western countries, several authors, mostly from Asian countries (Japan [83–86], Taiwan [87], and India [88]) but also from Germany [89], have revisited the nonsurgical treatment using intravenous or oral atropine for IHPS. Atropine sulfate is given daily for 1–8 days at various regimens [89] with increasing doses until vomiting stopped

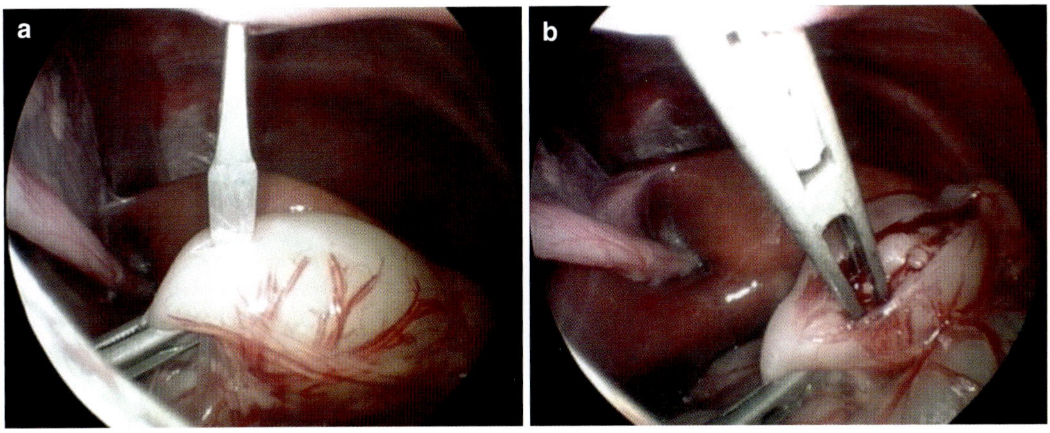

Fig. 14.4 Laparoscopic extramucosal plyloromytotomy. (**a**) Opening the serosa. Note the Johann grasper holding the duodenum just below the enlarged pylorus. The opening of the serosa is done with a disposable ophthalmologic knife in the avascular zone. (**b**) Splitting the muscle with a standard smooth dissector. The mucosa is already bulging proximally to the grasper

then maintained for 2 weeks. The rationale for atropine therapy is that the physiopathology of IHPS may be partially due to impaired function of acetylcholine and muscarinic receptors, thus releasing the pyloric muscle. Medical treatment may require 7 days or more of skilled nursing and careful follow-up. The results are fairly good with no significant complications. About 10–25 % patients require surgery for failure of medical treatment.

Conservative medical treatment with atropine is an option. To date there are no randomized controlled studies answering the question whether therapy with atropine can achieve sufficient resolution of IHPS to avoid surgery but only case series and a retrospective cohort study with low level of evidence [90]. Mercer studied ten relevant articles on the use of atropine for IHPS. The success rate of atropine therapy is about 85 %, whereas surgical EMP is >95 % [90]. Under a humoristic editorial title ("Medical Treatment of Idiopathic Hypertrophic Pyloric Stenosis: Should We Marinate or Slice the "Olive"?"), Rudolph, a pediatric gastroenterologist, advocates for the surgery arguing it solves the problem within 48–72 h with less than 1 % complications for a lower cost [91]. As per Aspelund, we believe conservative medical treatment with atropine should be considered as an alternative in infants with contraindications to anesthesia or surgery [92].

14.9 Other Gastric Outlet Obstructions

In infants, gastric outlet obstruction (GOO) is most often due to IHPS. However, several conditions other than IHPS may cause non-bilious vomiting in infants and children that we must be aware of (Table 14.1).

Gastric polyps may be either hyperplastic or adenomatous. Hyperplastic polyps are most common in children and account for 70–90 % of benign gastric polyps. A study at Johns Hopkins University reported that the prevalence of duodenal polyps in children was 0.4 % (22 of 5,766) of upper gastrointestinal endoscopies. Most of the duodenal polyps in that series were syndromic and were commonly associated with familial adenomatous polyposis [63, 94, 96]. However, sporadic cases have been described before or inside the pylorus [93].

An ectopic pancreas is not uncommon in children and the pyloric location has been described. Besides GOO, they can cause epigastric pain [101] and develop gastrointestinal bleedings or late malignant transformation. Thus surgical removal is suggested [100].

Even very unusual in infants, antral or pyloric malignancies have been reported and should always be considered as a possible etiology of a pyloric obstructive mass in older children [97, 105, 107]. The literature concerning such

Table 14.1 Gastric outlet obstructions non-IHPS

Anatomical anomalies	Treatment	Refs.
Prepyloric masses:		
Pyloric polyp	Endoscopic resection	[93–97]
Ectopic pancreas	Lap or open resection	[93, 97–102]
Tumors	Surgical resection, pyloroplasty	[97, 103–107]
Pyloric web	Endoscopic or lap pyloric opening	[63, 93, 108–113]
Pyloric atresia	Surgical resection	[114, 115]
Gastric volvulus	Lap gastropexy	[116]
Acquired gastric outlet obstructions		
Peptic ulcer disease (gastric or pyloroduodenal)	Medical TTT	[93, 117]
Brunner's glands hyperplasia	Lap pyloroplasty + medical	[118]
Eosinophilic gastritis	Surgical resection	[119]
Drug induced (ibuprofen)	Endoscopic pneumatic dilatation	[120]
Foreign bodies	Endoscopy	[121]

gastropyloric tumors in children is mainly limited to case studies. Gastrointestinal stromal tumor (GIST) [106], Burkitt's lymphoma, gastroblastoma [103], adenomyoma [104], and plasma cell granuloma [97] have been reported.

Prepyloric webs are unusual mucosal partial or total diaphragms that may cause GOO. Histologically, the web consists in normal mucosa and submucosa. It appears in the early infancy in most cases, but it has been reported in older children and even in adults. The treatments are either endoscopic or surgical resection [110–113].

Acute gastric volvulus in newborns and infants is known as a rare but life-threatening emergency that requires prompt recognition and treatment. The first description of this condition was made in 1866 by Berti based on the autopsy of a 61-year-old woman. Oltmann described the first pediatric patient in 1899. To date, more than 250 gastric volvulus in children have been described [116]. Gastric volvulus can be defined as torsion of more than 180° of the stomach around itself thus occluding the pylorus and inducing intermittent or persistent vomiting. The diagnosis is done by upper gastrointestinal contrast studies. The radiological signs include horizontalness of the stomach, the greater curvature being above the lesser one and crossing in front of the lower esophagus with the pylorus looking downward. Once recognized the surgical procedure is an anterior gastropexy with reinforcement of the esophagogastric angle performed by laparoscopy, without antireflux-associated procedure [116].

In the acquired conditions, children are older than the former one, i.e., after 1 year of age. Albeit unusual, peptic ulcers can occur in children and according to their sites may occlude the pylorus. Prior to proton pump inhibitors (PPI) and H2 blockers, peptic ulcer disease secondary to *Helicobacter pylori* was a more common cause of GOO than today. *Helicobacter pylori* are evidenced by urease test and medically treated. However, even at the era of PPI, persistent ulcer under adequate treatment can require for surgery [117].

The ingestion of foreign bodies is a common problem in infants, but fortunately the majority of them will pass through the digestive tract without any adverse effects. The peak incidence of foreign body ingestion is between 6 months and 3 years and coins are the most common. It has even been described in neonates (esophageal zipper in a 2 months old baby) [121, see also Chap. 16]. Most ingested foreign bodies remain entrapped in the esophagus at the level of its anatomic narrowing. However, some of them can be trapped in the antrum occluding the pylorus. There are no guidelines available to determine which type of object will pass safely. The size depends on the age of the child. The eventuality of foreign body impaction must always be considered in infants below 5 years of age and searched for.

References

1. Hildanus F (1646) Opera Omnia. Joh. Bejerus Ed, Frankfort
2. Blair P (1717) Philosoph Trans Royal Society, London 30 (353):631
3. Still GF (1923) A British Medical Association lecture on congenital hypertrophy of the pylorus. Br Med J 1:579–582, http://www.ncbi.nlm.nih.gov/pmc/articles/PMC2316051/pdf/brmedj06260-0003.pdf. Attested 11 Apr 2016

4. Still GF (1927) Place in family as a factor in disease. Lancet 2:795–853
5. Weber C (1758) Inaugural Thesis, Gottingen
6. Armstrong G (1767) An essay on the diseases most fatal to Infants. Cadell T Ed, London, p 61, https://books.google.ch/. Attested 11 Apr 2016
7. Ruhräh J (1930) Pediatric Biographies—Hezekiah Beardsley. Am J Dis Child 40:146
8. Beardsley H (1788) Congenital hypertrophic stenosis of the pylorus. In: Meigs F (ed) Cases and observations by the medical society of New Haven. New Haven, p 81
9. Kellett CE (1933) On the incidence of congenital Hypertrophic pyloric stenosis in the 17th and 18th centuries. Arch Dis Child 8:323–328, http://www.ncbi.nlm.nih.gov/pmc/articles/PMC1975288/
10. Simeon-Dawosky P (1842) Aus Meinen Tagenbusche: Hypertrophie des submueösen Zellgewebes am Pylorus eines 10 Wochen altgewordenen Kindes. Caspers Wchschr f d Ges Heilk 7:105–112, https://books.google.ch/. Attested 11 Apr 2016
11. Hirschsprung H (1888) Fälle von angeborener Pylorusstenose, beobachtet bei Säuglingen. Jahrb der Kinderh 28:61–88, https://archive.org/stream/b21714162/b21714162_djvu.txt. Attested 11 Apr 2016
12. Markowitz RI (2014) Olive without a cause: the story of the infantile hypertrophic pyloric stenosis. Pediatr Radiol 44(2):202–211
13. Beardsley H (1903) Congenital hypertrophic stenosis of the pylorus. Note by Prof. William Osier. Arch Pediatr NY 20:355
14. Loreta P (1887) Divulsioni del piloro e del cardias. Gazzete di Ospedalo Milano 8:803
15. DuFour H, Fredet P (1907) La sténose hypertrophique du pylore chez un nourrisson de deux mois traité avec succés par la pyloroplastie (présentation du malade). Bull Mem Soc Med Hop Paris 24:1221
16. Dufour H, Fredet P (1908) La Stenose Hypertrophique du Pylore chez le Nourrisson et son traitement chirurgical. Rev Chir 37:208–253
17. Weber W (1910) Ueber einen Technische neuerung bei der Operation der Pylorus Stenose des Säuglings. [Concerning an innovative operative technique for infantile pyloric stenosis]. Berlin Klin Wehschr 47:763
18. Rammstedt C (1912) Zur Operation der angeborenen Pylorusstenose. Med Klin Berl 8:1702–1705
19. Keys C, Johnson C, Teague W, MacKinlay G (2015) One hundred years of pyloric stenosis in the Royal Hospital for Sick Children Edinburgh. J Pediatr Surg 50(2):280–284
20. Applegate MS, Druschel CM (1995) The epidemiology of infantile hypertrophic pyloric stenosis in New York State, 1983 to 1990. Arch Ped Adolesc Med 149:1123–1129
21. Persson S, Ekbom A, Granath F et al (2001) Parallel incidences of sudden infant death syndrome and infantile hypertrophic pyloric stenosis: a common cause? Pediatrics 108(4):E70
22. Wang J, Waller DK, Hwang LY et al (2008) Prevalence of infantile hypertrophic pyloric stenosis in Texas, 1999–2002. Birth Defects Res A Clin Mol Teratol 82(11):763–767
23. Ranells JD, Carver JD, Kirby RS (2011) Infantile hypertrophic pyloric stenosis: epidemiology, genetics, and clinical update. Adv Pediatr 58(1):195–206
24. Dunn PM (2006) Sir Frederic Still (1868–1941): the Father of British Pediatrics. Arch Dis Child Fetal Neonatal Ed 91(4):F308–F310
25. Krogh C, Gørtz S, Wohlfahrt J et al (2012) Pre- and perinatal risk factors for pyloric stenosis and their influence on the male predominance. Am J Epidemiol 176(1):24–31
26. Nielsen JP, Haahr P, Haahr J (2000) Infantile hypertrophic pyloric stenosis. Decreasing incidence. Dan Med Bull 47:223–225
27. de Laffolie J, Turial S, Heckmann M, Zimmer KP, Schier F (2012) Decline in infantile hypertrophic pyloric stenosis in Germany in 2000–2008. Pediatrics 129(4):e901–e906
28. Svenningsson A, Svensson T, Akre O et al (2014) Maternal and pregnancy characteristics and risk of infantile hypertrophic pyloric stenosis. J Pediatr Surg 49(8):1226–1231
29. Mahalik S, Prasad A, Sinha A, Kulshrestha R (2010) Delayed presentation of hypertrophic pyloric stenosis: a rare case. J Pediatr Surg 45(2):e9–e11
30. Stark CM, Rogers PL, Eberly MD, Nylund CM (2015) Association of prematurity with the development of infantile hypertrophic pyloric stenosis. Pediatr Res 78(2):218–222
31. Cascio S, Steven M, Livingstone H et al (2013) Hypertrophic pyloric stenosis in premature infants: evaluation of sonographic criteria and short-term outcomes. Pediatr Surg Int 29(7):697–702
32. Georgoula C, Gardiner M (2012) Pyloric stenosis a 100 years after Ramstedt. Arch Dis Child 97:741–745
33. Yang G, Brisseau G, Yanchar NL (2008) Infantile hypertrophic pyloric stenosis: an association in twins? Paediatr Child Health 13(5):383–385
34. Krogh C, Fischer TK, Skotte L et al (2010) Familial aggregation and heritability of pyloric stenosis. JAMA 303:2393–2399
35. Carter CO (1961) The inheritance of congenital pyloric stenosis. Br Med Bull 17:251–254
36. Carter CO, Evans KA (1969) Inheritance of congenital pyloric stenosis. J Med Genet 6:233–254
37. Mitchell LE, Risch N (1993) The genetics of infantile hypertrophic pyloric stenosis. A reanalysis. Am J Dis Child 147:1203–1211
38. Capon F, Reece A, Ravindrarajah R et al (2006) Linkage of monogenic infantile hypertrophic pyloric stenosis to chromosome 16p12–p13 and evidence for genetic heterogeneity. Am J Hum Genet 79:378–382
39. Everett KV, Capon F, Georgoula C et al (2008) Linkage of monogenic infantile hypertrophic pyloric stenosis to chromosome 16q24. Eur J Hum Genet 16:1151–1154
40. Everett KV, Chioza BA, Georgoula C et al (2008) Genome-wide high-density SNP based linkage analysis of infantile hypertrophic pyloric stenosis identifies loci on chromosomes 11q14-q22 and Xq23. Am J Hum Genet 82:756–762

41. Everett KV, Chioza BA, Georgoula C et al (2009) Infantile hypertrophic pyloric stenosis: evaluation of three positional candidate genes, TRPC1, TRPC5 and TRPC6, by association analysis and re-sequencing. Hum Genet 126:819–831
42. Peeters B, Beninga MA, Hennekam RCM (2012) Infantile hypertrophic pyloric stenosis – genetics and syndromes. Nat Rev Gastroenterol Hepatol 9:646–660
43. San Fillippo JA (1976) Infantile hypertrophic pyloric stenosis related to ingestion of erythromycin estolate. J Pediatr Surg 11:177–180
44. Honein MA, Cragan JD (2014) Balancing competing risks: perinatal exposure to macrolides increases the risk of infantile hypertrophic pyloric stenosis. Evid Based Med 19(6):239–241
45. Eberly MD, Eide MB, Thompson JL, Nylund CM (2015) Azithromycin in early infancy and pyloric stenosis. Pediatrics 135(3):483–488
46. Wayne C, Hung JHC, Chan E et al (2016) Formula-feeding and hypertrophic pyloric stenosis: is there an association? A case–control study. J Pediatr Surg 51:779–782
47. Evans NJ (1982) Pyloric stenosis in premature infants after transpyloric feeding. Lancet 320(8299):665
48. Latchaw LA, Jacir NN, Harris BH (1989) The development of pyloric stenosis during transpyloric feedings. J Pediatr Surg 24(8):823–824
49. Panteli C (2009) New insights into the pathogenesis of infantile pyloric stenosis. Pediatr Surg Int 25:1043–1052
50. Vanderwinden JM, Mailleux P, Schiffmann SN et al (1992) Nitric oxide synthase activity in infantile hypertrophic pyloric stenosis. N Engl J Med 327:511–515
51. Huang PL, Dawson TM, Bredt DS et al (1993) Targeted disruption of the neuronal nitric oxide synthase gene. Cell 75:1273–1286
52. Abel RM (1996) The ontogeny of the peptide innervation of the human pylorus, with special reference to understanding the aetiology and pathogenesis of infantile hypertrophic pyloric stenosis. J Pediatr Surg 31(4):490–497
53. Ladd WE, Ware PF, Pickett LK (1946) Congenital hypertrophic pyloric stenosis. JAMA 131:647–651
54. White MC, Langer JC, Don S et al (1998) Sensitivity and cost minimization analysis of radiology versus olive palpation for the diagnosis of hypertrophic pyloric stenosis. J Pediatr Surg 33(6):913–917
55. Snoek AP (2015) Aspiration risk in pyloric stenosis. Paediatr Anaesth 25(9):966
56. Teele RL, Smith EH (1977) Ultrasound in the diagnosis of idiopathic hypertrophic pyloric stenosis. N Engl J Med 296:1149–1150
57. Mullassery D, Mallappa S, Shariff R et al (2008) Negative exploration of pyloric stenosis – is it preventable? BMC Pediatr 8:37–91
58. Rohrschneider WK, Mittnacht H, Darge K, Troger J (1998) Pyloric muscle in asymptomatic infants: sonographic evaluation and discrimination from idiopathic hypertrophic pyloric stenosis. Pediatr Radiol 28:429–434
59. Mollitt DL, Golladay ES, Williamson S et al (1987) Ultrasonography in the diagnosis of pyloric stenosis. South Med J 80:47–50
60. Lund Kofoed PE, Høst A, Elle B, Larsen C (1988) Hypertrophic pyloric stenosis: determination of muscle dimensions by ultrasound. Br J Radiol 61(721):19–20
61. Neilson D, Hollman AS (1994) The ultrasonic diagnosis of infantile hypertrophic pyloric stenosis: technique and accuracy. Clin Radiol 49:246–247
62. O'Keeffe FN, Stansberry SD, Swischuk LE et al (1991) Antropyloric muscle thickness at US in infants: what is normal? Radiology 178:827–830
63. Otjen JP, Iyer RS, Phillips GS, Parisi MT (2012) Usual and unusual causes of pediatric gastric outlet obstruction. Pediatr Radiol 42(6):728–737
64. Dalton BG, Gonzalez KW, Boda SR et al (2016) Optimizing fluid resuscitation in hypertrophic pyloric stenosis. J Pediatr Surg 51(8):1279–1282
65. Tan HL, Bianchi A (1986) Circumumbilical incision for pyloromyotomy. Br J Surg 73:399
66. Misra D, Mushtaq I (1998) Surface umbilical pyloromyotomy. Eur J Pediatr 8:81–82
67. De Caluwe D, Reding R, De Ville de Goyet J (1998) Intraabdominal pyloromyotomy through the umbilical route: a technical improvement. J Pediatr Surg 33(12):1806–1807
68. Donnellan WL, Cobb LM (1991) Intraabdominal pyloromyotomy. J Pediatr Surg 26:174–175
69. Gauderer MWL (2008) Experience with a nonlaparoscopic, transumbilical, intracavitary pyloromyotomy. J Pediatr Surg 43:884–888
70. Alain JL, Grousseau D, Terrier G (1990) Pyloromyotomie extramuqueuse par laparoscopie. Chir Pediatr 31(4–5):223–224
71. Alain JL, Grousseau D, Terrier G (1991) Extramucosal pyloromytomy by laparoscopy. J Pediatr Surg 26(10):1191–1192
72. Leclair MD, Plattner V, Mirallie E et al (2007) Laparoscopic pyloromyotomy for hypertrophic pyloric stenosis: a prospective, randomized controlled trial. J Pediatr Surg 42(4):692–698
73. Hall NJ, Pacilli M, Eaton S et al (2009) Recovery after open versus laparoscopic pyloromyotomy for pyloric stenosis: a double-blind multicentre randomised controlled trial. Lancet 373(9661):390–398
74. Yagmurlu A, Barnhart DC, Vernon A, Georgeson KE et al (2004) Comparison of the incidence of complications in open and laparoscopic pyloromyotomy: a concurrent single institution series. J Pediatr Surg 39(3):292–296
75. Sola JE, Neville HL (2009) Laparoscopic vs open pyloromyotomy: a systematic review and meta-analysis. J Pediatr Surg 44(8):1631–1637
76. Carrington EV, Hall NJ, Pacilli M et al (2012) Cost-effectiveness of laparoscopic versus open pyloromyotomy. J Surg Res 178(1):315–320
77. Scorpio RJ, Tan HL, Hutson JM (1995) Pyloromyotomy: comparison between laparoscopic and open surgical techniques. J Laparoendosc Surg 5:81–84

78. Van der Bilt JDW, Kramer WLM, van der Zee DC, Bax NMA (2004) Laparoscopic pyloromyotomy for hypertrophic pyloric stenosis. Impact of experience on the results in 182 cases. Surg Endosc 18(6):907–909
79. Andropoulos DB, Heard MB, Johnson KL et al (1994) Postanesthetic apnea in full-term infants after pyloromyotomy. Anesthesiology 80(1):216–219
80. Davis PJ, Galinkin J, McGowan FX et al (2001) A randomized multicenter study of remifentanil compared with halothane in neonates and infants undergoing pyloromyotomy. Emergence and recovery profiles. Anesth Analg 93(6):1380–1386, and 1387–1392
81. Kachko L, Simhi E, Freud E et al (2009) Impact of spinal anesthesia for open pyloromyotomy on operating room time. J Pediatr Surg 44(10):1942–1946
82. Perger L, Fuchs JR, Komidar L, Mooney DP (2009) Impact of surgical approach on outcome in 622 consecutive pyloromytomies at a pediatric teaching institution. J Pediatr Surg 44:2119–2125
83. Nagita A, Yamaguchi J, Amemoto K et al (1996) Management and ultrasonographic appearance of infantile hypertrophic pyloric stenosis with intravenous atropine sulfate. J Pediatr Gastroenterol Nutr 23(2):172–177
84. Yamataka A, Tsukada K, Yokoyama-Laws Y et al (2000) Pyloromyotomy versus atropine sulfate for infantile hypertrophic pyloric stenosis. J Pediatr Surg 35(2):338–341
85. Kawahara H, Takama Y, Yoshida H et al (2005) Medical treatment of infantile hypertrophic pyloric stenosis: should we always slice the "olive"? J Pediatr Surg 40(12):1848–1851
86. Takeuchi M, Yasunaga H, Horiguchi H et al (2013) Pyloromyotomy versus i.v. atropine therapy for the treatment of infantile pyloric stenosis: nationwide hospital discharge database analysis. Pediatr Int 55(4):488–491
87. Huang YC, Su BH (2004) Medical treatment with atropine sulfate for hypertrophic pyloric stenosis. Acta Paediatr Taiwan 45(3):136–140
88. Singh UK, Kumar R, Prasad R (2005) Oral atropine sulfate for infantile hypertrophic pyloric stenosis. Indian Pediatr 42(5):473–476
89. Meissner PE, Engelmann G, Troeger J et al (2006) Conservative treatment of infantile hypertrophic pyloric stenosis with intravenous atropine sulphate does not replace pyloromyotomy. Pediatr Surg Int 22:1021–1024
90. Mercer AE, Phillips R (2013) Question 2: Can a conservative approach to the treatment of hypertrophic pyloric stenosis with atropine be considered a real alternative to surgical pyloromyotomy? Arch Dis Child 98(6):474–477
91. Rudolph CD (1966) Medical treatment of idiopathic hypertrophic pyloric stenosis: should we marinate or slice the "olive"? J Pediatr Gastroenterol Nutr 23:399–401
92. Aspelund G, Langer JC (2007) Current management of hypertrophic pyloric stenosis. Semin Pediatr Surg 16(1):27–33
93. Yen JB, Kong MS (2006) Gastric outlet obstruction in pediatric patients. Chang Gung Med J 29(4):401–405
94. Attard TM, Abraham SC, Cuffari C (2003) The clinical spectrum of duodenal polyps in pediatrics. J Pediatr Gastroenterol Nutr 36:116–119
95. Wang LC, Lee HC, Yeung CY et al (2009) Gastrointestinal polyps in children. Pediatr Neonatol 50(5):196–201
96. Brooks GS, Frost ES, Wesselhoeft C (1992) Prolapsed hyperplastic gastric polyp causing gastric outlet obstruction, hypergastrinemia and hematemesis in an infant. J Pediatr Surg 27:1537–1538
97. Murphy S, Shaw K, Blanchard H (1994) Report of three gastric tumors in children. J Pediatr Surg 29:1202–1204
98. Ertem D, Tutar E, Cam S et al (2006) Severe gastric outlet obstruction in a child with ectopic pancreas: is there a role for Helicobacter pylori? J Pediatr Gastroenterol Nutr 43(3):385–387
99. Sharma SB, Gupta V (2004) Ectopic pancreas as a cause of gastric outlet obstruction in an infant. Indian J Gastroenterol 23(6):219
100. Strobel CT, Smith LE, Fonkalsrud EW et al (1978) Ectopic pancreatic tissue in the gastric antrum. J Pediatr 92:586–588
101. Özcan C, Çelik A, Gülü C et al (2002) A rare cause of gastric outlet obstruction in the newborn: pyloric ectopic pancreas. J Pediatr Surg 37:119–120
102. Lund DP, Compton CC, Scully RE et al (1999) A three-week-old girl with pyloric stenosis and an unexpected operative finding – pancreatic heterotopia involving the gastric pylorus, with acute pancreatitis. (Hypertrophic pyloric obstruction.). N Engl J Med 341(9):679–684
103. Shin DH, Lee JH, Kang HJ et al (2010) Novel epitheliomesenchymal biphasic stomach tumour (gastroblastoma) in a 9-year-old: morphological, ultrastructural and immunohistochemical findings. J Clin Pathol 63(3):270–274
104. Sanchez Garcia S, Rubio Solis D, Anes Gonzales D et al (2016) Gastric adenomyoma clinically simulating hypertrophic pyloric stenosis. Radiologia 58(2):148–151
105. Arellano CM, Kritsaneepaiboon S, Lee EY (2011) CT imaging findings of malignant neoplasms arising in the epigastric region in children. Clin Imaging 35:10–20
106. Kaemmer DA, Otto J, Lassay L et al (2009) The Gist of literature on pediatric GIST: review of clinical presentation. J Pediatr Hematol Oncol 31:108–112
107. Benesch M, Leuschner I, Wardelmann E et al (2011) Gastrointestinal stromal tumours in children and young adults: a clinicopathologic series with long-term follow-up from the database of the Cooperative Weichteilsarkom Studiengruppe (CWS). Eur J Cancer 47:1692–1698
108. Salah W, Baron TH Sr (2013) Gastric antral web: a rare cause of gastric outlet obstruction treated with endoscopic therapy. Gastrointest Endosc 78(3):450
109. Bing L, Wei-Bing C, Shou-Qing W et al (2013) Laparoscope-assisted diagnosis and treatment of

prepyloric web in children – report of three cases. J Pediatr Surg 48(7):1633–1636
110. Campbell DP, Vanhoutte JJ, Smith EI (1973) Partially obstructing antral web—a distinct clinical entity. J Pediatr Surg 8:723–728
111. Lui KW, Wong HF, Wan YL et al (2000) Antral web – a rare cause of vomiting in children. Pediatr Surg Int 16:424–425
112. Bell MJ, Ternberg JL, Keating JP et al (1978) Prepyloric gastric antral web: a puzzling epidemic. J Pediatr Surg 13:307–313
113. Johnson GM (1971) Gastric mucosal diaphragm in a child. Pediatrics 47:916–919
114. Hermanowicz A, Debek W (2015) Image in clinical medicine: single bubble – pyloric atresia. N Engl J Med 373(9):863
115. Muller M, Morger R, Engert J (1990) Pyloric atresia: report of four cases and review of the literature. Pediatr Surg Int 5:276–279
116. Darani A, Mendoza-Sagaon M, Reinberg O (2005) Gastric volvulus in children: myth or reality? J Pediatr Surg 40(5):855–858
117. Patel RA, Baker SS, Sayej WN, Baker RD (2011) Two cases of helicobacter pylori-negative gastric outlet obstruction in children. Case Rep Gastrointest Med 2011:Article ID 749850. Epub
118. El Faleh I, Lutz N, Reinberg O (2009) Gastric outlet obstruction by Brunner's gland hyperplasia in an 8-year-old child. J Pediatr Surg 44(4):E21–E24
119. Katiyar R, Patne SC, Dixit VK et al (2016) Primary eosinophilic gastritis in a child with gastric outlet obstruction. J Gastrointest Surg 20:1270–1271 [Epub ahead of print]
120. Gobbi D, Billi P, Fascetti Leon F, Alvisi P, Lambertini A, Lima M (2013) Pneumatic pyloric dilatation for the treatment of gastric outlet obstruction in a child. Pediatr Int 55(3):382–385
121. Hernot S, Yadav SP, Kathuria B et al (2015) An uncommon oesophageal foreign body in a neonate. Br Med J Case Rep e-pub Jan 30;2015. pii: bcr2014208719. doi: 10.1136/bcr-2014-208719

Congenital Duodenal Stenosis

15

David C. van der Zee

15.1 Introduction

Congenital duodenal stenosis or atresia is one of the more common neonatal intestinal obstructions, which is increasingly more often already detected by prenatal ultrasound, demonstrating a distended stomach and bulbus duodeni. In the past it would be the typical double bubble sign on abdominal X-ray in neonates presenting with bilious vomiting [1, 2].

The obstruction may present as a stenosis or web, or true atresia, and should be discriminated from malrotation with or without volvulus. In 20 % duodenal atresia is associated with malrotation; 30 % of the patients have Down syndrome. Sometimes the duodenal atresia is seen in conjunction with esophageal atresia [1, 3].

Classical management of duodenal atresia is a side-to-side and diamond-shaped anastomosis between the proximal bulbus and the distal duodenum, bypassing the obstruction that is usually located at the level or just below the pancreas.

With the onset of minimal invasive surgery and increasing experience, the laparoscopic management of duodenal atresia has come into scope [2, 4].

D.C. van der Zee
Department of Pediatric Surgery, Wilhelmina Children's Hospital, University Medical Center Utrecht, 85090, Utrecht 3508 AB, The Netherlands
e-mail: d.c.vanderzee@umcutrecht.nl

15.2 Preoperative Workup

After confirmation of the diagnosis, the patient can be planned for operative correction as an elective procedure. The patient is lined up with a nasogastric tube to decompress the stomach and bulbus duodeni, an i.v. for fluid administration, and an arterial line, if possible, for monitoring during the laparoscopy. Nowadays, patients are also monitored by means of near-infrared spectrometry, to secure sufficient cerebral blood flow during the laparoscopic procedure. Antibiotics are given for 24 h.

15.3 Positioning on the Operating Table

The patient is positioned at the lower end of a short operating table to allow comfortable access for the surgeon. The operating table sheet is wrapped over the flexed legs to secure the patient from sliding from the table when it is placed in anti-Trendelenburg position.

15.4 Trocar Positioning

The first 5-mm trocar is introduced in an open way in the sub-umbilical fold. With the use of a 3×0 Vicryl suture, that is placed in the fascia in a U-shape, the trocar can be fixed to prevent it from falling out. A silicone tubing around the shaft of

M. Lima (ed.), *Pediatric Digestive Surgery*, DOI 10.1007/978-3-319-40525-4_15

the trocar on the other hand can prevent the trocar from sliding in. The flow is maximized at 2–3 l/min and the maximum pressure is set to 5–8mmHg.

After insufflation two additional 3-mm trocars can be placed, one in the right lower quadrant and one in the left mid-abdomen. Beware not to place the trocar in the right lower quadrant too low, otherwise the freedom of moving the trocar is reduced. On the other hand, if the trocar is placed too high, it will lie above the level of the liver and duodenum and it will be difficult to handle the instrument. Therefore this trocar should be placed under direct vision to determine the best position.

15.5 Operative Procedure

The first step is to mobilize the right colonic flexure by blunt and/or sharp dissection. This should be sufficiently halfway to the transverse colon, in order to get a good access to the duodenum. If the bulbus duodeni is grossly distended, it is helpful to put a stay suture in the bulbus and extend it outside through the skin to pull away the bulbus from the pancreas and pars horizontalis in order to be able to sufficiently mobilize the distal duodenum. Bands and adhesions can be taken down by blunt traction. Try to avoid grasping the duodenum itself as much as possible to avoid damage to the duodenal wall. Determine carefully where the suspected obstruction is located; this may be an annular pancreas, a stenosis or a true atresia. By mobilizing the distal duodenum, a malrotation can be confirmed or excluded.

In case of a stenosis or a web, a longitudinal anti-mesenterial incision can be made over the stenosis or incisures. A stenosis can be simply closed transversely; a web should be exposed sufficiently to incise the web without damaging the Vater papilla. Liberally make use of stay sutures in the wall to be able to clearly discern all anatomic structures. The defect can be closed transversely.

In case of a pancreas annulare or true atresia, the distal duodenum can be incised longitudinally over 1–1.5 cm. approximately 1–2 cm away from the obstruction. Either a longitudinal or transverse incision is made over the bulbus duodeni (Fig. 15.1). The content of the bulbus is removed with a suction device. When making a diamond-shaped anastomosis, the first Vicryl 5×0 suture is laid from the right corner of the bulbus (Fig. 15.2) to halfway to the right side of the distal duodenum (outside-in, inside-out). The stay suture in the bulbus is released far enough to allow a tension-free tying of the knot of this suture (Fig. 15.3). The long end of the suture is led out through the abdominal wall to stabilize the intestine and suture line. A second suture is laid from the left corner of the bulbus to halfway to the left side of the distal duodenum (outside-in, inside-out). After tying this suture, the needle is passed into the inside of the intestinal wall, and a running suture can be made over

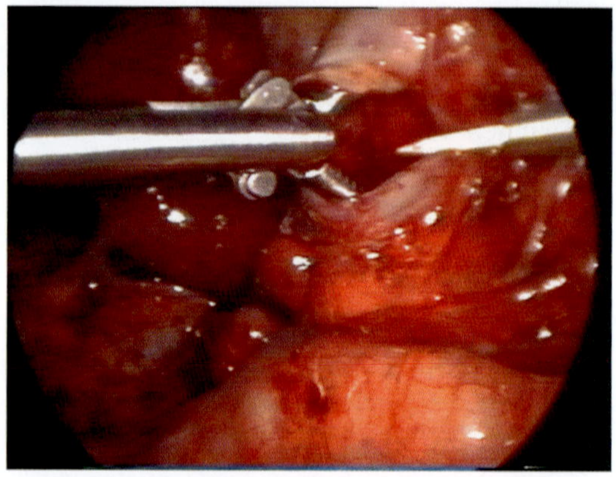

Fig. 15.1 Transverse incision in the bulbus duodeni

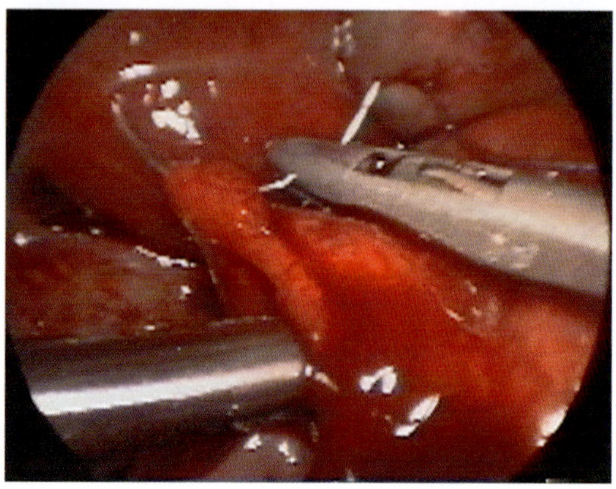

Fig. 15.2 First suture through the distal duodenum

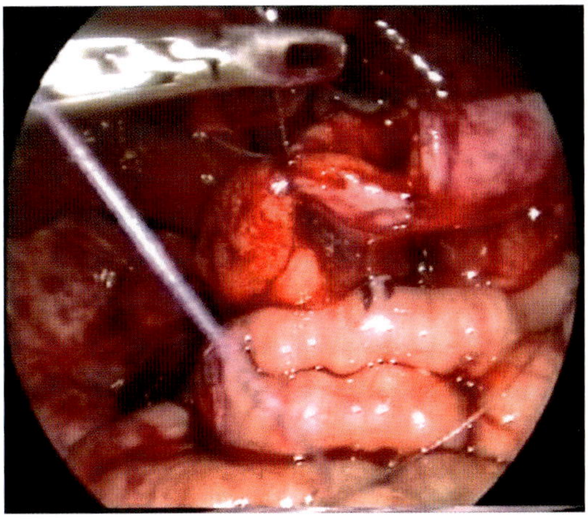

Fig. 15.3 Approximation of first suture from midway bulbus to superior edge of distal duodenum

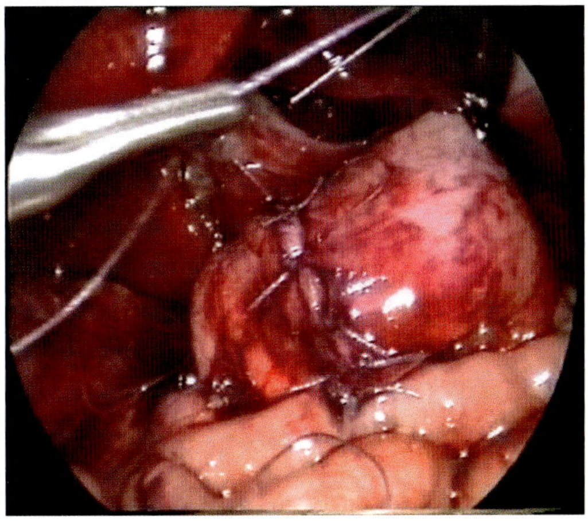

Fig. 15.4 Completion of anastomosis

the posterior wall from the inside. Usually by pulling on the short end of the left suture, the posterior wall will present itself nicely for the running suture. At the right end, the needle is led out and tied with the short end of the first suture. This same suture can usually be used to run back over the anterior wall and tied to the short end on the left side finishing the anastomosis (Fig. 15.4). There is no tapering of the bulbus duodeni. There is no exploration of the distal duodenum for other membranes or obstructions, as they are seldom [5]. The stay sutures are cut and all trocars are removed under direct vision. The U-shape suture in the umbilicus can be used to close this defect. The other fasciae are closed with a Vicryl 5×0 suture and Steri-Strips for the skin. No drain or any trans-anastomotic drain is left behind.

15.6 Postoperative Care

The patients are kept nil per mouth for 24 h, after which feeding is started with 8x10 ml, irrespective of any gastric retention. Feeding is extended according to age and weight over the following days. Retentions up to 30 cc are accepted and given back. It is better not to measure retentions, but observe the child clinically and adjust feeding regimen accordingly.

Feeding and admission times are usually more dependent on concomitant anomalies like cardiac abnormalities or Down syndrome.

15.7 Personal Experience

We described the first case of laparoscopic repair of duodenal atresia in 2001 [4]. In a first series from 2000 to 2005, 22 children were operated laparoscopically. In four cases the procedure was converted. In five patients there was leakage of the anastomosis. This was reason to stop the laparoscopic approach at that moment until the procedure was adjusted sufficiently to ban out any more leakage.

With increasing experience and changing to a running suture that secured the anastomosis, we picked up the procedure again. From 2008 to March 2015, another 22 children were operated laparoscopically without any more complications. All procedures could be completed laparoscopically [3].

15.8 Discussion

Repair of duodenal atresia is one of the most complex minimal invasive procedures. This is mainly because of the limited space available. In thoracoscopic repair of esophageal atresia, the rigid thoracic cage secures some space. In the abdomen with low pressures of 5–8 mmHg, the overlying liver and moving intestines, next to gas leakage along the trocars, leaves a limited space for moving around. Often an extra trocar is placed in the epigastrium to lift up the liver to give additional exposure. Also the liberal use of stay sutures gives more stability to the operating field. It helps if the assistant that holds the camera pulls on the umbilical trocar to give additional space. The major step forward in determining success was the use of running sutures that give an even tension along the whole anastomosis. Since adjusting this technique, we have seen no more incidents of leakage.

Another issue is the endoscope. In open surgery an incision is made directly over the underlying duodenum. In laparoscopy the view is fixed from the umbilicus, giving another angle at which the anomaly is approached. Good anatomical knowledge of the course of the duodenum is obligatory. Good exposure is important. Therefore the first step is to mobilize the overlying right colonic flexure sufficiently away, that is, it does not fall back constantly in front of the duodenum and pancreas head.

The second step is to identify the bulbus duodeni and pancreas head. It often is helpful when a stay suture is placed in the bulbus to lift it away from the pancreas head and distal duodenum.

When mobilizing the distal duodenum, try not to grasp the duodenal wall, but take down the bands and adhesions between two grasping forceps just adjacent to the duodenum. When the duodenum is sufficiently mobilized, a longitudinal incision can be made with straight scissors or a pylorotomy knife. In open surgery a diamond-shaped anastomosis is advocated, although some authors claim that a simple side-to-side anastomosis is just as well. A diamond-shaped anastomosis is well feasible in laparoscopy, but there is no objection to make a side-to-side anastomosis.

No effort is made to advance a trans-anastomotic tube or explore more distal membranes, because they occur only seldom, and if they do, they can be addressed in a separate procedure, or even by balloon dilatation under fluoroscopy if the membrane is not too thick [5].

Some authors advocate tapering of the bulbus duodeni [6]. In our view it is questionable if this will give any advantage to restoration of the passage of gastric contents. In our experience we have never had to taper the bulbus in any of our patients. Obviously the bulbus is distended and will always remain distended. However, if this does not lead to feeding problems, there is no reason to make a procedure more complicated than necessary. On the contrary, we start feeding the children as of the second postoperative day and accept retentions up to 30 cc, as there will always be some pooling of gastric and duodenal content in the distended bulbus. Usually, the children tolerate the feeding very well, and oral intake can usually be increased like in all neonates of their gestational age.

In conclusion the laparoscopic management of duodenal obstruction is feasible and has a good outcome. The procedure is technical demanding and usually requires an experienced laparoscopic surgeon.

References

1. Aguayo P, Ostlie DJ (2010) Duodenal and intestinal atresia and stenosis. In: Holcomb III GW, Murphy JP, Ostlie DJ Ashcraft's pediatric surgery, 5th ed. Elsevier Inc, Philadelphia
2. van der Zee DC, Bax NMA (2008) Laparoscopic treatment of duodenal and jejunal atresia and stenosis. In: Bax NMA, Georgeson KE, Rothenberg SS, Valla JS, Yeung CK (eds) Endoscopic surgery in infants and children. Springer, Berlin
3. van der Zee DC (2011) Laparoscopic repair of duodenal atresia: revisited. World J Surg 35:1781–1784
4. Bax NM, Ure BM, van der Zee DC, van Tuijl I (2001) Laparoscopic duodenoduodenostomy for duodenal atresia. Surg Endosc 15:217
5. St Peter SD, Little DC, Barsness KA, Copeland DR, Calkins CM, Yoder S, Rothenberg SS, Islam S, Tsao K, Ostlie DJ (2010) Should we be concerned about jejunoileal atresia during repair of duodenal atresia? J Laparoendosc Adv Surg Tech A 20:773–775
6. Adzick NS, Harrison MR, deLorimier AA (1986) Tapering duodenoplasty for megaduodenum associated with duodenal atresia. J Pediatr Surg 21:311–312

16 Caustic Ingestion and Foreign Bodies

Olivier Reinberg

16.1 Introduction

Their homes and surroundings can be dangerous places for children, particularly with regard to the possibility of unintentional swallowing of foreign bodies or potentially dangerous liquids.

Children are naturally curious, exploring in and around their homes. They develop their senses by physically interacting with the things around them, touching and placing them in their mouth. As a result, each year millions of calls are made to poison control centers or pediatric emergency rooms after unintentional swallowing of foreign bodies or potentially dangerous liquids. Most of these accidents could have been prevented. This chapter focuses on caustic and various foreign body ingestions [1].

16.2 Caustic Injuries

16.2.1 Epidemiology of Caustic Injuries

Ingestions of corrosive substances, alkalis or acids, are common both in low- or high-income countries in spite of prevention measures to minimize the hazards of household products and laws for containers with child-resistant closures. The majority of ingestions occurs in children younger than 5 years and could be preventable [2–4]. Ingestion in children older than 5 years is suspect and in adolescents, mainly in girls, is usually intentional with larger volumes swallowed [2]. In addition, there might be an unknown number of cases of abuse.

The true prevalence of these injuries is unknown. According to the report on pediatric trauma done by the World Health Organization and the UNICEF, more than 120,000 children under 6 years old suffered caustic injuries in the United States in 2004 [1, 5]. While most exposures to household products result in mild poisoning, cleaning agents, strong alkalis, and acids can lead to severe tissue damages. In the pediatric group, 70–90 % of burns are related to alkali substances and 10–30 % to acids [2–4, 6, 7].

Chemicals around the house to which children may have access contribute significantly to unintentional poisonings in childhood, both in developed countries and in low-income countries. Only the substances differ. In developed countries exposures to cleaning agents, such as ammonia, bleach, dishwasher, and laundry detergents, are most common, especially the dishwasher tablets that are the most frequent household products involved in injuries [2–4]. Dishwasher detergents are highly corrosive substances causing potentially life-threatening injuries and severe morbidity [4, 7, 8]. In most countries dishwasher tablets are not included in the regulations

O. Reinberg
Pediatric Surgery, Rochettaz 24, CH – 1009 Pully, Switzerland
e-mail: olreinberg@gmail.com

M. Lima (ed.), *Pediatric Digestive Surgery*, DOI 10.1007/978-3-319-40525-4_16

for child-resistant closures. Another concern is that liquid household products such as soaps, liquid soaps, and dishwasher and laundry detergents are packaged to imitate food or have other attributes that appeal to children (smell, color). Due to new trends in food marketing, the frontier between food products and cosmetics has been blurred. In 2011, the Scientific Committee on Consumer Safety of the European Commission stated that "Products which, although not foodstuffs, possess a form, odor, color, appearance, packaging, volume or size, so that is likely that consumers, especially children, will confuse them with foodstuffs and in consequence place them in their mouths, or suck or ingest them, which might be dangerous and cause, for example, suffocation, poisoning, or the perforation or obstruction of the digestive tract" [9]. These recommendations are fairly followed, as prevention does not carry much weight compared with the expected benefits.

This last decade, new concentrated laundry "pods" or capsules appeared on markets and are associated with more severe accidents compared to classic laundry detergents. Detergent "pods" are small, single-use doses of concentrated detergent encased in a water-soluble membrane (polyvinyl alcohol) to dissolve in wash water and release the detergent. They are colorful designed like candies. Compared to classic laundry detergents, the chemical composition of laundry pods has a higher concentration of surfactants and ethoxylated alcohols and a higher viscosity and hydrotropic power. They are filled under pressure, so when the child places the capsule in his mouth and bites it or sucks on it, thus dissolving the water-soluble membrane, the content explodes before the eyes or in the mouth with subsequent ingestion and/or inhalation. A spectrum of clinical effects from minor to serious injuries, even deaths, was seen with ingestions, inhalations, ocular exposures, or combinations of them. In the USA, from 2012 to 2013, 17,230 children exposed to laundry detergent pods were reported to US poison control centers [8, 10]. In Italy, laundry detergent pods have become the most commonly ingested household product since becoming available in 2010 [11]. From 2012 to 2015, 34 reports from different countries (France, Canada, the USA, Italy, the UK) came to the same conclusions and warn clinicians, parents, and caregivers. They all conclude that measures should be taken to avoid ingestions of these products, but nothing has been done to date to regulate their use and composition. "These publications, although commendable for resulting in positive outcomes, also serve to highlight previously identified weaknesses in the NPDS surveillance system (USA, but other national agencies as well)" [12].

In developing or lower-income countries, sodium hypochlorite or sodium hydroxide (lye, caustic soda), used to make soap, as a bleaching agent, to manufacture textiles, for washing or chemical peeling of fruits and vegetables, for cocoa processing, for olive softening or blackening (also with potassium hydroxide), or to prepare "medicines," is left reachable for children often on the ground.

16.2.2 Prevention of Caustic Injuries

The most obvious risk factor for ingestion of a substance is its presence in the domestic environment, within the reach of children. Dispensing them in containers without child-resistant closures increases the risk of poisoning. The use of appropriate labeling ("skull and crossbones") serves as parents' warning but not to children who are unlikely to recognize the significance of these signs. Subsequently, the best prevention is to keep them out of their reach. Bathroom cabinets and kitchen cupboards or locked drawers appear to be the safest storage places. Unfortunately, in modern houses, the bad habit is to store harmful products in the locker under the sink instead of putting them in a high place. Safe packaging cannot compensate for unsafe storage.

In high-income countries, dangerous products are required by law to be distributed in child-resistant packaging, i.e., requiring several complex actions such as turning while pushing downwards or squeezing. The common standards for tests adopted in most countries require that at least 85 % of children aged from 42 to 51 months must be unable to open the container within 5 min [13]. Child-resistant packaging is one of the best-documented successes in preventing the unintentional poisoning of children [1]. Unfortunately, rules for child-resistant packaging currently exist only in very few countries, such as Australia, Canada, New Zealand, the United States, and the European Union. Furthermore, no closure is perfect. Up to 20 % of children aged between 42 and 51 months may be able to overcome a child-resistant closure, and their parents are most often unaware [14].

An alternative approach is to lower the level of the toxicity or to make it repellent or uninteresting for children. Toxicity can be lowered by reformulation and many dangerous substances could be replaced. Color can play a role, as pink, purple, and yellow are attractive for children, while dark blue, violet, or brown-green are unappreciated colors. Children initially prefer sweet tastes and reject sour and bitter tastes. Therefore bittering agents have been used to prevent from ingestions and poisonings. The most commonly used aversive agent is the denatonium benzoate (Bitrex® or Aversion®), which has an unpleasant taste at very low concentrations unbearably bitter to most humans [15–17]. The problem with sodium hypochlorite or hydroxide is their lack of smell and their harmless appearance. The addition of <1 % ammoniac is enough to give them an unpleasant smell with a subsequent repellent effect on children, but unfortunately also on their mothers who will not buy such a product. Unfortunately there are no published data on the effectiveness of aversing agents in limiting the ingestion of household products.

In developing or lower-income countries, these dangerous products are freely bought on markets and diluted or transferred in beverage bottles at home where they are stored on the ground or in places reachable for children. As the manufacturing facilities are scarce, it could be cheap and easy to color sodium hypochlorite or hydroxide and to add ammoniac. During our numerous missions, we have frequently received interest from many governmental or nongovernmental authorities but without effects.

16.2.3 Physiopathology of Caustic Injuries

Both acids and bases can be defined as caustics, which cause significant tissue damages on contact with the esophagus. Most acids produce a coagulation necrosis by denaturing proteins, inducing a coating coagulum that protects the underlayers from deeper penetration. Bases induce more severe injuries known as liquefactive necrosis, i.e., the denaturation of proteins together with a saponification of fats, which penetrate deep through the esophageal wall and can go through it. The lesions are colonized by bacteria within 24–48 h worsening the tissue damages.

The severity of the damages is related to several factors, including the pH, the concentration, and the volume of the agent. The contact time is of little interest as a lesion occurs within a few seconds. The physical form of the agent plays a significant role: the ingestion of solid pellets results in prolonged local contact time with the esophagus, thus deeper localized burns, while liquids generate superficial but more extensive lesions. For this reason it is of major importance to refrain from drinking after pellet ingestion as it may induce both types of lesion. Vomitings – spontaneous or induced using emetic – worsen the lesions due to a repeated exposure.

Depending on the extent of burn, inflammation or necrosis may extend through the whole esophageal wall until perforation occurs either in the mediastinum with subsequent mediastinitis or in the trachea or bronchi. With the disappearance of the mucosa, the facing surfaces adhere to each other worsening the stenosis of the esophagus or occluding its lumen, moving toward a fistula. Like the skin, the long-term effect of caustic esophageal burns is a hypertrophic scarring process, which can result in stricture formation. Mucosal reepithelization is a slow process, usually not complete before 4–6 weeks. Not until a complete reepithelization, the inflammation continues, and granulation tissue comes to maturity when fibroblast proliferation replaces the submucosa and muscular layers, initiating strictures. Thus a stricture formation is detectable after 2 weeks and is definite by the fourth week. This is the best time to start dilatations. In a series of 80 pediatric patients, de Jong reports 29 % of early and late medical complications and 20 % that developed severe esophageal strictures requiring esophageal replacement in two-thirds of them [18]. Baskin reports 81 of which 16 % developed a stricture even in some cases of low grades [19].

If the muscular layers of the esophagus have been destroyed, they will not regenerate and be replaced by fibrous tissue. Even if the lumen has been kept open, the contraction waves will never overpass that point.

The caustic burn induces a shortening of the esophagus and a motility disorder resulting in reflux and poor esophageal clearance, which adds a peptic stenosis to a caustic one evidenced by histology (O. Reinberg, unpublished). For this reason all our patients under conservative treatment with dilatations receive proton pump inhibitors (PPI).

16.2.4 Diagnosis of Caustic Injuries

A suspicion of caustic ingestion requires a detailed questioning, asking for the nature of the product, its form, the amount, and the precise time of the injury. When receiving an emergency call, remind the parents or the caregivers to avoid drinking or eating (no emetic agent) and ask to bring the product and the packaging with them. This will help to identify the ingested substance and measure its pH.

There is a large variation of symptoms after caustic ingestion ranging from nothing to life-threatening conditions. Several studies have indicated that the clinical manifestations are poor predictors of the presence and the extent or depth of esophageal injury [3, 4, 18, 20]. Initial symptoms and clinical signs are mostly related to the edema. However, the presence of more than three symptoms or signs is associated with increased likelihood of esophageal injury [3]. Reversely, Gandreault wrote that 12 % of children with proven esophageal injuries had no significant esophageal or abdominal complaints [20]. Thus any suspected caustic ingestion should be referred to medical facilities to be investigated.

The most common symptoms are drooling, dysphagia, odynophagia, vomiting, and oral liquid refusal. Respiratory symptoms such as tachycardia, dyspnea, dysphonia, and stridor are evocating upper airway injury and may be seen immediately or delayed due to the progressive edema, but can be seen without airway involvement. Hematemesis is related to severe esophageal injuries, extensive or deep. Chest or abdominal pain and rigidity suggest profound injury and perforation of the esophagus or the stomach [3].

The oral cavity should be carefully inspected to look for lip swelling, tongue erythema, leukoplakia, or oral ulceration. Blind placement of a nasogastric tube should be avoided due to the increased risk of perforation.

Chest, lateral neck, and abdominal X-rays are systematically done to look for the presence of free air in the retropharynx, mediastinum, or peritoneum.

Contrast studies (UGI) are not helpful at early stages. They do not reveal mucosal injuries or overestimate the lesions showing mainly the edema. They represent a waste of time postponing the endoscopy. If done, the use of barium should be avoided in case of perforation, and hydrosoluble contrasts should be preferred. Delayed UGI are of great value to evaluate the number and the severity of stenosis when they occur, i.e., since the third week.

Upper endoscopy remains the cornerstone to define the extent and severity of the injury. Even if debated, as the absence of symptoms and signs does not exclude a serious injury, we believe that a panendoscopy should be done by a multidisciplinary team, under general anesthesia, using all available means, in every patient who is suspected of caustic ingestion. Endoscopy should be performed within 24–48 h of the injury before the esophageal wall begins to weaken [4, 21, 22]. The later it is performed, the higher is the risk of perforation. Rigid endoscopes give a better view of the upper airways, the trachea, and the esophageal omentum. The newest small diameter fiberscopes (ø 6 mm) allow for less traumatic exams of the body of the esophagus, down to the stomach including intra-stomachal version.

In any case, the initial endoscopic evaluation must include the larynx and the upper airways, as associated lesions are not unusual: 15 % in our experience. In the de Jong series, 5 % of patients had the hypopharynx primarily involved with no evidence of oral cavity injury. About 12–20 % of patients could have concurrent esophageal injury without any oral pathological finding. Reversely, in spite of some oral lesions, over 70 % of children are free of significant visceral involvement [3, 4, 18, 21, 22].

Practically based, prior to endotracheal intubation, an assessment of laryngotracheal injury is performed with a rigid endoscope. This initial evaluation should include vocal cord movements as paralysis can occur at the time of the caustic injury. Then the child is intubated and the upper esophagus is explored using first the rigid endoscope then the body of the esophagus and the stomach with a flexible fiberscope. If done earlier, the esophagoscopy should reach the stomach, but in case of delayed endoscopy, it is wise to stop at the level of the most proximal circumferential injury. The authors advocating complete esophagoscopy stress the high mortality rate associated with full-thickness necrosis of the lower esophagus and stomach requiring early recognition and intervention. This is true in adults who swallow large amounts of caustic for suicide but very unusual in children. The length of the intact proximal esophagus above the first stenosis should be carefully measured to anticipate swallowing problems. Under view control, a nasogastric tube has to be placed during the initial endoscopy.

Due to stagnation, lesions are more frequent and more serious at the level of anatomic narrowings of the esophagus (cricopharyngeal area, aortic arch left main bronchus and above the esophagogastric junction). Grading of the endoscopic lesions should be helpful to give a prognosis and define the treatment. Unfortunately, there is no common grading system and reported data are not comparable. Our concern is to assess the presence of a lesion, if it is partial or circular and to evaluate its length and depth. The former classification in four grades by Estrera has been implemented by Zargar, describing two subgroups in grade 2 and 3 (a and b), making a difference whether there are ulcers or pseudomembranes [23–25]. As Rossi, we consider that the classification proposed by the Italian Consensus on Not Bleeding Emergency Endoscopy (AIRONE 2008) summarizes most of them and is easily usable [3, 25, 26] (Table 16.1). To summarize, Grade 1 injuries are superficial, Grade 2 are transmucosal, and Grade 3 and 4 refer to transmural injuries. However, precise endoscopic description of the lesions must be very accurate and should be documented with photos and/or videos.

Patients with Grade 0 or 1 are unlikely to have a complicated course or develop complications.

The patients are usually observed for 24 h, fed under supervision, and once tolerated, are discharged.

However, they must be recontrolled on short and long terms. Should any dysphagia or other symptom occur, a UGI should be done to look for a delayed stenosis.

Patients with Grade 2 are treated the same way but more slowly and systematically have a UGI done between 4 and 6 weeks from injury as 50 % of patients of Grade 2b injury may develop strictures requiring dilatations [4].

There is no define treatment for more severe cases and they must be evaluated from case to case. If a NG tube has been placed during the initial endoscopy, it is used to start early enteral nutrition. However, we must consider the placement of a gastrostomy, as the treatment will last long (see below).

Recently, technetium-labeled sucralfate scan, as described by Millar, has been used as a useful and cost-effective screening method to confirm or exclude significant injury, thus avoiding endoscopy [27]. The sucralfate adheres to inflamed mucosa which is recorded on a scan. Patients without any significant adherence should not have a significant injury and could be discharged without follow-up [27, 28]. Computer tomography or magnetic resonance imaging is helpful to assess a perforation and precise its level.

Table 16.1 Classification for caustic injuries in children [25, 26]

Grade	Endoscopic features	Extent of lesions
0	No lesion	
1	Erythema of the mucosa	
2a	Pseudomembranes	Partial/noncircumferential
2b	Ulcer/necrosis	Partial/noncircumferential
3a	Pseudomembranes	Circumferential
3b	Ulcer/necrosis	Circumferential
4	Full-thickness changes/perforations	

16.2.5 Initial Treatment of Caustic Injuries

16.2.5.1 Antibiotics, Corticoids, PPI

In most teams, caustic ingestions are routinely given antibiotics, steroids, and H2 blockers (PPI) [2–4].

Antibiotics seem useless to prevent bacterial colonization of the esophageal lesions as it occurs in a devascularized tissue where microcirculation has been destroyed, so their routine use is debatable. They are indicated in case of perforation and respiratory involvement. Riffat suggests that there is evidence of a lower rate of stricture formation with the use of antibiotics: by decreasing bacterial counts in the necrotic tissue, superinfection is reduced which may lessen the stricture formation [2]. Occasionally, we have observed a peak of fever after dilatation in some children. As cerebral abscesses have been reported in such circumstances, those cases received a prophylactic dose of antibiotics before each dilatation without recurrence of fever [29].

The beneficial role of steroid on inflammation and scarring process is still debated. They could be used in first- and second-degree injuries but not in third degrees because of the potential increased risk of perforation. Some cases are reported who developed a gastric ulcer with associated hemorrhage after receiving systemic steroids [18]. A meta-analysis of 13 studies done by Fulton over 50 years has concluded that steroid use does not decrease the incidence of stricture formation following Grade 2 caustic ingestion, and therefore, the use of steroids was not advised [30]. Some reports, more specifically concerning infants and toddlers, have shown that the use of high dosage of corticosteroids, starting at the early phase of treatment, could be beneficial in decreasing the need for dilatations [31–33]. Our experience is that corticoids do not prevent from esophageal stenosis in serious caustic burns, but are helpful to achieve faster resolution of the edema, mainly on the airways.

The caustic burn induces a shortening of the esophagus and a motility disorder resulting in reflux with poor esophageal clearance, which adds a peptic stenosis to a caustic one as evidenced by histology (O. Reinberg, unpublished). For this reason, as many others, all our patients under conservative treatment with dilatations receive proton pump inhibitors (PPI) even if their efficiency has not been proven [2–4, 18].

16.2.5.2 Gastrostomy

Benign esophageal strictures usually produce dysphagia for solids, liquids, or both, with slow and insidious progression of weight loss and malnutrition. If the stenosis is important with subsequent dysphagia lasting for more than a month, a gastrostomy should be done to avoid long-lasting total parenteral nutrition with its potential complications. Most patients referred to us, even those with a previously done gastrostomy, were in poor nutritional conditions and must be placed under refeeding program before surgery.

Percutaneous endoscopic gastrostomy (PEG) is our favorite technique for feeding tube placement in children with inadequate nutritional intake. However, it is not feasible after caustic ingestion and a gastrostomy has to be performed. As most of our patients are in poor conditions, they require a gastrostomy including a gastropexy to avoid parietal disunion related to malnutrition. We have described a technique of a real Stamm gastrostomy performed by laparoscopy for these cases [34]. This laparoscopic technique combines the advantages of a minimal invasive procedure with the safety of an open operation and related gastric attachments to the abdominal wall.

The proper placement of the gastrostomy on the anterior stomach wall is a major concern. When intending to replace an esophagus, the surgeon never knows which transplant can be used: if the gastrostomy has been placed too close from the greater curvature, he may face an interruption of the gastroepiploic artery and a gastric tube cannot be achieved. When performing a gastrostomy for caustic stenosis, it is wise to place it far away from the great curvature, just in case a tube could be done.

Gastrostomies are our first choices of surgical access to the bowel, better than jejunostomies. However, if the stomach has been involved in the caustic injury, we must refrain from using it and then perform a jejunostomy.

In some cases, we used an interesting artifice suggested in 1974 by Papahagi and Popovici: when performing the gastrostomy, these authors ligated the middle colonic artery and sometimes the right one to stimulate the development of the left one, anticipating a transverse isoperistaltic colonic replacement [35].

16.2.5.3 Dilatations

About a month after caustic ingestion, once the edema has gone, the diagnosis of stenosis can be assessed by an esophagogram and an endoscopy. Then, according to the severity of the stenosis, a dilatation program can be started. The rate of stricture formation reported in literature varies from 2 to 63 % (!). Isolated short stenosis of the esophagus, i.e., 1–2 cm, can be treated by dilatations with good results. Long ones (more than 3 cm), multiple stenosis (more than two), or those with a tracheoesophageal fistula cannot be solved by dilatations and require an esophageal replacement [36, 37]. However, the decision should not be precipitated.

Of the various methods to dilate, we use three of them: the Tucker-Rehbein bougie on a never-ending loop, the Savary-Gillard bougie on an atraumatic guidewire (M. Savary was our Chief of ENT in Lausanne, Switzerland), or the balloon dilators similar to angioplasty. The Tucker-Rehbein bougie has the advantage of being done without endoscopy or chest X-rays control, with a very low risk of perforation. It requires placing a string from the nose, down into the esophageal lumen, and externalized through the gastrostomy. It can be used both ways, antegrade or retrograde. To dilate, the Tucker-Rehbein bougie is tied to either ends of the string and pushed or pulled using progressively larger dilators. When using balloon dilatators, a radial pressure on the stricture is performed that is thought to be better than a longitudinal direction of dilatations as done with the other methods. But balloon dilatation is not as safe as described, as it can be difficult to control the strength of expansion when the balloon inflates suddenly. For this reason the Savary or the Tucker-Rehbein's techniques are softer and more progressive. Our belief is that all different techniques should be available in a team caring with caustic burns and be adapted to each case and dilatation.

The optimal frequency of dilatation is not well established in the literature, and our practice was to use a symptom-based approach, but an interval of 3 weeks seems appropriate in most cases. We encourage normal eating as soon as possible, as pieces are good self-dilatators, but with a high risk of entrapment. The scarring process of the esophagus is long, and the evolution of a stenosis must be confirmed by repeated esophagograms. An important apparent stenosis related to the inflammatory process can last for months before its disappearance. On the other hand, a dilatation program without significant improvement after a year can be considered as a failure. For these reasons we do not continue a dilatation program more than 1 year. However, some teams persist in dilating patients for years, up to 15 years [18]. Dilatation should be continued as long as a progressive increase in esophageal diameter is noted, along with the recovery of a normal feeding. Even after, dilatation has to be continued from time to time. Without improvement at 12 months, we consider doing an esophageal replacement. Indications for esophageal replacements and their timing vary widely. As a result, children are often subjected to prolonged courses of dilatations prior to esophageal replacement or, conversely, may be exposed to unnecessary surgery [36]. A strong predictor of poor outcome was the delay from ingestion to beginning of dilatations [36, 38].

16.2.5.4 Stents

The early insertion of stents was first proposed by Salzer in 1920 and later advocated by Fell [39, 40]. Early reports fell into disfavor because the strictures soon reformed after removal of the stent [18]. However, Coln as well as Estrera wrote that after stenting, the frequency of recurrences decreased and the strictures were easier to dilate [23, 41]. The use of a self-expanding esophageal stent for malignant strictures is well documented first on animals and now applied in human cases of malignant and recalcitrant benign strictures [42–45]. It has evolved toward early endoscopic esophageal stenting using removable plastic or metallic self-expandable stent [46], or better using biodegradable stents [47, 48]. These techniques are under evaluation and the new materials available are promising. They could play an interesting role to prevent stenosis; however, many migrations or displacements are described [3, 46]. Recently, Okata published the histology of a removed esophagus after self-expandable biodegradable stenting and was able to compare the histology of the esophageal wall under the stent and at distance from its ends. The resected specimens showed thickened scar formation at the level of the stricture, while the degree of esophageal wall damage, both at the proximal and distal ends of the stricture, was slight [48, 49].

The idea is that the stent prevents the adhesion of the facing surfaces of the esophagus, thus minimizing the stenosis, but they cannot restore the defect of the muscular layers. Even if the lumen remains open, a rigid, nonpropulsive segment of the esophagus will be left. Until now we refused to use them as we have been referred 11 children with major complications after esophageal stenting: migrations in the mediastinum and in the left bronchus and posterior erosion of the trachea; one of them 7 years old having had 42 previous procedures.

16.2.5.5 Other Treatments

Many agents have been tried as adjuvant therapies in order to prevent excessive granulation tissue formation.

Mitomycin C is an antibiotic-cytostatic drug derived from *Streptomyces caespitosus* similar to antialkylating agents. It inhibits DNA and protein synthesis by inducing cross-linking, thus fibroblast proliferation. It is used in multidrug regimen in oncology for disseminated carcinoma as well as for transitional cell tumor of genitourinary tract, but it has a poor antimitotic effect. However, its properties have led to its use as an agent for reducing scar formation in ophthalmology for the treatment of pterygium surgery since 1963 and of refractory glaucoma since 1983, and it is commonly used today in those fields even in children. It has been used by ENT surgeons for recurrent laryngeal or tracheal stenosis both in adult and children. We first presented the use of mitomycin C in recurrent esophageal strictures in children in 2001 at the 33rd annual meeting of the Canadian Association of Paediatric Surgeons [50], followed by Afzal who published the first pediatric cases [51]. The use of mitomycin C is still limited in this indication with some cases or very small series reported [52–54]. In our team, first we dilate the stenosis with Tucker-Rehbein or Savary bougies, then the mitomycin C is applied by the ENT surgeons through a rigid esophagoscope. Two ml of mitomycin C Kyowa® solution 2 mg/ml are applied for 2 min using a peanut positioned on the area uncovered with mucosa under visual control. We have the experience of 25 pediatric cases treated with 1 to 4 topical application of mitomycin C after dilatation either for recurrent esophageal stenosis or for stenosis of the upper anastomosis after esophageal replacement with a success rate of 82 %. Other authors came to the same conclusions (El-Asmar 2015, 21 children, 86 % success [55]).

Hyaluronic acid is used in many clinical situations as diverse as neurosurgery and wound healing. A study showed that hyaluronic acid treatment could be effective in treating damage and preventing strictures after experimental caustic esophageal burn on rats [56]. Several other different chemical agents (heparin, vitamin E, caffeic acid phenethyl ester, tamoxifen, 5-fluorouracil) have also been used experimentally, but only a few of these have been added to clinical treatments. Most of these agents impair collagen metabolism and inhibit fibroblastic proliferation either by direct or indirect routes. Physical treatments have also been used such as argon plasma coagulation, but they remain anecdotal [57].

Surgical segmental resections followed by end-to-end anastomosis have a very high rate of failure even after adding enlargement procedures. Unlike the resection of a congenital esophageal stenosis where the anastomosis is performed in normal tissue on both sides of the malformation, the resection of a caustic stenosis is always done in an injured pathologic tissue and leads to recurrence of the stenosis as done under tension in a poorly vascularized tissue.

16.3 Foreign Bodies

16.3.1 Ingested Foreign Bodies (FBs)

The ingestion of foreign bodies (FBs) is a common problem in infants, but fortunately the majority of them will pass through the digestive tract without any adverse effects. The peak incidence of FB ingestion is between 6 months and 3 years, and coins are the most common with an occurrence of >125,000 ingestions per year (2007) and 20 deaths reported in the United States during a 10-year period [58–60]. It has even been described in neonates (esophageal zipper in a 2 months old baby) [61]. Some kids continue to put unbelievable objects in their mouths after infancy. Coins, toys, crayons, and ballpoint pen caps are most often ingested during the childhood [62, 63]. Food impactions are not as frequent as in adults but not unusual [63].

The dangerous FBs are those who remain entrapped in the esophagus at the level of anatomic narrowings: esophageal omentum, aortic arch and left major bronchus, and above the esophagogastric junction. There are no guidelines available to determine which type of object will pass safely. The size depends on the age of the child. A study done by Tander on 62 ingestions in children tries to correlate the sizes of the FB with the ages: up to 5 years of age entrapments occurred for objects between 17 and 23 mm, and after 5, objects from 23 to 26 mm were involved [64].

A FB impacted in the esophagus leads to a pressure lesion and local necrosis resulting in stenosis or perforation. Once in the stomach, it may pass through the pylorus and be eliminated in the stools. But it can be retained anywhere along the bowel at places of anatomical narrowing or angulation such as duodenojejunal flexure or ileocecal valve causing mechanical obstruction. If the object has irregular or sharp edges, it may lodge anywhere in the GI tract. If the objects are elongated, they can become trapped in the appendix or ileocecal valve.

16.3.2 Management of FBs

After ingestion, children can be asymptomatic at the time of presentation. If present, common symptoms include drooling, gagging, dysphagia, odynophagia, decreased appetite, food refusal, neck pain, chest pain, abdominal pain, cough, stridor, wheezing, and respiratory distress. Esophageal FBs often present with respiratory complaints. In most patients physical examination is normal [59, 63].

The priority is to assess the presence of a FB.

Chest radiographs including the neck, and a supine abdominal one, should be obtained to rule out ingestion. Two orthogonal projections are mandatory, because some FBs, especially those of discoid shape, could be shown only in one view [59, 62]. Limited chest radiograph not including the upper thoracic inlet may miss a higher-up foreign body. Radiological visualization depends on radiopacity. Radiograph detects as much as 80 % of all FBs [62]. Objects of metal, except aluminum, most animal bones, and glass are opaque on radiographs. Objects composed of plastic and most fish bones are radiolucent structures, and their diagnosis may be challenging.

Careful attention should be placed on the edges of a presumed coin to exclude the double halo typical of a button battery, which may easily be mistaken for a coin. Regarding FBs, such as fish bones, chicken bones, and toothpicks, an X-ray has a sensitivity that ranges from 23 to 55 % for the first two and 9 % for the latter. In case of toothpicks, even other imaging studies have a low sensitivity, 15 % for MDCT and 29 % for ultrasound (US). But they are the methods of choice in the diagnosis of a FB that migrated from the GI tract and retained in the soft tissues [62, 65].

An expert panel from the North American Society for Pediatric Gastroenterology Hepatology and Nutrition (NASPGHAN) was convened and produced the following guidelines for practical clinical approaches to the pediatric patient with a variety of FB ingestions [63].

Symptomatic FBs impacted in the esophagus have to be removed urgently. Asymptomatic FBs in the esophagus should be removed within 24 h to reduce the risk of significant esophageal injury or erosion into neighboring structures.

Once in the stomach, FBs can generally be managed expectantly in asymptomatic patients. Parents should be instructed to monitor the stools for passage of the FBs. X-rays should be obtained every 1–2 weeks until clearance can be documented. If the FB is still retained in the stomach after 2–4 weeks of observation, elective endoscopic removal may be considered. Children with underlying anatomic or surgical changes, such as previous pyloromyotomy, have an increased risk for retained FBs [63, 66, 67]. Just before removal of a retained gastric FB, X-rays should be repeated to make sure that the FB has not passed just before.

The gold standard is endoscopic removal under general anesthesia. Most ingested FBs are best treated with flexible endoscopes, which allow retrograde exploration of the gastric fundus. However, rigid esophagoscopy may be helpful for proximal foreign bodies impacted at the level of the upper esophageal sphincter or hypopharyngeal region. Various retrieval devices are used, including rat-tooth and alligator forceps, polypectomy snares, polyp graspers, Dormier baskets, retrieval nets, magnetic probes, etc. Before endoscopy, practicing grasping test on an object similar to the ingested one may help to determine the most appropriate available retrieval device and in what fashion the object has to be seized.

However, nonendoscopic methods have been successfully used. The very high esophageal FBs can be retrieved with forceps under direct laryngoscopy. We have a good experience with the use of a Foley catheter under fluoroscopic guidance to “sweep” out coins lodged in the esophagus, while the patient is maintained in the prone Trendelenburg position [68–71]. It can be done without anesthesia in selected patients. The positioning of the Foley catheter can be helped with some contrast in the balloon. Esophageal bougienage is another technique that uses a blunt Hurst dilator to push down an esophageal FB into the patient’s stomach [72–74]. It is safe and cost-effective compared with endoscopic removal. The disadvantage is that direct inspection of the esophagus for underlying pathology is not done as well as inability to retrieve the FB, which “falls” in the stomach.

16.3.3 Particular Cases

16.3.3.1 Button Batteries

Button batteries represent a special category of pediatric ingested foreign body because of their potential for severe morbidity and mortality particularly if impacted in the esophagus [75–81]. The number has increased by 80 % between 1998 and 2008 due to their large use in toys and electronic devices [81–83]. Ingested button batteries have been reported to cause esophageal stricture and perforation [75, 76, 79], vocal cord paralysis [80], tracheoesophageal fistulas, and even deaths [63, 78, 81].

Button battery cells generally contain a heavy metal like mercury, manganese, silver, and lithium and a strong hydroxide of sodium or potassium. The quality of the sealing between anode and cathode is highly variable. Some of them can resist hours in gastric acid. Reversely, others are quickly dissolved with a leak of the potentially toxic or corrosive content leading to intoxication or mucosal damage by ulceration, which may further lead on to perforation and secondary stricture formation [80]. The damage can also be due to electrical discharge leading to low-voltage burns, and pressure necrosis especially in the esophagus [81]. These very severe complications can occur within a few hours as experienced on animals and be proven in toddlers (transmural necrosis of the esophagus within 3 h) [81, 84].

Once in the stomach, batteries rarely cause any harm to the gastric wall, and its spontaneous passage through the pylorus is expected. Subsequently, conservative management is a generally accepted alternative. However, gastric perforation has already been described 2 days after ingestion [85]. Even after conservative management, these patients have to be followed up as distal bowel disturbances have been described such as Meckel's diverticulum perforation or impaction in the ileocecal valve [86].

Consequently, overall consensus is that batteries lodged in the esophagus should be removed immediately. Opinions differ on the management of those located in the stomach in children. We follow the protocol suggested by Eisen [87], waiting to see whether the battery will spontaneously pass through the pylorus within 24 h, as long as the patient manifests no sign of injury to the stomach. When batteries are retained longer in the stomach and/or the patient becomes symptomatic, we attempt endoscopic removal.

16.3.3.2 Magnets

Pediatric magnet ingestions have received increasing attention over the past 10 years. Although most of those small smooth ingested FBs will pass spontaneously through the gastrointestinal tract, multiple magnets are a danger of being able to attract each other through different loops of bowel, arresting their movement, and causing transmural pressure necrosis. This can lead to bowel perforation, fistula formation, volvulus, obstruction, intra-abdominal sepsis, and death [88–90].

The US Centers for Disease Control and Prevention has reported one death and 20 surgeries for bowel perforations related to magnet ingestions between 2002 and 2006 [91]. In 2011 there were 30 publications on such cases with more than 100 bowel perforations in children. The US National Electronic Injury Surveillance System showed that the rate of magnet-related injury had increased dramatically over the period from 2002 to 2011 [90, 92], as did the Consumers' Federation of Australia [92], the Hospital for Sick Children in Toronto, Canada [88], and the Surgical Section of the American Academy of Pediatrics [93]. These changes are related to the documented technological shift from ferrite magnets to neodymium-iron-boron magnets that are approximately 10–20 times more powerful. They are often sold as sets of multiple spheres approximately 5 mm in diameter or as parts of toy construction kits. In 2013, Health Canada issued a recall of neodymium-iron-boron magnet sets marketed as desk toys [94]. The United States Consumer Product Safety Commission established a mandatory standard to prevent magnets detaching from toys. This standard also prohibits magnets and loose magnet components in toys for children under age 14 years [95]. Unfortunately, hundreds of thousands of magnet sets have already been sold, and despite these regulations, vendors via the Internet continue to sell these products. The North American Society for Pediatric Gastroenterology, Hepatology, and Nutrition released survey results in 2012 demonstrating that despite increasing warning labels, these labels were ineffective at preventing ingestion [96].

The median age at ingestion is between 2 and 5 years of age. But parents and caretakers should counsel teenagers and young adults of the hazards of fake body piercings that use small magnet backs. Consumer Product Safety Commission reported instances of teenagers swallowing magnets unintentionally when placed on the opposite sides of tongue jewelry to mimic body piercings [97].

Most patients are asymptomatic. A plain abdominal radiograph is recommended at admission if magnet ingestion is suspected as they are radiopaque FBs. However, X-rays and computed tomography lack the sensitivity to determine the number of magnetic objects, thus making management decision difficult. Some authors consider that any ingestion should be treated as though multiple magnets were ingested [98].

If case of ingestion of an attested single magnet and if its size is small enough to pass spontaneously, the child could be managed by observation only. If multiple magnets are ingested or if their actual number cannot be determined as it occurs in most cases, intervention is required. If the magnetic FB remains in the esophagus or in the stomach, it should be removed by endoscopy or using a magnetic probe. Once multiple magnets have passed the pylorus and remain in the duodenum, an attempt of endoscopic removal could be done. In case of failure to remove multiple magnets endoscopically or if they are already in the jejunum or below, surgical intervention is required to avoid further complications. This can be done by laparoscopy with umbilical extraction or by laparotomy [93, 98–100].

16.3.3.3 Sharp and/or Long Objects

Ingestion of large and/or long objects is also an issue of special concern. The reported incidence of FBs causing perforation of the GI tract is less than 1 %, with the objects being elongated or sharp in most of the cases, such as toothpicks, pins, fish, or chicken bones [59]. Furthermore, long, narrow, and pointed ingested FBs >5 cm in length (3 cm in young children) are unlikely to clear the duodenal sweep and, if they do, are equally unlikely to pass through the ileocecal valve [59, 63]. Subsequently, large or long objects, even though they are blunt, should be removed from the stomach. Given the low risk of endoscopy and albeit rare but significant risk of severe morbidity and mortality from swallowed sharp objects, removal of all of them within the reach of the endoscope is recommended [63].

References

1. Peden M, Oyegbite K, Ozanne-Smith J et al (2008) World report on child injury prevention. World Health Organization/UNICEF, Geneva
2. Millar AJ, Cox SG (2015) Caustic injury of the oesophagus. Pediatr Surg Int 31:111–121
3. Rossi A (2015) Acute caustic ingestion: state of the art and new trends. J Gastroenterol Hepatol Res 4(3):1501–1506
4. Riffat F, Cheng A (2009) Pediatric caustic ingestion: 50 consecutive cases and a review of the literature. Dis Esophagus 22:89–94
5. Watson W et al (2005) Annual report of the American Association of Poison Control Centers Toxic Exposure Surveillance System. Am J Emerg Med 23:589–666
6. Janousek P, Kabelka Z, Rygl M et al (2006) Corrosive injury of the oesophagus in children. Int J Pediatr Otorhinolaryngol 70(6):1103–1107
7. Arevalo-Silva C, Eliashar R, Wohlgelernter J et al (2006) Ingestion of caustic substances: a 15-year experience. Laryngoscope 116:1422–1426
8. Bertinelli A, Hamill J, Mahadevan M et al (2006) Serious injuries from dishwasher powder ingestions in small children. J Paediatr Child Health 42:129–133
9. Scientific Committee on Consumer Safety of the EU (2011) Opinion on the potential health risks posed by chemical consumer products resembling food and/or having child-appealing properties. Characteristics of CPRF and CAP 8:18–22. doi:10.2772/31904
10. Valdez AL, Casavant MJ, Spiller HA (2014) Pediatric exposure to laundry detergent pods. Pediatrics 134:1127–1135
11. Bramuzzo M, Amaddeo A, Facchina G et al (2013) Liquid detergent capsule ingestion: a new pediatric epidemic? Pediatr Emerg Care 29(3):410–411
12. Scharman EJ (2012) Liquid “laundry pods”: a missed global toxicosurveillance opportunity. Clin Toxicol (Phila) 50(8):725–726
13. Durham G (1998) Code of practice for child-resistant packaging of toxic substances. Ministry of Health, Wellington. http://www.moh.govt.nz. ISBN 0-478-22836-8 (Internet) Accessed 20 Dec 2015
14. Chien C et al (2003) Unintentional ingestion of over the counter medications in children less than 5 years old. J Paediatr Child Health 39:264–269
15. Berning CK, Griffith JF, Wild JE (1982) Research on the effectiveness of denatonium benzoate as a deterrent to liquid detergent ingestion by children. Fundam Appl Toxicol 2:44–48
16. Sibert JR, Frude N (1991) Bittering agents in the prevention of accidental poisoning: children’s reactions to denatonium benzoate (Bitrex). Arch Emerg Med 8:1–7
17. Hansen SR, Janssen C, Beasley VR (1993) Denatonium benzoate as a deterrent to ingestion of toxic substances: toxicity and efficacy. Vet Hum Toxicol 35(3):234–236
18. de Jong AL, Macdonald R, Ein S et al (2001) Corrosive esophagitis in children: a 30-year review. Int J Pediatr Otorhinolaryngol 57:203–211
19. Baskin D, Urganci N, Abbasoglu L et al (2004) A standardised protocol for the acute management of corrosive ingestion in children. Pediatr Surg Int 20(11–12):824–826
20. Gaudreault P, Parent M, McGuigan MA et al (1983) Predictability of esophageal injury from signs and

symptoms: a study of caustic ingestion in 378 children. Pediatrics 71:767–770
21. Temiz A, Oguzkurt P, Ezer SS et al (2012) Predictability of outcome of caustic ingestion by esophagogastroduodenoscopy in children. World J Gastroenterol 18(10):1098–1103
22. Crain EF, Gershel JC, Mezay AP (1984) Caustic ingestion. Symptoms as predictors of esophageal injury. Am J Dis Child 138(9):863–865
23. Estrera A, Taylor W, Mills LJ et al (1986) Corrosive burns of the esophagus and stomach: a recommendation for an aggressive surgical approach. Ann Thorac Surg 41:276–283
24. Zargar SA, Kochhar R, Mehta S et al (1991) The role of fiberoptic endoscopy in the management of corrosive ingestion and modified endoscopic classification of burns. Gastrointest Endosc 37:165–169
25. Arcidiacono R, Rossi A, Grosso C et al (1992) Proposition d'une nouvelle classification endoscopique des lesions par ingestion de caustiques. Acta Endosc 22(4):413–418
26. Betalli P, Falchetti D, Giuliani S et al (2008) Caustic ingestion in children: is endoscopy always indicated? The results of an Italian multicenter observational study. Gastrointest Endosc 68(3):434–439
27. Millar AJ, Numanoglu A, Mann M et al (2001) Detection of caustic oesophageal injury with technetium 99 m-labelled sucralfate. J Pediatr Surg 36(2):262–265
28. Mittal BR, Bhoil A, Kashyap R et al (2013) (99m) Tc-pertechnetate scintigraphy and endoscopy in assessment of caustic-induced gastric mucosal injury. Clin Nucl Med 38(3):e146–e147
29. Angel C, Wrenn E, Lobe T (1991) Brain abscess—an unusual complication of multiple esophageal dilatations. Pediatr Surg Int 6(1):42–43
30. Fulton JA, Hoffman RS (2007) Steroids in second degree caustic burns of the esophagus: a systematic pooled analysis of fifty years of human data: 1956–2006. Clin Toxicol (Phila) 45(4):402–408
31. Cadranel S, Scaillon M, Goyens P et al (1993) Treatment of esophageal caustic injuries— experience with high-dose dexamethasone. Pediatr Surg Int 8(2):97–102
32. Boukthir S, Fetni I, Mazigh Mrad S et al (2004) High doses of steroids in the management of caustic esophageal burns in children. Arch Pediatr 11:13–17
33. Usta M, Erkan T, Cokugras FC et al (2014) High doses of methylprednisolone in the management of caustic esophageal burns. Pediatrics 133(6):E1518–E1524
34. Vasseur Maurer S, de Buys Roessingh A, Reinberg O (2015) Laparoscopic technique to perform a true Stamm gastrostomy in children. J Pediatr Surg 50(10):1797–1800
35. Papahagi E, Popovici Z (1974) Procédé pour améliorer l'irrigation de la plastie dans l'oesophagoplastie par le côlon transverse et le côlon ascendant isopéristaltique. J Chir (Paris) 108:229–240
36. Panieri E, Rode H, Millar AJW et al (1998) Oesophageal replacement in the management of corrosive strictures: when is surgery indicated? Pediatr Surg Int 13:336–340
37. Reinberg O (2014) Les oesophagoplasties chez l'enfant. E-Mem Acad Natl Chir 13(2):011–022
38. Arul GS, Parikh D (2008) Oesophageal replacement in children. Ann R Coll Surg Engl 90(1):7–12
39. Salzer H (1920) Early treatment of corrosive esophagitis. Wein Klin Wochensch 33:307
40. Fell SC, Denize A, Becker MH et al (1966) The effect of intraluminal splinting in the prevention of caustic stricture of the esophagus. J Thorac Cardiovasc Surg 52(5):675–681
41. Coln D, Chang J (1986) Experience with esophageal stenting for caustic burns in children. J Pediatr Surg 21(7):588–591
42. Grundy A (1994) The Streckes esophageal stent in the management of esophageal strictures: technique of insertion and early clinical experience. Clin Radiol 49:421–424
43. Song H, Choi K, Kwon H et al (1992) Esophageal strictures: treatment with a new design of modified Gianturco stent. Radiology 184(3):729–734
44. Lange B, Kubiak R, Wessel LM et al (2015) Use of fully covered self-expandable metal stents for benign esophageal disorders in children. J Laparoendosc Adv Surg Tech A 25(4):335–341
45. Bethge N, Sommer A, Vakil N (1995) Treatment of esophageal fistulas with a new polyurethane covered, self-expanding mesh stent: a prospective study. Am J Gastroenterol 90(12):2143–2146
46. Zhang J, Ren L, Huo J et al (2013) The use of retrievable fully covered self-expanding metal stent in refractory postoperative restenosis of benign esophageal stricture in children. J Pediatr Surg 48(11):2235–2240
47. Bychkova OV, Lazyuk I (2009) Bio-degradable stents? A new approach to the treatment of caustic stenoses in children. Folia Gastroenterol Hepatol 7(1):1–6
48. Karakan T, Utku OG, Dorukoz O et al (2013) Biodegradable stents for caustic esophageal strictures: a new therapeutic approach. Dis Esophagus 26(3):319–322
49. Okata Y, Hisamatsu C, Bitoh Y et al (2014) Efficacy and histopathological esophageal wall damage of biodegradable esophageal stents for treatment of severe refractory esophageal anastomotic stricture in a child with long gap esophageal atresia. Clin J Gastroenterol 7(6):496–501
50. Reinberg O, Yazbeck S (2001) Use of mitomycin C in the conservative treatment of short esophageal stenosis. In: Paper presented at the 33rd annual meeting of the Canadian Association of Paediatric Surgeons, Winnipeg, 13–16 Sept 2001
51. Afzal NA, Albert D, Thomas AL et al (2002) A child with oesophageal strictures. Lancet 359(9311):1032

52. Olutoye OO, Shulman RJ, Cotton RT (2006) Mitomycin C in the management of pediatric caustic esophageal strictures: a case report. J Pediatr Surg 41:e1–e3
53. Uhlen S, Fayoux P, Vachin F et al (2006) Mitomycin C: an alternative conservative treatment for refractory esophageal stricture in children? Endoscopy 38:404–407
54. Heran MK, Baird R, Blair GK et al (2008) Topical mitomycin-C for recalcitrant esophageal strictures: a novel endoscopic/fluoroscopic technique for safe endoluminal delivery. J Pediatr Surg 43(5):815–818
55. El-Asmar KM, Hassan MA, Abdelkader HM et al (2015) Topical mitomycin C can effectively alleviate dysphagia in children with long-segment caustic esophageal strictures. Dis Esophagus 28(5):422–427
56. Cevik M, Demir T, Karadag CA et al (2013) Preliminary study of efficacy of hyaluronic acid on caustic esophageal burns in an experimental rat model. J Pediatr Surg 48(4):716–723
57. Boxberger F, Maiss J, Amann K et al (2008) Severe high grade stenosing hyperkeratosis of the esophagus after ingestion of alkali: successful treatment by argon plasma coagulation. Endoscopy 40(Suppl 2):E260–E261
58. Bronstein AC, Spyker DA, Cantilena LR Jr et al (2008) 2007 Annual Report of the American Association of Poison Control Centers' National Poison Data System (NPDS): 25th Annual Report. Clin Toxicol (Phila) 46:927–1057
59. A-Kader HH (2010) Foreign body ingestion: children like to put objects in their mouth. World J Pediatr 6(4):301–310
60. Chen X, Milkovich S, Stool D et al (2006) Pediatric coin ingestion and aspiration. Int J Pediatr Otorhinolaryngol 70:325–329
61. Hernot S, Yadav SP, Kathuria B et al (2015) An uncommon oesophageal foreign body in a neonate. Br Med J Case Repe-pub Jan 30;2015. pii: bcr2014208719. doi: 10.1136/bcr-2014-208719.
62. Grassi R, Faggian A, Somma F et al (2015) Application of imaging guidelines in patients with foreign body ingestion or inhalation: literature review. Semin Ultrasound CT MR 36(1):48–56
63. Kramer RE, Lerner DG, Lin T et al (2015) Management of ingested foreign bodies in children: a clinical report of the NASPGHAN Endoscopy Committee. J Pediatr Gastroenterol Nutr 60(4):562–574
64. Tander B, Yazici M, Rizalar R et al (2009) Coin ingestion in children: which size is more risky? J Laparoendosc Adv Surg Tech A 19(2):241–243
65. Webb W (1995) Management of foreign bodies of the upper gastrointestinal tract: update. Gastrointest Endosc 41(1):39–51
66. Stringer MD, Kiely EM, Drake DP (1991) Gastric retention of swallowed coins after pyloromyotomy. Br J Clin Pract 45:66–67
67. Fleisher AG, Holgersen LO, Stanley-Brown EG et al (1986) Prolonged gastric retention of a swallowed coin following pyloromyotomy. J Pediatr Gastroenterol Nutr 5:811–813
68. Kelley JL, Leech MH, Carr MG (1993) A safe and cost-effective protocol for the management of esophageal coins in children. J Pediatr Surg 28(7):898–900
69. Harned RK, Strain JD, Hay TC et al (1997) Esophageal foreign bodies: safety and efficacy of Foley catheter extraction of coins. Am J Roentgenol 168:443–446
70. Gasior AC, Knott EM, Sharp SW et al (2013) Predictive factors for successful balloon catheter extraction of esophageal foreign bodies. Pediatr Surg Int 29(8):791–794
71. Heinzerling NP, Christensen MA, Swedler R (2015) Safe and effective management of esophageal coins in children with bougienage. Surgery 158(4):1065–1070
72. Dahshan AH, Kevin Donovan G (2007) Bougienage versus endoscopy for esophageal coin removal in children. J Clin Gastroenterol 41:454–456
73. Arms JL, Mackenberg-Mohn MD, Bowen MV et al (2008) Safety and efficacy of a protocol using bougienage or endoscopy for the management of coins acutely lodged in the esophagus: a large case series. Ann Emerg Med 51:367–372
74. Allie EH, Blackshaw AM, Losek JD et al (2014) Clinical effectiveness of bougienage for esophageal coins in a pediatric ED. Am J Emerg Med 32(10):1263–1269
75. Litovitz T, Schmitz BF (1992) Ingestion of cylindrical and button batteries: an analysis of 2382 cases. Pediatrics 89:747–757
76. Samad L, Ali M, Ramzi H (1999) Button battery ingestion: hazards of esophageal impaction. J Pediatr Surg 34:1527–1531
77. Yardeni D, Yardeni H, Coran AG et al (2004) Severe esophageal damage due to button battery ingestion: can it be prevented? Pediatr Surg Int 20:496–501
78. Imamoğlu M, Cay A, Koşucu P et al (2004) Acquired tracheo-esophageal fistulas caused by button battery lodged in the esophagus. Pediatr Surg Int 20:292–294
79. Raboei EH, Syed SS, Maghrabi M et al (2009) Management of button battery stricture in 22-day-old neonate. Eur J Pediatr Surg 19:130–131
80. Hamilton JM, Schraff SA, Notrica DM (2009) Severe injuries from coin cell battery ingestions: 2 case reports. J Pediatr Surg 44:644–647
81. Kimball SJ, Park AH, Rollins MD et al (2010) A review of esophageal disc battery ingestions and a protocol for management. Arch Otolaryngol Head Neck Surg 136(9):866–871
82. American Association of Poison Control Centers (2015) American Association of Poison Control Centers Advises Public on Poison Hazards this Holiday Season Reports. http://www.aapcc.org/press/52/. 10 Dec 2015. Accessed 20 Dec 2015
83. Litovitz TL, Klein-Schwartz W, White S et al (2001) 2000 annual report of the American Association of

Poison Control Centers Toxic Exposure Surveillance System. Am J Emerg Med 19:337–395
84. Soccorso G, Grossman O, Martinelli M et al (2012) A 20 mm lithium button battery causing an oesophageal perforation in a toddler: lessons in diagnosis and treatment. Arch Dis Child 97(8):746–747
85. Honda S, Shinkai M, Yoshiko Usui Y et al (2010) Severe gastric damage caused by button battery ingestion in a 3-month-old infant. J Pediatr Surg 45:E23–E26
86. Karaman A, Karaman I, Erdoğan D et al (2007) Perforation of Meckel's diverticulum by a button battery: report of a case. Surg Today 37:1115–1116
87. Eisen GM, Baron TH, Dominitz JA et al (2002) Guideline for the management of ingested foreign bodies. Gastrointest Endosc 55:802–806
88. Strickland M, Rosenfield D, Fecteau A (2014) Magnetic foreign body injuries: a large pediatric hospital experience. J Pediatr 165(2):332–335
89. Naji H, Isacson D, Svensson J, Wester T (2012) Bowel injuries caused by ingestion of multiple magnets in children: a growing hazard. Pediatr Surg Int 28(4):367–374
90. Bowel injuries caused by ingestion of multiple magnets in children: a growing hazard (2006) Gastrointestinal injuries from magnet ingestion in children – United States, 2003–2006. Morb Mortal Wkly Rep 55 (48):1296–300
91. Agbo C, Lee L, Chian V et al (2013) Magnet-related injury rates in children. J Pediatr Gastroenterol Nutr 57:14–17
92. Consumers' Federation of Australia. ACT: ban on small high powered magnets. 30 Aug 2012. Available at: http://consumersfederation.org.au/act-ban-on-small-high-powered-magnets/. Accessed 20 Dec 2015
93. Waters AM, Teitelbaum DH, Thorne V et al (2015) Surgical management and morbidity of pediatric magnet ingestions. J Surg Res 199:137–140
94. Health Canada. Health Canada is taking action to have small, powerful magnet sets removed from the marketplace. Health Canada Advisory. 22 May 2013;RA-31619. Available at: http://www.healthycanadians.gc.ca/recall-alert-rappel-avis/hc-sc/2013/31619a-eng.php. Accessed 20 Dec 2015
95. Commission, U. S. C. P. S. Magnet Information Center. Available from: http://www.cpsc.gov/Safety-Education/Safety-Education-Centers/Magnets. Accessed 20 Dec 2015
96. North American Society for Pediatric Gastroenterology, Hepatology and Nutrition. Warning labels ineffective at preventing high-powered magnet ingestions. Available from: http://www.naspghan.org/files/documents/pdfs/advocacy/2012/Final%20NOLA%20Press%20Release.pdf. Accessed 20 Dec 2015
97. Commission, U. C. P. S. CPSC Warns High-Powered Magnets and Children Make A deadly mix. Available from: http://www.cpsc.gov/en/Newsroom/News-Releases/2012/CPSCWarns-High-Powered-Magnets-and-Children-Make-a-Deadly-Mix/. Accessed 20 Dec 2015
98. Butterworth J, Feltis B (2007) Toy magnet ingestion in children: revising the algorithm. J Pediatr Surg 42(12):e3–e5
99. Michaud L, Bellaïche M, Olives JP; Groupe francophone d'hépatologie, gastroentérologie et nutrition pédiatriques (GFHGNP) (2009) Ingestion of foreign bodies in children. Recommendations of the French-Speaking Group of Pediatric Hepatology, Gastroenterology and Nutrition. Arch Pediatr 16 (1):54–61
100. Vijaysadan V, Perez M, Kuo D (2006) Revisiting swallowed troubles: intestinal complications caused by two magnets: a case report, review and proposed revision to the algorithm for the management of foreign body ingestion. J Am Board Fam Med 19(5):511–516

17 Disorders of Intestinal Rotation and Fixation

Anastasia Mentessidou and Amulya K. Saxena

17.1 Embryology

17.1.1 Normal Intestinal Rotation

In the fourth week of fetal life, the primitive intestine is a relatively straight tube with a slight anterior bulge in the central portion. The superior mesenteric artery arising from the posterior wall enters the center of this anterior bulge. During the next 6 weeks, the intestine grows faster than the coelomic cavity, and as a result it is forced to herniate within the umbilical cord (Fig. 17.1a). The intestine enters the umbilical cord at a point corresponding to the duodenojejunal junction and leaves it at a point corresponding to the primary colonic flexure. The cranial part of the herniation, lying cranial to the superior mesenteric artery, corresponds to the jejunum and ileum as distal as the omphalomesenteric duct, while the caudal part to the terminal ileum and colon. After the tenth week, the coelomic cavity has grown sufficiently and the intestine returns in the abdomen.

Normal intestinal rotation includes a 270° anticlockwise rotation of both the duodenojejunal loop and the cecocolic loop around the axis of the superior mesenteric artery. As a result, the duodenojejunal loop passes from a position above the superior mesenteric artery to a position below and finally to the left side of the artery, while the cecocolic loop passes from a position below the superior mesenteric artery to a position above and finally to the right of the artery (Fig. 17.1a–c).

The process of intestinal rotation has been traditionally divided in three stages. Stage I includes the initial 90° anticlockwise rotation, which will result in positioning of the duodenojejunal loop to the right of the superior mesenteric artery and the positioning of the cecocolic loop to the left of the artery (Fig. 17.1b). This stage occurs during the extracelomic phase of intestinal development. Stage II corresponds to the next 180° anticlockwise rotation, which takes place while the intestine returns into the abdomen and is completed by the end of the 12th week. These further 180° will complete the total 270° rotation, which will finally position the duodenum below the superior mesenteric artery and the duodenojejunal junction to the left of the superior mesenteric artery, as well as the colon above the superior mesenteric artery and the cecocolic loop to the right of the artery (Fig. 17.1c). Stage III constitutes the final 90° anticlockwise rotation of the cecocolic loop, which is usually completed until birth and results in the descent of the cecum from the right hypochondrium below the liver to its final position in the right iliac fossa. Stage III is attributed to dif-

A. Mentessidou, MD • A.K. Saxena, MD, PhD, DSc(hon), FRCS(Glasg) (✉)
Department of Pediatric Surgery, Chelsea Children's Hospital, Chelsea and Westminster Hospital NHS Fdn Trust, Imperial College London, London, UK
e-mail: amulya.saxena@nhs.net

M. Lima (ed.), *Pediatric Digestive Surgery*, DOI 10.1007/978-3-319-40525-4_17

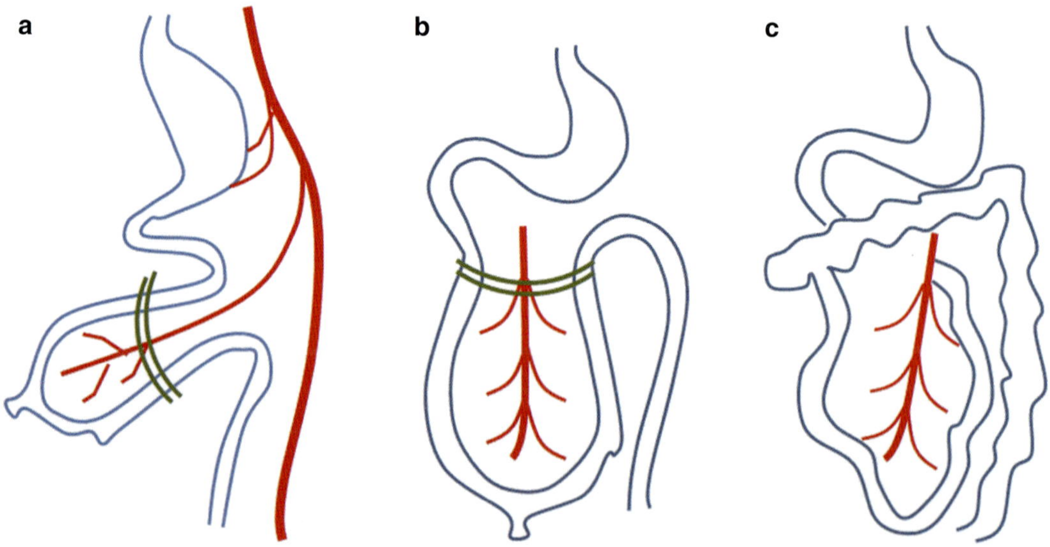

Fig. 17.1 Normal rotation of fetal intestine. (**a**) Orientation of the bowel in the umbilical cord before rotation starts. (**b**) Initial 90° anticlockwise rotation (stage I). (**c**) Further 180° anticlockwise rotation (stage II), which brings the duodenojejunal loop below and to the left of the superior mesenteric artery and cecocolic loop above and to the right of the superior mesenteric artery (From Lister J (1990) Malrotation and volvulus of the intestine. In: Lister J, Irving IM (eds) Neonatal surgery, 3rd edn. Butterworth & Co, London)

ferential growth. It must be highlighted that the staging of intestinal rotation serves only for understanding purposes, while the intestinal rotation is, in reality, a continuous process and should be conceived as such.

After normal rotation and fixation will be completed, the normal mesenteric attachment will extend from the ligament of Treitz, at the level of the pylorus, to the cecum. The second and third portion of the duodenum, as well as the ascending and the descending colon, will be fixed retroperitoneally [1–5].

17.1.2 Disorders of Intestinal Rotation and Fixation

17.1.2.1 Complete Non-rotation

The term refers to the absence of any intestinal rotation. It is characterized by a small and large bowel coursing vertically and a common longitudinal mesentery.

17.1.2.2 Incomplete Rotation

The term refers to the absence of stage II and III rotation, i.e., after the initial 90° anticlockwise rotation of the duodenojejunal and cecocolic loop around the superior mesenteric artery axis, no further rotation has occurred. As a result, the duodenum and small bowel are located on the right side of the artery and the cecum and colon on the left. Congenital adhesive bands between the bowel loops and the parietal peritoneum are often encountered.

17.1.2.3 Malrotation

The term refers to abnormalities occurring during stage II rotation and might include several different types based on the degree of rotation accomplished. In the commonest type, the intestinal rotation has stopped at some point just before the 180°, and, thus, the duodenojejunal loop has failed to cross the midline and lies to the right of the superior mesenteric artery (Fig. 17.2). Similarly, the cecocolic loop has rotated for almost 180° but no further and lies anterior to the duodenum and to the superior mesenteric artery or slightly to the left. Congenital adhesive bands, traditionally known as Ladd's bands, course from the cecum to the parietal peritoneum usually obstructing the second part of the duodenum.

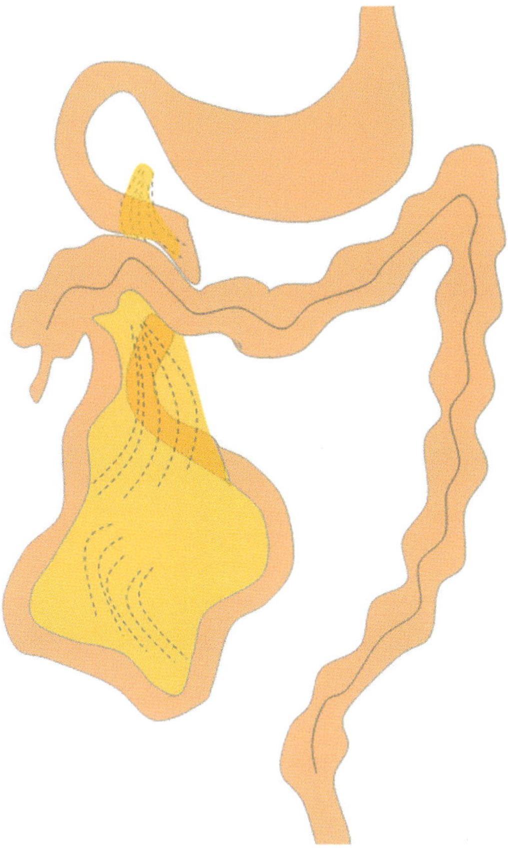

Fig. 17.2 Commonest type of malrotation. Anticlockwise rotation of duodenojejunal and cecocolic loops has stopped at 180° (From Lister J (1990) Malrotation and volvulus of the intestine. In: Lister J, Irving IM (eds) Neonatal surgery, 3rd edn. Butterworth & Co, London)

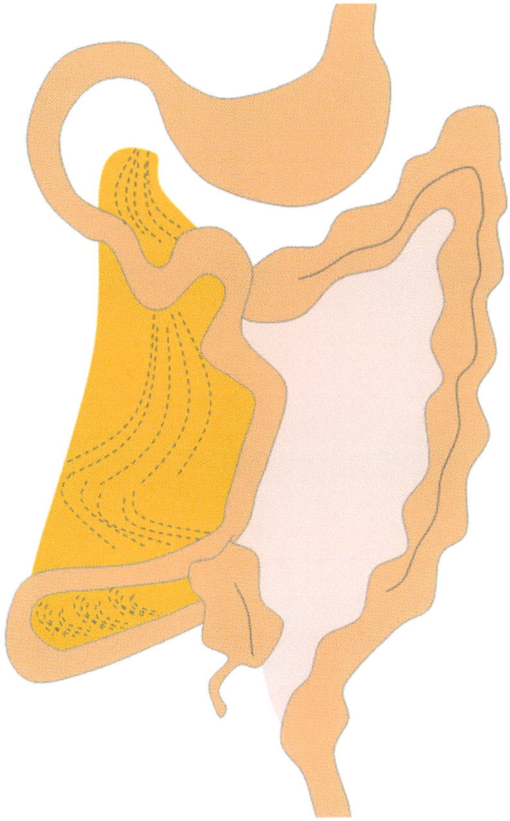

Fig. 17.3 Reverse rotation following the initial anticlockwise 90° rotation of stage I. The 90° clockwise intestinal rotation (From Lister J (1990) Malrotation and volvulus of the intestine. In: Lister J, Irving IM (eds) Neonatal surgery, 3rd edn. Butterworth & Co, London)

17.1.2.4 Reverse Rotation

It refers to less common types of malrotation, in which the first 90° anticlockwise rotation (stage I) is followed by further 90–180° in the clockwise direction. As a result, the duodenum lies anterior to the superior mesenteric artery. The position of the cecum varies, based on the degree of its rotation. It might descend in the lower abdomen behind the small bowel mesentery, after a 90° clockwise rotation (Fig. 17.3), or it might cross the midline behind the superior mesenteric vessels and reach the right iliac fossa—after a 180° clockwise rotation (Fig. 17.4).

17.1.2.5 Atypical Malrotation or Malrotation Variant

The intestinal rotation has been interrupted at some point between 180 and 270°. As a result, the ligament of Treitz is to the left of the midline but lower than the level of the pylorus.

In most cases of abnormal intestinal rotation and fixation, the small intestine has a narrow mesenteric base and, therefore, is prone to twist around the mesenteric vessels on a clockwise direction causing midgut volvulus. Other causes of intestinal obstruction in malrotation are the kinks and compression of the lumen caused by the congenital bands.

The lack of normal fixation of the right or left colon might result in the formation of potential spaces within the mesocolon, like hernial sacs, in which the small intestine might be entrapped causing right or left mesocolic hernias (Fig. 17.5) [6]. These internal hernias might cause recurrent partial obstruction of the small bowel or might eventually result in complete obstruction and strangulation [7–16].

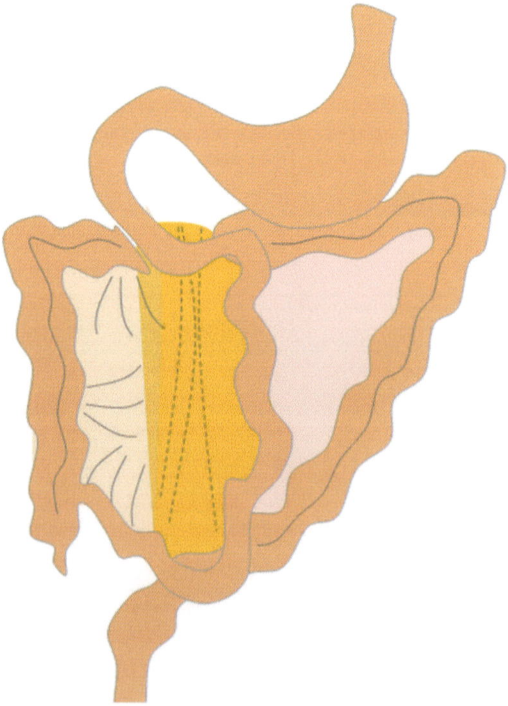

Fig. 17.4 Reverse rotation following the initial anticlockwise 90° rotation of stage I. Complete clockwise intestinal rotation through 180° (From Lister J (1990) Malrotation and volvulus of the intestine. In: Lister J, Irving IM (eds) Neonatal surgery, 3rd edn. Butterworth & Co, London)

17.2 Epidemiology and Associated Malformations

Intestinal malrotation is seen in up to 1:6000 live births. Most patients with volvulus (52–64 %) present in the first month of life and the majority of them (70 %) within the first week of life. Sporadic cases occur throughout life. Associated anomalies are found in 30–60 % of cases of malrotation. These include diaphragmatic hernias, exomphalos and gastroschisis, complete duodenal atresia or duodenal webs, jejunal atresia, Hirschsprung's disease, anorectal malformations, and mesenteric cysts. Rotation and fixation abnormalities are also known to coexist with heterotaxy, with 70 % of these patients having malrotation [9, 10, 17, 18].

17.3 Clinical Manifestations

The primary symptom is the sudden onset of forceful vomiting, usually bilious and less commonly yellowish, in a previously healthy infant. Vomiting might be due to duodenal obstruction caused by Ladd's bands, in the absence of volvulus, or might be the result of an acute obstruction caused by midgut volvulus. Crampy abdominal pain is also common. The obstruction might not be complete, so meconium and stool may be passing. Blood-stained emesis and passage of blood per rectum suggest bowel strangulation and are ominous signs.

Abdominal distention may or may not be present. Sometimes, the upper abdomen might appear distended and the lower abdomen scaphoid. Generalized distention is usually indicative of gangrenous volvulus and is a late sign. Tenderness on palpation is not a constant finding and, like abdominal distention, might be a late sign. Dehydration secondary to vomiting and/or intestinal ischemia, metabolic acidosis, and sepsis develop rapidly.

Intermittent or partial chronic midgut volvulus usually presents in children older than 2 years with symptoms of chronic vomiting, usually bilious, intermittent colicky abdominal pain, hematemesis, diarrhea, constipation, failure to thrive, and protein-calorie malnutrition.

In the rare types of reverse rotation, in which the colon lies behind the superior mesenteric artery, symptoms associated with partial or complete colonic obstruction might present later in adult life [19–21].

17.4 Radiologic Diagnosis

A plain abdominal film showing gaseous distention of the stomach (Fig. 17.6a), and sometimes of the proximal duodenum as well (Fig. 17.6b), and a relatively gasless pattern in the rest of the abdomen is typical of midgut volvulus. Such a film might be all what is required to make the diagnosis in an infant with bilious vomiting, who is not stable enough to undergo an upper GI contrast study. However, plain abdominal radiog-

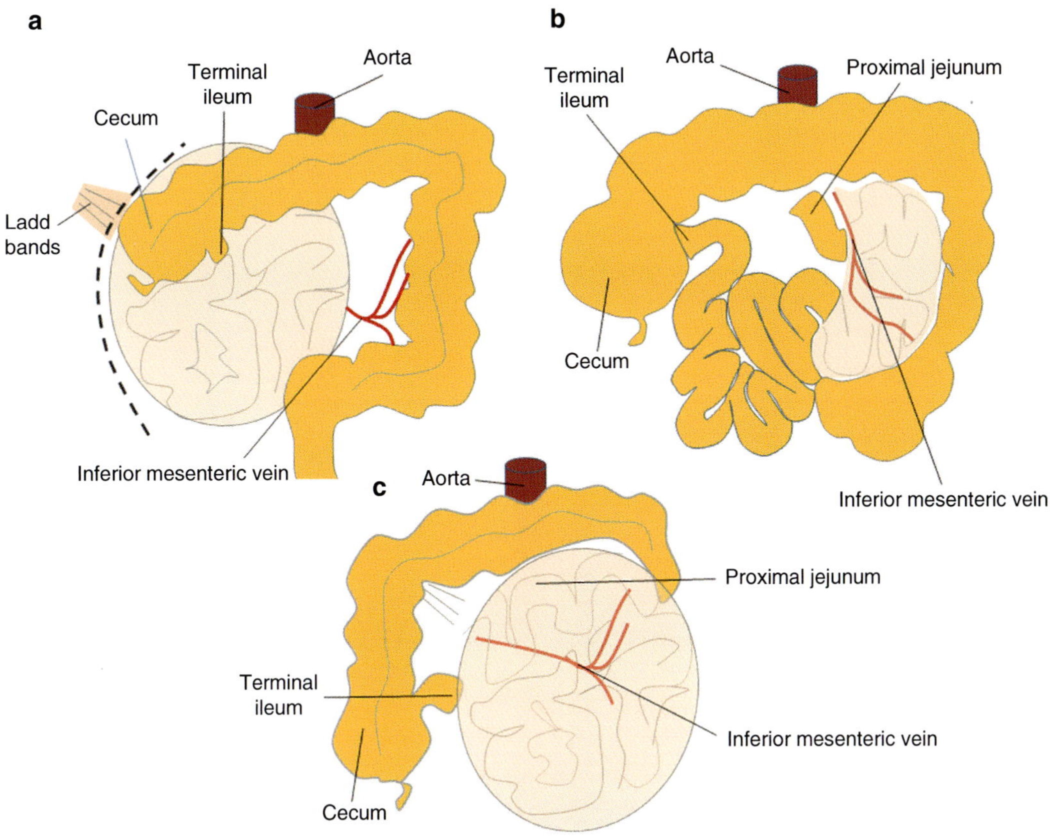

Fig. 17.5 *Right* (**a**) and *left* (**b**, **c**) mesocolic hernias. The interrupted line in (**a**) shows the surgical incision at the area of the lateral peritoneal reflection used to reduce the herniated small bowel from the mesocolon. Note that the inferior mesenteric vein delineates the right margin of the left mesocolic hernias in (**b**) and (**c**) (From Willwerth BM et al. (1974) Congenital mesocolic (paraduodenal) hernia: embryologic basis of repair. Am J Surg 128:358)

raphy may not always be diagnostic, and, thus, an upper GI contrast study should always be considered in a bilious vomiter with a normal abdominal film.

The upper GI contrast study is the investigation of choice for the evaluation of a patient with suspected abnormalities of intestinal rotation. In normal intestinal rotation, the duodenum descends to the right of the midline, courses transversely to the left, and then ascends to the left of the midline up to duodenojejunal junction at the level of the pylorus; the loops of the proximal jejunum are subsequently seen on the left of the midline.

In malrotation, the duodenum descends to the right of the midline and fails to course transversely to the left of the midline (Fig. 17.7a). Instead of crossing the midline, the contrast medium is seen to fill the jejunal loops on the right of the midline (Fig. 17.7b). Delay in the passage of the contrast into the jejunal loops and the characteristic spiral configuration of the proximal jejunum, known as "corkscrew" sign, indicate obstruction because of midgut volvulus (Fig. 17.8). In atypical malrotation, the duodenojejunal junction is demonstrated at the midline or to the left of the midline but lower than the level of the pylorus (Fig. 17.9).

Although contrast enema is considered of low diagnostic value and is in present times rarely used, it has historically been used and can theoretically demonstrate the displaced cecum. However, 20–30 % of the cases with malrotation have a normally sited colon, and, furthermore, the mobile cecum is frequently seen in the right

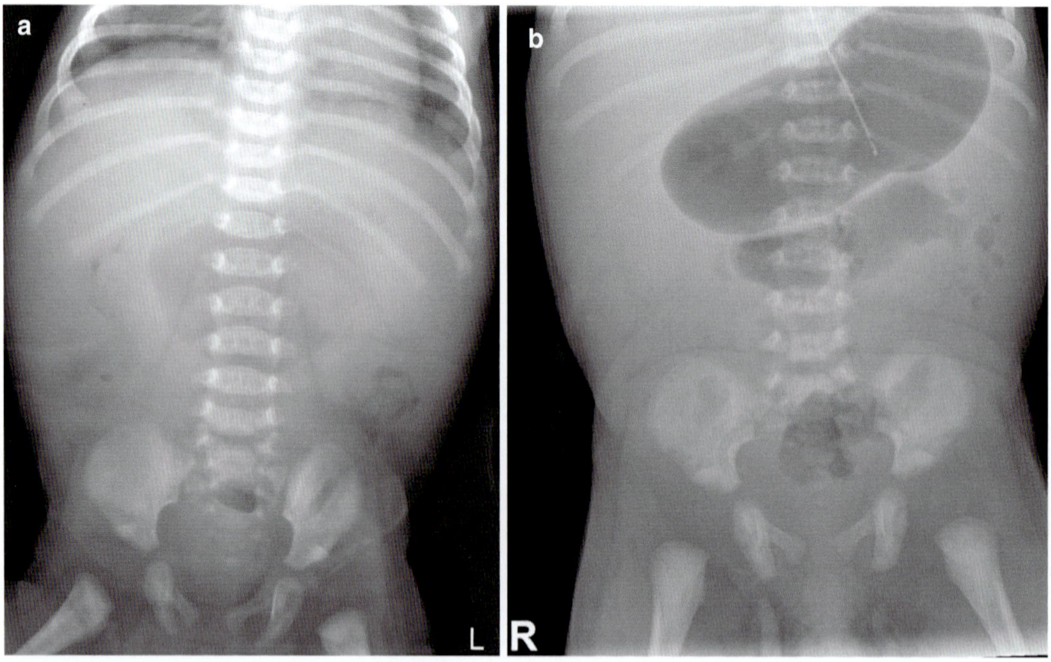

Fig. 17.6 Plain radiographs of infants with midgut volvulus, showing gaseous distention of the (**a**) stomach and of the (**b**) stomach and duodenum, with a paucity of gas distally

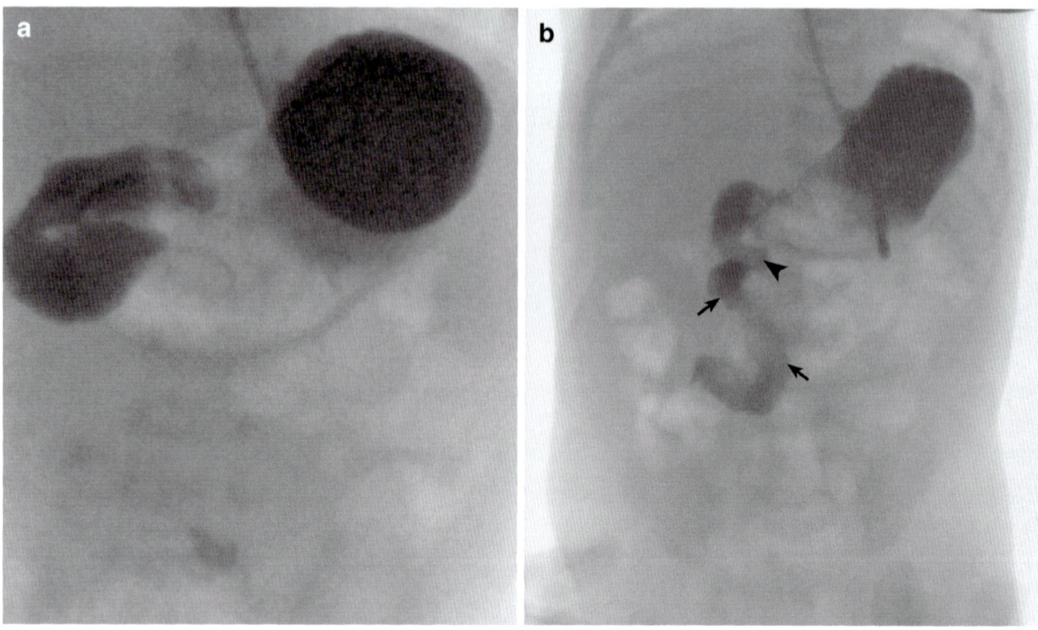

Fig. 17.7 Images from contrast studies of infants showing malrotation. (**a**) The duodenum descends to the right of the midline and then fails to course transversely to the left. (**b**) The duodenojejunal flexure (*arrowhead*) lies to the right of the midline, and the contrast is seen passing from the duodenum to the proximal jejunum (*arrows*) to the right of the midline

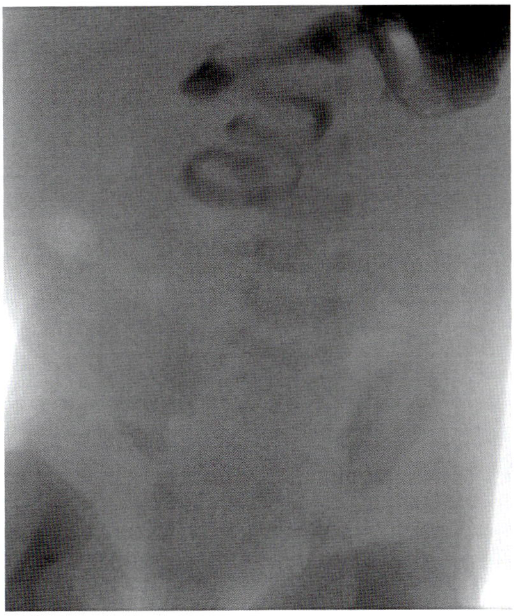

Fig. 17.8 Contrast study of an infant with midgut volvulus. The proximal jejunum courses inferiorly, to the right of the midline, in a spiral configuration

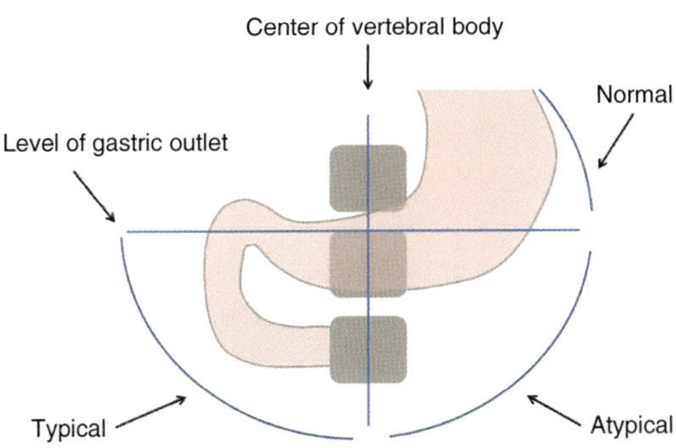

Fig. 17.9 Classification of malrotation as typical and atypical on the basis of the location of the ligament of Treitz (and duodenojejunal flexure) in relation to the midline, as indicated by the vertebral body, and to the level of the gastric outlet (From Dassinger MS, Smith SD (2012) Ch 86. Disorders of intestinal rotation and fixation. In: Coran AG et al. (eds) Pediatric surgery, 7th edn. Elsevier Saunders, Philadelphia)

iliac fossa. The converse is also true, with the position of the cecum in normal individuals being variable [22, 23].

Sonography has lately become popular and is increasingly used to demonstrate abnormalities of intestinal rotation by showing an abnormal relationship of the superior mesenteric vein to the superior mesenteric artery. The inversion in the superior mesenteric artery and vein relationship, with the superior mesenteric artery on the right and superior mesenteric vein on the left, anterior to the abdominal aorta, on color Doppler imaging is diagnostic of malrotation. In some cases of malrotation, however, the orientation between the vessels is normal. Additional sonographic signs are a fluid-filled dilated duodenum and transverse intraperitoneal duodenum. The swirling appearance of the mesentery and superior mesenteric vein around the superior mesenteric artery, known as "whirlpool" sign, on color Doppler imaging is suggestive of midgut volvulus [24, 25].

17.5 Management

Rapid intravenous fluid resuscitation, initiation of parenteral broad-spectrum antibiotics, placement of a nasogastric tube, and expeditious laparotomy are essential.

17.5.1 Ladd's Procedure

The abdomen is opened through a supraumbilical right transverse incision. Ladd's procedure consists of the following steps: (1) exteriorization of the bowel and inspection of the bowel and the mesenteric root in order to recognize the type of the malrotation, (2) counterclockwise derotation of the volvulus, (3) division of the Ladd's bands and straightening of the duodenum, (4) appendicectomy, and (5) placement of the small bowel in the right abdomen and of the cecum in the left lower quadrant.

Exteriorization of the entire bowel is necessary, avoiding traction to the mesentery, in order to understand the anatomy. The volvulus is usually untwisted in 180° turns until the transverse colon and cecum are brought into view anterior to the superior mesenteric pedicle. The bowel is covered with warm moist packs until its pink color returns. Common findings suggestive of malrotation include Ladd's bands extending from the terminal ileum, cecum, and/or right colon to the duodenum, fixation of the duodenum and/or proximal jejunum to the cecum and/or right colon, and abnormal positioning and mobility of the cecum and/or the duodenum. In the commonest type, the cecum is found in the right hypochondrium, fixed by Ladd's bands passing over the second and third parts of the duodenum (Fig. 17.2). The duodenum should be adequately freed from all adhesive bands until it is straightened and seen to course freely downward to the right side of the abdomen (Fig. 17.10). Dissection is carried out close to the serosa of the duodenum with careful attention to the superior mesenteric vessels. All additional adhesive bands between intestinal loops or between loops and the parietal peritoneum should be meticulously divided until the whole intestine from the duodenum to the sigmoid colon is free of kinks, in order to avoid recurrence of obstructive symptoms. Appendicectomy should not be performed if the cecum appears severely cyanotic.

It is important to prove that no associated intrinsic duodenal obstruction is present. For this reason, passing a nasogastric tube through the duodenum or a feeding tube through a gastrotomy is recommended.

In reverse rotation, it is sometimes possible to move the colon from behind the mesenteric vessels to a position anterior to them by a 360° anticlockwise rotation of the midgut. However, freeing the duodenum and the underlying mesenteric vessels from the colonic wall is usually sufficient to release the colonic obstruction.

In the presence of a mesocolic hernia, the hernial sac should not be resected, because this might cause devascularization of the colon. In the right mesocolic hernia, the entrapped small bowel is freed by incising the avascular lateral peritoneal reflection of the right colon (Fig. 17.5a). In the left mesocolic hernia, particular attention should be drawn to retain the inferior mesenteric vein, which courses along the right margin of the hernial sac (Fig. 17.5b, c). The small intestine is sometimes easily reduced through the neck of the sac without the need for further dissection.

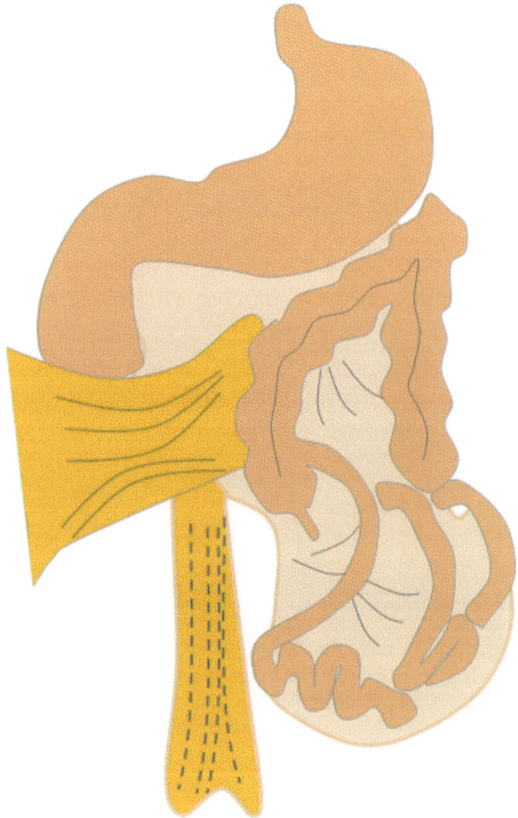

Fig. 17.10 Division of Ladd's bands in order to release and straighten the duodenum (From Lister J (1990) Malrotation and volvulus of the intestine. In: Lister J, Irving IM (eds) Neonatal surgery, 3rd edn. Butterworth & Co, London)

However, it is occasionally required to mobilize the inferior mesenteric vein and/or even make an incision to the right of the vein in order to widen the neck of the sac. After reduction of the mesocolic hernias, the peritoneum of the sac is sutured to the posterior wall to obviate recurrence.

When there is a localized gangrenous segment, then segmental resection and primary anastomosis should be performed. When, however, there are multiple areas of questionable viability or when the entire midgut appears nonviable, the tendency should be on the side of underresection rather than over-resection. A relook laparotomy 12–24 h later, when recovery of the affected bowel loops and/or demarcation of necrotic bowel segments will be clearly evident, is recommended. Preserving the minimum length of the intestine required for survival, preferably including the ileocecal valve, should be the highest priority.

Operative correction of asymptomatic patients found to have atypical malrotation has been recently questioned. Atypical malrotation is less likely to be complicated with volvulus or internal hernias in comparison to typical malrotation (2 vs. 16 % and 7 vs. 21 %). Moreover, patients with atypical malrotation more commonly present with persistent symptoms post-Ladd's procedure in comparison to patients with typical malrotation (21 vs. 12 %) [26, 27].

17.5.2 Laparoscopic Approach

Minimally invasive techniques can be used for both diagnosis and management of malrotation and might be particularly useful in cases with doubtful diagnosis. The comparative studies between the open and laparoscopic approach are limited by their retrospective nonrandomized design. Theoretically, although laparoscopy has well-recognized benefits, it is also believed to cause fewer adhesions and, as a result, to be possibly related with a higher risk of recurrent volvulus. No significant differences in terms of postoperative complications between the laparoscopic and open approach have been revealed to date. Prospective trials with long-term follow-up are required to make safe conclusions [28–31].

17.5.3 Postoperative Complications

The dilatation of the duodenum and the vascular compromise of the bowel might cause prolonged postoperative ileus even up to 5–7 days. This is managed with expectant policy, continuous gastric aspiration through a nasogastric tube, and intravenous fluids. Patients with extensive bowel injury and short bowel syndrome will need special management with long-term total parenteral nutrition.

The incidence of postoperative intussusception is 3.1 % (vs. 0.05 % in other laparotomies). It usually presents with abdominal distention and bilious vomiting 5–8 days postoperatively [32]. The incidence of postoperative adhesive ileus is 4 %. The incidence of recurrent volvulus is low (0.5–1.3 % in reported series).

Mortality rate has reduced significantly over the last 60 years. However, it is still at least 65 % when more than 75 % of the bowel is necrotic.

17.5.4 Management of Asymptomatic Malrotation

Controversy exists over the management of asymptomatic, typical or atypical, malrotation, which has usually been diagnosed incidentally during the evaluation for nonspecific complaints or prior to reflux surgery. Moreover, atypical malrotation is at a significantly lower risk of volvulus and internal hernia in comparison with typical malrotation and is associated with increased incidence, as high as 13 %, of persistent symptoms postoperatively—when symptomatic—and increased incidence, as high as 22 %, of postoperative complications [33].

17.5.5 Management of Malrotation in Heterotaxy Syndrome

Management of asymptomatic malrotation in heterotaxy syndrome remains also controversial. Because of the high incidence of malrotation in heterotaxy, screening of all these patients and prophylactic Ladd's procedure in the presence of malrotation are the standard of care in many centers. However, high complication rates up to 14 %, including a 10 % incidence of small bowel obstruction, have been reported after Ladd's procedure in heterotaxy patients. On the basis of findings of increased morbidity and mortality after Ladd's procedure in heterotaxy patients, some authors now suggest that routine screening of asymptomatic heterotaxy patients for malrotation should be abandoned. Others have suggested that patients with left atrial isomerism are less likely to be malrotated than patients with right atrial isomerism, and, therefore, they should be offered expectant management if they are asymptomatic [34, 35].

References

1. Grob M (1957) Lehrbuch der Kinderchirurgie. Georg Thieme Verlag, Stuttgart
2. His W (1980) Anatomie menschlicher embryome. FCN Vogel, Leipzig
3. Mall FP (1898) Development of the human intestine and its position in the adult. Johns Hopkins Hosp Bull Balt 9:197
4. McIntosh R, Donovan EJ (1939) Disturbances of rotation of the intestinal tract. Am J Dis Child 57:116
5. Snyder WH, Chaffin L (1954) Embryology and pathology of the intestinal tract. Ann Surg 140:368
6. Willwerth BM et al (1974) Congenital mesocolic (paraduodenal) hernia: embryologic basis of repair. Am J Surg 128:358
7. Berdon WE et al (1970) Midgut malrotation and volvulus. Radiology 96:365
8. Chang J et al (1993) Intestinal rotation and fixation abnormalities in heterotaxia: early detection and management. J Pediatr Surg 28:1281
9. Curry J, Lakshminarayanan B (2013) Malrotation. In: Spitz L, Coran A (eds) Operative pediatric surgery, 7th edn. CRC Press Taylor & Francis Group, Boca Raton
10. Dassinger MS, Smith SD (2012) Ch 86. Disorders of intestinal rotation and fixation. In: Coran AG et al (eds) Pediatric surgery, 7th edn. Elsevier Saunders, Philadelphia
11. Dott NM (1923) Anomalies of intestinal rotation. Br J Surg 11:251
12. Fraser JE, Robbins RH (1915) On the factors concerned in causing rotation of the intestine in man. J Anat Physiol 50:75
13. Janik JS, Ein SH (1979) Normal intestinal rotation with nonfixation: a cause of chronic abdominal pain. J Pediatr Surg 14:670
14. Kluth D, Lambrecht W (1994) Disorders of intestinal rotation. In: Freeman NV et al (eds) Surgery of the newborn. Churchill Livingstone, New York
15. Stewart DR et al (1976) Malrotation of the bowel in infants and children: a 15-year review. Surgery 79:716
16. Lister J (1990) Malrotation and volvulus of the intestine. In: Lister J, Irving IM (eds) Neonatal surgery, 3rd edn. Butterworth & Co, London
17. Bentley JFR (1959) Mesenteric cysts with malrotated intestine. BMJ 2:223
18. Hill SJ et al (2014) Heterotaxy syndrome and malrotation: does isomerism influence risk and decision to treat. J Pediatr Surg 49:934
19. Dott NM (1927) Volvulus neonatorum. Br Med J 1:230
20. Howell CG et al (1982) Malrotation, malnutrition and ischemic bowel disease. J Pediatr Surg 17:469
21. Lewis JE (1966) Partial duodenal obstruction with incomplete duodenal rotation. J Pediatr Surg 1:47
22. Simpson AJ et al (1972) Roentgen diagnosis of midgut malrotation: value of upper gastrointestinal radiographic study. J Pediatr Surg 7:243
23. Tackett JJ et al (2014) Malrotation: current strategies navigating the radiologic diagnosis of a surgical emergency. World J Radiol 6:730–736
24. Pracros JP et al (1992) Ultrasound diagnosis of midgut volvulus: the 'whirlpool' sign. Pediatr Radiol 22:18
25. Zhou LY et al (2015) Usefulness of sonography in evaluating children suspected of malrotation: comparison with an upper gastrointestinal contrast study. J Ultrasound Med 34:1825
26. Ladd WE (1932) Congenital obstruction of the duodenum in children. N Engl J Med 206:277
27. Ladd WE (1937) Congenital duodenal obstruction. Surgery 1:878
28. Bass KD et al (1998) Laparoscopic Ladd's procedure in infants with malrotation. J Pediatr Surg 33:279
29. Bax NM, van der Zee DC (1988) Laparoscopic treatment of intestinal malrotation in children. Surg Endosc 12:1314
30. Fraser JD et al (2009) The role of laparoscopy in the management of malrotation. J Surg Res 156:80
31. Ooms N et al (2016) Laparoscopic treatment of intestinal malrotation in children. Eur J Pediatr Surg 26: 376–381
32. Kidd J et al (2000) Intussusception following Ladd's procedure. Arch Surg 135:713
33. Mehall JR et al (2002) Management of typical and atypical intestinal malrotation. J Pediatr Surg 37:1169
34. Elder CT et al (2014) The role of screening and prophylactic surgery for malrotation in heterotaxy patients. J Pediatr Surg 49:1746
35. Landisch R et al (2015) Observation versus prophylactic Ladd for asymptomatic intestinal rotational abnormalities in heterotaxy syndrome: a systematic review. J Pediatr Surg 50(11):1971–1974

18 Alimentary Tract Duplications

Noemi Cantone and Mario Lima

18.1 Introduction

Enteric duplications are rare development malformations that can occur anywhere along the alimentary tract from the tongue to the anus. To date, there is no unique classification that can explain their extremely variable onset, size, and location. Calder was the first to publish a report of alimentary tract duplications, back in 1773, describing a duodenal duplication. The term "intestinal duplication" was used for the first time by Fitz in 1884 but was not widely used until it became commonly used in 1937, thanks to Ladd and a further classification by Gross in 1953 [1–3]. Several terms had been used before then to describe such anomalies such as giant diverticula, enterogenous cyst, or unusual Meckel's diverticula. The current nomenclature, as suggested by Ladd and Gross, depends on the anatomic location of the duplication in relation to the normal gastrointestinal tract.

18.2 Epidemiology

Gastrointestinal duplications are observed in 1 every 4500 births, representing 0.1–0.3 % of all congenital malformations, with a slight predominance in white males [1, 4]. Most duplications are diagnosed in children, prenatally or within the first two years of life in approximately two thirds of the cases; less than 30 % of all lesions are detected in adults [1,5]. They are generally single, but in 10–20 % of cases, they are multiple; if one duplication is diagnosed, it is therefore advisable to search for other ones. About 75 % of the lesions are found in the abdomen and 20 % in the thoracic cavity, and in a small percentage, they are located in the thoracoabdominal region. The small bowel, in particular the ileum, is the site where they mostly occur; jejunal and ileal lesions are most common (50–53 %), followed by esophageal and mediastinal (15–21 %), colonic (12–15 %), gastric (6–9 %), duodenal (4–7 %), rectal (4–5 %), thoracoabdominal (2–4 %), and cervical (1 %) lesions (Fig. 18.1 and Table 18.1). Although the embryologic site of origin is uncertain, duplication is commonly referred to as foregut, midgut, or hindgut derived, depending on its location; almost half of all duplications occur in the midgut, while a third is located in the foregut [1,6,7]. Associated anomalies have been observed in about 30–50 % of patients: spinal and vertebral malformation in thoracic or thoracoabdominal duplications, intestinal malrotation, atresia and anorectal malformation in abdominal lesions, and urogenital tract anomalies in midgut and hindgut malformations. Congenital heart diseases and pulmonary airway malformations are rarely associated with foregut duplications [5,6].

N. Cantone (✉) • M. Lima
Pediatric Surgery, S. Orsola-Malpighi Hospital, Bologna University, via Massarenti 11, Bologna 40138, Italy
e-mail: noemicantone@hotmail.it

M. Lima (ed.), *Pediatric Digestive Surgery*, DOI 10.1007/978-3-319-40525-4_18

18.3 Embryology

The embryologic site of origin and the pathophysiology of these anomalies are unknown. Several theories have been proposed, but none of them, if considered individually, can explain all the different combinations of type, location, and associated anomalies of duplications.

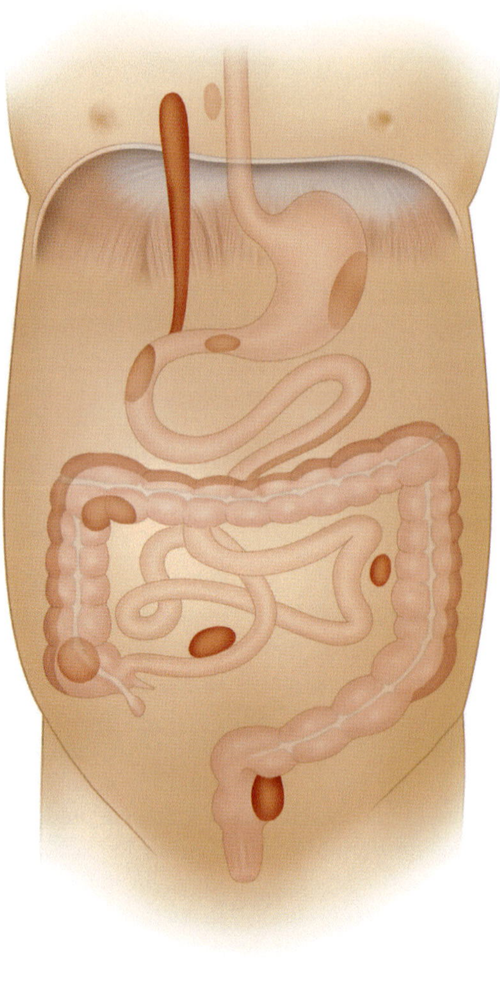

Fig. 18.1 Distribution of duplications by location and frequency

There are four major theories concerning the origin of enteric duplications:

The partial or abortive twinning theory states that alimentary tract duplications are the result of incomplete twinning. This hypothesis can apply in particular for the foregut and hindgut duplications that are associated with doubling of the mouth, genitourinary tract, and lower bowel. The extent of the twinning depends on the moment the process starts [8].

The aberrant luminal recanalization theory, postulated by Bremer in 1944, proposed that duplication is due to the persistence of outpouching of the fetal bowel. This theory may apply to those duplications of the segment of the gastrointestinal tract that goes through a "solid stage," such as the esophagus, small bowel, and colon. After this phase, which occurs between 6 and 8 weeks of intrauterine life, the progressive craniocaudal growth allows the development of a lumen. According to Bremer's theory, duplication may be the result of an incomplete or defective vacuolization of the intestine and/or the persistent embryological diverticula with the formation of two channels, either communicating with each other or not. This theory can apply to simple duplications, i.e., not associated with other anomalies, and provides a functional explication of the highest occurrence of duplications in the ileal tract, which is the main site of diverticula; however, it does not provide proper explanation for the heterotopic mucosa found in some duplications and why the lesions are located more frequently on the mesenteric side while most of diverticula are found instead on the antimesenteric side [9].

Bentley and Smith in 1960 proposed *the split notochord theory* to describe the duplications that develop in the chest and are associated with spinal defects and skin anomalies. During the third to fourth week of gestation, the notochord starts to

Table 18.1 Distribution of duplications by location and frequency

Foregut duplications	Midgut duplications	Hindgut duplications
Esophageal: 15–21 %	Jejunal: 10–18 %	Colonic: 12–15 %
Thoracoabdominal: 2–4 %	Ileal: 35–40 %	Rectal: 4–5 %
Gastric: 6–9 %	Cecal: 3–5 %	
Duodenal: 4–7 %		

close and separate from the endoderm. If an error occurs during the separating phase, an abnormal adhesion between the neural tube ectoderm and the gut endoderm forms, with the development of a gap and a secondary herniation of endodermal cells; furthermore, endodermic tissue can act as a barrier to the anterior fusion of the vertebral mesoderm resulting in vertebral defect. This mechanism may explain the long duplication cysts and foregut duplication, their dorsal location, and the association with spinal malformation (15 % of the cases). It does not explain, however, the entire range of abnormalities (such as heterotopic gastric mucosa) [10].

The environmental factors theory suggests that stress, hypoxia, and trauma can be involved as cause factors of the malformation as described by Mellish and Koop in 1961. Although the actual mechanism that induces the malformation is not clear, an intrauterine vascular accident and/or a compression from nearby organs could explain the anomalies and the association with other malformations as intestinal atresia [11].

Foregut duplications need to be discussed separately. Foregut duplications include a wide spectrum of anomalies, the esophageal, the bron-chogenic, and the neurenteric cysts, subdivided according to their embryologic origin, the anatomopathological characteristics, and the anatomical district concerned. It is believed that bronchogenic and the esophageal duplication cysts result from an altered budding of the embryonic foregut between the fifth and the eighth week of gestation; notochord subdivision alterations can explain the origin of the neurenteric cysts. About 50–60 % of foregut duplications are bronchogenic; they are usually located close to the trachea but can be found in many locations (mediastinum, intraparenchymal, paraesophageal, paratracheal, perihilar) and are frequently associated with congenital pulmonary airway malformations (congenital cystic adenomatoid malformations, pulmonary sequestration), forming hybrid lesions. An enteric cyst may be lined by ciliated respiratory epithelium, but the presence of bronchial wall structures, particularly cartilage, but also smooth muscle and glands, is necessary for diagnosis of bronchogenic cyst; a neurenteric cyst can also be lined by enteric-type mucosa and has a pedicle that extends to the spinal canal [12, 13].

18.4 Anatomical Pathology

As described by Ladd, enteric duplications have three characteristics: (1) an intimate anatomical connection with any part of the gastrointestinal tract, (2) an epithelial lining representing some portion of the alimentary tract, and (3) a well-developed coat of smooth muscle [3]. The lesion tends to locate on the antimesenteric side of the alimentary tract with which it frequently shares the muscular coat and blood supply. The epithelial lining is usually the same as the mucosa native to the lesion, but in 35 % of the cases, an ectopic tissue is present, most commonly gastric followed by pancreatic mucosa, which predisposes to complication as ulceration, hemorrhage, and perforation; rarely, in the thoracic duplication, a respiratory epithelial lining can be present. Generally duplications are classified as two entities, the tubular and the cystic type. Cystic lesions are more common (65–90 %); they are more frequently found in the small intestine and can have big size; and they are closed at their two ends and normally covered with the same mucosa as the native intestine. They do not usually communicate with the intestinal lumen. The tubular type (10–35 %) can often be remarkably long; it may communicate with the adjacent alimentary tract, usually in the caudal end or at both ends, and can contain heterotopic mucosa more frequently than the cystic type [1, 5, 14].

Li et al. have classified small intestinal duplications in two types based on the vascular pattern (Fig. 18.2).

Type 1 lesion or parallel type (74.4 %): the duplication develops in one side of the mesentery, and there are two separated blood vessels, one perfusing duplication and one native bowel.

Type 2 lesion or intramesenteric type (24.6 %): the duplication is located between the two layers of mesentery and vessels from both sides of the mesentery cross the duplication to reach the native bowel.

In their study, Li and colleagues found that vertebral defects were more frequently associated with the type 2 lesion (91.6 %) than the type 1 lesion (5.5 %), hypothesizing a different embry-

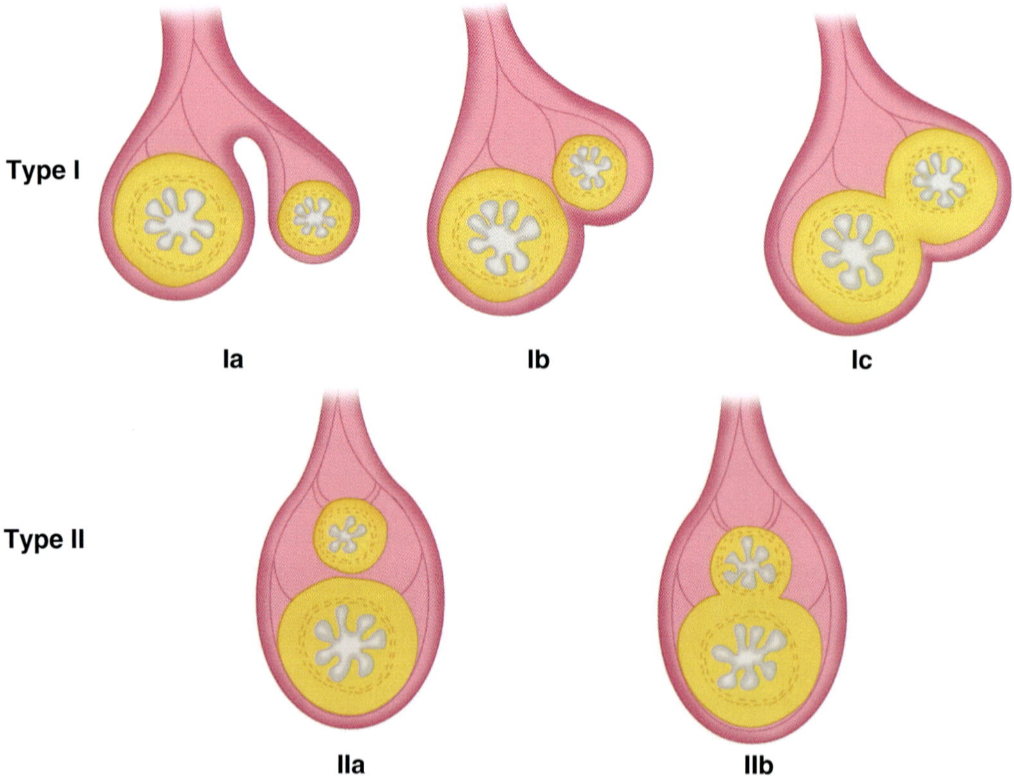

Fig. 18.2 Classification of small intestinal duplications based on their blood supply. In *type 1*, the duplication is located on one side of the mesentery, and the main artery of the duplication is parallel to the main artery of the bowel. *Type 1a*, the duplication has a separate mesentery; *type 1b*, the duplication shares common mesentery with the gut; and *type 1c*, the duplication shares common muscular coat with the gut. In *type 2*, the lesion is located between the two layers of the mesentery and supplied by vessels from both sides of the mesentery that pass over from both surfaces of the duplication to reach the native bowel. *Type 2a*, the duplication is separate from the bowel, and *type 2b*, the duplication shares common muscular coat with the bowel

ologic cause as the origin of the two anomalies. Furthermore, their study shows how the knowledge of the vascular anatomy of small intestinal duplications may have a surgical implication, allowing excision of these lesions without resection of the adjacent bowel. The type 1 duplication could be excised by dividing the mesentery; the type 2 duplication may be enucleated by tying off the short branches from the main vessels [15].

18.5 Clinical Manifestations

Clinical manifestations are extremely variable, depending on the site, type, and size of the duplication and if it contains gastric mucosa. Most duplications (80%) are detected in the first two years of age, in particular in half of the cases in the first six months of age. They are frequently asymptomatic and diagnosed incidentally on routine X-ray or ultrasound examination performed for other malformations or rarely may be an incidental intraoperative finding. In recent years the diagnosis has been increasingly made with prenatal ultrasonography.

When located in the mediastinum, they could lead to pneumonia, wheezing, cough, or dysphagia. Symptoms such as respiratory distress and failure to thrive are more common in small infants, whereas chest pain occurs more frequently in older children.

The most common presentations of an abdominal duplication are abdominal pain and distension, vomiting, and abdominal mass. Complications include bleeding and perforation due to an ectopic gastric mucosa, with peptic ulceration or intestinal occlusion due to the development of volvulus, intussusception, or extrinsic compression frequently for an acutely enlarged cystic mass. Other rare complications are pancreatitis and cholecystitis in the gallbladder, duodenal and pancreatic duplication, cyst infection, and malignancy, the latter more frequent in adulthood and in hindgut duplications. Volvulus and intussusceptions are more frequent in midgut duplications, whereas in hindgut duplications symptoms by mass effect with obstruction of both the urinary tract and the bowel tract prevail. Bleeding, hemorrhage with melena, and perforation are frequent both in midgut and hindgut duplications [4, 14, 16].

18.6 Diagnosis

The high resolution modern imaging techniques allow physicians to identify enteric duplications in the prenatal age, in particular those located in the chest and in the upper abdomen, in approximately 30 % of cases. Since duplications are often associated with other malformations, if an enteric duplication is found during a prenatal ultrasound, a fetal magnetic resonance imaging (MRI) is advisable. The fetal MRI also allows physicians to identify fetuses at risk who might require invasive procedures (i.e., thoraco-amniotic shunt for fetal hydrops or mediastinal shift) and to establish the best therapeutic strategy in the postpartum so as to avoid complications [14, 16].

The clinical history and the physical examination are the first step for the diagnosis of a duplication, whereas the laboratory exams may detect only anemia in case of bleeding due to heterotopic mucosa or higher serum amylase and lipase levels in the rare case of pancreatitis.

Postnatally ultrasound can be useful to demonstrate the nature (solid or cystic) and the location of the mass as well as to evaluate any connection with the adjacent intestine. The cystic lesion appears as an anechoic structure (in case of no bleeding) surrounded by a 2–3 mm thick wall that determines a characteristic and pathognomonic echogenic signal defined as "gut signature" or "double layer," which is made up of an hyperechoic inner mucus layer and a hypoechoic muscular outer layer.

An abdominal X-ray can show a mass effect in the event of a large cyst or signs of intestinal obstruction or perforation in complicated cases. A thorax X-ray can show a mass usually located in the medium or posterior mediastinum and eventually associated vertebral anomalies.

Computerized axial tomography scan (CT scan) and MRI are more accurate in showing the anatomical features and the relationship with nearby organs; MRI is advisable in the childhood and useful to detect any spinal involvement.

Gastrointestinal contrast studies can demonstrate a filling defect as the duplication does not usually communicate with the intestinal lumen. The endoscopic ultrasonography, the esophagogastroduodenoscopy, and the wireless capsule endoscopy can show ulcers or stenosis and can help defining better the anatomy before a surgery. The endoscopic ultrasound (EUS) can provide further information, detecting the cystic nature of the lesion with its characteristic wall, its location, and its anatomical relationships with adjacent structures; it can also be useful as a guide for fine needle aspiration, which is used only in selected cases.

In the case of a patient presenting anemia and lower gastrointestinal bleeding, a scintigraphy with technetium-99m pertechnetate can be useful to identify ectopic gastric mucosa and make a differential diagnosis with the Meckel's diverticulum.

Definitive diagnosis is based on histopathological findings after surgical excision.

Differential diagnosis includes intrathoracic mass or tracheoesophageal fistula in the foregut duplications, appendicitis, Meckel's diverticulum and other causes of intussusception in the small bowel duplications, and constipation or Hirschsprung's disease in colonic and hindgut duplication. In the rare case of a gastric or duodenal duplication, the sign and symptoms can mimic a hypertrophic pyloric stenosis or a gastroesophageal reflux [1, 4, 8, 14].

18.7 Management

Management depends on the presentation. Intestinal duplications often require an urgent surgical intervention due to the onset of complications such as perforation, intestinal occlusion, or severe bleeding. This is why, although the treatment of asymptomatic lesions remains controversial, most authors currently recommend surgery even with no symptoms in order to avoid any complication at a later moment [16, 17]. The type of surgery varies depending on the cases [6, 7]:

- Enucleation of the intestinal duplication only where possible.
- Resection of the duplication along with the adjacent intestinal segment and end-to-end anastomosis in the event of small cystic or short tubular duplications.
- Total excision of the duplication through extramucosal dissection according to Wrenn procedure, which includes stripping of the entire mucosa through a series of multiple incisions; this technique applies to extended tubular duplications or large cystic ones where an intestinal resection would cause a short bowel syndrome [18, 19].
- Drainage procedure, like fenestration or marsupialization of the duplication into the lumen after total or partial resection or puncture of the lesion, in the cases where removal is difficult, i.e., in the duodenal duplication, mediastinal duplication, or duplication near biliary or pancreatic tracts; this intervention has a high risk of recurrence.

18.8 Classification and Treatment by Location

18.8.1 Oropharyngeal Duplications

Oropharyngeal duplications are very rare, being 1 % of all duplications. The most common location is the floor of the mouth and they may contain gastric or colonic mucosa. In most cases they are asymptomatic; sometimes, however, failure to thrive may be the presenting symptom. The treatment consists in an oral approach with cyst resection and oral mucosa reposition [1, 14].

18.8.2 Cervical Duplications

Esophageal duplications starting from the cervical area are extremely rare, are usually cystic, and are strictly adherent to the esophagus. Symptoms include a palpable mass and/or symptoms due to compression of the adjacent structures; this is why the diagnosis is usually made during the first months of life. The CT scan is the gold standard for diagnosis to evaluate any anatomical connections. The differential diagnosis includes lymphatic malformations, cysts of the airway, branchial apparatus cysts, thyroglossal cysts, cervical lymphadenopathies, and esophageal diverticula. Treatment consists in complete excision, if possible, or partial excision with mucosa removal through a supraclavicular approach [1, 14].

18.8.3 Thoracic Duplications

Thoracic duplications are the second most common site of duplications, accounting for approximately 15–21 % of alimentary tract duplications; the foregut duplication is the second cause of mediastinal mass after neurogenic tumors. Although esophageal duplications may develop throughout the length of the esophagus, two thirds of these lesions are found in its lower third and one third in the upper/middle third of the esophagus. They are typically located in posterior mediastinum, more commonly in the right side. They are usually cystic and do not share a muscular wall or communicate with the esophageal lumen. In 80 % of the cases, they are diagnosed in childhood and are more frequent in male patients. The clinical presentation includes symptoms secondary to extrinsic tracheal and esophageal compression up to respiratory distress; the upper esophageal duplication can cause stridor, tirage, and cough, while duplication in the middle or lower esophagus can cause dysphagia, epigastralgia, chest pain, or vomiting. Furthermore, gastric mucosa is present in about 30–50 % of all esophageal duplications, with possible bleeding and secondary hematemesis, melena, or hemoptysis as a manifestation of fistula formation with bronchial tree. Other rare manifestations include cardiac arrhythmia, retrosternal and thoracic back pain, and cyst rupture with mediastinitis. Additionally, they are very frequently associated with vertebral anomalies (20–50 %) and thus defined neurenteric cyst, including hemivertebra or spinal dysraphism, with possible neurological problems (in 20 % of cases, a communication with the spinal cord is described); other anomalies found in a lower percentage of cases include diaphragmatic hernia and esophageal atresia. A clinical suspicion, if not raised prenatally, may arise with a thorax X-ray, a contrast study of the upper gastrointestinal tract, and eventually an endoscopy. Endoscopically they cannot be distinguished from a lipoma, a leiomyoma, a gastrointestinal stromal tumor, or a submucosal lesion. With EUS the duplication appears as an anechoic cyst with the characteristic multilayered wall structure; the EUS-guided fine needle aspiration is possible but usually reserved for lesions of indeterminate appearance, atypical or suspected for malignancy, also due to the high risk of post-aspiration infections. The best imaging technique to define anatomic details is CT scan or MRI; the latter is the gold standard for defining neurenteric cysts. An abdominal ultrasound is required to exclude any associated intestinal duplications which are found up to a third of the cases [4, 14].

The treatment of choice consists of the exeresis or enucleation, if possible, through a thoracotomy or a thoracoscopic procedure; other authors suggested the surveillance with EUS of some asymptomatic lesions.

The approach used in the intrathoracic cysts is a posterolateral thoracotomy with the patient positioned on the opposite site with respect to the lesion location. The muscle-sparing technique ensures a gentle separation and a rapid cicatrization. Resection of the cyst must be close to the esophagus and must include the removal of the residual mucosa. If the cyst is in the contest of the esophagus wall and does not communicate with the esophageal lumen, the duplication must be removed by opening the wall of the esophagus and performing an extramucosal excision, leaving the mucosa intact. Any communication with the esophageal lumen must be closed, repairing the muscular defect also with an edge of duplication and checking the mucosal integrity by air or fluid insufflation through a nasogastric tube. In some cases it might be useful to perform the surgery under the guide of a flexible endoscope.

Video-assisted thoracoscopic resection is possible in many cases (Fig. 18.3). The patient is placed in a lateral position on the healthy flank. The homolateral arm is raised above the head, the hemithorax is elevated by axillary roll, and the body is rotated into a near-prone position to expose the posterior part of the thorax. The optic (5–10 mm/0–30°) is inserted with an open technique in the V intercostal space, along the middle axillary line, inferior to the tip of the scapula. Two or more 3–5 mm instrumental ports are introduced to create a triangulation of the instruments. Single-lung ventilation with collapse of the ipsilateral lung can help the surgical removal of the cyst. The mass is exposed with blunt dissection and cauterization; after dissection, the mass is aspirated for decompression, if required, and extracted through a trocar site. If the cyst cannot be removed completely due to the risk of damaging the esophagus or the airways, the borders of the cyst can be left and ablated using electrocauterization. At the end of the procedure, it is important to check and close any leak in the esophageal wall which might pose the risk of an esophageal perforation or a pseudodiverticulum formation. Usually an apical chest drainage is left.

In the case of neurenteric cysts, a surgery with the aid of neurosurgeons is required; resection of the bone and laminectomy, if required, are usually the first step, with subsequent exeresis of the thoracic mass. Mortality in these cases may be high [12, 13].

18.8.4 Thoracoabdominal Duplications

Thoracoabdominal duplications are 2–4 % of all duplications. They are generally the tubular type, can communicate with the intestinal lumen, and frequently have ectopic gastric mucosa. They go down to the right of the esophagus, go over the

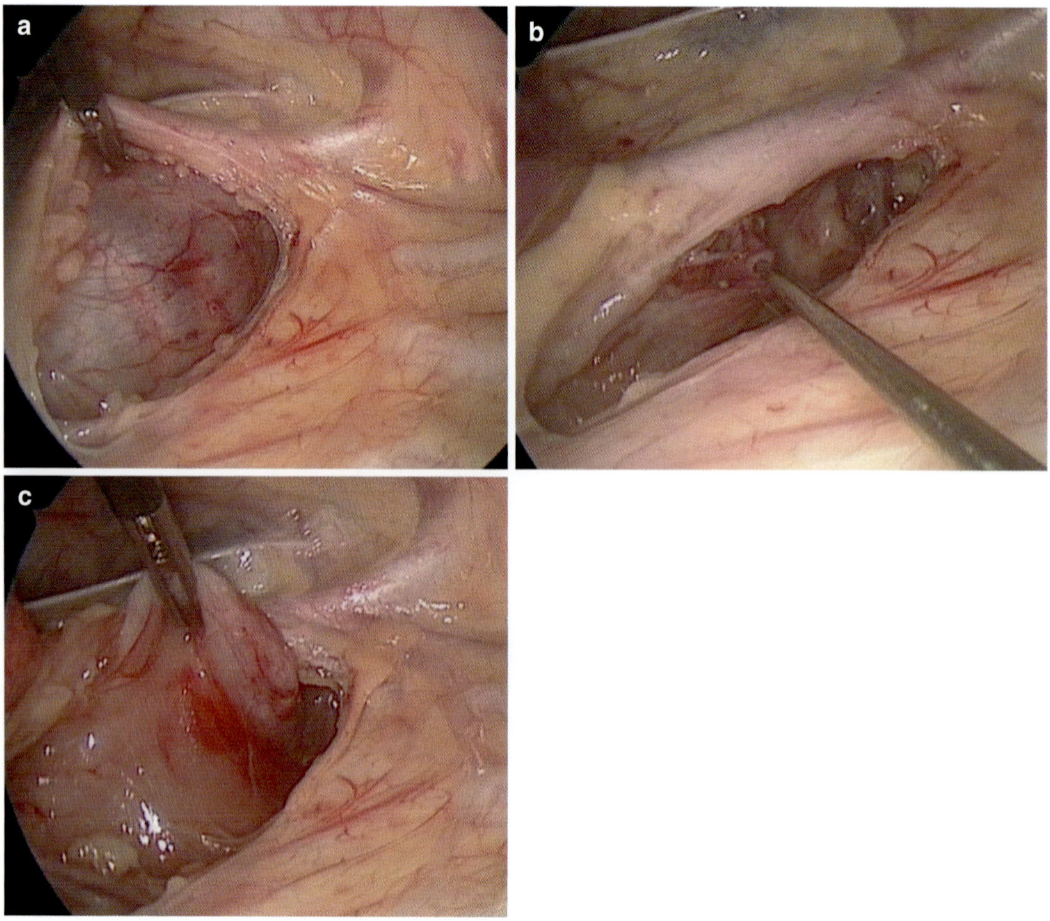

Fig. 18.3 Thoracoscopic excision of an esophageal duplication. (**a**) Thoracoscopic identification of the duplication. (**b**) The lesion is aspirated to facilitate the removal. (**c**) After blunt dissection, the mass is extracted through a trocar site by an endobag or a finger glove

diaphragm near the right pillar or through the esophageal or aortic orifice, and extend along the greater curvature of the stomach and the mesenteric side of the duodenum and jejunum. Clinical picture is similar to that of the thoracic duplications, with the association of abdominal symptoms such as recurrent abdominal pain or palpable mass; neurological symptoms may also be present as they are frequently associated with rachis malformations in the thoracic area. The diagnostic investigations required are the same as those for the thoracic duplications: thoracic and abdominal CT scan and MRI are required before performing any surgery. The treatment consists in one-stage combined thoracoabdominal approach; occasionally a laminectomy is also necessary in the case of intraspinal lesions. After removing the rachis component, the duplication is separated from the esophagus and is removed up to the diaphragmatic defect and then sutured; alternatively, the thoracic portion is pulled into the abdomen through the diaphragm and then removed. The duplication is finally removed through an abdominal approach, by means of an excision or following Wrenn's surgical principles [1, 5].

18.8.5 Gastric Duplications

Gastric duplications account for 5–9 % of all duplications. Unlike other duplications, they appear to be more frequent in females. They are more often cystic and noncommunicating lesion and are located along the greater curvature, although they can be found in any part of the stomach. The lining mucosa is usually the gastric type, although intestinal or colonic mucosa may be found; gastric duplications may also contain pancreatic mucosa or ciliated cells and can rarely communicate with the pancreatic duct system. These patients usually become symptomatic in the first months of life. The symptoms are usually related to the mass effect and include vomiting, abdominal pain, epigastric pain, weight loss and failure to thrive, and sometimes pancreatitis; if a communication with the lumen is present, a peptic ulceration can result in a hemorrhage with hematemesis and melena or perforation.

Diagnostic evaluation includes an abdominal ultrasound in order to differentiate a gastric duplication from a hypertrophic pyloric stenosis, of which it can mimic the symptoms, and from pancreatic pseudocysts and choledochal cysts which are included in the differential diagnosis of these duplications as well. A barium swallow, an endoscopy, or an EUS can provide further information, but an abdominal CT scan is usually necessary to define better the anatomy and identify any synchronous lesions [15, 16].

The treatment of the gastric duplication should be complete resection. Most duplications can be easily removed by an extramucosal dissection, suturing the muscular defect, and checking, at the end of the procedure, the integrity of the gastric wall by insufflating air through a nasogastric tube; the excision can be performed via laparoscopy (Fig. 18.4). In other cases, the duplication is removed via a partial gastrectomy (wedge resection)

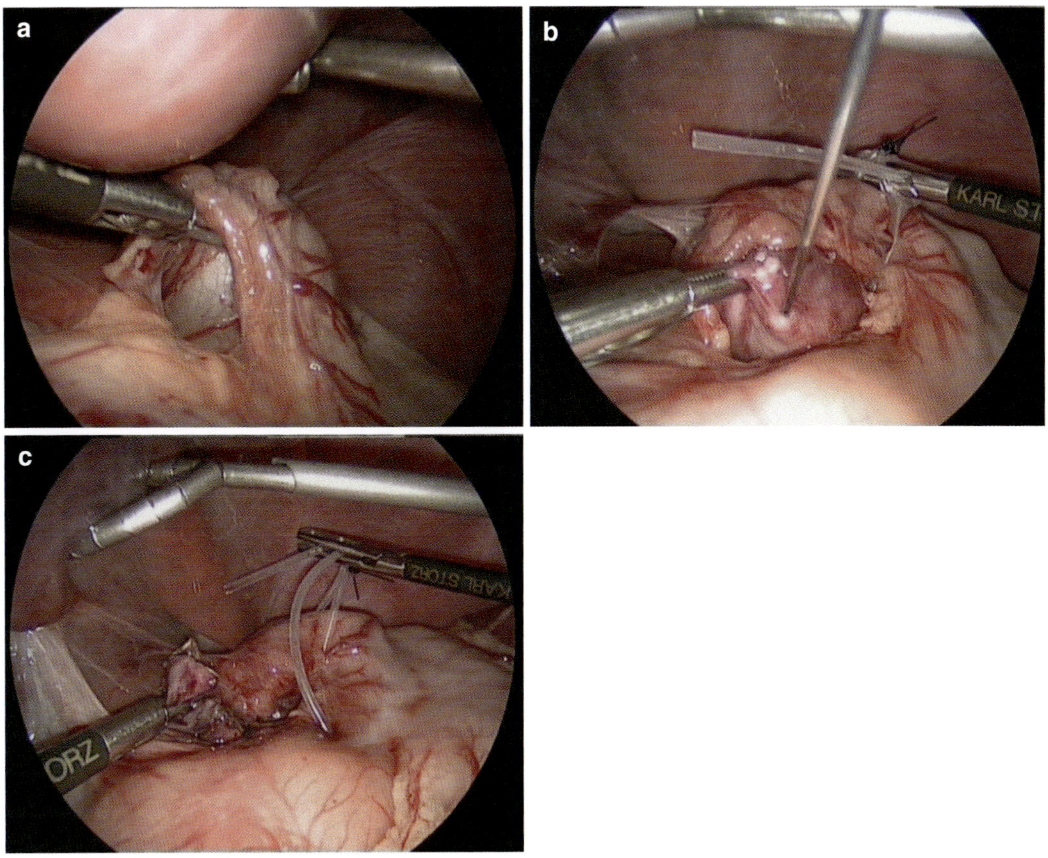

Fig. 18.4 Laparoscopic removal of a gastric duplication. (**a**) Laparoscopic identification of the gastric duplication. (**b**) The cystic lesion is emptied before the enucleation. (**c**) The lesion is removed by an endobag. Gastric duplications, as well as duodenal and colonic duplications, need a purely laparoscopic approach

or, in case of a long duplication, by partial resection and stripping of the residual mucosa. An alternative procedure is to divide the septum between the gastric duplication and the gastric lumen with a linear stapler, with a high risk of complication if the ectopic mucosa is left in situ [6, 20, 21].

18.8.6 Duodenal Duplications

The duodenum is a rare location for duplications and accounts for 4–7 % of all duplications. They are frequently the cystic type, may occasionally communicate with the duodenal lumen, and are covered by duodenal mucosa in most cases or more rarely by pancreatic, gastric, or intestinal mucosa. They are located in the medial or posterior portions of the first or the second part of the duodenum with a possible communication with the pancreatic or common bile duct. The clinical picture is usually not specific, with abdominal pain or distension or failure to thrive, up to an intestinal obstruction with a palpable mass; pancreatitis, jaundice, and hemorrhage due to peptic ulceration may be the onset. An abdominal ultrasound can show a cystic mass, the position of which, in association with the clinical picture, often creates difficulties with the differential diagnosis with a pancreatic cyst and pseudocyst and choledochal cysts; an upper gastrointestinal contrast study can show an extrinsic compression of the duodenum with alterations of the C-shaped duodenal convexity. A CT scan, an endoscopic retrograde cholangiopancreatography (ERCP), and an MRI cholangiography are useful to evaluate the connections with the adjacent structure, in particular with the pancreas and biliary tree. Due to their location and close anatomical relations with the duodenum, biliary tree, and pancreas, the complete exeresis with division of any ductal communication can be very difficult; if an exeresis cannot be performed, partial excision with mucosectomy or endoscopic or percutaneous drainage is possible, although internal drainage is preferable. Marsupializations of the cyst to the duodenum or to a Roux-en-Y loop of the intestine are possible techniques; rarely a pancreaticoduodenectomy is required (Whipple procedure). In any case it is advisable to perform an intraoperative cholangiography to evaluate any connection with the biliary tree; in the case of gastric mucosa diagnosed through an intraoperative biopsy, it is highly recommended to remove it completely even with mucosal stripping only [7, 21].

18.8.7 Gallbladder and Pancreatic Duplications

These types of duplications are very rare.

Pancreatic duplications are more frequently located in the head of the pancreas (51 %), whereas the remaining ones are placed with the same frequency in the body or the tail. Symptoms and radiologic examinations are the same as with duodenal duplications. Treatments include duplication excision, cystojejunostomy, pancreaticoduodenectomy, or partial pancreatectomy; the differential diagnosis between pancreatic duplications and pancreatic pseudocysts can be made with a histological examination [8, 14].

Gallbladder duplications look like double gallbladders and duplicated cystic ducts. According to Boyden's classification, gallbladders may share a common cystic duct (vesica fellea divisa or bilobed gallbladder) or more frequently may have two cystic ducts (vesica fellea duplex or true duplication); the true duplication is subclassified into "H-shaped type," in which two separate gallbladders and cystic ducts enter separately into the common bile duct, and "Y-shaped type," where the two cystic ducts unite before entering into the common bile duct [22]. The clinical presentation can be like an acute cholecystitis or may include bleeding due to the presence of heterotopic gastric mucosa. The diagnosis of gallbladder duplication is often made intraoperatively. ERCP and intraoperative cholangiography are the most accurate tests in displaying the biliary tract anatomy of gallbladder duplications and have been recommended to define the biliary tract anatomy clearly before surgical intervention. Simultaneous removal of both gallbladders by both open and laparoscopic techniques is recommended to avoid cholecystitis and symptomatic gallstones in the remaining organ [6, 7].

18.8.8 Small Bowel Duplications

They are the most common intestinal duplications (50–53 % of all duplications). The most common location is the ileum. They may be the noncommunicating cystic type or the tubular type, frequently communicating, and are located on the mesenteric side. A third of the duplications is diagnosed in the neonatal period, and in about 70 % of the cases, the onset is within the first two years of life. The clinical picture can include a palpable mass, recurrent abdominal pain, or symptoms secondary to a complication such as intussusception, volvulus, small bowel obstruction, peptic ulcer, and perforation due to the presence of ectopic gastric mucosa. If not diagnosed prenatally, radiological investigations to be performed postnatally include an abdominal ultrasound, which can show the typical cystic aspect of duplications with "double layer" and can be sufficient to diagnose a duplication; the technetium-99m pertechnetate scintigraphy in patients who have bleeding, which ensures a differential diagnosis with Meckel's diverticulum; and CT scan and MRI in case of diagnostic doubts. The differential diagnosis includes mesenteric or omental cyst, ovarian cyst, and Meckel's diverticulum, which is conversely located on the antimesenteric side of the bowel [5, 6, 8, 14].

The diagnosis is frequently intraoperative. Recently, laparoscopy has been suggested as a diagnostic and therapeutic method as it reduces hospitalization and post-surgery pain; in small intestinal duplications, a video-assisted procedure may be performed because the bowel is easily extracted from the umbilicus (Fig. 18.5). In laparoscopic procedure, the patient is in a supine lithotomic position. An umbilical trocar for the optic is inserted; a 5 mm is usually used for small bowel and cecal duplications, while a 10 mm Hasson-type trocar is recommended for video-assisted procedure. Two or more 3–5 mm instrumental ports are introduced to create a triangulation of the instruments; in the video-assisted procedure, only one instrumental trocar is necessary, usually positioned in the left flank. Pneumoperitoneum is created (8–10 mmHg of pressure, 0.5–1 lt/min of flow). The procedure is performed in a laparoscopic way in the gastric, duodenal, and colonic duplications, while in the small intestinal duplication, a video-assisted procedure may be used. Small intestinal cystic duplications can be enucleated without resection of the adjacent bowel, according to the principles of Li and colleagues (see above). If it is not possible, a resection of both duplications and native bowel after ligation and division of associated mesenteric vessels with primary end-to-end anastomosis can be performed [16, 17, 20, 21].

Very long tubular duplications represent a greater surgical challenge for the high risk of short bowel syndrome secondary to massive resection. The extramucosal dissection envisages the stripping of the mucosal lining through a series of longitudinal seromuscular incisions and the resection of the two ends of the duplication, which usually communicate and are possible sites of bleeding ulcers due to the presence of ectopic gastric mucosa [18, 19]; this operation may be performed by video-assisted procedure (Fig. 18.6) [21]. Alternatively, a marsupialization with creation of a large window proximally and distally between the duplication and the adjacent intestinal lumen may be performed to allow the drainage of the duplication, however, with the risk of retained gastric mucosa. During surgery it is important to check the whole bowel in order to exclude the presence of multiple lesions and any association in the newborn period with intestinal atresia or malrotation.

18.8.9 Hindgut Duplications

Colonic and rectal duplications account for about 16–20 % of all duplications. The hindgut duplication may be classified in three types. The first type is the cystic or short tubular duplication, frequently located in the mesenteric side, with clinical and imaging features similar to the small bowel duplications. The second type includes the mass located in the midline, in front of the sacrum or coccyx, and behind the rectum; they are usually cystic masses that frequently share the rectum vascularization and can be difficult to remove. The last type is the side-to-side rectal and

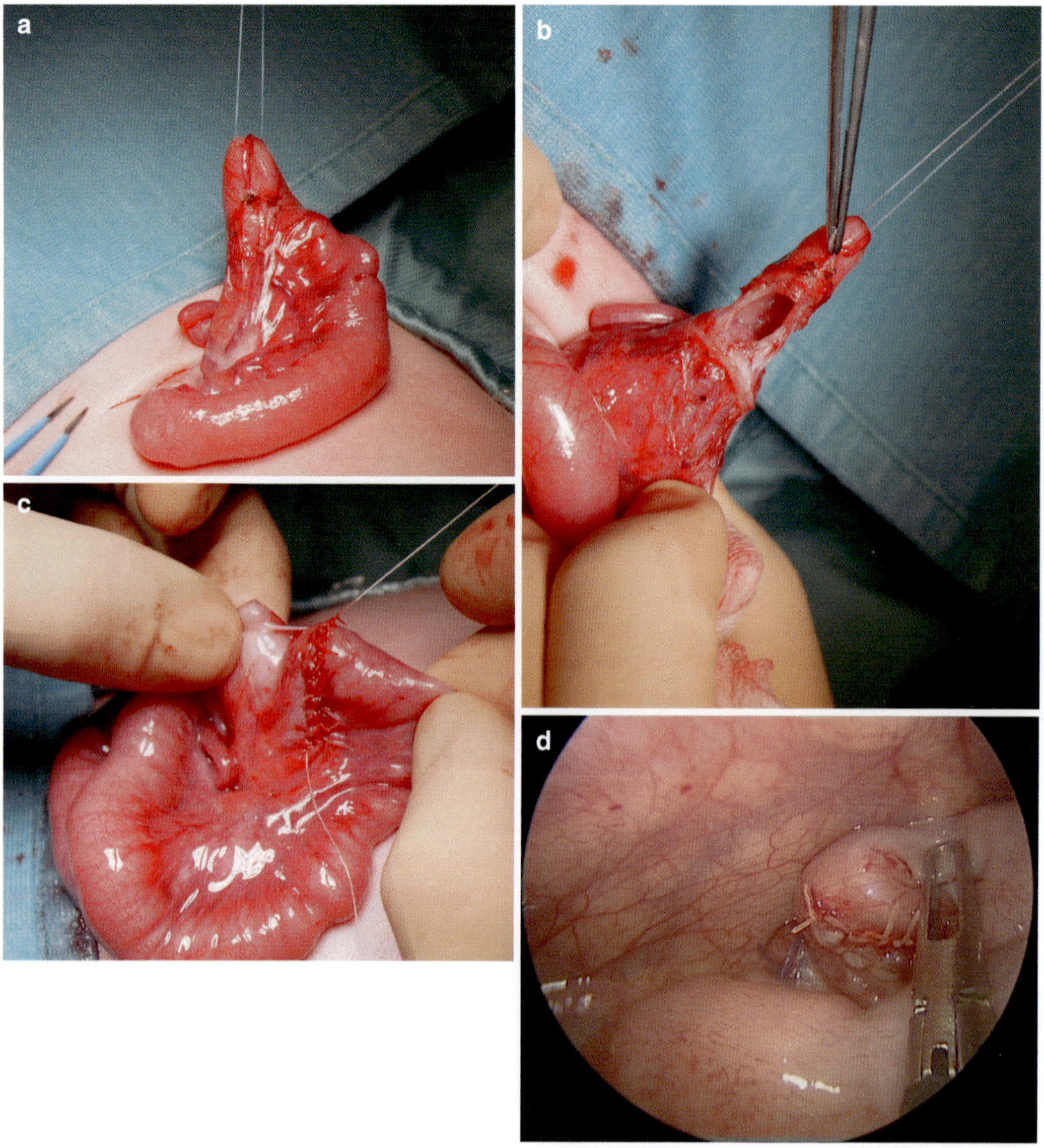

Fig. 18.5 Video-assisted procedure for small intestinal duplications. (**a**) After laparoscopic identification of the ileal duplication, the ileum is exteriorized through the umbilical wound. (**b**) The small intestinal cystic duplication is enucleated in an open way without a need of resection of the adjacent bowel. (**c**) The residual muscular defect is repaired. (**d**) At the end of the procedure, a laparoscopic control is performed to check the suture or anastomosis and to exclude bleeding

colonic duplication; they are tubular, located on the mesenteric or antimesenteric side, and usually communicate with the intestinal lumen; they can develop throughout the entire colon and open up in the perineum. The last type is twice more frequent in females and may be associated with rectogenital or rectourinary fistula, duplication of internal or external genitalia, or vertebral anomalies (abortive twinning anomalies). The clinical picture varies and includes abdominal pain, constipation, and obstruction symptoms; in the case of urogenital fistula, gas or stool can pass through the vagina or with urine; urinary obstruction or retention and bleeding are very rare symptoms. Rectal duplications are typically the cystic type and located in the retrorectal space. They can

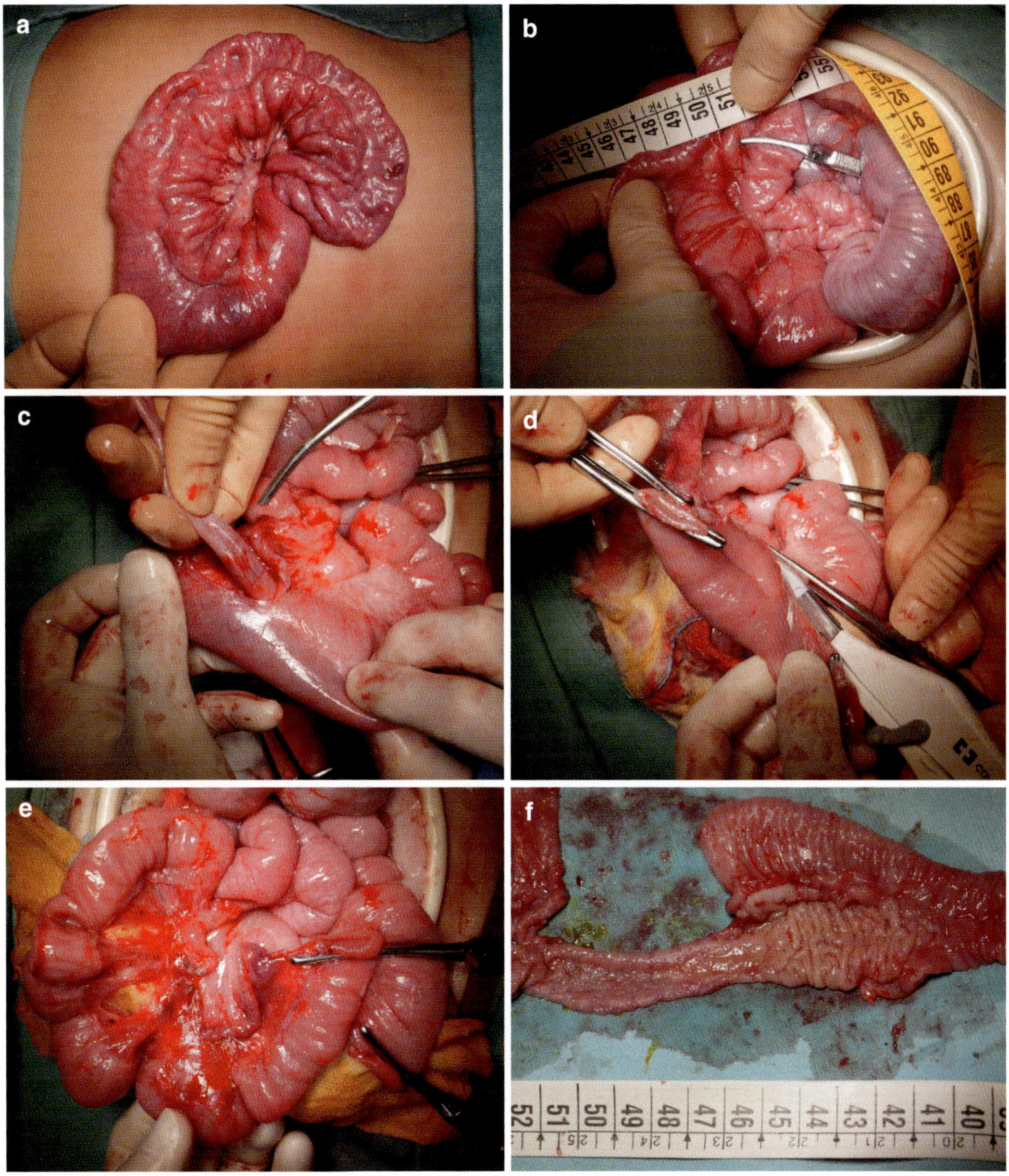

Fig. 18.6 Surgical approach for long tubular duplications. (**a**) After laparoscopic identification of the long tubular duplication, the ileum is extracted through the umbilical wound, using an Alexis retractor. (**b**) The resection of the entire tubular duplication can lead to short bowel syndrome. (**c**) A mucosal stripping is performed. (**d**) The junctions of duplicated and normal bowel are resected, due to the frequent presence of heterotopic gastric mucosa in these sites. (**e**) The ileum aspect at the end of the procedure. (**f**) The duplication aspect after resection (mucosa lining and distal communication segment)

dislocate or compress the rectum, the bladder, or the ureters, thus causing stypsis or fecal incontinence, hydronephrosis, or perianal fistula in the case of communication with the rectal lumen; prolapse is very rare. Other congenital anomalies are rarely associated; the differential diagnosis must be made with ovarian cyst, rhabdomyosarcoma, or sacrococcygeal teratoma. Pelvic ultrasound, barium enema, fistulography, and CT scan or MRI are the investigations that can be performed in order to diagnose hindgut duplications; a voiding cystourethrogram must be performed in the forms with genitourinary fistula [1, 7, 8, 14].

Treatment of colon duplications varies according to their type, extension, and form. Cystic duplications can be removed by enucleation or resection. For tubular duplications the approach consists of resection, if possible, or marsupialization or fenestration, creating a large communication between the duplication and the colon, both proximally and distally, with dissection of the distal part of the duplication, if there is an opening into the perineum or in the urogenital system.

Treatment of rectal duplications varies from exeresis via a sagittal posterior approach or endorectally to marsupialization via a transanal approach up to separation of the septum between the duplication and rectum.

As colon and rectal duplications rarely contain ectopic mucosa, stripping of the mucosa is not usually performed. The incidence of neoplastic changes (mainly adenocarcinoma) in hindgut duplications is anyway higher than in other locations [1, 8, 21].

References

1. Dennis PL (2006) Chapter 88. Alimentary tract duplications. In: Grosfeld JL, Neil JA O, Fonkalsrud EW, Coran AG (eds) Pediatric surgery, vol 1, 6th edn. Mosby Elsevier, Philadelphia, pp 1389–1398
2. Gross RE (1953) Surgery of infancy and childhood. WB Saunders, Philadelphia
3. Ladd WE (1937) Duplications of alimentary tract. South Med J 30:363–371
4. Azzie G, Beasley S (2003) Diagnosis and treatment of foregut duplications. Semin Pediatr Surg 12(1):46–54. Review
5. Iyer CP, Mahour GH (1995) Duplications of the alimentary tract in infants and children. J Pediatr Surg 30(9):1267–1270
6. Schalamon J, Schleef J, Höllwarth ME (2000) Experience with gastro-intestinal duplications in childhood. Langenbecks Arch Surg 385(6):402–405
7. Stern LE, Warner BW (2000) Gastrointestinal duplications. Semin Pediatr Surg 9(3):135–140. Review
8. Puligandla PS, Nguyen LT, St-Vil D, Flageole H, Bensoussan AL, Nguyen VH, Laberge JM (2003) Gastrointestinal duplications. J Pediatr Surg 38(5): 740–744
9. Bremer JL (1944) Diverticula and duplications of the intestinal tract. Arch Pathol 38:132–140
10. Bentley JF, Smith JR (1960) Developmental posterior enteric remnants and spinal malformations: the split notochord syndrome. Arch Dis Child 35:76–86
11. Mellish RW, Koop CE (1961) Clinical manifestations of duplication of the bowel. Pediatrics 27:397–407
12. Randi B, Tursini S, Destro F (2013) Thoracic foregut duplications. In: Lima M (ed) Pediatric endoscopic and minimally invasive surgery. Clueb, Bologna. pp 79–89
13. Ruggeri G, Destro F, Gregori G, Lima M (2013) Foregut duplications. In: Lima M (ed) Pediatric thoracic surgery. Springer, Milan, pp 269–278
14. Macpherson RI (1993) Gastrointestinal tract duplications: clinical, pathologic, etiologic, and radiologic considerations. Radiographics 13(5):1063–1080. Review
15. Li L, Zhang JZ, Wang YX (1998) Vascular classification for small intestinal duplications: experience with 80 cases. J Pediatr Surg 33(8):1243–1245. Review
16. Laje P, Flake AW, Adzick NS (2010) Prenatal diagnosis and postnatal resection of intraabdominal enteric duplications. J Pediatr Surg 45(7):1554–1558
17. Patiño Mayer J, Bettolli M (2014) Alimentary tract duplications in newborns and children: diagnostic aspects and the role of laparoscopic treatment. World J Gastroenterol 20(39):14263–14271
18. Dòmini R, Appignani A, Ceccarelli PL, Lima M (1986) Duplication of the entire small intestine: a case report. Z Kinderchir 41(6):371–374
19. Wrenn EL (2000) Alimentary tract duplications. In: Holder (ed) Pediatric surgery. WB Saunders Co, Philadelphia
20. Lima M, Molinaro F, Ruggeri G, Gargano T, Randi B (2012) Role of mini-invasive surgery in the treatment of enteric duplications in paediatric age: a survey of 15 years. Pediatr Med Chir 34(5):217–222
21. Randi B, Maffi M, Destro F (2013) Intestinal duplications. In: Lima M (ed) Pediatric endoscopic and minimally invasive surgery. Clueb, Bologna. pp 241–252
22. Boyden EA (1926) The accessory gallbladder-an embryological and comparative study of aberrant biliary vesicles occurring in man and domestic mammals. Am J Anast 38:177–231

Meckel's Diverticulum

19

François Varlet, Sophie Vermersch, Nasser Bustangi, Manuel Lopez, and Aurélien Scalabre

19.1 Introduction

Described since 1598 by Wilhelm Fabricius Hildanus, this intestinal diverticulum was known as Meckel's diverticulum (MD) because Johann Friedrich Meckel demonstrated in 1809 in chicken embryos the connection between primitive small bowel and yolk sac, and he was the first to describe the diverticulum as a remnant of the omphalomesenteric or vitelline duct [1]. The MD is the commonest congenital abnormality of the gastrointestinal tract and is present in approximately 1–2% of the population [2–7]. Clinical presentations of MD are extremely wide from total latency to severe complications as obstruction, bleeding, peritonitis, hernia, or tumor. The lifetime risk of complication is estimated around 4–6%, decreasing with age [3]. Of the patients developing complications, 60% are less than 2 years of age and over one third are less than 1 year of age [4]. The preoperative diagnosis remains a challenge, whereas the treatment is nearly codified.

F. Varlet (✉) • S. Vermersch • N. Bustangi
M. Lopez • A. Scalabre
Department of Pediatric Surgery, Centre Hospitalier Universitaire, 42055, Saint-Etienne Cedex 2, France
e-mail: francois.varlet@chuse.fr

19.2 Embryology

As a result of cephalocaudal and lateral folding of the embryo from the 14th day, a portion of the endoderm-lined yolk-sac cavity is incorporated into the embryo to form the primitive gut (Fig. 19.1). Two other portions of the endoderm-lined cavity remain outside the embryo: yolk sac and allantois (Fig. 19.2).

The middle part of the primitive gut, or midgut, remains temporally connected to the yolk sac by the vitelline duct or yolk stalk (Fig. 19.3). Progressively, the vitelline duct regresses and disappears between fifth and eighth weeks, but sometimes its total or partial persistence induces omphalomesenteric abnormalities: fistula, band, cyst, sinus, and diverticulum. The diverticulum, corresponding to a failure of regression of the intestinal part of the duct, is named MD.

Then the intraembryonic portion of the MD, future basis of the diverticulum, comes from the midgut, and the extraembryonic portion corresponds to the tip of the diverticulum coming from the yolk-sac components. The yolk-sac cells are pluripotent and can produce a non-ileal mucosa or heterotopic tissue, as gastric, duodenal, or pancreatic mucosa, with a risk of complications, especially bleeding when gastric or pancreatic tissues are present [8–10]. This hypothesis can account for the reason that the distal part of MD is the most likely to contain ectopic mucosa. According to Mukai, when the MD is long, with a height-to-diameter (HD) ratio

M. Lima (ed.), *Pediatric Digestive Surgery*, DOI 10.1007/978-3-319-40525-4_19

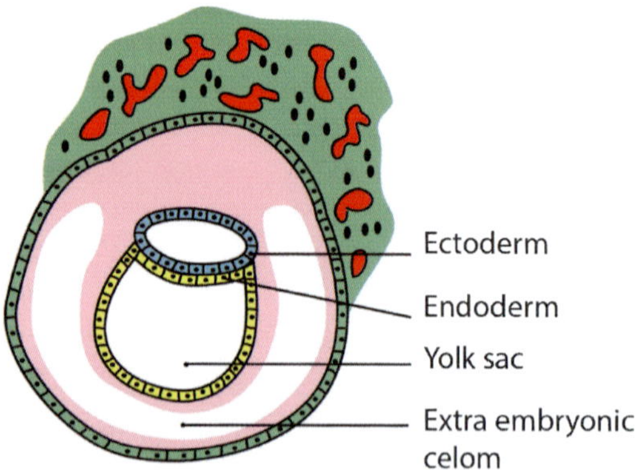

Fig. 19.1 Embryo day 13

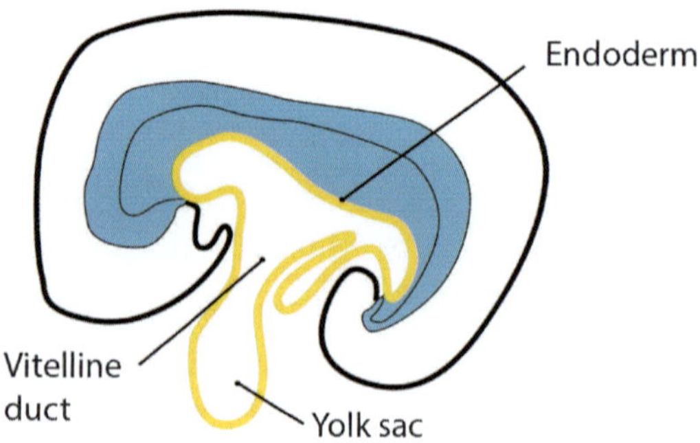

Fig. 19.2 Embryo day 28

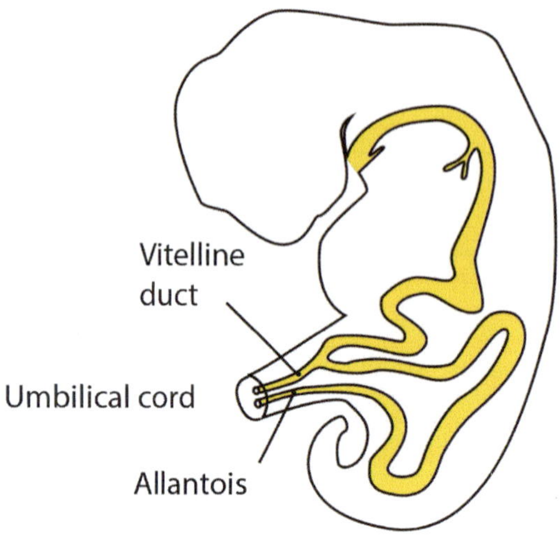

Fig. 19.3 Embryo day 35

upper than 1.6, the ectopic mucosa is only in the tip of MD, while short diverticula (less than 1.6 HD ratio) have ectopic tissue in almost all areas [9, 10].

19.3 Anatomy and Histology

MD is unique on the antimesenteric border and located at the end of superior mesenteric artery, when intestinal vascular arcades are replaced by straight arteries, and MD is usually supplied by the vitellointestinal artery originating from the ileal branches of superior mesenteric artery. MD is a true diverticulum localized to within 100 cm from ileocecal valve and composed of normal intestinal wall. Its form is usually vermicular, but sometimes its basis is spread out. Most of MD appear as a 3–5 cm fingerlike structure, but occasionally present less than 2 cm long or as a larger saccular lesion with 5–10 cm diameter. The diverticulum can be laid on a side of the mesentery, and during a bowel examination, it is mandatory to explore the two sides of the mesentery to avoid a missed MD. Another type of MD is the "inverted diverticulum," where the fingerlike structure is inside the bowel. MD is free in the peritoneal cavity in 73.8 % [11] or fixed by a congenital band to the umbilicus or to the mesentery of terminal ileum; this can lead small bowel obstruction with or without volvulus.

MD has an ileal mucosa, but heterotopic mucosa can be found, and then 80–85 % of the ectopic tissue is gastric mucosa, sometimes associated with pancreatic tissue. Isolated pancreatic tissue or duodenal mucosa can be present in MD. Heterotopic tissue is usually identified in symptomatic diverticula, but it can be present in asymptomatic MD. From a series of 583 patients with symptomatic MD reported in 1978, 93 had heterotopic tissue within the diverticulum, especially gastric mucosa (65/93, 69.8 %) and pancreatic tissue (22/93, 23.5 %) [12]. Another series reported 71 heterotopic tissues from 180 symptomatic MD in adult patients (39.4 %), with 59 gastric mucosa (83.1 %) and 9 pancreatic tissues (12.6 %) [13]. Nevertheless, the histology from 806 resected asymptomatic MD in adult was gastric tissue in 67 (8.3 %), pancreatic tissue in 22 (2.7 %), carcinoid tumor in 17 (2.1 %), diverticulitis in 26 (3.2 %), other pathology findings in 16 (2 %), and no abnormalities in 658 (81.6 %). Then, the presence of gastric and pancreatic tissue in MD is predictive to complications, especially bleeding [8, 9]. No relationship to *Helicobacter pylori* "gastritis" and bleeding was demonstrated [14].

19.4 Epidemiology

MD is the most prevalent congenital anomaly of the alimentary tract. The rule of two traditionally describes its characteristics, such as a prevalence rate of 2 % in the general population, a male-to-female ratio of 2:1, an incidence rate of 2 % for symptomatic MD, the presence of symptoms before the age of 2 years, a location at a distance of 2 ft to the ileocecal valve, a diverticular length of 2 in., and two types of common ectopic tissues [15].

From autopsy studies, a MD was found in 386 autopsies of 31,499 performed, resulting in a prevalence of 1.23 %, and the current mortality from MD was 0.001 % [16]. From the Pediatric Hospital Information System (PHIS) database in the United States, there were 2389 children with a diagnosis code of MD over a 9-year period (2004–2012) from 4,338,396 children admitted during the study interval (1/1816). Among them, 945 children had a symptomatic MD (1/4590 hospital admissions) [17]. The incidence decreased with age: 56.4 % were under 6 years of age, 26.8 % between 6 and 12 years of age, and 16.8 % were older than 12 years of age. In this study, 74 % were male with a male-to-female ratio of 3:1 [18]. This prevalence confirms the male-to-female ratio for symptomatic MD in the pediatric population reported previously, between 2 and 3:1 [12, 13, 18]. The ratio is similar for asymptomatic MD [13]. Caucasians are overrepresented (63.4 %), while African-Americans were disproportionately less often affected (16.4 %) in the study population [17].

Male predisposition is observed in peptic ulcer disease which may share a similar pathogenesis with bleeding MD. CDX2 is a homeobox transcription factor, and recent studies demonstrated a close relationship between lack of CDX2 expression and differentiation of ectopic gastric tissues in MD. In addition, methylation of CDX2 with downregulation of gene expression is found to be increased in males. Then, sex and specific gene expression may be involved in embryonic gut differentiation into ectopic gastric mucosa and activity of gastric gland cells. More studies are required to confirm this hypothesis, but it seems interesting in trying to explain the male prevalence [19–21].

19.5 Clinical Manifestations

The risk of developing a complication from a MD should be about 4 % between 0 and 5 years of age. The most common presentations of symptomatic MD are obstruction, intussusception, bleeding, and diverticulitis (Table 19.1).

Table 19.1 Meckel's diverticulum complications

	Yamaguchi (1978) [12]	Grapin (1990) [5]	Kusumoto (1992) [18]	Park (2005) [13] <11 year	>11 year	Total	%
Bleeding	71	599	215	18	69	972	*29.8*
Obstruction	219	275	146	11	37	766	*23.5*
Volvulus	19		42	8	9		
Intussusception	82	201	98	4	10	395	*12.1*
Non-perforated diverticulitis	76	440	47	10	32	758	*23.2*
Perforated diverticulitis	44		84	7	18		
Littré hernia	28	200	12		2	242	*7.4*
Umbilical pathology	10	57				67	*2.1*
Tumor	19	34	8		3	64	*1.9*
Total	568	1806	652	238		3264	100

Table 19.2 Meckel's diverticulum obstructions

	Yamaguchi [12]	Kusumoto [18]	Park [13]	Total	%
Obstruction	219	146	48	413	60.3
Intussusception	82	98	14	194	28.3
Volvulus	19	42	17	78	11.4
Total	320	286	79	685	100

Intestinal obstruction is the most common complication and was found in 35.6 % of patients, children and adults, due to inflammation, congenital band between the umbilicus and MD or mesodiverticular band and MD (60.3 %), intussusception (28.3 %), or volvulus (11.4 %) (Table 19.2). They are found out during the operation, and in the case of late diagnosis, a small bowel ischemia can require resection concerning sometimes about 1 meter long, with a risk of a postoperative malabsorption. Usually intussusception on MD leads to a severe obstruction and is difficult to reduce, even during surgical procedure.

Rectal bleeding is the second most common symptom (29.8 %). Bleeding can present as hematochezia and melena or, rarely in child, with occult blood loss. Most often, hemorrhage can be brisk presenting with painless bright red blood in stools with or without hypovolemia. The rate of hemoglobin at admission is often lower than 8 mg/dL and requires transfusion frequently [6]. Such cases are usually associated with a MD containing ectopic gastric or pancreatic mucosa with peptic ulceration. Every hematochezia should call forth MD in children.

Peritoneal symptoms or peritonitis can disclose a MD (23.2 %) and the diagnosis of appendicitis is often done. In case of normal appendix during sonography, CT scan, or surgical procedure, the search of MD is mandatory.

In 7.4 % of cases, the child has an inguinal hernia (Littré hernia), and its painless and nonreducible characters have to catch the eye because adhesions between MD and processus vaginalis are frequent. But the diagnosis is most often done during an operation for hernia.

Umbilical flow may reveal a patent omphalomesenteric duct (2.1 %), especially when a failure of cauterization occurs. Then a MD has to be looked for as when there is umbilical sinus or granuloma.

Uncommonly, presentations are enterolith or foreign body within MD [12, 22]. Tumors of MD are also rare in children as leiomyoma, desmoplastic tumor, or lymphoma [23–25].

19.6 Imaging and Diagnosis of MD

The preoperative diagnosis of MD is uncommon, and this is often an intraoperative discovery during treatment of small bowel obstruction, intussusception, or peritonitis. Yamaguchi et al. reported that preoperative diagnosis was done in only 34 of 600 patients (5.6 %) in 1978 [12]. But now MD is more often evocated in the preoperative period with improvement of imaging [26, 27].

Plain radiographs are not usually helpful in making the diagnosis of MD, and they are normal in the majority or show nonspecific signs such as small bowel obstruction or perforation. Uncommonly, enteroliths may be seen on plain film, typically triangular and flat, but they are not specific and can be identified in other pathologies: appendicitis, intestinal tubular duplication, urolithiasis or within ovarian dermoid cyst.

Ultrasound is not the most sensitive radiologic examination but can help when a Meckel's diverticulitis occurs. Nevertheless, in a series of ten patients with diverticulitis who underwent preoperative ultrasound, six were wrongly diagnosed with appendicitis [28].

Contrast studies can detect a MD, and the classical appearance is a blind-ending tubular or saccular structure arising from the antimesenteric border of the distal ileum. The base of MD is spotted by a "mucosal triangular plateau" when the bowel is distended and by a triradiate fold pattern when the bowel is collapsed. Sometimes, mucosal irregularity may be noted, due to ectopic gastric mucosa or filling defects from clots in a bleeding MD. This barium enema seems a less sensitive investigation than small bowel enema, or enteroclysis, for detection of MD, but needs to intubate the duodenum with discomfort and increases the radiation dose [26, 27]. A study reviewing 415 enteroclysis included 13 patients who had a confirmed histological diagnosis of MD, and 11 were correctly identified on enteroclysis with only one false-positive result [29]. In a Japanese study, about 776 patients included 118 barium enemas, 55 (47 %) had a correct diagnosis of MD, but they seem more useful in adult than in pediatric population [18].

CT scan is very useful in diagnosing and assessing the MD complications, particularly for intra-abdominal abscess, obstruction, perforation, or tumor. From 40 patients with MD reported recently (8 children and 32 adults), 26 were asymptomatic and 14 symptomatic. MD was detected on CT scan in 11 of 26 asymptomatic patients (42.3 %) and in 8 of 14 symptomatic patients (57.1 %) presenting small bowel obstruction, diverticulitis, hernia, or bleeding. The amount of peritoneal flat at the level of MD was related to its detection [30]. CT scan is able to identify bleeding from a MD with active extravasation of intravenously injected contrast medium [31]. Recent studies have suggested that CT scan enterography is a useful method for diagnosis of MD [32].

Mesenteric angiography can be used to investigate gastrointestinal hemorrhage with a MD. In the absence of bleeding, a MD can be recognized by demonstrating a persistent vitellointestinal artery [26]. In a study of 16 patients with bleeding, the feeding vitellointestinal artery was identified in 11 of the patients [33]. Angiodysplasia associated with MD was reported, and this association is important to know because it may cause further gastrointestinal bleeding following MD resection [34].

MRI is not yet used for diagnosis of MD and the experience with it remains limited. MR enteroclysis is an alternative to CT enteroclysis and has been used to successfully identify a MD [35]. The advantages are to reduce the dose of ionizing radiation and to evaluate small bowel function through MR fluoroscopy [36].

Technetium 99m pertechnetate scintigraphy is known to accumulate in the mucin-secreting cells in the gastric mucosa, and it is used to visualize symptomatic MD which often contains heterotopic gastric epithelium. The sensitivity of technetium 99m pertechnetate scintigraphy is 85 % in children, decreasing to 54 % in adults [13, 37]. The sensitivity can be increased by administering pentagastrin, glucagon, or H2 antagonist or by imaging with single-photon emission computed tomography (SPECT) allowing a better localization of MD. The reported incidence of ectopic mucosa in MD varies from 15 to 50 %, according to the number of non-symptomatic incidental cases included in each series. False-positive results are due to the presence of ectopic gastric mucosa elsewhere in the bowel, such as duodenal or jejunal duplication, intussusception, volvulus, inflammatory bowel disease as ulcerative colitis, or Crohn's disease, and in postoperative patients [38]. False-negative results are frequent due to the absence of ectopic gastric mucosa, but other causes have been identified such as the presence of barium from previous radiological examination which can attenuate gamma radiation, and then scintigraphy should not be performed if there is residual contrast medium within the abdomen [39]. Sometimes, it is also possible to have abundant gastric mucosa in a MD with a negative scintigraphy because technetium 99m pertechnetate is taken up by specific cells within gastric mucosa, especially fundic mucosa, not always present when only antral mucosa is within the MD [40]. Then, repeat technetium 99m pertechnetate scintigraphy can improve the results with appropriate preparation [41]. Despite these results, technetium 99m pertechnetate scintigraphy remains helpful in evaluating patients with a suspected MD, especially in children with evidence of gastrointestinal bleeding. Recently, the sensitivity and specificity for ectopic gastric mucosa were reported as 94 and 97 %, respectively [42]. Scintigraphy with tagged red blood cells to detect active hemorrhage may be also useful in detecting and localizing a bleeding MD, but it is not specific [26, 27].

Capsule endoscopy is another alternative in the investigation of non-identified intestinal bleeding, but requires further experience because only a few isolated cases have been reported in this indication [43]. In adult series of 47 patients with obscure gastrointestinal bleeding, the capsule endoscopy showed the source of bleeding in 74.4 % of all patients, and only one had a MD [44]. A potential complication may be the retention of capsule within the MD or in their digestive tract, but the risk is low, about 1 % [45].

Double-balloon enteroscopy seems to get a good visualization of bleeding Meckel's diverticulum and can be associated with minimal invasive surgery; 14 children were diagnosed and treated by such management with success [46].

In summary, the widespread utilization of various imaging modalities has led to a worked improvement in preoperative diagnosis of MD. CT scan and technetium 99m pertechnetate scintigraphy remain the principal imaging means. CT or MR enterography and direct visualization by endoscopic techniques will be developed in the future.

19.7 Treatment

The treatment of a symptomatic MD is resection. Conventional surgical management has been laparotomy for diverticulectomy, wedge excision or segmental ileal resection, and anastomosis. During the past decades, there has been a tremendous development of minimal invasive surgery in children, and the number of reports on laparoscopy increased dramatically, demonstrating good efficiency for diagnosis and treatment of MD, shorter hospitalization, less postoperative pain, and good cosmetic results [47–49].

Concerning surgical procedure, the aim is to remove all the diverticulum with all the heterotopic gastric or pancreatic mucosa to avoid recurrence of bleeding particularly. Then the safer procedure is segmental ileal resection and anastomosis. Wedge resection is less used because postoperative stenoses were described. But diverticulectomy has also been shown to have lower morbidity than segmental resection [50]. The external appearance of MD can help to choose the surgical procedure according to the HD ratio. When the MD is long, with a HD ratio upper than 1.6, heterotopic mucosa is not in the proximal part of the diverticulum, close to the ileum, and a diverticulectomy can be performed safely. When the MD is short with a risk of heterotopic mucosa close to the ileum or spreading within the ileum, ileal resection is required [9, 10]. These criteria seem to be convincing. Macroscopic thickening could indicate the presence of heterotopic mucosa, but Varcoe et al. demonstrated it has only 54 % chance of containing gastric or pancreatic tissues, making this an unacceptable method of detection [10].

Laparoscopic approach is now well admitted and two laparoscopic procedures can be performed. The first one is the three-port procedure allowing a good exploration of small bowel, diagnosis, and treatment of MD inside the peritoneal cavity or outside through the umbilicus. The second procedure is single-incision laparoscopic surgery (SILS), also called trans-umbilical laparoscopic-assisted approach, where a 10 mm lens with operative channel allows an overview of the peritoneal cavity. Sometimes the MD is identified quickly and can be grasped and delivered through the umbilicus. When it is not possible, one or two other ports are required, in left and right iliac fossa. An important issue of this extracorporeal technique is the enlargement of the umbilical opening before MD delivery to allow easy exteriorization of the bowel and to facilitate the replacement of the bowel in the abdomen, because intestinal edema and congestion frequently occur during time of the anastomosis [49]. Sometimes, the laparoscopic approach cannot be performed and open surgery is required, especially when a small bowel obstruction leads an abdominal distension hindering a good laparoscopic exploration.

Diverticulectomy can be performed extracorporeally or intracorporeally by inserting a linear stapling device along the antimesenteric border when the MD is long. Segmental ileal resection can be done laparoscopically but leads a longer operation, even when performed by skilled laparoscopic surgeons. Finally, extracorporeal resection and anastomosis seem to be more simple and safe [49, 51–56]. The postoperative course is

Table 19.3 Postoperative complications

Author (cases)	Wound infection	Small bowel obstruction	Ileus	Fistula	Intra-abdominal abscess	Other infections	Eventration	Bleedi
St-Vil [6] (164)	1	7	0	1	0	1 septicemia	1	0
Bani-Hani [56] (68)	2	1	1	0	0	0	0	0
Shalaby [52] (33)	0	0	0	0	0	0	0	0
Park [13] (100)	3[a]	7	0	0	1	0	1	1 coliti
Sai Prasad [53] (36)	0	3	0	0	0	0	0	0
Chan [51] (18)	1	0	0	0	0	0	0	0
Alemayehu [54] (14)	0	2	0	0	0	0	0	0
Paparella [49] (17)	0	0	0	0	0	1	0	0
Duan [55] (55)	0	0	0	0	0	0	0	1[b]
Total (505)	*7*	*20*	*1*	*1*	*1*	*2*	*2*	*2*
%	1.38	3.96	0.19	0.19	0.19	0.39	0.39	0.39

[a]Three incidental Meckel's diverticulum during treatment of prostatic or colonic cancer
[b]One bleeding after diverticulectomy

usually uneventful, but complications may occur, especially small bowel obstruction requiring surgery most often (Table 19.3).

An unresolved question is the management of incidental MD. Although many authors classically proposed a resection of incidental MD to avoid future complications [56–58], Soltero et al. first proposed to respect incidental MD, demonstrating that there was only a small chance of an asymptomatic MD causing disease in later life [3]. A selective approach was also recommended for patients in whom the rate of complications is higher, patients younger than 50 years of age, male patients, MD length greater than 2 cm, and detection of an abnormal feature within the diverticulum [13]. But Zani et al. demonstrated from a meta-analysis that 132 of 2975 patients had postoperative complications after incidental MD resection (4.4 %), and they had a significantly higher early complication rate than leaving in situ: 5.3 % of the resected compared with 1.3 % of the nonresected MD. These authors reviewed also four studies which reported long-term follow-up of patients with incidentally detected MD left in situ, and no complications occurred from 91 patients. Moreover, they demonstrated that 758 resections of incidental MD are required to prevent one death. For them, leaving an incidental MD in situ reduces the risk of postoperative complications without increasing late complications, and there is no compelling evidence to support prophylactic resection of incidentally detected MD during surgery, even in young children [16].

When a life-threatening lower gastrointestinal bleeding occurs, emergency mesenteric angiography and embolization of the bleeding point can be performed. This management is only the first step of treatment because a few days after angiography, the risk of bleeding recurrence or small bowel obstruction is high [59, 60]. MD resection remains mandatory in these cases.

Conclusions

MD is a common intestinal abnormality in general population, but finally the risk of complication is low. It is more frequent in male patients. The diagnosis of MD must be called forth in a wide range of abdominal manifestations as pain, obstruction, rectal bleeding, or hernia.

Technetium 99m pertechnetate scintigraphy and CT scan can detect the diverticulum, but there are false-positive and false-negative results. Still today, the surgical indication is often set without the diagnosis of MD, and it is identified during the operation, especially when a small bowel obstruction occurs. Laparoscopic-assisted diverticulectomy and segmental ileal resection are the main procedures to treat MD, but open surgery is sometimes mandatory. When incidental MD is identified, no prophylactic resection is recommended today.

References

1. Meckel JF (1809) Uber die divertikel am darmkanal. Arch Physiol 9:421–453
2. Rambaud P, Varloteaux CH, Bessard G (1974) Le diverticule de Meckel chez l'enfant. Med Infant 5:445–451
3. Soltero MJ, Bill AH (1976) The natural history of Meckel's diverticulum found in King County, Washington, over a fifteen year period. Am J Surg 132:168–173
4. Benson CD (1979) Surgical implications of Meckel's diverticulum. In: Ravitch MM, Welch KJ, Benson CD, Aberdeen E, Randolph JG (eds) Pediatric Surgery. 3rd edn. Year Book Medical Publishers, Inc, Chicago/London, pp 955–960
5. Grapin C (1990) Diverticule de Meckel et pathologie omphalomésentérique. In: P Hélardot, J Bienaymé, F Bargy (eds) Chirurgie Digestive de l'Enfant. Doin Edn, Paris, pp 449–461
6. St-Vil D, Brandt ML, Panic S et al (1991) Meckel's diverticulum in children: a 20-year review. J Pediatr Surg 26:1289–1292
7. Carlioz P (2007) Le diverticule de Meckel. De l'embryologie à la chirurgie. Sauramps Medical. Montpellier
8. Sadler TW (1995) Langman's medical embryology, 7th edn. Williams & Wilkins, Baltimore, pp 242–271
9. Mukai M, Takamatsu H, Noguchi H, Fukushige T, Tahara H, Kaji T (2002) Does external appearance of a Meckel's diverticulum assist in choice of the laparoscopic procedure? Pediatr Surg Int 18:231–233
10. Varcoe RL, Wong SW, Taylor CF, Newstead GL (2004) Diverticulectomy is inadequate treatment for short Meckel's diverticulum with heterotopic mucosa. ANZ J Surg 74:869–872
11. Soderlund S (1959) Meckel's diverticulum. A clinical and histologic study. Acta Chir Scand Suppl Suppl 248:1–233
12. Yamaguchi M, Takeuchi S, Awazu S (1978) Meckel's diverticulum. Investigation of 600 patients in Japanese literature. Am J Surg 136:247–249
13. Park JJ, Wolff BG, Tollefson MK, Walsh EE, Larson DR (2005) Meckel diverticulum. The Mayo Clinic experience with 1476 patients (1950-2002). Ann Surg 241:529–533
14. Finn LS, Christie DL (2001) Helicobacter pylori and Meckel's diverticula. J Pediatr Gastroenterol Nutr 32:150–155
15. Poley JR, Thielen TE, Pence JC (2009) Bleeding Meckel's diverticulum in a 4-month-old infant: treatment with laparoscopic diverticulectomy. A case report and review of the literature. Clin Exp Gastroenterol 2:37–40
16. Zani A, Eaton S, Rees CM, Pierro A (2008) Incidentally detected Meckel diverticulum. To resect or not to resect? Ann Surg 247:276–281
17. Alemayehu H, Hall M, Desai AA, St. Peter S, Snyder CL (2014) Demographic disparities of children presenting with symptomatic Meckel's diverticulum in children hospitals. Pediatr Surg Int 30:649–653
18. Kusumoto H, Yoshida M, Takahashi I, Anai H, Maehara Y, Sugimachi K (1992) Complications and diagnosis of Meckel's diverticulum in 776 patients. Am J Surg 164:382–383
19. Martin E, Vanier M, Tavian M et al (2010) CDX2 in congenital gut gastric-type heteroplasia and intestinal-type Meckel diverticula. Pediatrics 126:e723–e727
20. Huang CC, Lai MW, Hwang FM et al (2014) Diverse presentations in pediatric Meckel's diverticulum: a review of 100 cases. Pediatr Neonatol 55:369–375
21. Yuasa Y, Nagasaki H, Akiyama Y et al (2005) Relationship between CDX2 gene methylation and dietary factors in gastric cancer patients. Carcinogenesis 26:193–200
22. Clark JK, Paz DA, Ghahremani GG (2014) Imaging of Meckel's diverticulum in adults: pictorial essay. Clin Imaging 38:557–564
23. Calone P, Rivosecchi M (1978) Tumors of Meckel's diverticulum. Minerva Chir 33:487–492
24. Al-Dabbagh AI, Salih SA (1985) Primary lymphoma of Meckel's diverticulum. J Surg Oncol 28:17–20
25. Qureshi SS, Ramadnar MR, Viswanatham S et al (2007) Desmoplastic small round cell tumor in Meckel's diverticulum. J Clin Oncol 25:3372–3374
26. Thurley PD, Halliday KE, Somers JM, Al-Daraji WI, Ilyas M, Broderick NJ (2009) Radiological features of Meckel's diverticulum and its complications. Clin Radiol 64:109–118
27. Kotha VK, Khandelwal A, Saboo SS et al (2014) Radiologist's perspective for the Meckel's diverticulum and its complications. Br J Radiol 87:20130743
28. Baldisserotto M, Maffazzoni DR, Dora MD (2003) Sonographic findings of Meckel's diverticulitis in children. AJR Am J Roentgenol 180:425–428
29. Malginte DDT, Elmore MF, Isenberg M, Dolan PA (1980) Meckel diverticulum: radiologic demonstra-

tion by enteroclysis. AJR Am J Roentgenol 134: 925–932
30. Kawamoto S, Raman SP, Blackford A, Hruban RH, Fishman EK (2015) CT detection of symptomatic and asymptomatic Meckel diverticulum. AJR Am J Roentgenol 205:281–291
31. Danzer D, Gervaz P, Platon A, Poletti PA (2003) Bleeding Meckel's diverticulum diagnosis: an unusual indication for computed tomography. Abdom Imaging 28:631–633
32. Elsayes KM, Menias CO, Harvin HJ, Francis IR (2007) Imaging manifestations of Meckel's diverticulum. AJR Am J Roentgenol 189:81–88
33. Mitchell AW, Spencer J, Allison DJ, Jackson JE (1998) Meckel's diverticulum: angiographic findings in 16 patients. AJR Am J Roentgenol 170:1329–1333
34. Katz MD, Teitelbaum GP (1991) Angiodysplasia associated with Meckel's diverticulum: case report. Cardiovasc Intervent Radiol 14:188–190
35. Akman C, Korman U, Ogut G et al (2005) A combination of small bowel imaging methods: conventional enteroclysis with complementary magnetic resonance enteroclysis. Clin Radiol 60:778–786
36. Umschaden HW, Gasser J (2003) MR enteroclysis. Radiol Clin North Am 41:231–248
37. Sfakianakis GN, Conway JJ (1981) Detection of ectopic gastric mucosa in Meckel's diverticulum and in other aberrations by scintigraphy. 1. Pathophysiology and 10-year clinical experience. J Nucl Med 22:647–654
38. Diamond IR, Hayes-Jordan A, Phillips MJ, Langer JC (2008) Crohn's disease in a Meckel's diverticulum: report of a case. Pediatr Surg Int 24:361–363
39. Kiratli PO, Aksoy T, Bozkurt MF, Ohran D (2009) Detection of ectopic gastric mucosa using 99^{m}Tc pertechnetate: review of literature. Ann Nucl Med 23:97–105
40. Ariga M, Suga K, Matsunaga N et al (2001) Failure to detect a huge Meckel's diverticulum with abundant ectopic gastric mucosa on gastric mucosal scintigraphy with Tc-99m pertechnetate. Clin Nucl Med 26:470–471
41. Vali R, Daneman A, McQuattie S, Shammas A (2015) The value of repeat scintigraphy in patients with high clinical suspicion for Meckel diverticulum after a negative or equivocal first Meckel scan. Pediatr Radiol 45:1506–1514
42. Sinha CK, Pallewatte A, Easty M et al (2013) Meckel's scan in children: a review of 183 cases referred to two paediatric surgery specialist centres over 18 years. Pediatr Surg Int 29:511–517
43. Desai SS, Alkhouri R, Baker SS (2012) Identification of Meckel's diverticulum by capsule endoscopy. J Pediatr Gastroenterol Nutr 54:161
44. Hartmann D, Schmidt H, Bolz G et al (2005) A prospective two-center study comparing wireless capsule endoscopy with intraoperative enteroscopy in patients with obscure bleeding. Gastrointest Endosc 61:826–832
45. Mylonaki M, MacLean D, Fritscher-Ravens A, Swain P (2002) Wireless capsule endoscopic detection of Meckel's diverticulum after nondiagnostic surgery. Endoscopy 34:1018–1020
46. Qi S, Huang H, Wei D, Lv C, Yang Y (2015) Diagnosis and minimally invasive surgical treatment of bleeding Meckel's diverticulum in children using double-balloon enteroscopy. J Pediatr Surg 50:1610–1612
47. Valla JS, Steyaert H, Leculée R, Peybere B, Jordana F (1998) Meckel's diverticulum and laparoscopy of children. What's new? Eur J Pediatr Surg 8:26–28
48. Chan KW, Lee KH, Mou JW, Cheung ST, Tam YH (2008) Laparoscopic management of complicated Meckel's diverticulum in children: a 10-year review. Surg Endosc 22:1509–1512
49. Paparella A, Nino F, Noviello C et al (2014) Laparoscopic approach to Meckel's diverticulum. World J Gastroenterol 20:8173–8178
50. Pinero A, Martinez-Barba E, Canteras M, Rodriguez JM, Castellanos G, Parilla P (2002) Surgical management and complications of Meckel's diverticulum in 90 patients. Eur J Surg 168:8–12
51. Chan KW, Lee KH, Wong HYV et al (2014) Laparoscopic excision of Meckel's diverticulum in children: what is the current evidence? World J Gastroenterol 20:15158–15162
52. Shalaby RY, Soliman SM, Fawy M, Samaha A (2005) Laparoscopic management of Meckel's diverticulum in children. J Pediatr Surg 40:562–567
53. Sai Prasad TR, Chui CH, Singaporewalla FR et al (2007) Meckel's diverticular complications in children: is laparoscopy the order of the day? Pediatr Surg Int 23:141–147
54. Alemayehu H, Stringel G, Lo IJ, Golden J, Pandya S, McBride W, Muensterer O (2014) Laparoscopy and complicated Meckel diverticulum in children. JSLS 18:e2014.00015
55. Duan X, Ye G, Bian H et al (2015) Laparoscopic vs. laparoscopically assisted management of Meckel's diverticulum in children. Int J Clin Exp Med 8:94–100
56. Bani-Hani KE, Shatnawi NJ (2004) Meckel's diverticulum: comparison of incidental and symptomatic cases. World J Surg 28:917–920
57. Cullen JJ, Kelly KA, Moir CR (1994) Surgical management of Meckel's diverticulum. An epidemiologic population-based study. Ann Surg 220:564–568
58. Arnold JF, Pellicane JV (1997) Meckel's diverticulum: a ten-year experience. Am Surg 63:354–355
59. Bevernage C, Maleux G, De Hertogh G, Miserez M (2010) Life-threatening lower gastrointestinal bleeding in a 2-year-old boy treated by transcatheter embolization: uncommon features of a complicated Meckel diverticulum. Pediatr Radiol 40:1702–1705
60. De Beule T, Op de Beeck K, De Hertogh G, Sergeant G, Maleux G (2014) CT diagnosis of a post-embolization ischemic diverticulitis of Meckel. Acta Radiol Short Rep 3:2047981614531954

20 Acute Appendicitis

Michela Maffi and Mario Lima

20.1 Introduction

Acute appendicitis is the most common cause for emergency abdominal surgery in children. Early diagnosis and treatment are mandatory to avoid complications especially in younger children. Several factors influence clinical manifestation in pediatric population: symptoms can be aspecific, not well explained because of the age, or voluntarily increased or decreased because of fear. Familial background can also influence patient's capability to demonstrate symptoms. For these reasons, diagnosis of acute appendicitis could be more challenging in children than in adults.

20.2 Epidemiology

Acute appendicitis is the diagnosis of 1–8 % of children evaluated at the emergency department for abdominal pain [1, 2]. The estimated incidence ranges from 1 to 6/10,000 between birth and 4 years of age and from 19 to 28/10,000 between 5 and 14 years of age. Boys are more frequently affected than girls [3–5].

Patients younger than 6 years of age most often present advanced disease (about 57 % of cases) [6]. This is probably due to the higher presence of nonspecific symptoms in these patients.

The finding of advanced disease up to perforation correlates both with duration of symptoms and age, being higher in small patients (neonates and children <5 years) [7].

20.3 Anatomy

The appendix is a blind-end tubular structure raising from the cecum and located in the right iliac fossa in most of people. In patients affected by congenital anomalies of intestinal position such as omphalocele, gastroschisis, diaphragmatic hernia, malrotation, or situs inversus viscerum, the appendix could be found in upper abdominal quadrant or in the left iliac fossa [8]. In most of cases, these patients already underwent complementary appendectomy during abdominal surgery. If not, anamnestic data could help diagnosis.

The base of appendix is invariably situated at the end of the free *taenia* of the cecum, while the tip position and artery origin could widely vary (Figs. 20.1 and 20.2).

We cannot forget that a child is an evolving person. Some anatomic features of appendix can change during development and correlate with incidence and presentation of appendicitis. For example, the appendix is funnel shaped during the first year of life making it difficult to be

M. Maffi (✉) • M. Lima
Pediatric Surgery, S. Orsola-Malpighi Hospital, Bologna University, Via Massarenti 11, Bologna 40138, Italy
e-mail: michela.maffi@libero.it; mario.lima@unibo.it

M. Lima (ed.), *Pediatric Digestive Surgery*, DOI 10.1007/978-3-319-40525-4_20

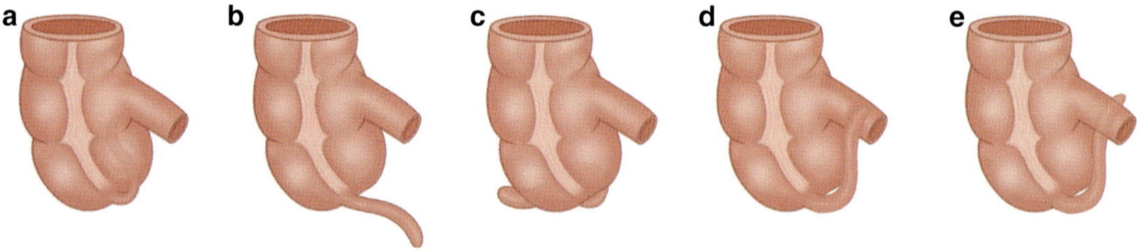

Fig. 20.1 Appendiceal tip position can widely vary. Here the most frequent positions in which it is possible to find the appendix are illustrated. (**a**) Ascending into the retrocecal recess (65 %). (**b**) Descending into the iliac fossa (31 %). (**c**) Transverse retrocecal position (about 2.5 %). (**d**) Ascending paracecal, preileal position (1 %). (**e**) Ascending paracecal, retroileal position (about 0.5 %)

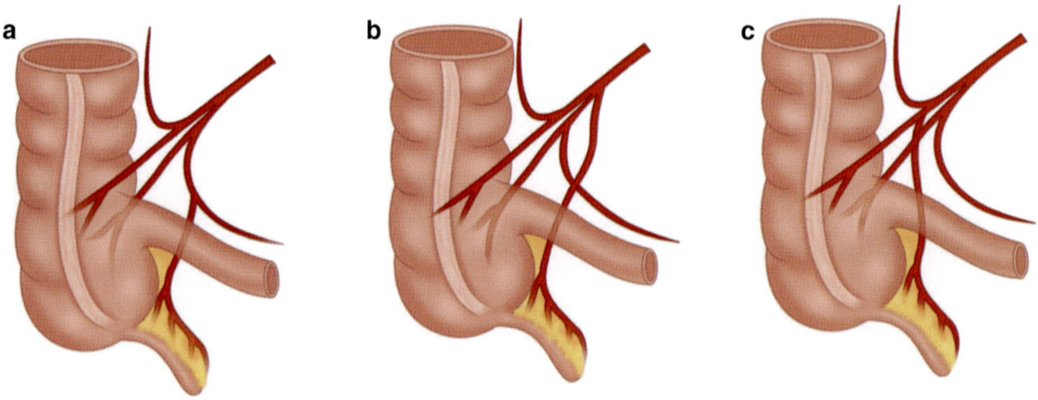

Fig. 20.2 Variations of appendicular artery. (**a**) Origin of the appendicular artery from an "ileal branch" of ileocolic artery (35 %). (**b**) Origin of the appendicular artery from ileocolic artery immediately before it divides into its terminal branches (28 %). (**c**) Origin of the appendicular artery from anterior cecal artery (20 %)

obstructed. The omentum is underdeveloped in younger children making easier a rapid diffusion of intra-abdominal infections. This feature could explain the quick clinical evolution and worsening of acute appendicitis in younger patients.

Furthermore, the appendiceal epithelium contains lymphoid follicle that may obstruct the lumen. These structures reach their maximal size during adolescence correlating with the peak incidence of acute appendicitis [9].

20.4 Pathophysiology

Obstruction of the appendiceal lumen is the first pathogenetic moment [9, 10]. Fecal material, foreign bodies, hypertrophic lymph node, bands, and torsion can be the causes. As a consequence the patient feels colic pain poorly localized in the periumbilical region.

The lack of physiologic washout of the lumen causes distension of the lumen, wall thickness, and bacterial overgrowth. Mucosal barrier is overwhelmed, leading to bacterial invasion of the wall, inflammation, ischemia, gangrene, and eventually perforation [9, 10].

Involved microorganisms belong to the normal bacterial flora, both aerobic and anaerobic: *E. coli*, *Peptostreptococcus* sp., *Bacteroides Fragilis*, and *Pseudomonas* sp. [11].

Inflammation of the wall finally involves appendiceal peritoneum leading to localized tenderness on abdominal evaluation.

Risk of perforation increases with time passed from the onset of symptoms, being rare during the first 12 h and occurring more likely after 72 h.

Intra-abdominal dissemination of the infection is prevented by omentum and intestinal loops, which migrate in the involved site confining the disease. If this barrier is insufficient, as it happens in small children, bacteria rapidly spread in the abdominal cavity leading to a diffuse peritonitis.

20.5 Clinical Manifestation

The clinical presentation of acute appendicitis classically includes the following symptoms [9]:

- Anorexia
- Periumbilical pain at the onset
- Migration of pain in the lower right quadrant (commonly in the first 24 h)
- Vomiting (after the pain onset)
- Fever, commonly mild
- Right lower tenderness
- Signs of peritoneal irritation

This classical pattern is less common in pediatric age: specific findings could be difficult to elicit; typical symptoms are not always present and may vary with age.

20.5.1 Newborns

Appendicitis in neonates is a rare condition, often correlated with quite high mortality (28 %), principally due to challenging diagnosis [12, 13]. Symptoms orient toward abdominal disease but are often aspecific: abdominal distension and tenderness, decrease in feeding intake, vomiting, lethargy or irritability, and temperature instability [12].

20.5.2 Children Younger Than 5 Years

Appendicitis is uncommon in pre-scholar age. In the history, there are aspecific findings such as fever, vomiting, diffuse abdominal pain with tenderness, and rebound. Diarrhea is quite common and makes difficult to differentiate appendicitis from gastroenteritis. Difficulty with or refusal to ambulate may also be present and due to right hip pain [14].

20.5.3 Children Between 6 and 12 Years of Age

Appendicitis is common in this age. Clinical findings belong to the typical ones: fever, early periumbilical pain and subsequent migration to the lower right quadrant with localized tenderness and rebound, anorexia, vomiting, pain with percussion, hopping, or coughing [15]. Diarrhea and dysuria may also be present and reflect low peritoneum irritation.

20.5.4 Adolescent

Clinical findings are those of the adulthood. The onset of pain typically occurs before vomiting, being a sensitive indicator for acute appendicitis. In pubertal girls, attention must be paid to gynecologic conditions that may have similar clinical presentation.

20.6 Diagnosis

The diagnosis of appendicitis is made clinically and should be suspected in all children with abdominal pain and tenderness on physical examination.

20.6.1 History

The history is characterized by the recent onset of pain, initially periumbilical or diffuse, which subsequently migrates into the right iliac fossa where it remains dull and constant or gets progressively worse. The child with acute appendicitis usually refuses food and complains nausea or has vomiting, also repeated. Patients usually prefer to lie still with one or both hips flexed. Abdominal movements during breath are reduced due to peritoneal irritation. Limp or difficulty with ambulation may be present.

20.6.2 Abdominal Evaluation

Local tenderness in the right lower quadrant and in particular in the McBurney's point is the most reliable clinical sign of abdominal appendicitis and is called McBurney's sign.

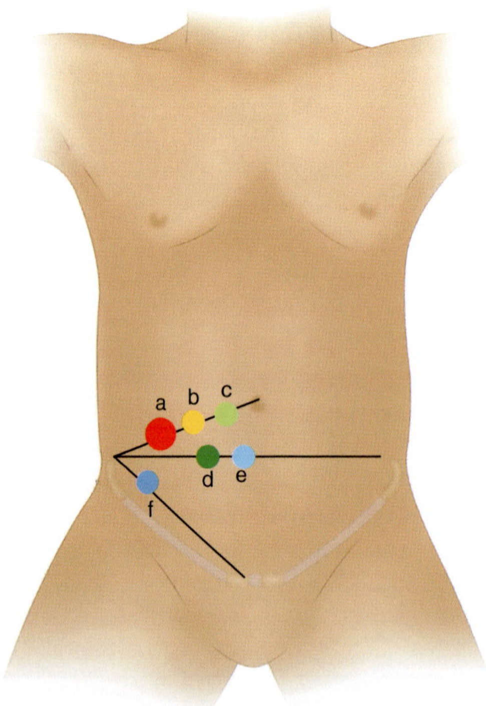

Fig. 20.3 (*a*) *McBurney's point*: a point that lies one-third of distance laterally on a line drawn from the umbilicus to the right anterior superior iliac spine. (*b*) *Morris' point*: a point an inch and a half from the umbilicus in a line drawn from the navel to the right anterior superior spine of the ilium. (*c*) *Munro's point*: a point at the right edge of the rectus abdominis muscle, between the umbilicus and the anterior superior spine of the ilium. (*d*) *Lanz point*: it is situated on a line connecting the two anterior superior iliac spines one-third of the distance from the right spine. (*e*) *Clado point*: a point at the right edge of the rectus abdominis muscle on a line connecting the two anterior superior iliac spines. (*f*) *Jalaguier point*: it is located in the middle of the line connecting the right anterior superior iliac spine and the pubic tubercle

Many are the historically described points where it's possible to evoke pain and appreciate tenderness on palpation (Fig. 20.3).

Peritoneal irritation makes it possible to elicit pain during particular maneuvers [9]:

- Blumberg sign or rebound tenderness: increased pain with release of manual pressure in the right iliac fossa
- Rovsing sign: pain in the right lower quadrant during palpation of the left side by cecal distension
- Obturator sign: pain on flexion and internal rotation of the right hip caused by a pelvic appendix which irritates the obturator internus muscle
- Iliopsoas sign: pain on extension of the right hip caused by a retrocecal appendicitis.
- Rotter sign: pain during rectal exploration caused by endopelvic appendicitis

20.6.3 Laboratory Testing

The value of the laboratory tests is limited to detect a bacterial infection. The information received by them must necessarily be integrated with clinical data.

Classically, the following tests are the most useful:

- White blood cell count (WBC)
- Absolute neutrophil count (ANC)
- C-reactive protein (CRP)

WBC and ANC are elevated in 96 % of patients with acute appendicitis, and WBC values <9000/ml are associated with acute appendicitis in less than 10 % of patients with this suspected diagnosis [6, 16].

Elevated CRP is less sensitive in the first 24 h from the onset of symptoms, but is more sensitive than WBC in patients with symptoms for 24–48 h [17].

When WBC and CRP are elevated, specificity for appendicitis reaches 90 %, but sensitivity remains low (40 %) [18].

Further test may help the differential diagnosis:

- Urinalysis: to exclude urinary tract infections
- Liver transaminases and bilirubin: to exclude cholestasis and cholecystitis
- Lipase and amylase: to exclude acute pancreatitis
- Electrolytes: to investigate and eventually correct imbalances

20.6.4 Risk Estimation

History, physical examination, and laboratory results are used from several scores to estimate risk of appendicitis. Alvarado score is the most

Table 20.1 Pediatric appendicitis score (PAS)

Items	Score
Anorexia	1
Nausea or vomiting	1
Migration of pain	1
Fever>38°	1
Pain with cough, percussion, or hopping	2
Right lower quadrant tenderness	2
WBC>di 10,000/ml	1
ANC>di 7500/ml	1
Total	*10*

known in adult patients but does not have adequate accuracy in children.

Pediatric appendicitis score (PAS) (Table 20.1) [19] achieves acceptable diagnostic accuracy and may guide decision-making. PAS is a ten-item score that permits risk stratification.

- PAS ≤2 or 3 suggests a low risk for appendicitis (0–2 %) and suggests to discharge the patient as long as the caretakers (properly instructed regarding signs of appendicitis) note a persistent pain or onset of additional symptoms that require a further evaluation.
- PAS ≥7 or 8 indicates a high risk for appendicitis (78–96 %). In clinical practice, these patients undergo surgical consult and appendectomy in most of the cases preceded or not by imaging evaluation.
- PAS of 3–6 or 7 indicates intermediate risk (8–48 %). These patients should undergo serial abdominal evaluation, diagnostic imaging, and observation in the hospital [20–24].

20.6.5 Imaging

20.6.5.1 Ultrasonography (US)

US is the first-line imaging tool in children with atypical or equivocal clinical findings for appendicitis. It is available in most of the centers and allows to investigate alternative diagnosis such as ovarian torsion or cyst, cholecystitis or cholelithiasis, urinary tract dilatations, and abdominal masses. In our practice, all girls with suspected diagnosis of appendicitis undergo US to exclude gynecologic anomalies.

Unfortunately, diagnostic accuracy depends upon experience and skills of the sonographer. Therefore, a negative US in the case of persistent symptoms is not sufficient to exclude appendicitis, and the examination may be made difficult by pain and anxiety or in the case of overweight children.

Despite this, the following findings may support the diagnosis of appendicitis:

- Diameter>6 mm
- Wall thickness of the appendix>2 mm
- Noncompressible tubular structure in the right lower quadrant
- Intraluminal fecalith
- Thickening of the mesentery
- Localized tenderness with graded compression
- Free fluid in the lower right quadrant
- Localized collection in the lower right quadrant (abscess)

In case of persistent symptoms and equivocal findings on US, the patient should undergo serial evaluations (both clinical and instrumental), till the clinical features become clearer. In the case of progressive clinical worsening with no clear diagnosis, second-level imaging investigation can be done [25].

20.6.5.2 Computed Tomography (CT) and Magnetic Resonance Imaging (MRI)

CT has high specificity and sensitivity for the diagnosis of acute appendicitis (94–100 % and 93–100 %, respectively) [26, 27].

Despite this, CT does not appear to reduce the negative appendectomy rate (NAR). The only exception is in children younger than 5 years of age where CT significantly reduces NAR [28]. If CT is performed, it should be a contrast-enhanced CT with intravenous contrast.

CT has the disadvantage of ionizing radiation exposure. In centers with adequate experience in interpreting MRI and rapid availability, it may be preferable to CT because of similar diagnostic accuracy without radiation exposure.

20.6.5.3 Plain Abdominal Radiographs

Abdominal X-ray has a poor value in diagnosis of appendicitis. It may reveal a fecalith and signs of obstruction or perforation or may exclude alternative diagnosis such as a basilar pneumonia.

20.6.6 Differential Diagnosis

Acute appendicitis in children often presents with atypical symptoms; moreover, many diseases can mimic appendicitis. The principal diseases involved in differential diagnosis are summarized in Table 20.2.

20.7 Treatment

Appendectomy is the standard treatment in the case of acute appendicitis and may prevent progression to sepsis and septic shock.

Laparoscopic approach, when well-trained surgeons are available, should be attempted. According to the literature, mini-invasive treatment significantly reduces hospital length stay, risk of wound infections, and late bowel obstruction [29, 30].

Mini-invasive appendectomy can be performed using a three-port or a single-incision technique [31].

20.7.1 Timing

Children with estimated early appendicitis could receive antibiotics and undergo appendectomy during the next 24 h according to the operative and professional resources. According to the literature, there is no increase in the frequency of complex appendicitis in patients who had a delay of 12–24 h after admission [32].

In the case of advanced appendicitis, i.e., when a gangrene or perforation is suspected, the patient should undergo urgent appendectomy rather than a delayed appendectomy.

Table 20.2 Differential diagnosis

Disease	Clinical and instrumental findings
Emergent surgical diagnoses	
Bowel obstruction	Previous surgery
	Bilious vomiting
	Abdominal X-ray: distended loops, air-fluid levels, pneumoperitoneum
Intestinal malrotation	Signs of bowel obstruction (see above)
	Upper digestive tract X-ray: duodenal compression
	US: abnormal position of major intestinal vessels
Intussusception	Intermittent episodic abdominal pain with vomiting
	Blood in the stool
	Palpable sausage-shaped mass in right quadrants
	US: target image
	Contrast enema: stop of contrast progression
Meckel's diverticulitis	Clinically indistinguishable
	Intraoperative diagnosis in most of the cases
Ovarian torsion	Localized pain
	Vomiting
	US: absence of blood flow with Doppler ultrasounds, enlarged ovary
Ectopic pregnancy	Amenorrhea
	Vaginal bleeding
	US: ectopic pregnancy
Testicular torsion	Scrotal pain that may radiate to the flank
	US: absence of blood flow with Doppler ultrasounds
Omental torsion	Localized pain
	Obese patient
	Fever or vomiting less prominent
Emergent nonsurgical diagnoses	
Hemolytic uremic syndrome	Vomiting
	Abdominal pain
	Diarrhea
	Acute renal failure
	Microangiopathic hemolytic anemia, thrombocytopenia
Diabetic ketoacidosis	Polyphagia, polydipsia, polyuria
	Anorexia, vomiting, abdominal pain
	Hyperglycemia, metabolic acidosis, glycosuria, ketonuria

Table 20.2 (continued)

Disease	Clinical and instrumental findings
Primary peritonitis	Underlying chronic condition
	Ascites
Other nonsurgical diagnoses	
Sickle cell disease	Anemia
	History
Henoch-Schönlein purpura	Colicky pain
	Purpuric rush over legs and buttocks
Nephrolithiasis	Colicky flank pain
	Hematuria
	US: echogenic foci with acoustic shadowing
Urinary tract infection	Dysuria
	Nitrites
	Bacteria and WBC in urinalysis
Pelvic inflammatory disease	Diffuse lower abdominal pain
	Fever
	Purulent endocervical discharge
Ovarian cyst	Localized pain
	Anorexia and vomiting less common
	US: ovarian cyst
Mittelschmerz	Recurrent midcycle pain
	Typically mild and unilateral
Streptococcal pharyngitis	Sore throat
	Abdominal pain
	Vomiting
	Cervical nodes
	Exudative pharyngitis
Pneumonia	Cough, fever, tachypnea
	Rales on auscultation
	Chest X-ray: presence of infiltrates
Gastroenteritis	Diffuse abdominal pain
	Diarrhea
	Vomiting
Mesenteric lymphadenitis	US finding: nonspecific indicator of infection, inflammation
	Etiology: bacterial gastroenteritis, inflammatory bowel disease, lymphoma

Some authors propose interval appendectomy in the case of well-appearing patients with appendiceal mass or abscess. These patients are initially managed nonoperatively with intravenous antibiotics, pain management, and eventual CT-guided drainage of the abscess followed by interval appendectomy after 10–12 weeks later [33]. The aim of this delay is to avoid the morbidity of immediate appendectomy while treating the underlying appendicitis. Indication for intervention includes lack of clinical improvement after 24–48 h, continued fever, worsening of tenderness, and increased mass dimension.

20.7.2 Preoperative Care

Children with acute appendicitis need fluid therapy, antibiotic, and pain control.

Fever, vomiting, and inflammation lead to fluid and electrolyte loss, so rehydration with isotonic crystalloid is mandatory to establish and maintain euvolemia.

A prophylactic dose of a broad-spectrum antibiotic focused on intestinal flora should be administered 30–60 min before the incision is made.

Acceptable antibiotics include ceftriaxone and metronidazole, piperacillin and tazobactam, cefoxitin, cefotetan, gentamicin, and either clindamycin or metronidazole in patients with allergy to penicillins and cephalosporins.

Pain control should be assessed on pain severity and in pediatric age can be achieved with intravenous paracetamol 15 mg/kg/dose.

20.7.3 Technical Details

20.7.3.1 Transumbilical Laparo-assisted Appendectomy (TULAA)

The patient lies in supine position. A single subumbilical or transumbilical incision is performed for a 12 mm Hasson trocar. A 10 mm telescope with inbuilt working channel is inserted to explore abdominal cavity. Atraumatic grasper is used to move bowel loops and find the appendix. Adhesions can be removed with a laparoscopic swab and eventual free collections are aspirated. The appendix is exteriorized through the umbilical incision and removed as in the standard open technique (Fig. 20.4).

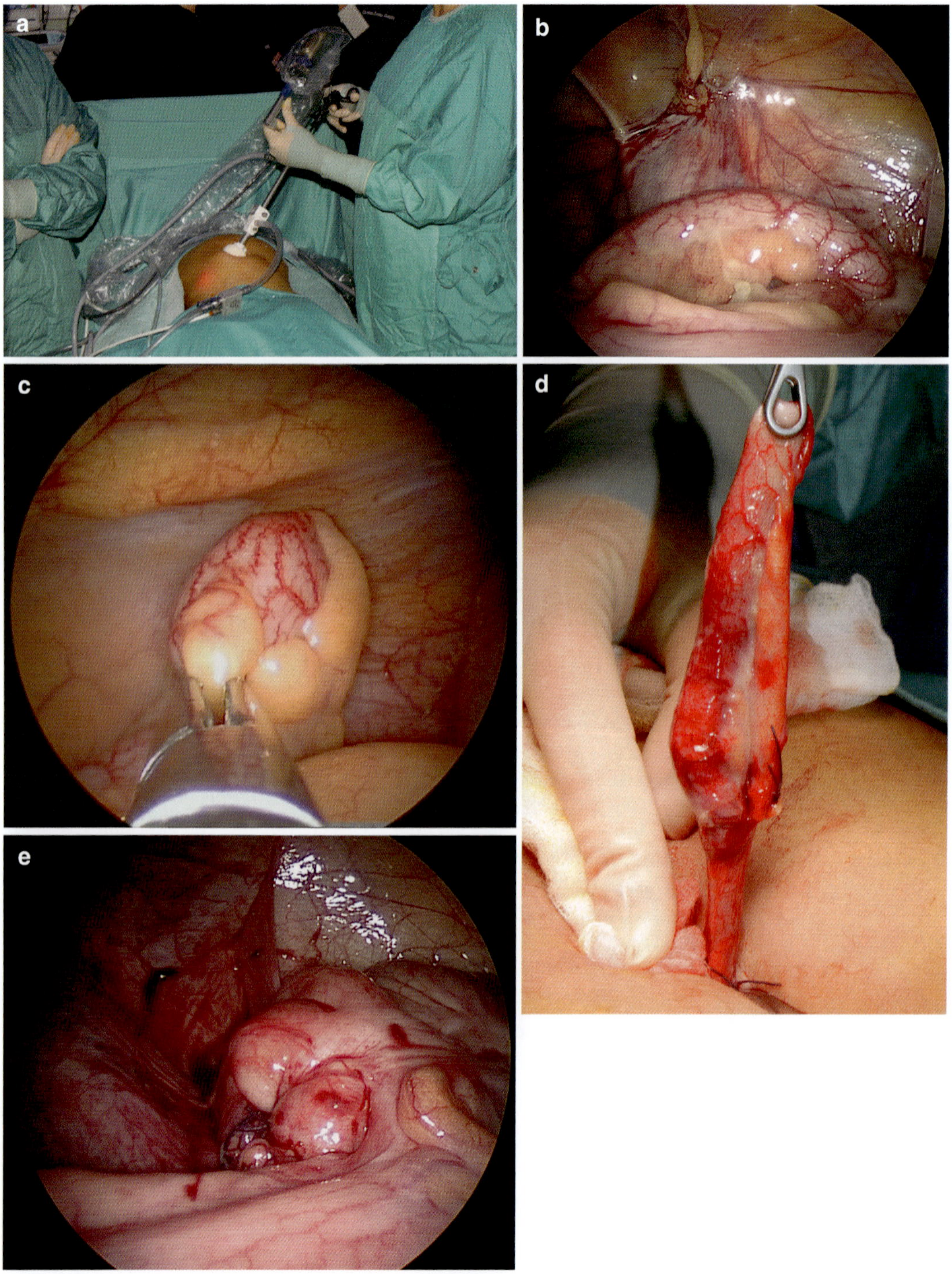

Fig. 20.4 Transumbilical laparo-assisted appendectomy. A 10 mm telescope with inbuilt operative channel is inserted in the umbilical trocar (**a**). The appendix is isolated from eventual adhesion (**b**), handled with an atraumatic grasper (**c**), and exteriorized through the umbilical incision where it can be skeletonized (**d**). At the end of the procedure, the right iliac fossa and the stump are checked (**e**)

20.7.3.2 Totally Laparoscopic Appendectomy

The patient lies in supine position. A single sub-umbilical or transumbilical incision is performed for a 12 mm Hasson trocar. A 10 mm telescope is inserted to explore abdominal cavity. Two further 5 mm trocars are positioned according to the suspected position of the appendix (Fig. 20.5). The appendix can be isolated by coagulation of the blood supply and removed after tying the base with one or two endoloops according to the surgeon's habits. In any case, the stump must be as short as possible to avoid recurrences. The closure of feeding vessels can be performed with different instruments: monopolar hook, bipolar coagulator, LigaSure®, etc. Once cut, the appendix is removed through the umbilical incision. If purulent collections are present, abdominal cavity should be irrigated with saline until the return fluid becomes clear (Fig. 20.6).

20.7.3.3 Open Appendectomy

The patient lies in supine position. Several incisions have been described to be suitable for appendectomy, but McBurney incision is still the most used. Muscles are split in the direction of their fibers and the peritoneum is opened. Once the appendix is found, its mesentery is divided and the appendiceal base is clamped and ligated. Stump inversion is usually performed but it does not seem to be necessary according to the literature. If purulent collection is present, it must be aspirated and the cavity should be irrigated. Abdominal wall is close in layers.

20.7.4 Intraoperative Considerations

In the case of normal appendix, attention must be paid to exclude other surgical causes of abdominal pain such as Meckel's diverticulitis or gynecologic anomalies (cysts, appendages) and

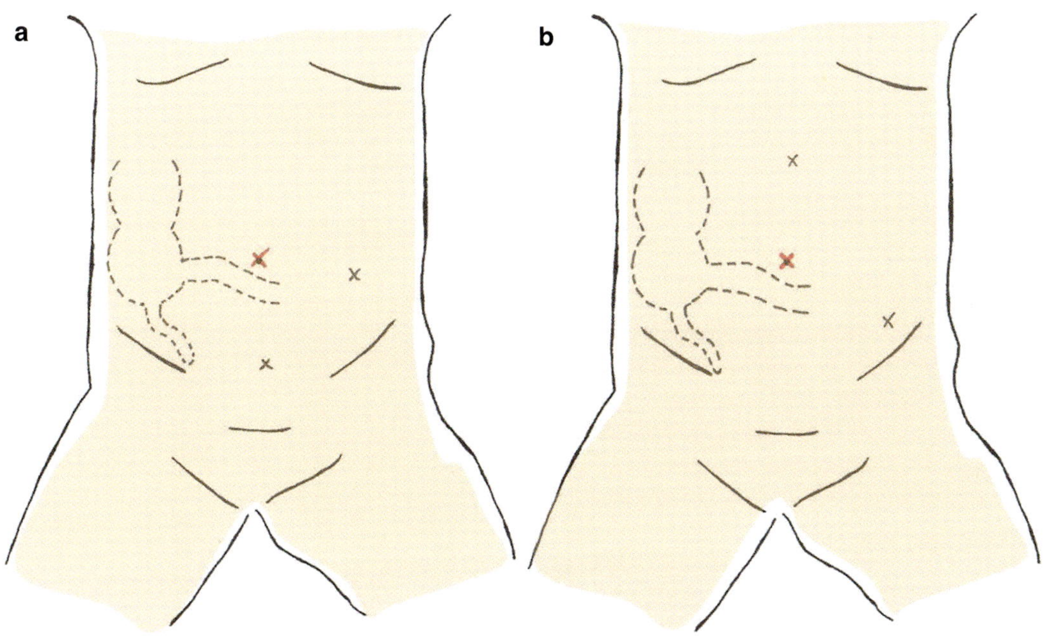

Fig. 20.5 Operative trocars can be positioned according to the suspected position of the appendix and to the most suitable position for the surgeon. (**a**) Operative trocars are placed in the left iliac fossa and in the epigastrium, respectively; (**b**) operative trocars are placed in the left iliac fossa and in suprapubic position (useful if appendiceal tip is in the right flank or subhepatic)

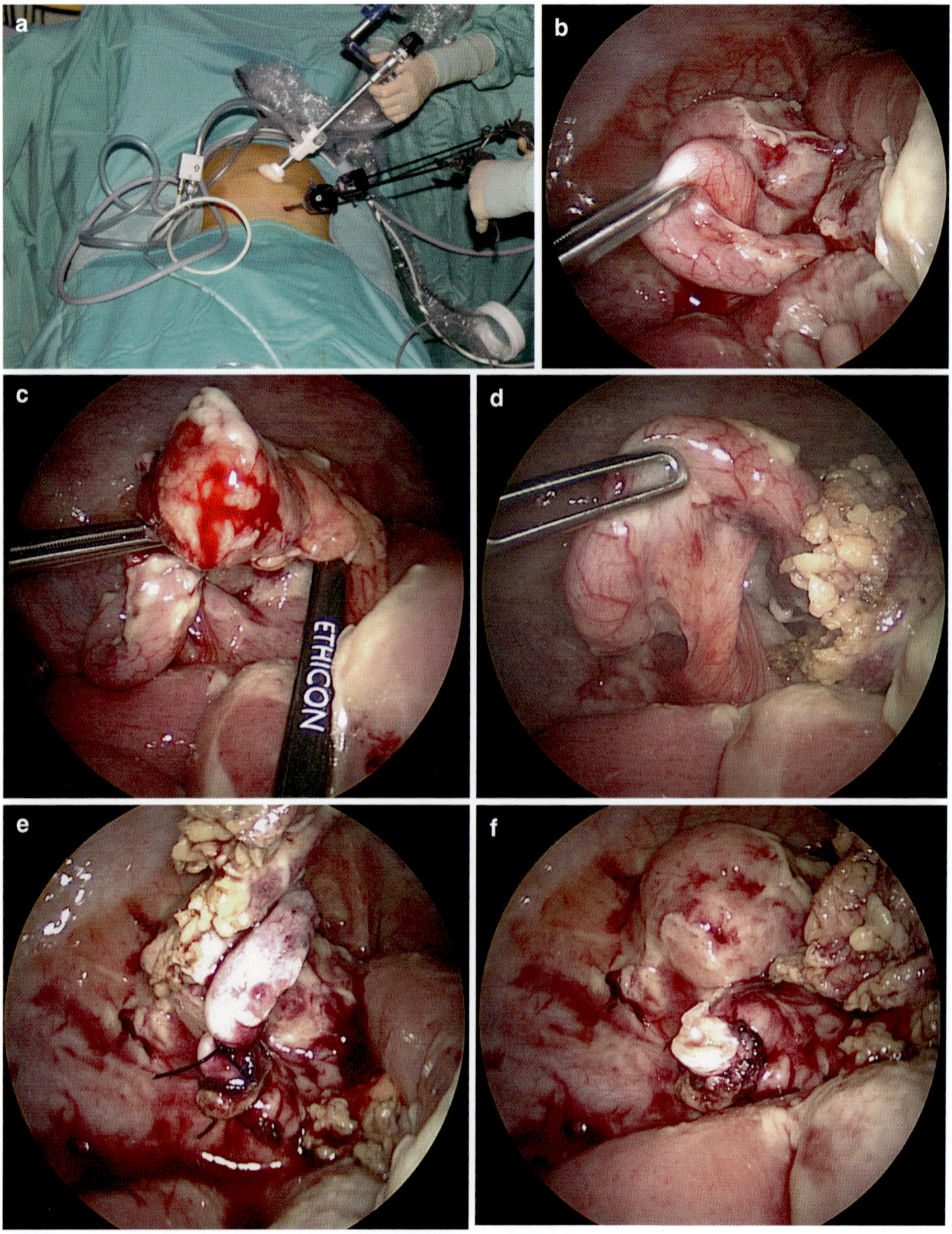

Fig. 20.6 Laparoscopic appendectomy. In our clinical practice, we always start with a single-incision technique. In the case of tight adhesions, two 5 mm operative trocars are placed in the left iliac fossa and in suprapubic position (**a**) to easily handle the appendix (**b**). Omental adhesions may be present and can be removed with the use of the monopolar hook (**c**) that is also useful to divide the mesentery (**d**). The appendiceal base is tied with an endoloop and exteriorized (**e**). At the end of the procedures, the residual stump is checked (**f**)

omental torsion. In our practice, an apparently normal appendix is removed because histology could reveal microscopic inflammation or intraluminal diseases.

If a carcinoid tumor is noted, simple appendectomy is sufficient in most of the cases. Right hemicolectomy is indicated if the tumor is greater than 2 cm in diameter, if it invades through the appendiceal wall, and if lymph nodes are involved.

In the case of grossly perforated appendix, eventual fecalith should be searched in the pelvis especially if described on preoperative imaging.

Abdominal drain is not recommended in early and uncomplicated appendix. Some authors reported no benefit for prophylactic drainage also in the case of complicated appendicitis (local peritonitis without perforation, with perforation, or with periappendicular abscess) [34]. Abdominal drain maintains a role in the case of tenuous closure of the appendiceal base and of risk for bleeding.

20.7.5 Postoperative Care

Intravenous antibiotics should be administered until the absence of fever, return of bowel function, resolution of pain, and normalization of WBC according to the American Pediatric Surgical Association [35].

Oral intake can be started as the patient appreciates bowel movements. Patients with complicated appendicitis often have a paralytic ileus, and placement of a nasogastric tube can be necessary. In these cases, oral fluids can be reintroduced once intraperitoneal inflammation and infection have improved and the ileus has resolved and can be slowly followed by solid foods as tolerated.

Pain control should be assessed on the patient and can be usually achieved with paracetamol 15 mg/kg/dose every 6 h and NSAID for the first 24 h and opiates as needed. According to a recent report [36], intraoperative rectus sheath block (eventually added to port site infiltration) significantly reduces postoperative pain in the case of laparoscopic approach.

20.7.6 Complications

- Wound infection is the most common early complication. With adequate technique, disinfection, and antibiotic therapy, the current rate of wound abscess ranges between 2 and 9 % of cases with gangrenous or perforated appendix [37, 38]. The treatment consists of wound opening and repeated irrigations and disinfections.
- Intra-abdominal abscess should be suspected in patients who remain febrile, complain abdominal pain, and are unable to tolerate regular diet after 5 or 7 days from surgery. Initial treatment consists of broad-spectrum antibiotics followed by drainage in the case of no response.
- Postoperative adhesions may cause mechanical bowel obstruction with an estimated incidence of less than 1 % of children [39]. Treatment requires surgical adhesiolysis.
- Stump appendicitis refers to inflammation of residual appendiceal tissue [40, 41]. It may occur if a too long stump is left or if the appendiceal base is tied with two ligatures too far apart during appendectomy.

References

1. Scholer SJ, Pituch K, Orr DP, Dittus RS (1996) Clinical outcomes of children with acute abdominal pain. Pediatrics 98:680
2. Reynolds SL, Jaffe DM (1992) Diagnosing abdominal pain in a pediatric emergency department. Pediatr Emerg Care 8:126
3. Addiss DG, Shaffer N, Fowler BS, Tauxe RV (1990) The epidemiology of appendicitis and appendectomy in the United States. Am J Epidemiol 132:910
4. Ohmann C, Franke C, Kraemer M, Yang Q (2002) Status report on epidemiology of acute appendicitis. Chirurg 73:769
5. Anderson JE, Bickler SW, Chang DC, Talamini MA (2012) Examining a common disease with unknown etiology: trends in epidemiology and surgical management of appendicitis in California, 1995–2009. World J Surg 36:2787
6. Rothrock SG, Pagane J (2000) Acute appendicitis in children: emergency department diagnosis and management. Ann Emerg Med 36:39
7. Rothrock SG, Skeoch G, Rush JJ, Johnson NE (1991) Clinical features of misdiagnosed appendicitis in children. Ann Emerg Med 20:45

8. Akbulut S, Ulku A, Senol A et al (2010) Left-sided appendicitis: review of 95 published cases and a case report. World J Gastroenterol 16:5598
9. Bundy DG, Byerley JS, Liles EA et al (2007) Does this child have appendicitis? JAMA 298:438
10. Rabah R (2007) Pathology of the appendix in children: an institutional experience and review of the literature. Pediatr Radiol 37:15
11. Bennion RS, Baron EJ, Thompson JE Jr et al (1990) The bacteriology of gangrenous and perforated appendicitis – revisited. Ann Surg 211:165
12. Schwartz KL, Gilad E, Sigalet D et al (2011) Neonatal acute appendicitis: a proposed algorithm for timely diagnosis. J Pediatr Surg 46:2060
13. Karaman A, Cavuşoğlu YH, Karaman I, Cakmak O (2003) Seven cases of neonatal appendicitis with a review of the English language literature of the last century. Pediatr Surg Int 19:707
14. Sakellaris G, Tilemis S, Charissis G (2005) Acute appendicitis in preschool-age children. Eur J Pediatr 164:80
15. Colvin JM, Bachur R, Kharbanda A (2007) The presentation of appendicitis in preadolescent children. Pediatr Emerg Care 23:849
16. Bates MF, Khander A, Steigman SA et al (2014) Use of white blood cell count and negative appendectomy rate. Pediatrics 133:e39
17. Kharbanda AB, Cosme Y, Liu K et al (2011) Discriminative accuracy of novel and traditional biomarkers in children with suspected appendicitis adjusted for duration of abdominal pain. Acad Emerg Med 18:567
18. Gavela T, Cabeza B, Serrano A, Casado-Flores J (2012) C-reactive protein and procalcitonin are predictors of the severity of acute appendicitis in children. Pediatr Emerg Care 28:416
19. Samuel M (2002) Pediatric appendicitis score. J Pediatr Surg 37:877
20. Goldman RD, Carter S, Stephens D et al (2008) Prospective validation of the pediatric appendicitis score. J Pediatr 153:278
21. Hatcher-Ross K (2009) Sensitivity and specificity of the Pediatric Appendicitis Score. J Pediatr 154:308
22. Bhatt M, Joseph L, Ducharme FM et al (2009) Prospective validation of the pediatric appendicitis score in a Canadian pediatric emergency department. Acad Emerg Med 16:591
23. Ebell MH, Shinholser J (2014) What are the most clinically useful cutoffs for the Alvarado and Pediatric Appendicitis Scores? A systematic review. Ann Emerg Med 64:365
24. Zúñiga RV, Arribas JL, Montes SP et al (2012) Application of Pediatric Appendicitis Score on the emergency department of a secondary level hospital. Pediatr Emerg Care 28:489
25. Mittal MK, Dayan PS, Macias CG et al (2013) Performance of ultrasound in the diagnosis of appendicitis in children in a multicenter cohort. Acad Emerg Med 20:697
26. Doria AS, Moineddin R, Kellenberger CJ et al (2006) US or CT for diagnosis of appendicitis in children and adults? A meta-analysis. Radiology 241:83
27. Lowe LH, Penney MW, Stein SM et al (2001) Unenhanced limited CT of the abdomen in the diagnosis of appendicitis in children: comparison with sonography. AJR Am J Roentgenol 176:31
28. Bachur RG, Hennelly K, Callahan MJ et al (2012) Diagnostic imaging and negative appendectomy rates in children: effects of age and gender. Pediatrics 129:877
29. Aziz O, Athanasiou T, Tekkis PP et al (2006) Laparoscopic versus open appendectomy in children: a meta-analysis. Ann Surg 243:17
30. Sauerland S, Jaschinski T, Neugebauer EA (2010) Laparoscopic versus open surgery for suspected appendicitis. Cochrane Database Syst Rev. (1):CD001546.
31. St Peter SD, Adibe OO, Juang D et al (2011) Single incision versus standard 3-port laparoscopic appendectomy: a prospective randomized trial. Ann Surg 254:586
32. Bhangu A, United Kingdom National Surgical Research Collaborative (2014) Safety of short, in-hospital delays before surgery for acute appendicitis: multicentre cohort study, systematic review, and meta-analysis. Ann Surg 259:894
33. St Peter SD, Aguayo P, Fraser JD et al (2010) Initial laparoscopic appendectomy versus initial nonoperative management and interval appendectomy for perforated appendicitis with abscess: a prospective, randomized trial. J Pediatr Surg 45:236
34. Allemann P, Probst H, Demartines N et al (2011) Prevention of infectious complications after laparoscopic appendectomy for complicated acute appendicitis – the role of routine abdominal drainage. Langenbecks Arch Surg 396(1):63–68. doi:10.1007/s00423-010-0709-z. Epub 2010 Sep 10
35. Lee SL, Islam S, Cassidy LD, et al (2010) Antibiotics and appendicitis in the pediatric population: an American Pediatric Surgical Association Outcomes and Clinical Trials Committee systematic review. J Pediatr Surg 45:2181
36. Hamill JK, Liley A, Hill AG (2015) Rectus sheath block for laparoscopic appendicectomy: a randomized clinical trial. ANZ J Surg 85(12):951–956. doi:10.1111/ans.12950
37. Lee SL, Yaghoubian A, Kaji A (2011) Laparoscopic vs open appendectomy in children: outcomes comparison based on age, sex, and perforation status. Arch Surg 146:1118
38. Lee SL, Yaghoubian A, de Virgilio C (2011) A multi-institutional comparison of pediatric appendicitis outcomes between teaching and nonteaching hospitals. J Surg Educ 68:6
39. Tsao KJ, St Peter SD, Valusek PA et al (2007) Adhesive small bowel obstruction after appendectomy in children: comparison between the laparoscopic and open approach. J Pediatr Surg 42:939
40. Liang MK, Lo HG, Marks JL (2006) Stump appendicitis: a comprehensive review of literature. Am Surg 72:162
41. Mangi AA, Berger DL (2000) Stump appendicitis. Am Surg 66:739

Intussusception

21

Francesca Destro, Michela Maffi, and Mario Lima

21.1 Definition

The term intussusception derives from the Latin words *intus* (within) and *suscipere* (to receive), and it refers to the invagination of the part of the intestine into the adjacent segment [1]. It is one of the most common causes of acute abdomen in children [2]. It can involve any tract of the mesenteric intestine.

21.2 Classification

We can recognize different types of intussusception based on the following aspects:

- General = permanent (fixed, 80 % of cases) and transient (reduced spontaneously that happens in 20 % of cases; this form is frequently underestimated because the clinical symptoms develop during gastroenteritis)
- Specific = idiopathic (without a pathologic lead point – PLP, 95 %), with PLP (Meckel's diverticulum, appendix, polyps, carcinoid tumor, Schonlein-Henoch purpura, foreign body, duplication of the bowel, cystic fibrosis, etc.) and postoperative intussusception
- Anatomic = ileocolic (85 %), ileoileocolic (10 %), appendicocolic, cecocolic or colocolic (2.5 %), jejunojejunal, ileoileal (2.5 %)
- Other types = recurrent forms

F. Destro • M. Maffi (✉) • M. Lima
Pediatric Surgery, S. Orsola-Malpighi Hospital, Bologna University, Via Massarenti 11, 40138 Bologna, Italy
e-mail: francesca_destro@hotmail.com; michela.maffi@libero.it; mario.lima@unibo.it

21.3 Incidence, Age, and Sex

The incidence is 2–4 cases/1000 live births. There is a seasonal variation with peaks during spring and in the middle of winter when gastroenteritis and respiratory infections that lead to lymphatic hypertrophy are more common.

Idiopathic intussusception is more frequent within the first 2 years of age (also in premature babies) with most cases presenting at around 6 months of age. Males are affected more than females (M:F = 2:1).

Symptomatic intussusception with a PLP can occur at any age, especially in older patient (also in adults).

21.4 Etiopathogenesis

The affection has not usually a cause ("idiopathic intussusception"), and it is rarely related to a PLP ("symptomatic intussusception") [3].

Idiopathic intussusception seems to be related to an intestinal dysmotility after weaned or

M. Lima (ed.), *Pediatric Digestive Surgery*, DOI 10.1007/978-3-319-40525-4_21

gastrointestinal/respiratory infections. The lead point could be a thickened lymphoid tissue of the bowel wall (Peyer's patches). In fact the lymphoid tissue, which is more represented in babies and children than in adults (adenoids, tonsils, and lymph nodes), increases during infection processes. *Adenovirus* and *Rotavirus* have been identified in 50% of children with gastroenteritis who develop intussusceptions. Sometimes the intussusception sets up shortly after abdominal surgery when peristalsis is still uncoordinated (1% of cases). In utero intussusception has been associated to the development of intestinal atresia.

Involved intestinal segments are the terminal ileum and cecum that enter in the ascending colon (ascending intussusception) or the terminal ileum that enters the ascending colon without the cecum that remains fixed (ileocolic intussusception). Mixed forms (ileocecocolic) are common.

PLP intussusception (5–10% of cases) happens not only in babies, and it is typical of children in scholar age. It has not a typical intestinal site (it may be jejunojejunal, ileoileal, ileocecal, ileocolic, colocolic). It is caused by the presence of an intestinal structure into the lumen (focal or diffuse lesions, such as intussuscepted Meckel's diverticulum or appendix, polyp – especially in case of Peutz-Jeghers polyposis, duplication cyst, Schonlein-Henoch purpura, ectopic pancreatic node, lymphoma, and other neoplasias) that acts as foreign body stimulating peristalsis and pushed forward together with the intestinal wall.

The caudal portion of the intussuscepted segment is the "head of the intussusception." The invaginated bowel is called intussusceptum, and the recipient bowel is the intussuscipiens. The prograde bowel peristalsis leads to the angulation and compression of the mesenteric vessels that are carried into the recipient bowel together with the intussusceptum. The effects are a local edema, venous compression, stasis, and congestion. When the arterial supply is compromised, there is local ischemia and bowel necrosis with risk of perforation.

21.5 Clinic

Idiopathic intussusception occurs in well-fed babies who have always been well. The baby is suddenly in pain and starts crying with painful face, legs abducted on the abdomen. The clinical picture improves after a few minutes, the baby falls asleep or starts playing again, and everything returns normal. Symptoms represent soon after (15–30 min intervals) abdominal pain, vomit (alimentary and biliary), and rectal bleeding. The presence of mucus-hematic feces ("red currant jelly stool") alarms parents who take the baby to the emergency room.

General physical conditions deteriorate if there is not a prompt diagnosis (dehydration, hypothermia, shock).

The abdomen is normal between the attacks of pain. Sometimes it is possible to appreciate an abdominal mass (sausage-like) whose location varies depending on the level reached by the intussusception (spiral pathway around the belly): right iliac fossa, hepatic flexure, above, at the left, and below the umbilicus. Sometimes the intussuscepted segment passes distally, and it is palpated on rectal examination. This situation should be distinguished from the rectal prolapse. The presence of diarrhea does not exclude intussusception. On examination the baby may be febrile and dehydrated. The classic triad of symptoms (incessant cry related to abdominal pain, red currant jelly stool, and palpable mass) is not always present in children >2 years of age who often present with symptoms of the underlying disease (PLP).

21.6 Diagnosis

The clinical history and the examination suggest the diagnosis.

The abdominal x-ray shows an abnormal gas distribution throughout the small intestine with an absence of cecal gas (ileocecal forms) and elements suggestive of a right-sided soft tissue mass. Air fluid levels and dilated bowels are present in case of intestinal obstruction. However

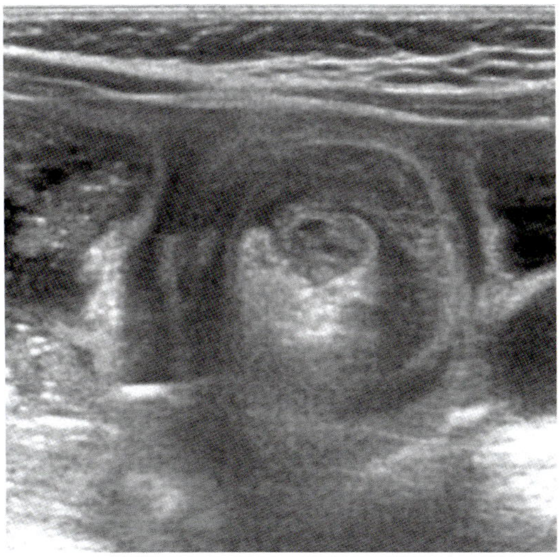

Fig. 21.1 US showing a target sign: two rings of low echogenicity with an intervening hyperechoic ring

intussusception signs are nonspecific, and the role of x-rays remains controversial.

Ultrasounds (US) are the first-level investigation for the diagnosis [3] with a reported accuracy of 100 %: there are pathognomonic features such as 3–5 cm (diameter) mass with the resemblance of a donut or target sign (two rings of low echogenicity with an intervening hyperechoic ring similar to a donut) (Fig. 21.1). Contrast enema is the gold standard for the diagnosis and can be therapeutic. The mean of contrast stops when it meets the intussusception, and the rounded barium column becomes concave forming a meniscus that flattens out when the intussusception is displaced (Fig. 21.2). The disadvantage is related to the fact that it is an invasive procedure.

21.7 Treatment

The first therapeutic measure is the fluid resuscitation of the baby together with nasogastric tube placement if there is vomit. The intussusception can be reduced by radiologic contrast enema or by intervention. The removal of the PLP is required in case of "secondary forms." Medical treatment can be used before, along with, and after radiologic reduction, and it consists of steroid administration in case of lymphoid hyperplasia and Schonlein-Henoch purpura. Steroids seem to modulate intestinal immunological activity and reduce the bowel edema in acute forms.

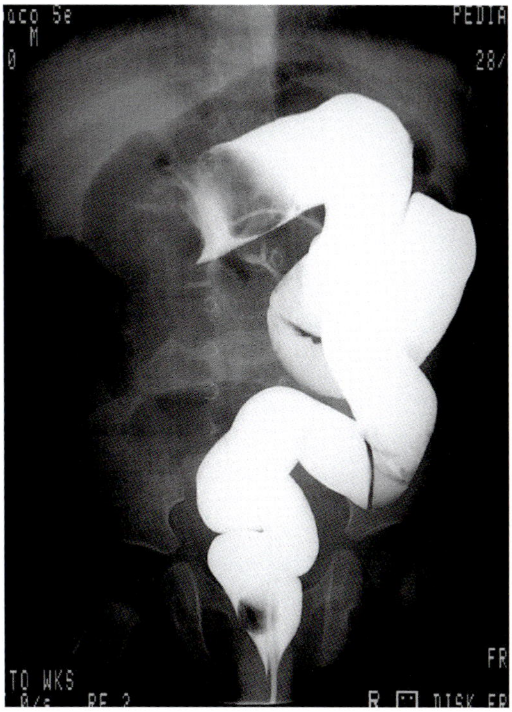

Fig. 21.2 Contrast enema. The column of contrast stops at the head of the intussusception

Patients who do not need immediate surgery (signs of intestinal perforation, peritonitis, or free intra-abdominal air) are eligible for enema reduction (hydrostatic or pneumatic). Radiologic reduction is effective in 90 % of cases [4, 5]. Pneumoenema is safe, quick, and easy to perform and should be attempted in all children with intussusception. It is performed with a Foley catheter inserted into the rectum with the balloon inflated. The buttocks are taped, and air is used to create a pressure of 120 mmHg for 5 min. The procedure has been effective where the air fills into the terminal ileum even if sometimes the passage of air is not associated with complete reduction. Hydrostatic barium enema reduction under fluoroscopic guidance is the preferred option in many centers. Barium enema shows the

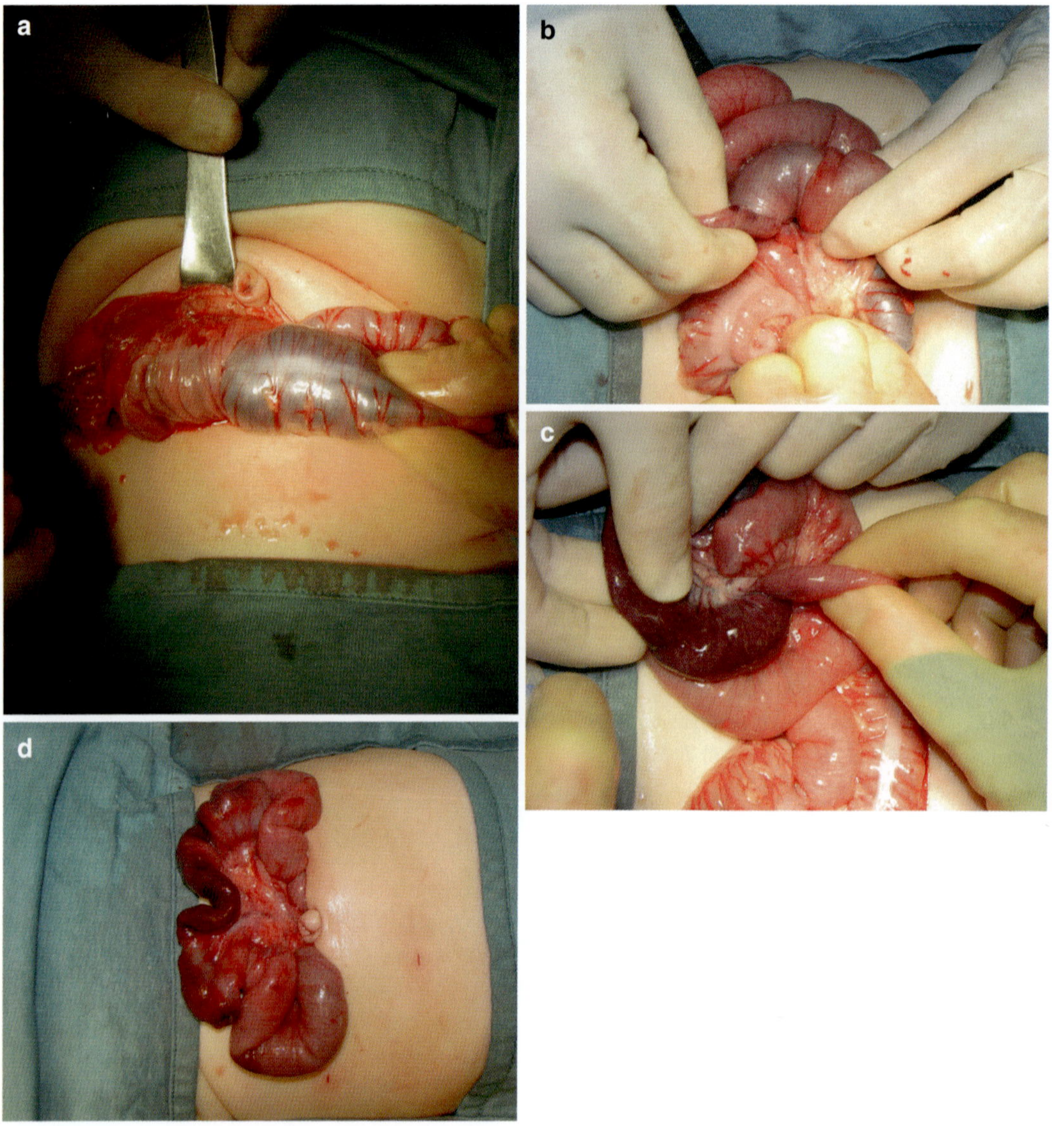

Fig. 21.3 Laparotomic reduction of the invagination. The invaginated tract is exteriorized (**a**) and progressively squeezed (**b**) until complete resolution of the invagination (**c**). In this case the intussusception was due to the presence of Meckel's diverticulum (**d**)

"crab's claw sign" related to the passage of contrast between the layers of the intussusception. Once again, the column of barium exerts a pressure of 120 mmHg that is held for 3–5 min. The passage of barium in the terminal ileum indicates successful reduction. The risk of intestinal perforation exists for both the procedures (<1 %) with the difference that barium in the peritoneal cavity leads to intense inflammatory response.

After the reduction, the baby should be kept for observation in hospital for some time with intravenous fluids. Antibiotics should be continued in case of difficult reduction or fever. When there is intestinal obstruction, the nasogastric tube is kept until gas passes freely through the intestine.

Recurrent intussusception is described in 5–10 % of cases after enema reduction, mostly

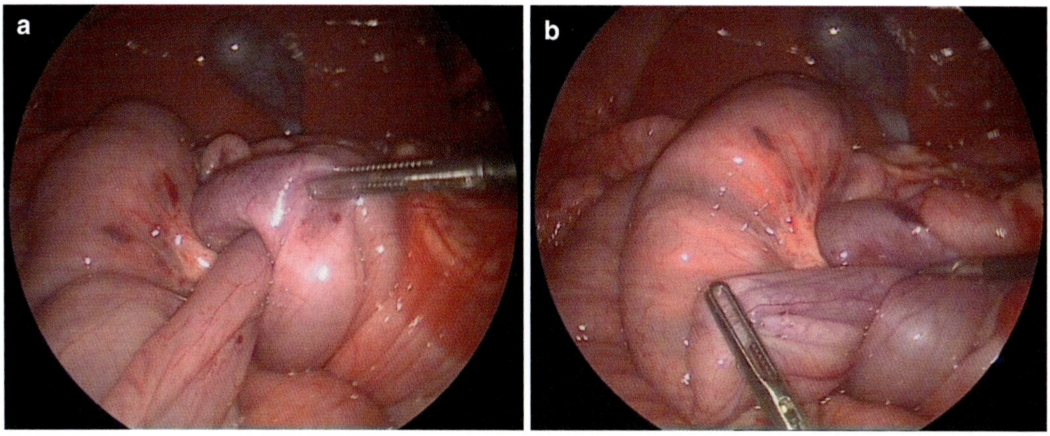

Fig. 21.4 Laparoscopic reduction of the invagination. Once the neck of the intussusception is identified (**a**), a gentle manipulation of both intussusceptum and intussuscipiens helps to reduce invagination (**b**)

within 72 h [4]. Some authors suggest performing maneuvers to improve radiologic reduction rates: steroid administration, smooth muscle relaxants and sedation, transabdominal manipulation, and delayed repeat enema. The rationale for repeat enema lies in the evidence that 10 % have already been reduced at surgery and 40 % are easily reduced. Criteria for delayed enema (after 2–4 h) are onset of symptoms <36 h, temperature <38°C, pulse rate <150/min, the movement of the intussusception, and asymptomatic patients.

Surgery is required when enema reduction fails. Classical operation is performed by laparotomy (small right-sided transverse incision). The intussusception mass is palpated and is brought outside the wound, and the reduction is attempted by exerting gentle and persistent pressure at its distal end (constant pinching, squeezing like a tube of toothpaste, or milking backward in retrograde fashion through the wall of the intussuscipiens) (Fig. 21.3). The index finger can be inserted into the intussusception to enlarge the space between the intussuscipiens and intussusceptum. The intestine appears edematous, but its aspect improves with irrigation with warm saline solution. Ischemic segments should be removed avoiding long resections (reduction should be always attempted as much as possible). Some colleagues at the end of the manual reduction perform appendectomy. Laparoscopic reduction has been described as an effective alternative with reduced scarring, adhesions, pain, and hospitalization length although its role is still questioned (Fig. 21.4) [6, 7]. Feeding is resumed shortly after surgery in cases without resections. Antibiotic prophylaxis is recommended. Surgical complications are described in 14 % of cases: wound infection and dehiscence, intestinal obstruction for adhesions, and perforation. Delay in diagnosis is the main factor related to morbidity and mortality. The latter has rapidly declined to less than 1 % in developed countries.

References

1. Jiang J, Jiang B, Parashar U, Nguyen T, Bines J, Patel MM (2013) Childhood intussusception: a literature review. PLoS One 8(7):e68482. doi:10.1371/journal.pone.0068482.Print2013. PubMed PMID: 23894308, PubMed Central PMCID: PMC3718796, Review
2. Shah S (2013) An update on common gastrointestinal emergencies. Emerg Med Clin North Am 31(3):775–793. doi:10.1016/j.emc.2013.05.002. Review
3. Charles T, Penninga L, Reurings JC, Berry MC (2015) Intussusception in children: a clinical review. Acta Chir Belg 115(5):327–333. Review
4. Gray MP, Li SH, Hoffmann RG, Gorelick MH (2014) Recurrence rates after intussusception enema reduction: a meta-analysis. Pediatrics 134(1):110–119. doi:10.1542/peds.2013-3102. PubMed PMID: 24935997, Epub 2014 Jun 16. Review

5. Bekdash B, Marven SS, Sprigg A (2013) Reduction of intussusception: defining a better index of successful non-operative treatment. Pediatr Radiol 43(6):649–656. doi:10.1007/s00247-012-2552-6. PubMed PMID: 23254683, Epub 2012 Dec 20. Review
6. Sklar CM, Chan E, Nasr A (2014) Laparoscopic versus open reduction of intussusception in children: a retrospective review and meta-analysis. J Laparoendosc Adv Surg Tech A 24(7):518–522. doi:10.1089/lap.2013.0415. Review
7. Apelt N, Featherstone N, Giuliani S (2013) Laparoscopic treatment of intussusception in children: a systematic review. J Pediatr Surg 48(8):1789–1793. doi:10.1016/j.jpedsurg.2013.05.024. Review

22 Hirschsprung's Disease

Matthew W. Ralls, Arnold G. Coran, Daniel H. Teitelbaum, Francesca Destro, and Mario Lima

22.1 Definition

Hirschsprung's disease (HD) or "congenital megacolon" is a congenital developmental disorder characterized by the absence of ganglion cells in the distal intestine with variable proximal extension.

22.2 Classification

The proximal extension of the aganglionic tract starting from the internal anal sphincter is useful to classify the different forms of HD.

The most common form is the rectosigmoid, "short segment" or classical form (74–80 % of cases), which involves the rectum or rectosigmoid tract. The second most common form is the "long segment" (12–22 % of cases) that extends up to the splenic flexure or up to the transverse colon. In 4–13 % of cases, there is a total colonic aganglia in which the aganglia extends to the entire colon and usually reaches the terminal ileum.

The exact incidence of the "ultrashort" form is unknown: according to several authors, it represents 9–25 % of the cases [1].

22.3 Embryogenesis

Ganglion cells of the alimentary canal are derived from the neural crest, and they migrate through the caudal fibers of the vagus nerve. The process of migration follows a proximal to distal direction through the gastrointestinal tract. The first neuroblasts are found in the esophagus from the fifth week of gestation. The migration is completed by 13 weeks postconception. The mature nerve plexus ("myenteric") includes the submucosal plexus that is divided into superficial (Meissner) and deep (Henle) and the intramuscular plexus of Auerbach. The three plexuses form the "enteric nervous system." The ganglion cells are absent in all three plexuses in HD patients. The lack of such cells is attributed to an arrest in the neuroblast migration process along the alimentary canal.

22.4 Etiology

In infants with HD, the ganglion cell migration process is disturbed. The theory of the arrest of the neuroblast migration justifies the presence of a distal pathologic tract with variable proximal extension (the earlier the arrest, the greater the extent of the aganglionic tract). The primary cause

M.W. Ralls • A.G. Coran • D.H. Teitelbaum
C.S. Mott Children's Hospital, University of Michigan Hospital and Health Systems, Ann Arbor, MI, USA

F. Destro • M. Lima (✉)
Pediatric Surgery, S. Orsola-Malpighi Hospital, Bologna University, Via Massarenti 11, Bologna 40138, Italy
e-mail: mario.lima@unibo.it

M. Lima (ed.), *Pediatric Digestive Surgery*, DOI 10.1007/978-3-319-40525-4_22

of HD is related to cellular and molecular anomalies in the nervous system development and neural crest migration along the alimentary canal.

The increased risk of HD in siblings of affected individuals, compared to the remaining population, and the different incidence in males and females, the association of HD with other syndromes/chromosomal abnormalities, and the existence of animal models with Mendelian inherited colonic aganglionosis suggest the presence of genetic factors. Moreover, mutations in the receptor tyrosine kinase (RET) proto-oncogene have been convincingly demonstrated.

HD is a classic example of a complex genetic disease with multifactorial etiology. In fact, the high incidence of sporadic cases (80–90 %), the variable expressivity (variable extension of the aganglionic tract), and the incomplete penetrance suggest a complex pattern of inheritance (multifactorial disease) and the involvement of multiple genes.

22.5 Physiopathology

The HD is characterized by a state of functional intestinal obstruction followed by the dilation of the normal innervated upper intestine, from which derives the term "megacolon."

Between the pathological aganglionic segment that is classically narrow and the healthy normal intestine, typically dilated, there is an area where the ganglionic nerves are present but to a lesser degree than normal: this area is known as "transition area" and it has a characteristic "funnel" shape.

The innervation of the alimentary canal has an intrinsic component, the enteric nervous system (submucosal and intramuscular plexuses), and an extrinsic component composed by the parasympathetic and orthosympathetic fibers that connect to the central nervous system. The parasympathetic system is excitant, while the sympathetic one is inhibitory, although there are numerous exceptions to this rule.

The intestinal peristaltic activity depends on the enteric nervous system. In fact, the intestinal peristalsis is not abolished by the section of the nerves distributed to the bowel wall but disappears when the bowel wall is covered with local anesthetic.

The peristaltic reflexes and muscle relaxation are expected to be abolished in case of HD as the ganglia of the enteric nervous system are absent. However, the aganglionic segment is characterized by a state of tonic contraction of unknown origin.

It is important to enlighten the difference between aganglia and denervation. The HD is characterized by aganglia and not denervation. In fact, numerous studies have shown that the intestinal aganglionic segment has an increased number of adrenergic and cholinergic fibers.

The concentration of acetylcholine, compared to normal, is two to nine times higher, and the concentration of catecholamine is at least three times higher. The absence of gangliar cells could prevent the physiological peristalsis, allowing the parasympathetic fibers to form the sacral plexus, to directly stimulate the smooth muscle cells, causing an uncontrolled contraction.

Actually the cause of the tonic contraction of the aganglionic segment remains unknown, but it is responsible for the state of functional occlusion and subsequent dilatation of the upper normoganglionic intestine normogangliare.

22.6 Incidence

The HD affects approximately 1/5000 live births and is more common in males (M:F = 4:1).

22.7 Associated Anomalies

The incidence of associated abnormalities in patients with HD varies according to different case studies, from 11 to 30 %:

- Trisomy 21 (7 %)
- Neurocristopathies and eye abnormalities (12 %), explained by the common embryological origin
- Congenital heart disease (2–8 %) or septal defects and patent ductus arteriosus
- Gastrointestinal abnormalities, anorectal malformations (2.5 %), and intestinal atresia (exceptional)

- Disganglionosis, with variable incidence depending on the series (0.3–62 %)

22.8 Clinical Presentation

Most children with HD (50–90 %) are diagnosed in the neonatal period. Typically, the infant with HD is born at term and present with failure to pass meconium.

The meconium passage in term infants usually occurs within 24–48 h after birth. In 60–90 % of patients with HD, the meconium passage is delayed beyond 24 h.

The clinical picture of HD is also characterized by abdominal distension, bilious vomiting (less frequent), and feeding intolerance that suggest a distal intestinal obstruction. When the disease is not suspected, rectal signs may solve spontaneously or with rectal stimulations with subsequent onset of chronic constipation.

Dietary changes and the use of laxatives and enemas may lead to a relative comfort for months/years. These patients present later in childhood with chronic constipation. The presence of severe chronic constipation with a history of intestinal disorders from the first days of life characterizes the clinical picture of an infant or a child suffering from HD. These children are "often sick" and have significant abdominal distension, anorexia, dystrophies, anemia, dysproteinemia, and recurrent episodes of infection.

The most feared complication is the onset of an enterocolitis (Hirschsprung-associated enterocolitis – HAEC). The HAEC is related to fecal stasis and bacterial overgrowth that determine necrotizing alterations of the intestinal mucosa and secondary infection. The HAEC can characterize the onset of the disease (one-third of HD cases) and may arise in a patient waiting for surgery but also after the surgical correction. The risk of HAEC determines the importance of early diagnosis of HD. Indeed, it is demonstrated that there is a greater frequency of HAEC in case of late diagnosis. Clinically, it is characterized by smelly diarrhea, fever, and worsening abdominal distension. If not properly treated, the HAEC can develop into a septic shock referred to as "toxic megacolon."

22.9 Diagnosis

When there is a clinical suspicion of HD, diagnostic investigations to be performed include radiologic evaluation (plain radiographs, barium enema), anorectal manometry, rectal full-thickness biopsy or serum muscle, and/or rectal biopsy by suction (rectal suction biopsy – RSB).

In the last three decades, the rectal biopsy by suction, with the demonstration of the high physical activity of submucosal acetylcholinesterase (AChE), has become the gold standard for the diagnosis of HD.

The first step investigation in case of intestinal occlusion or sub-ileus is the abdominal x-ray (Fig. 22.1). Plain radiographs show colonic gaseous distension that does not involve the distal colon (aganglionic) that is instead uninhabited.

The barium contrast enema is simple and exhaustive in the case of evident transition zone ("funnel" aspect) between the two segments (the

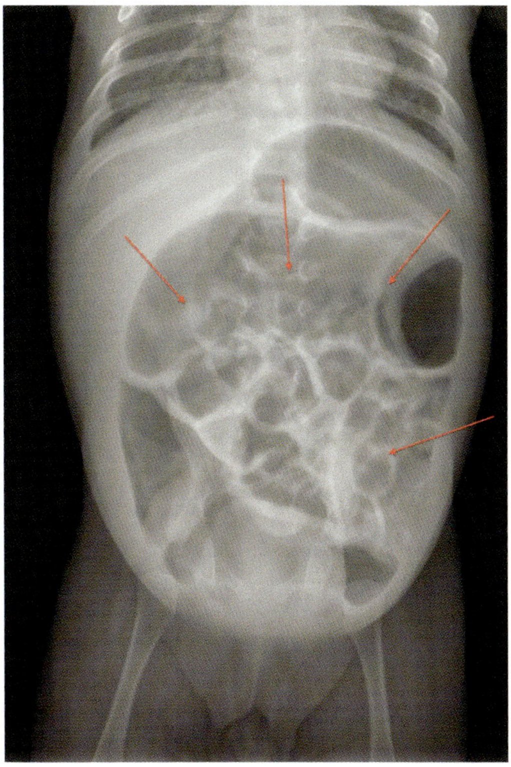

Fig. 22.1 Important colic distension (*red arrows*) on the x-ray with lack of air in the recto-sigma x

narrow aganglionic distal segment and the proximal dilated one) (Fig. 22.2). Another finding that is suggestive for HD is the retention of contrast in the colon on a 24-h post-evacuation film. In case of total colic aganglia, it is characteristic the presence of the microcolon associated with massive ileal reflux of contrast mean.

Anorectal manometry in affected patients shows the presence of a high-pressure rectal baseline reflex at rest and the absence of the recto-anal inhibitory reflex (RAIR).

Physiologically there is a reflex relaxation of the internal anal sphincter in response to recto-anal inhibitory reflex (RAIR). In patients with HD, the rectal baseline pressure is higher than normal, and the recto-anal inhibitory reflex is absent (negative RAIR). This technique has yielded good results when used in children, but it is not widely available for neonates.

The rectal biopsy (full-thickness biopsy) directly demonstrates the absence of ganglion cells in the myenteric plexus and the presence of cholinergic AChE-positive fibers in the hypertrophic submucosa. It is the most sensitive and specific investigation for the diagnosis of HD but also the most invasive because it requires a surgical procedure (Fig. 22.3). The suction biopsy was introduced in order to reduce this invasiveness. The procedure does not involve the colonic mucosa incision, as it is unnecessary for the diagnosis. The rectal suction biopsy with the immunochemical demonstration of acetylcholinesterase has become the gold standard for the diagnosis of HD. The procedure can be performed in an outpatient clinic. The rectal suction biopsy (RSB) is performed with the transanal Noblett clamp. Three samples are taken from 2 to 5 cm above the dentate line, and all samples must include a fragment of submucosa. The samples are taken at different points of the rectal circumference ("3, 6, and 9 h").

The immunochemical diagnosis is based on the HD physiopathology. In recto-colic aganglionic segments, there is a significant increment of the parasympathetic cholinergic elements from the sacrum. The cholinergic fibers in AChE-positive patient with HD are thick and intricate nervous trunks that cross the muscularis mucosa and as hypertrophied nerves in the submucosa. The immunochemical examination looks for the increment in cholinergic AChE-positive fibers in the submucosa.

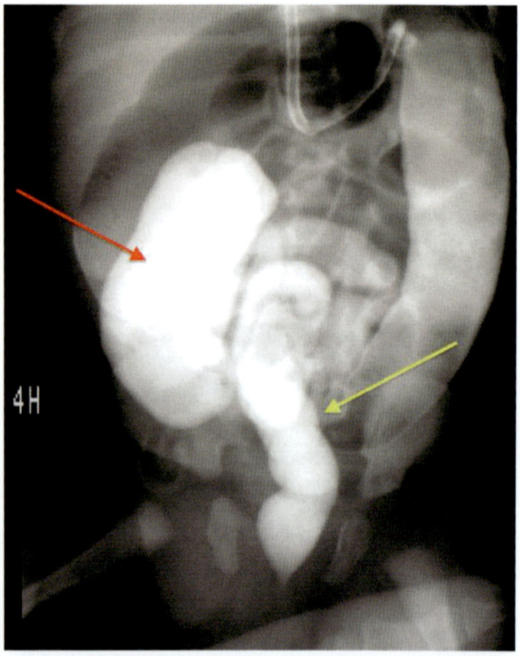

Fig. 22.2 Barium contrast enema showing a distal narrow aganglionic segment (*yellow arrow*) and a proximal dilated segment (*red arrow*)

22.10 Management

When there is a clinical suspicion of HD, the first therapeutic measure consists of performing rectal stimulations or irrigations in order to keep the colon clean and decompressed and avoid the onset of HAEC.

The irrigations are performed with physiological solution (approximately 10–20 cm^3/kg) to be repeated two to three times a day. Once the diagnosis is confirmed, the surgical timing depends on the patient's age. The majority of the diagnosis is performed in newborns, and the operation is planned between 2 and 4 months of life. In older patients, surgery is performed once the diagnosis has been confirmed. The "one-stage" correction has emerged as the procedure of choice, thanks to

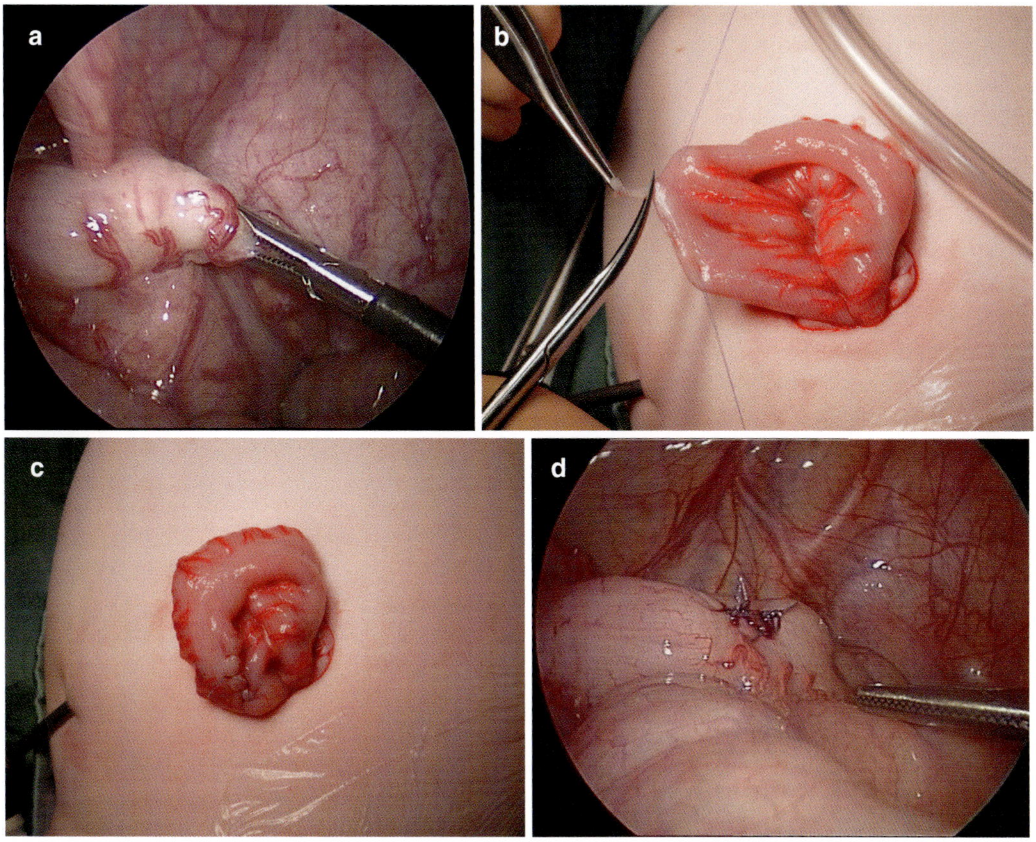

Fig. 22.3 Laparoscopic-assisted biopsy. The intestinal segment is chosen and exteriorized through the umbilical wound (**a**). The biopsy is performed outside the abdomen (**b**, **c**). Laparoscopic control at the end of the procedure (**d**)

the proven effectiveness of the "conservative bowel management" and the proven benefits of a neonatal intervention, reducing the role of the colostomy that today remains indicated for total colonic aganglia (ileostomy) and recurrent HAEC.

There are numerous surgical techniques described for the treatment of HD. The goals of surgery are the removal of the aganglionic bowel and the lowering (pull-through) of the normally innervated intestinal tract down to the anus, preserving the sphincter function.

The most commonly performed, and therefore considered "the major pull-through procedures," are:

- Swenson rectosigmoidectomy
- Duhamel retrorectal transanal pull-through
- Rehbein pull-through with anterior colorectal anastomosis
- Soave rectosigmoidectomy with aseptic endorectal colon pull-through

The Swenson procedure consists of removing the entire aganglionic colon and performing an end-to-end anastomosis above the anal sphincter after the perineal eversion of the aganglionic rectum. The procedure is associated with high risk of injuring the pelvic nerves, vessels, and other pelvic structures.

The Duhamel technique provides for the creation of a retrorectal pull-through (between the rectum and the sacrum) with subsequent anastomosis between the normally innervated bowel (posterior) and the aganglionic segment (anterior). Although the less pelvic dissection makes the procedure safer, there can be problems related to the persistence of aganglionic segments.

The Soave technique is largely used, thanks to the effectiveness and safety of the endorectal dissection. The technique involves an abdominal and a perineal step.

The abdominal step classically requires a laparotomy (left pararectal or sovrapubic incision according to Pfannenstiel) to access the abdominal cavity. The procedure starts from the determination of the distal normally ganglionic segment: the region is visually identified above the transition zone ("funnel zone") and confirmed performing a seromuscular biopsy in the colon next to the suspected transition zone. The sample is sent for histological examination. The mesocolon of the aganglionic segment (distal to the intestinal biopsy) is dissected once the presence of ganglia has been confirmed. Then the seromuscular layer is circumferentially separated from the rectal mucosa.

The perineal step provides for the transanal eversion of the rectal mucosal cylinder maintaining the seromuscular layer inside the pelvis. In other words, the pull-through bowel is lowered within a "cuff" made of aganglionic muscle. Once the everted mucosa has been resected, the aganglionic colon is lowered outside the perineum until the normally ganglionic region is reached. The aganglionic colon is removed, and the remaining mucosa of the colon is anastomosed with the residual anal mucosa.

At the end of the pull-through, the neorectum consists of a double muscular layer. The outer shell is the rectal native musculature ("cuff") located in anatomical continuity with the external sphincter, responsible for the physiological continence mechanisms. The internal muscular layer is represented by the musculature of the lowered normally ganglionic bowel whose function is to ensure the normal fecal progression.

In recent years, the evolution in the treatment of HD has permitted the use of laparoscopic surgery that gained acceptance becoming the technique of choice for the treatment of almost all type of HD.

In 1995, Keith E. Georgeson described "the primary laparoscopic-assisted transanal endorectal colon pull-through for Hirschsprung's disease." The procedure described by Georgeson may be defined as a "minimally invasive Soave-type operation" because it is based on the same surgical principles of the Soave technique with few differences: the section of the mesocolon is performed laparoscopically and the endorectal dissection is completed through the anus (transanal) and not through the abdominal cavity.

The technique has a first laparoscopic step and a subsequent perineal step. The laparoscopic step starts with the identification of the transition zone (by laparoscopic biopsy). Once the presence of ganglia has been confirmed, the mesocolon of the distal aganglionic bowel is dissected until you reach the peritoneal rectal reflection (Fig. 22.4).

The rectum is then dissected starting from the circumferential section of the peritoneal reflection. The rectal isolation proceeds with blunt dissection adjacent to the rectal walls (Fig. 22.5).

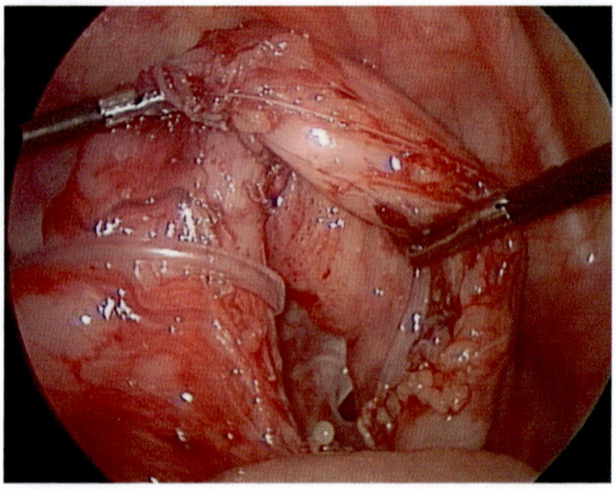

Fig. 22.4 Laparoscopic mesocolon dissection of the aganglionic bowel, performed distally to the biopsy

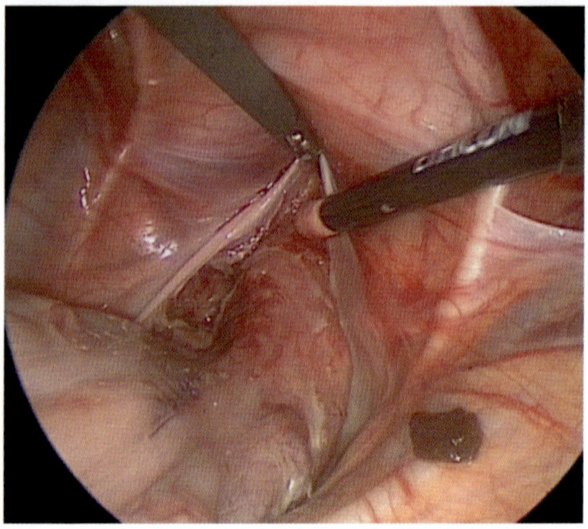

Fig. 22.5 Section of the rectal peritoneal reflection

The perineal step involves the dissection of the rectal mucosa and the subsequent pull-through of the colon. The transanal mucosal rectal dissection starts with a mucosal incision performed 0.5–1 cm above the dentate line (Fig. 22.6).

The blunt approach permits the identification of a submucosal plane of dissection (Fig. 22.7). The mucosectomy proceeds proximally for 10–15 cm until the plane of the rectal dissection (performed laparoscopically) has been reached. At this point, the rectum "prolapses" outside.

The rectal muscular layer ("cuff") is sectioned at its distal part, and it is reintroduced into the pelvis after the section of the anterior and posterior edges (Fig. 22.8).

The next step is the lowering of the colon inside the rectal muscular cuff until the normally ganglionic region (where there the biopsy was performed) is identified (Fig. 22.9).

The aganglionic bowel is resected and the colo-anal anastomosis is performed (Fig. 22.10) [2, 3].

22.11 Postoperative Care

A nasogastric tube is maintained for 12–24 h. The patient continues broad-spectrum antibiotic therapy for 5–7 days. The patient can be fed once

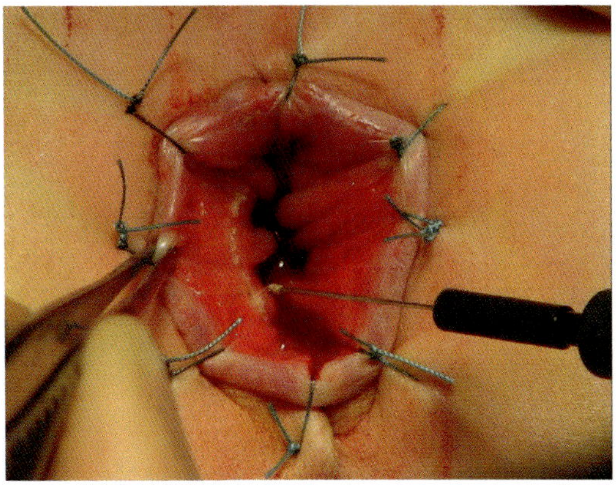

Fig. 22.6 Circumferential mucosal incision, 5–10 mm above the pectinate line

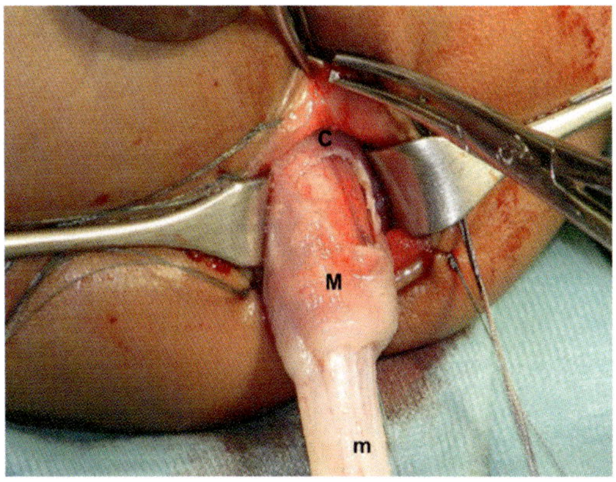

Fig. 22.8 Mucosectomy proceeds until the rectum prolapses (once the point of the laparoscopic isolation has been reached). The rectal muscular wall without the mucosa is sectioned and reintroduced into the pelvis (*m* mucosa, *M* muscle, *C* muscular cuff)

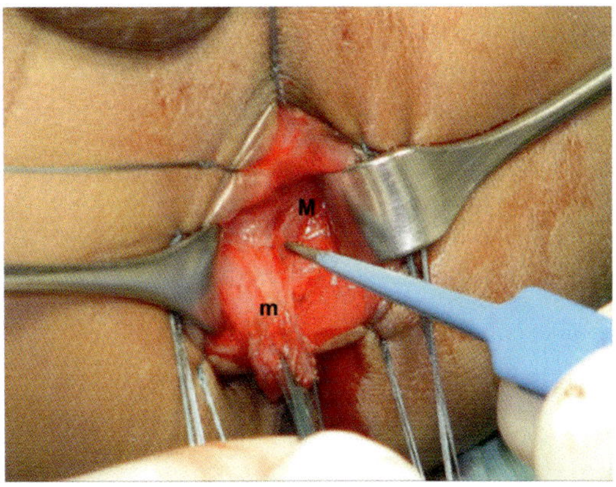

Fig. 22.7 A submucosal dissection plane is identified by blunt dissection (*m* anal mucosa with traction stitches, *M* muscular cuff)

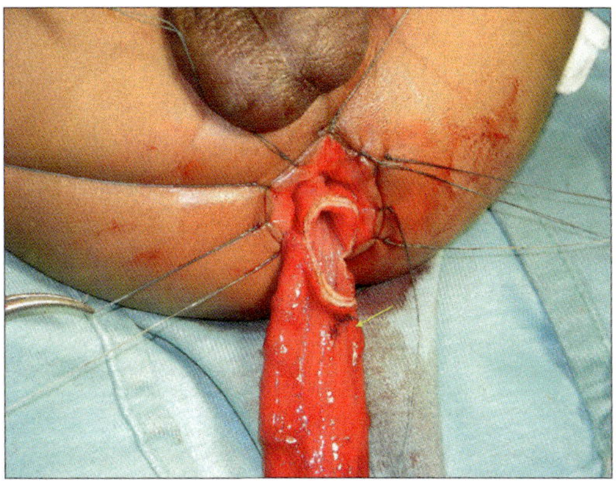

Fig. 22.9 Pull-through of the aganglionic colon inside the muscular cuff until the site of the biopsy (yellow arrow) is reached

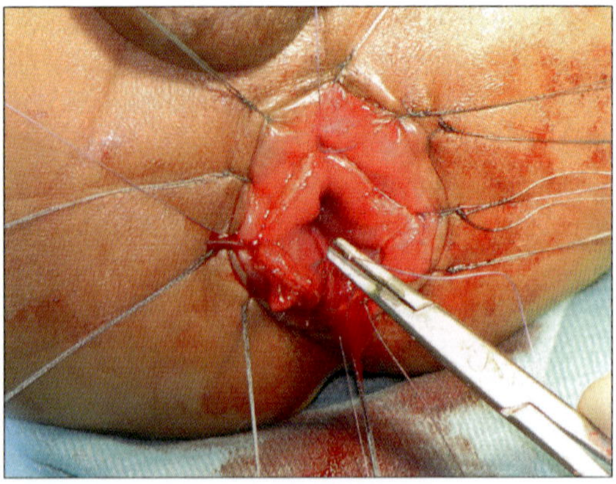

Fig. 22.10 Ano-colic anastomosis

bowel movements resume and discharged once full fed is reached. Two weeks after surgery, the anal anastomosis is dilated to avoid strictures. Anal dilatations continue for about 1 year.

22.12 Complications

The most frequent early postoperative complication is represented by colo-anal anastomosis dehiscence (3.2 %) which, if not massive, is solvable conservatively.

Late postoperative complications are more frequent:

- HAEC (2–40 %) treated by intensive bowel irrigations, broad-spectrum antibiotics, and, in severe unresponsive cases, packaging colostomy.
- Colo-anal anastomosis stenosis (0–20 %): a risk factor in the onset of a stenosis is its previous dehiscence; conservative treatment with anal dilatation is usually sufficient to resolve the stenosis.

22.13 Redo Pull-Through for Hirschsprung's Disease

22.13.1 Introduction

Härold Hirschsprung first described congenital aganglionosis and the associated clinical features in 1886. While Swenson is credited for the first successful treatment of Hirschsprung's disease (HD) [4] in 1948, there are descriptions of the disease process dating back several centuries [5]. Over the last 65 years, many modifications to the surgical repair of HD have been proposed. The operative principles remain the same in that the aganglionic bowel is resected and healthy, and ganglionated bowel is sutured or stapled low in the anal canal above the dentate line, known as a pull-through (PT). The most common techniques performed today are a transanal approach with or without laparoscopic assistance, a modified endorectal PT, and a Duhamel retrorectal PT.

Regardless of the technique, repair most often leads to satisfactory results. However, some children experience long-term postoperative complications [6]. These problems can present with a wide array of stooling disorders after an apparent successful PT procedure. These disorders can range from intermittent enterocolitis to far more significant issues such as severe stool retention, intestinal obstruction, as well as incontinence [7]. Many of these disorders can be managed medically or may even be self-limiting, but on rare occasions (<3 % of children from our own group of primary-PT cases), the child may require a redo-PT procedure.

22.13.2 Redo Pull-Through Data

There is a lack of data with respect to outcomes following redo PT for HD, and while studies have suggested that approach is superior, there is no consensus as to which is the superior approach [8–10]. Specific gaps in data include indications and timing for redo-PT surgery, surgical procedure for redo PT, and stooling outcomes. The University of Michigan recently published their experience over 40 years with PTs for Hirschsprung's disease, including 467 primary pull-through procedures [11]. Nine (2 %) of these eventually underwent redo PT. An additional 37 patients were referred after primary PT elsewhere required redo PT for a total of 46 individuals (52 % male) who underwent redo PT. Since that publication, five additional redo-PT cases have been performed. The child's primary PT was performed for varying levels of aganglionosis, with 59 % having rectosigmoid, 13 % left-sided, and 9 % mid-colon or right-sided (including one patient with total colonic) disease. For 19 % of patients, no recorded length of involved aganglionosis was documented. Open endorectal PT (ERPT) was the most frequent primary PT (41 %), followed by transanal ERPT (22 %), Swenson (17 %), Duhamel (11 %), and unknown operation (9 %).

22.13.2.1 Outcomes After Primary Pull-Through

Common and serious long-term complications after definitive treatment for HD are divided into three groups. These include soiling/incontinence, persistent problems with the passage of stool (e.g., constipation), and recurrent Hirschsprung-associated enterocolitis (HAEC) [12]. Factors contributing to these problems are either pathologic or anatomic. Pathologic causes comprise residual aganglionosis or transitional zone pathology. The anatomic causes involve stricture, with or without anastomotic leak, retained dilated segment, obstructing Duhamel pouch/Soave cuff, or twisted pull-through.

The complications were similar in the Michigan review of redo-PT patients. Early complications after the patient's primary PT occurred in 44 % of all cases that eventually underwent a redo PT. This rate was higher than a historical cohort of patients not requiring a redo PT (16 % $P=0.01$) [13]. These early complications included anastomotic leak (19 %), obstruction (9 %), twisted PT (4 %), and enterocolitis (6 %). Late complications in those children eventually requiring a redo PT included obstructive symptoms (87 %) of which functional constipation made up the majority (54 %). Obstruction was caused by stricture in 22%, and 9 % had a specific technical cause for constipation, including obstructing Duhamel pouch ($n=3$) and a twisted PT segment ($n=1$).

22.13.2.2 Indications for Redo PT and Pathology

Forty-one percent of patients underwent an ostomy creation prior to redo PT. This was due to a dilated colon ($n=10$), stricture ($n=3$), anastomotic leak ($n=3$), or other miscellaneous reasons ($n=3$). Twenty-eight percent of patients at our institution underwent intervention in an attempt to alleviate obstructive symptoms prior to redo PT as per our previously published algorithm [14]. These included anal dilations (two patients), posterior myotomy or myectomy (POMM; seven patients), or Botox® (Allergan, Inc. Irvine, CA) injection into the anal sphincters. The indications for POMM or dilations were stricture or tight cuff. However, five of seven were subsequently found to have retained aganglionosis either by biopsy or upon final review of pathology after redo PT. An additional child was found to have a twisted segment during redo PT.

Indication for redo PT in the recent review was most commonly for a retained aganglionosis/transition zone pathology (RA/TZP; 71 % overall). Other indications included stricture/obstructing Duhamel pouch (19 %), excessively tight cuff (8 %), and twisted PT (4 %), but none for recurrent enterocolitis alone (0 %). A small percentage of the reviewed patients had no listed indication for redo PT. The finding of RA/TZP causing the majority of problems highlights the importance of appropriate pathologic evaluation of the PT segment at the initial operation. Another interesting finding was that timing between primary PT and redo PT was suggestive of the indication for operation. Three groups were established. The immediate re-operative group (those performed within 6 months after the primary PT) all had gross anatomical indications (twisted segment, obstructing Duhamel pouch, or stricture) for their redo PT. The early (<3 years) and late (>3 years) redo-PT groups showed 40 and 70 % of patients having RA/TZP, respectively.

The primary PT pathology slides of the nine redo PTs that had the initial operation at Michigan were pulled from the archives and reviewed with a pediatric pathologist with expertise in HD. In eight of the nine, the proximal margin of the original PT segment had normal ganglion cells and lacked hypertrophic nerves at the time of the primary PT. Interestingly, the redo-PT specimen from each of these eight cases showed findings consistent with RA/TZP. There was a variable length of aganglionic bowel at the site of the anastomosis. This strongly suggests that an acquired aganglionic segment developed after the time of the primary PT. Of note, the last patient in this group was found to have a misread frozen section and an inappropriate and aganglionic segment of bowel used for the PT. Eventually, this patient was found to have total colonic aganglionosis (TCA), and a redo PT was performed 11 months after the initial surgery.

22.13.3 Operative Approach of Redo Pull-Through

Performing a redo PT is difficult in many respects. This is true both in the operating room and also in the initial workup and decision tree. Only experienced pediatric surgeons following an appropriate algorithm should take on these cases. Determination that redo PT is necessary is the first step. However, the redo operation carries risks far greater than the original surgery, and each patient should be approached on an individual basis, and an operative intervention should be planned according to its presentation, type of complication, underlying pathology, and previous surgical history. Because of this, operative approach can vary widely and is heavily dependent on these factors as well as surgeon preference as to the type of repair.

In our experience, an open ERPT was the most commonly performed redo-PT procedure (38 %). This was followed by a Swenson (25 %), Duhamel (13 %), and transanal ERPT (7 %). A small proportion of patients will have a frozen pelvis secondary to several previous attempts at redo PT. Distal dissection may not be possible. An end-to-end anastomosis (EEA) can be performed using a circular EEA stapling device.

22.13.4 Outcomes from Redo Pull-Through

Although complex and difficult, patients undergoing redo PT can achieve very good outcomes. Although the number of patients analyzed is small, it appears that there is no correlation with the type of initial or redo PT performed and the long-term outcomes. Complications are quite similar after redo PT compared to primary PT in experienced hands. Early complications include wound infection, anastomotic breakdown or leaks, abscess, perforation, and HAEC. There was, however, no difference in the redo-PT patients' early complication rate when compared to a matched cohort of children undergoing a primary PT (17 vs. 16 %, respectively, $P=0.7$). Late complications are also comparable. The overall rate of late complications was similar to those found in our primary-PT patients (40 vs. 32 %, respectively, $P=0.65$). These late complications comprise constipation, HAEC, stricture, obstruction, and fistula. Only constipation was found to be significantly higher ($P<0.05$) in the redo-PT group.

Of the 51 patients in our series, 32 remained current in our system, thus allowing long-term follow-up. A stooling survey (Kim et al.) was completed through a telephone interview [13] or through scoring based on recent clinic notes. Stooling scores comprised a composite evaluation of stooling pattern (e.g., excessively loose or explosive stooling), continence, and/or evidence of enterocolitis. Eleven patients were lost to follow-up; four were not yet toilet trained (all <3 years of age) or had stomas. The remaining 17 patients and/or families were interviewed. Mean follow-up was 224.5 ± 157.6 months (range 6.3–491.6 months). All these children had their stooling outcomes assessed. Total stooling scores are shown in Table 22.1. Stooling scores are listed in three categories. These are continence, stooling pattern, and enterocolitic complaints and are based on a previously established scoring system [13]. Lower scores denote better outcomes. Total scores were significantly worse in the redo-PT patients compared to the historically matched group of children undergoing a primary PT for HD (5.5 ± 1.2 vs. 12.2 ± 1.4, $P<0.05$). Stooling pattern scores (1.0 ± 0.2 vs. 4.1 ± 0.4, $P=0.001$) and enterocolitis scores (2.0 ± 0.4 vs. 4.2 ± 0.4, $P=0.001$) were statistically worse in the redo-PT group. Continence scores were not different. While slightly higher (worse) in the redo-PT

Table 22.1 Summary of Stooling Survey Outcomes. The Primary PT group is an historical group matched for sex, mental development delay and length of involved segment to the RedoPT group [10]. Stooling scores are broken down into 3 categories, continence, stooling pattern and enterocolitic complaints. A lower score denotes better outcome

Stooling Survey	Primary PT(n=45)	Redo PT (n=17)	P value
Total (0–40)	5.5±1.2	12.2±1.4	0.003*
Continence (0–21)	2.5±0.7	3.9±1.0	*NS*
Stooling pattern (0–9)	1.0±0.2	4.1±0.4	0.001*
Enterocolitis (0–10)	2.0±0.4	4.2±0.4	0.001*

group, continence was not statistically different from those undergoing a primary PT (2.5 ± 0.7 vs. 3.9 ± 1.0 $P=0.33$). In fact, daytime continence of redo-PT children was found to be 81 %. This was similar to the rate of daytime continence in the primary-PT control group of 86 % ($P=0.6$). Only 25 % of redo-PT patients had complaints of occasional nighttime soiling.

22.13.5 Principles of Redo PT

Definitive operative management of HD usually has favorable outcomes. However, with quality-of-life measures, there is a growing appreciation of stooling disorders which HD children present with after an otherwise successful PT procedure [15–17]. These disorders can range from intermittent enterocolitis to severe stool retention, intestinal obstruction, as well as incontinence [7]. Such disorders may be self-limiting, but on rare occasions (<3 % of children from our own group of primary PT cases), the child may be found to benefit from a redo-PT procedure.

With redo PT, stooling outcomes are significantly worse compared to those after a primary PT. Importantly, continence is still retained in the majority of children. In agreement with previous reports on redo PTs, the present study was unable to find a correlation in outcomes based on the type of PT, either at primary PT or redo PT [18–21]. This highlights the fact that the management of complex or recurrent HD requires expert evaluation. Each individual patient's situation should be handled by an experienced team of pediatric surgical specialists. The tailoring of an operative plan on a case-by-case basis is perhaps more important than the specific technique of choice. Nevertheless, several general principles should be followed. The critical step is for the surgeon and team to understand the etiology of the failed PT. For instance, for children with sphincteric spasm or a tight endorectal cuff, the transanal endorectal approach may be most appropriate [19]. In those infants who undergo an initial ERPT, often a redo PT (28 %) using an ERPT approach may be used. Either may be suitable for those patients with a relatively short segment of RA/TZP. Often, laparoscopy may be needed to assist with colonic mobilization and to perform confirmatory seromuscular biopsies if the segment length is in question.

The transabdominal approach is preferred for cases with long-segment aganglionosis, twisted PT, or stricture due to ischemia or leak. This allows for clear identification of the anatomy and complete mobilization of the bowel. Moreover, dissection through the likely dense scar can require an open operation. A twisted segment may be managed in several ways. An endorectal approach may be appropriate, but the child may do better with either a Duhamel or Swenson procedure. The Duhamel approach, as advocated by Langer, is also an option [19]. If this is done, the surgeon must consider the thickness of the tissue layers within the stapler. If an ERPT was the original procedure, the anastomosis will involve a new segment of ganglionic bowel and the original aganglionic muscularis propria, as well as various amounts of scar tissue. A thicker load, as large as the green load (4.5 mm) stapler, may be needed should the operative plan include a stapled anastomosis. In cases where scarring is severe, the authors have occasionally performed a full-thickness mobilization of the rectum as far distally as possible, transecting the diseased portion and then performing an end-to-end stapled anastomosis using an EEA-type stapling device with good results. This technique is useful in patients in whom the pelvis is too frozen to permit complete endorectal dissection or eversion of the distal rectum onto the perineum, but two points are important to emphasize. First, the surgeon should maintain a protective colostomy after the redo PT. In these cases, the EEA anastomosis needs to be intermittently dilated prior to ostomy closure to prevent stricture. Secondly, if the pelvis is frozen, a small length of residual aganglionosis may be left, and this may have to be secondarily dealt with using a more aggressive bowel regimen. The details of operative choices with given clinical situations can be found in greater detail in a chapter previously written by our group [14].

On the day of redo PT, it is imperative that experienced pediatric pathology support is available during the procedure. Although several technical errors have been identified (anastomotic leak and twisted PT segment) as problems leading to symptoms requiring redo PT, the majority of the patients who eventually required redo PT were found to have a pathologic cause for recurrent symptoms in our recent series of 51 individuals undergoing redo PT. This cause of treatment failure has been recently established by two large reviews. In a meta-analysis of 555 redo-PT patients, RA/TZP was cited as a major cause of failure [22]. Another [6] recent publication reported that 63 % of patients requiring redo PT had RA/TZP pathology. The term RA/TZP is used in our report whether the etiology was due to a pathology error at the time of the original PT or due to an acquired, secondary aganglionic segment. This finding is similar to a finding of transition zone pathology predicting problems by several other authors and emphasizes the need for experienced pathology support [6, 23].

Finding RA/TZP at redo PT can only be explained by a few scenarios. The first explanation is that a portion of aganglionic or transition zone bowel was used for the PT segment at the primary PT procedure. This should not happen in experienced hands. Several techniques should be utilized to avoid this misadventure. Full-thickness biopsies done circumferentially should be performed. A ring of tissue should be examined from the colon just distal to the planned pull-through segment prior to completing the anastomosis. This is the only way to assure oneself that the PT segment is entirely ganglionic because transition zones vary from mesenteric to antimesenteric sides as transition zones. Only sending a ring of colon will fully allow proper assessment of the pull-through specimen [6, 24, 25]. The second scenario is incorrect reading of the frozen section by an inexperienced pathologist, which argues for this type of surgery being done at major institution with expert pathology [26].

Even when using the aforementioned methods, the most experienced surgeons at high-volume centers can experience operative failure due to RA/TZP. Our experience has been similar. The original pathology slides of all patients who had both the primary PT and redo PT at our institution were rereviewed. In eight of nine, the proximal margin of the original PT segment had normal ganglion cells and lacked hypertrophic nerves. The ninth was recognized as a pathologic misread and redo was performed early. The redo-PT specimen from each of the remaining eight cases showed findings consistent with RA/TZP. This phenomenon supports a concept of an acquired segment of aganglionosis. Some authors have postulated that this may be a variant form of HD [27]. Others hypothesize that secondary aganglionosis may be due to neuronal cell death from an ischemic insult on the distal PT [28]. Review of the pathology showed no evidence of ischemia in the redo-PT pathology. The acquisition of this aganglionic segment may come from the child's own growth, potentially in association with an upward tension on the PT segment. This would lead to a stretching of the remaining aganglionic segment. Additionally, chronic constipation might contribute to elongation of the segment. These initial observations require more data to validate this speculative theory.

These redo-PT procedures are technically quite challenging and require expertise in all types of pull-through procedures for HD. We would advocate that these cases be evaluated and operated upon by an experienced pediatric surgeon with the necessary surrounding clinical support. It is of interest to note that our series had very few children requiring a redo PT due to a tight cuff or HAEC. This is at variance with other recent redo-PT series [24]; this may be due to an increasing appreciation and avoidance of these problems during the primary PT [29]. It may also be due to the fact that we have good success with a posterior myomectomy (POMM) procedure in children with these disorders [29]. The number of patients undergoing interventions for obstructive symptoms in this redo-PT group was three times higher than what we previously reported in our primary-PT patients (9 %) after their initial PT. This suggests that this group of patients would not have been cured without a redo PT. POMM can be successful when used in selected situations, e.g., recurrent enterocolitis or tight cuff, but is inappropriate with RA/TZP or mechanical complications.

Success rates vary widely after redo PT depending on the definitions of good outcomes [23, 24, 30]. Some series have reported very low fecal continence rates (50 % range) [31], but this may be due to injuries incurred at the primary PT. Others report a high cure rate after redo PT (over 91 %); however, these authors do not report a functional assessment of these patients [20]. Lawal et al. report that 85 % of patients had some degree of continence after redo PT [24]. Though a detailed score is not given, the results are similar to our own report of 81 % of patients remaining continent. The stooling pattern of our patients was quite good. Nevertheless, we found our stooling outcomes to be significantly worse than those in our own primary-PT patients. This emphasizes the fact that this group of children should be approached carefully by an experienced team. Aggressive prevention of functional constipation after anatomic repair is important in avoiding recurrent symptoms of large bowel obstruction.

In conclusion, re-operative HD surgery is complex. This begins with the workup after initial presentation following primary PT to the definitive surgical correction with redo PT. There is no best operative approach for a redo PT, and the decision tree can be variable with each patient. The operating pediatric surgeon must be able to utilize different operations to treat this problem and the treatment options available. While lesser procedures may provide relief in a select population, those with RA/TZP or mechanical problems will likely require a redo PT. Thus the diagnostic workup, treatment plan, and definitive surgical care should be coordinated and executed by an experienced, specialized team at a pediatric referral center.

References

1. Holschneider AM, Puri P (2000) Hirschsprung's disease and allied disorders, 2nd edn. Springer, New York
2. Georgeson KE, Robertson DJ (2004) Laparoscopic-assisted approaches for the definitive surgery for Hirschsprung's disease. Semin Pediatr Surg 13:256–262
3. Ruggeri G, Libri M, Randi B (2012) Morbo di Hirschsprung. In: Lima M (ed) Chirurgia Endoscopica e Mini-Invasiva Pediatrica. Clueb, Bologna
4. Swenson O, Bill AH Jr (1948) Resection of rectum and rectosigmoid with preservation of the sphincter for benign spastic lesions producing megacolon; an experimental study. Surgery 24(2):212–220
5. Raveenthiran V (2011) Knowledge of ancient Hindu surgeons on Hirschsprung disease: evidence from Sushruta Samhita of circa 1200–600 BC. J Pediatr Surg 46(11):2204–2208
6. Coe A, Collins MH, Lawal T, Louden E, Levitt MA, Pena A (2012) Reoperation for Hirschsprung disease: pathology of the resected problematic distal pull-through. Pediatr Dev Pathol Off J Soc Pediatr Pathol Paediatr Pathol Soc 15(1):30–38
7. Levitt MA, Dickie B, Pena A (2012) The Hirschsprungs patient who is soiling after what was considered a "successful" pull-through. Semin Pediatr Surg 21(4):344–353
8. Minford JL, Ram A, Turnock RR, Lamont GL, Kenny SE, Rintala RJ et al (2004) Comparison of functional outcomes of Duhamel and transanal endorectal coloanal anastomosis for Hirschsprung's disease. J Pediatr Surg 39(2):161–165; discussion –5
9. Saleh W, Rasheed K, Mohaidly MA, Kfoury H, Tariq M, Rawaf AA (2004) Management of Hirschsprung's disease: a comparison of Soave's and Duhamel's pull-through methods. Pediatr Surg Int 20(8):590–593
10. Craigie RJ, Conway SJ, Cooper L, Turnock RR, Lamont GL, Baillie CT et al (2007) Primary pull-through for Hirschsprung's disease: comparison of open and laparoscopic-assisted procedures. J Laparoendosc Adv Surg Tech A 17(6):809–812
11. Ralls MW, Freeman JJ, Rabah R, Coran AG, Ehrlich PF, Hirschl RB et al (2014) Redo pull-through for Hirschsprung disease: a single surgical group's experience. J Pediatr Surg 49(9):1394–1399
12. Murphy F, Puri P (2005) New insights into the pathogenesis of Hirschsprung's associated enterocolitis. Pediatr Surg Int 21(10):773–779

13. Kim AC, Langer JC, Pastor AC, Zhang L, Sloots CE, Hamilton NA et al (2010) Endorectal pull-through for Hirschsprung's disease-a multicenter, long-term comparison of results: transanal vs transabdominal approach. J Pediatr Surg 45(6):1213–1220
14. Ralls MW, Coran AG, Teitelbaum DH (2012) Reoperative surgery for Hirschsprung disease. Semin Pediatr Surg 21(4):354–363
15. Engum SA, Grosfeld JL (2004) Long-term results of treatment of Hirschsprung's disease. Semin Pediatr Surg 13(4):273–285
16. Ieiri S, Nakatsuji T, Akiyoshi J, Higashi M, Hashizume M, Suita S et al (2010) Long-term outcomes and the quality of life of Hirschsprung disease in adolescents who have reached 18 years or older – a 47-year single-institute experience. J Pediatr Surg 45(12):2398–2402
17. Rintala RJ, Pakarinen MP (2012) Long-term outcomes of Hirschsprung's disease. Semin Pediatr Surg 21(4):336–343
18. Dasgupta R, Langer JC (2008) Evaluation and management of persistent problems after surgery for Hirschsprung disease in a child. J Pediatr Gastroenterol Nutr 46(1):13–19
19. Langer J (1999) Repeat pull-through surgery for complicated Hirschsprung's disease: indications, techniques, and results. J Pediatr Surg 34:1136–1141
20. Weber TR, Fortuna RS, Silen ML, Dillon PA (1999) Reoperation for Hirschsprung's disease. J Pediatr Surg 34(1):153–156; discussion 6–7
21. Moore SW, Albertyn R, Cywes S (1996) Clinical outcome and long-term quality of life after surgical correction of Hirschsprung's disease. J Pediatr Surg 31(11):1496–1502
22. Friedmacher F, Puri P (2011) Residual aganglionosis after pull-through operation for Hirschsprung's disease: a systematic review and meta-analysis. Pediatr Surg Int 27(10):1053–1057
23. Schweizer P, Berger S, Schweizer M, Holschneider AM, Beck O (2007) Repeated pull-through surgery for complicated Hirschsprung's disease – principles derived from clinical experience. J Pediatr Surg 42(3):536–543
24. Lawal TA, Chatoorgoon K, Collins MH, Coe A, Pena A, Levitt MA (2011) Redo pull-through in Hirschsprung's [corrected] disease for obstructive symptoms due to residual aganglionosis and transition zone bowel. J Pediatr Surg 46(2):342–347
25. White FV, Langer JC (2000) Circumferential distribution of ganglion cells in the transition zone of children with Hirschsprung disease. Pediatr Devel Pathol 3(3):216–222
26. Shayan K, Smith C, Langer JC (2004) Reliability of intraoperative frozen sections in the management of Hirschsprung's disease. J Pediatr Surg 39(9):1345–1348
27. Puri P, Gosemann JH (2012) Variants of Hirschsprung disease. Semin Pediatr Surg 21(4):310–318
28. West KW, Grosfeld JL, Rescorla FJ, Vane DW (1990) Acquired aganglionosis: a rare occurrence following pull-through procedures for Hirschsprung's disease. J Pediatr Surg 25(1):104–108; discussion 8–9
29. Wildhaber B, Pakarinen M, Rintala R, Coran A, Teitelbaum D (2004) Posterior myotomy/myectomy for persistent stooling problems in Hirschsprung's disease. J Ped Surg 39(6):920–926
30. van Leeuwen K, Teitelbaum DH, Elhalaby EA, Coran AG (2000) Long-term follow-up of redo pull-through procedures for Hirschsprung's disease: efficacy of the endorectal pull-through. J Pediatr Surg 35(6):829–833; discussion 33–4
31. Pena A, Elicevik M, Levitt MA (2007) Reoperations in Hirschsprung disease. J Pediatr Surg 42(6):1008–1013; discussion 13–4

Inflammatory Bowel Disease

23

Giovanni Di Nardo, Andrea Pession, Luca Bertelli, Sara Isoldi, Rita Cozzali, Michela Maffi, and Mario Lima

Inflammatory bowel disease (IBD) includes two classic entities, Crohn's disease (CD) and ulcerative colitis (UC), and a third undetermined form (IBD-U), characterized by a chronic relapsing course resulting in a high rate of morbidity and impaired quality of life. In this chapter, we will describe the current knowledge in management options for children with IBD, emphasizing the unique aspects of the pediatric condition.

G. Di Nardo (✉)
Pediatric Gastroenterology Unit, International Hospital Salvator Mundi, Via Della Mura Gianicolesi 67, 00152 Rome, Italy,
e-mail: giovanni.dinardo3@alice.it

A. Pession
Pediatric Unit, S. Orsola-Malpighi Hospital, University of Bologna, Bologna, Italy

L. Bertelli
Pediatric Unit, S. Orsola-Malpighi Hospital, Bologna, Italy

S. Isoldi
Pediatric Gastroenterology Unit, Sapienza - University of Rome, Rome, Italy

R. Cozzali
Pediatric Gastroenterology Unit, Foligno Hospital, Foligno (PG), Italy

M. Maffi • M. Lima
Pediatric Surgery, S. Orsola-Malpighi Hospital, Bologna University, Bologna, Italy
e-mail: mario.lima@unibo.it

23.1 Ulcerative Colitis

23.1.1 Introduction

Ulcerative colitis is an idiopathic IBD affecting primarily the mucosal layer of the colon. UC is more frequent between ages 15 and 35 (20 % of patients are younger than 20 years old), even if it has been reported in every decade of life. The disease extent is variable; inflammation can be restricted either to the distal rectum or to the entire colon. Usually, early-onset disease (<5 years old) is more aggressive than adolescence or adult onset. Pediatric onset of disease is characterized by delayed skeletal maturation and a delayed onset of puberty. Hence, as well as gastrointestinal and extraintestinal complications, growth and nutrition are key priorities in the management of adolescents with UC, together with psychosocial implications [1].

23.1.2 Epidemiology and Pathogenesis

The incidence of UC in children has remained almost constant over the past five decades. Incidence rates are noted to be increased recently in countries where IBD was previously uncommon. According to Scandinavian, North American, and UK studies, UC incidence in children ranges from 2.1 to 4.2 cases/year/100,000 population. This disease is more common in

M. Lima (ed.), *Pediatric Digestive Surgery*, DOI 10.1007/978-3-319-40525-4_23

industrialized countries and in urban population. This peculiar distribution suggests that environmental factors may be fundamental to the development of such disease. Of course, genetic predisposition is crucial: higher rates are reported in Jewish population than non-Jewish, and they are even higher in the same ethnic population moved from low-risk geographic region to high-risk one. Concordance rates among monozygotic twins are about 16.5 % and among dizygotic twins about 2 %. Therefore, the pathogenesis of such disease seems to imply genetic, environmental, and immunologic factors. Precisely, the interaction between the intestinal microflora and the host innate immune system may lead to a deregulated immune response and consequently to inflammation. Antibiotic usage, especially early in childhood, and dietary habits may trigger UC by modifying microbiome. However, there is no data to support whether microflora alteration is the cause or the result of intestinal inflammation [2].

23.1.3 Clinical Features

UC is a chronic inflammatory bowel disease characterized by flare-ups and remissions. Clinical presentation of pediatric UC depends on disease extension, severity, and patient age. Most common symptoms include rectal bleeding, abdominal pain, and diarrhea. If the disease involves the rectum only (proctitis), common symptoms are tenesmus and urgency, together with bloody stools. Otherwise, left-sided colitis and pancolitis generally present with abdominal pain and diarrhea with blood and mucus. Systemic symptoms, such as low-grade fever, weight loss, anemia, lethargy, and growth retardation, may be present. Several studies have reported more extensive colonic involvement in childhood-onset compared to adult-onset disease. Furthermore, about 35 % of children with UC required immunomodulators within 12 months of diagnosis, and the median time to first surgery was shorter in patients with childhood-onset than in adult-onset patients. Although most of pediatric patients will present with a mild form of the disease, about 10–15 % of them will present with an acute and severe one (fulminant colitis). In adults this pattern is defined as the presence of six or more bloody stools per day along with one of the following: anemia, tachycardia, fever, and elevated ESR. This classification has never been validated in children, because of age-dependent hemoglobin values and pulse rate; moreover, fever is not so common in children with severe colitis. Therefore, a noninvasive, continuous scoring for pediatric UC activity evaluation has been proposed, which is the pediatric UC activity index (PUCAI). It is based on six variables, which are abdominal pain, rectal bleeding, stool consistency, nocturnal stools, number of stools each 24 h, and interruption to normal activities, and it is adequate to quantify the degree of disease severity. Cutoff scores for remission and mild, moderate, and severe disease have been identified and validated: PUCAI 0–9 indicates remission, 10–34 mild activity, 35–64 moderate activity, and 65–85 severe activity. PUCAI has been proven to correlate closely with physician's global assessment and endoscopic score. Acute severe UC is considered as a life-threatening condition, with risk of various complications. The mortality rate is about 1 %, and most common severe complications are massive hemorrhage, toxic megacolon, perforation, and intestinal infections. Potential complications of long-standing UC include dysplasia, colon cancer (CRC), and rarely strictures. A meta-analysis reported that the cumulative risk of CRC in patients with UC was 2 % at 10 years, 8 % at 20 years, and 18 % at 30 years. The risk is increased by specific factors, such as disease duration, extensive mucosal involvement, concomitant primary sclerosing cholangitis, family history of CRC, and early onset of UC. ECCO guidelines published in 2013 recommend a screening colonoscopy 8 years after the onset of colic symptoms. Ongoing surveillance should be repeated every 1, 3, or 5 years depending on the risk factors.

23.1.4 Extraintestinal Manifestations

Extraintestinal manifestations of UC may occur in 25–30 % of children with CU. It may present at diagnosis in about 6–23 % of children, with higher frequency in those >6 years. Many symptoms seem to be independent on disease activity, such as pyoderma gangrenosum, uveitis, axial arthropathy, autoimmune hepatitis, and primary sclerosing cholangitis. In particular, the latter affects 3–7.5 % of children with UC, and it is responsible for the destruction of biliary ducts that is most of the cases irreversible and refractory on medical treatment and often leads to liver transplantation. Symptoms such as peripheral arthritis, episcleritis, erythema nodosum, and aphthous stomatitis, on the contrary, usually come out or exacerbate parallel to intestinal inflammatory activity and extension. Several studies have reported an increased risk for venous thromboembolism (VTE) in IBD population, especially during flare-ups. For this reason, it is useful to verify the presence of additional risk factors for VTE, such as thrombophilia, chronic presence of antiphospholipid antibody, obesity, smoking, the use of oral contraceptives, and other medications with increased risk of thrombosis, in patients with UC.

23.1.5 Diagnosis

The diagnosis of UC relies on exhaustive anamnesis, the presence of gastrointestinal and extraintestinal manifestation, family history, and physical examination, together with endoscopic and histological characteristic features. It is essential to exclude other causes of intestinal inflammation, such as Crohn's disease and infectious colitis. In infancy, a common cause of bloody diarrhea with cramping is allergic colitis. In infancy, other causes of bloody diarrhea should be considered, such as necrotizing enterocolitis, Hirschsprung's enterocolitis, and intussusception. Differential diagnosis for early-onset colitis includes immunodeficiency; the most common are chronic granulomatous disease and IL10 receptor deficiency. In older children, polyps and Meckel's diverticulum should be considered. Physical examination consists primarily of abdomen and perianal region examination. Signs of abdominal distention, tenderness, and mass should be checked. Perianal abnormalities include fissures, skin tags, fistulas, or abscess. Eventual extraintestinal manifestations of IBD should be documented. Then, assessment of height, weight, and nutrition is useful [1].

23.1.5.1 Laboratory Assessment

The initial work-up consists in collection of multiple stool samples for microscopy and culture in order to exclude an enteric infection. Most frequent microbic agents that can mimic UC are *Shigella*, *Salmonella*, *Campylobacter*, *Enteropathogenic Escherichia coli*, *Yersinia*, and *Clostridium difficile*. Exclusion of enteric infection is fundamental, but we have to take into account that infective agents may trigger a first episode of flare of UC. Hence, the identification of an enteric infection does not necessarily exclude a diagnosis of UC. Stool inflammatory markers are helpful to assess bowel inflammation: fecal calprotectin and lactoferrin are generally increased in active UC. Fecal biomarkers may be useful as screening test, because they are noninvasive and they have a high sensitivity; however, they are largely nonspecific, since they cannot distinguish UC from CD or from any other inflammatory bowel conditions, including enteric infections. Routine laboratory studies may reveal a nonspecific inflammatory state with leukocytosis, thrombocytosis, hypoalbuminemia, and elevated C-reactive protein (CRP) and erythrocyte sedimentation rate (ESR). Nevertheless they have low specificity and sensitivity for gut inflammation, because in most cases (about 54 % of children with mild disease) they are quite normal at the time of diagnosis.

Even if results are often negative, two serological markers may be useful in differential diagnosis between CD and UC: the presence of antineutrophil cytoplasmic antibodies (ANCA) is more common in UC (60–70 %) than in CD (20–25 %), whereas anti-*Saccharomyces cerevisiae* antibodies (ASCA) are more frequently found in CD (50–70 %) than in UC (10–15 %). These markers may be useful to orientate the diagnosis in cases of chronic colitis not referable to UC nor CD despite extensive work-up.

23.1.5.2 Endoscopic and Histologic Evaluation

Colonoscopy and ileoscopy with biopsies play a pivotal role in the diagnostic process of UC. Typical endoscopic appearance of UC is diffuse uniform inflammation extending proximally from the rectum for a variable length. Common findings are erythema, granularity and increased

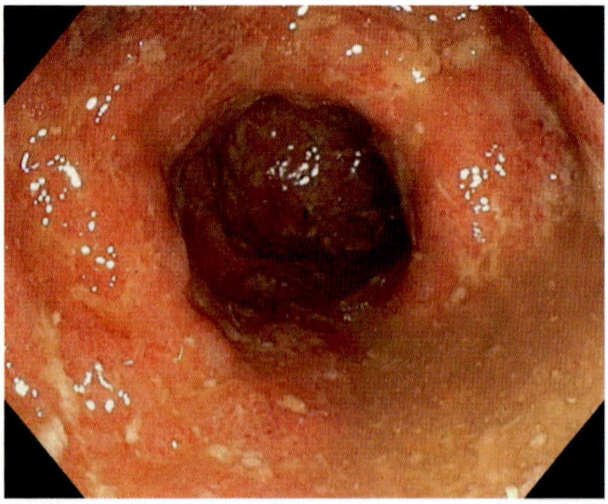

Fig. 23.1 Typical endoscopic findings of ulcerative colitis characterized by friability of colonic mucosa and the presence of erosions and minute ulcers

friability of colonic mucosa, loss of normal vascular pattern, and the presence of erosions and minute ulcers (Fig. 23.1). In case of severe disease, deeper ulcerations may be present, and, rarely, strictures have been described. Pseudopolyps are characteristic of a long-standing disease. If pancolitis is present, the inflammation may involve the terminal ileum that may exhibit a nonerosive erythema and edema of the mucosa ("backwash ileitis"). Ileal inflammation correlates with the degree of inflammation of the right colon. Typical histological findings of UC are a continuous pattern of acute and chronic inflammation limited to mucosal layer, with basal plasmacytosis, crypt distortion, crypt abscesses, and goblet cell depletion. Generally, inflammation progressively decreases from distal to proximal colon. The absence of granulomas helps to exclude CD. The adult-based Montreal disease classification system for IBD includes three types of UC: proctitis (E1), left-sided disease (E2), and disease proximal to the splenic flexure (E3). Recently, Paris classification has modified the Montreal system for pediatric UC by the addition of E4 (disease proximal to hepatic flexure) and S1 (severe UC).

In children five atypical features of UC have been reported:

1. Rectal sparing: 5–30 % of untreated pediatric patients exhibit a macroscopic, though not microscopic, normal rectal mucosa. This feature is more frequent in younger children.
2. Short duration: in young children with short duration of disease, biopsies may show a focal inflammation or absence of typical architectural distortion.
3. Cecal patch: about 2 % of children with left-sided colitis exhibit an area of cecal inflammation. Histopathologic examination reveals a nonspecific inflammation without granulomas.
4. Upper gastrointestinal endoscopy: 4–8 % of children present an upper gastrointestinal involvement, with diffuse or focal inflammation and mild ulcerations.
5. Acute severe colitis: children with acute pancolitis may have histopathology findings similar to CD, such as transmural inflammation and deep ulcers. However, lymphoid aggregates are absent, and ulcers are typically V-shaped, differently from CD.

Hence, in addition to ileocolonoscopy, the ESPGHAN Revised Porto Criteria for IBD recommend to perform esophagogastroduodenoscopy with biopsies in all children, when IBD is suspected, irrespective of the presence or absence of upper gastrointestinal symptoms.

23.1.5.3 Small Bowel Imaging

Small bowel evaluation is essential if IBD is suspected. The ESPGHAN Revised Porto Criteria for IBD recommend to perform it during the diagnostic work-up, in order to evaluate the extent or the presence of small bowel CD and to aid the diagnosis in patients with atypical UC; it can be delayed in patients with typical UC. Magnetic resonance imaging is an accurate radiation-free test useful to ascertain the extent and the degree of the disease. In order to better evaluate the lumen, distention of intestinal loops may be produced by polyethylene glycol solution administration, given by mouth or by nasogastric tube. Ultrasound may also be useful in IBD evaluation because it is a noninvasive, low-cost, widespread available tool. However interobserver variability is very high. Small intestine contrast US, consisting in using of an oral anechoic contrast, increases its sensitivity and reduces interobserver variability.

Alternative methodologies in the assessment of small bowel disease are capsule endoscopy (CE) and balloon-assisted enteroscopy (BAE). The first is a high-sensitivity and well-tolerated tool, although it does not consent to take biopsies, and has a high number of false-positive features. If stricture is suspected, patency capsule should precede CE, because of the risk of retention. BAE may be very useful in small bowel evaluation, because of the possibility to biopsies taken. However, it is indicated in selected cases. Radiological tools, such as plain abdominal radiograph and abdominal/pelvic CT scans, may be useful to detect UC complications, like toxic megacolon and perforation [3].

23.1.6 Management

Management of children with UC consists not only in inducing and maintaining remission; considering that chronic diseases influence growth and psychological aspects of children, in this population, it is necessary to optimize growth and to ensure pubertal development and physiologic well-being. Treatment options depend on the extent and severity of disease. Medical treatment should be proposed first. Surgery should be reserved to patients with severe and/or refractory disease or with serious pharmacological side effects.

23.1.6.1 Mild-to-Moderate Colitis

The first-line therapy in children with mild-to-moderate colitis is oral aminosalicylates, which can be combined with topical aminosalicylates to increase remission rate, if tolerated. Aminosalicylates are used in induction and maintenance treatment of UC. The aminosalicylates of choice are mesalazine and sulfasalazine. Their effectiveness is quite similar, but sulfasalazine is considered superior to mesalazine in patients with associated arthropathy, although dose-dependent adverse events (headaches, nausea, and fatigue) are more frequent. Oral mesalazine dosage for pediatric population is 60–80 mg/kg/day in one or two daily doses with a maximal dose of 4, 8 g/daily. Rectal mesalazine is dosed 25 mg/kg up to 1 g once daily. Sulfasalazine is dosed 40–70 mg/kg/day in one or two daily doses up to 4 g/day. To minimize side effects, sulfasalazine may be started at a dose of 10–20 mg/kg/day with a gradual dose increase over a 2-week period. In addition, sulfasalazine impairs folic acid absorption, so its supplementation is recommended to prevent anemia. Maintenance dose of mesalazine is the same as used for induction therapy. Because of their safety profile, they could be continued indefinitely. Dosage may be reduced after a long period of complete remission. Serious side effects are uncommon, and they usually resolve when the medication is stopped. Acute intolerance to aminosalicylates may mimic a flare of colitis, and it precludes any further usage of that drug. Patient's response to medication may be evaluated 2 weeks after onset of therapy. If no response is seen then, rectal therapy (if not started already) or oral steroids should be offered.

23.1.6.2 Proctitis/Left-Sided Colitis

Left-sided colitis and proctitis are usually managed with topical mesalazine or topical steroids. Mesalazine is available as enema and suppositories. They can be used for induction and maintenance remission. Suppositories are useful for proctitis, while left-sided colitis is treated with enemas, as long as they can reach the left colon. Corticosteroids enema or suppositories are useful for induction therapy, but prolonged treatment may cause systemic side effects. Often, oral aminosalicylates are added to the topical therapy in patients with moderate left-sided colitis.

23.1.6.3 Moderate Colitis

Oral steroids are useful in inducing remission in pediatric patient with moderate colitis and systemic symptoms. Because of their well-known side effects (e.g., weight gain, fluid retention, growth retardation, mood disorders, osteopenia, aseptic necrosis, glaucoma, cataracts), corticosteroids should be tapered shortly after remission is achieved. Standard corticosteroids therapy involves oral prednisone or prednisolone, which are dosed 1 mg/kg up to 60 mg/day once daily. Beclomethasone dipropionate is an alternative steroid that may be used orally or rectally in mild-to-moderate colitis, with fewer systemic steroids side effects.

23.1.6.4 Severe Colitis

Severe acute colitis is a potentially life-threatening condition, defined by PUCAI greater than 65. It requires hospitalization for further evaluation and management. Assessment of vital sign and key blood test evaluation are essential. Stool samples should be collected for culture and *Clostridium difficile* toxin detection. Severe UC first-line therapy is intravenous corticosteroids. Methylprednisolone is dosed 1–1.5 mg/kg/day up to 60 mg/day in one or two doses daily. In addition, supportive treatment may be required: fluid rehydration, correction of electrolytes imbalance, blood transfusion, and albumin infusion. PUCAI score should be evaluated daily. A score of greater than 45 on day 3 of admission is predictive of lack of response to corticosteroids. A score of greater than 70 on day 5 guided the start of rescue therapy. There is no agreement about intravenous corticosteroid therapy duration; 7–14 days of therapy are usually enough to obtain a good clinical response. Recently, a consensus statement for managing acute severe ulcerative colitis in children from ECCO, ESPGHAN, and the Porto IBD Group of ESPGHAN has been published. Key points of this document are the following:

1. Stool evaluation should include standard culture and specific screening for *C. difficile*.
2. In children with steroid-resistant disease, CMV infection should be excluded endoscopically.
3. Disease activity should be monitored frequently during admission, with regular assessment of vital signs, daily PUCAI score evaluation, and monitoring of key blood tests (ESR, full blood count, albumin, and electrolytes) at admission and at subsequent intervals.
4. First-line therapy is intravenous corticosteroids with methylprednisolone.
5. Antibiotics are not recommended routinely but should be considered when infection is suspected or when toxic megacolon is present.
6. There is no evidence for the routine use of prophylactic heparin to prevent thromboembolic events.
7. Aminosalicylate therapies should be interrupted at admission, and in naive patients, its introduction should be delayed.
8. Regular diet should be continued. If oral intake seems inadequate, nutritional support (enteral or parenteral) should be considered. Oral intake should be ceased when surgery appears imminent and it is contraindicated in toxic megacolon.
9. Children with increasing or severe abdominal pain should be investigated for complication onset, such as perforation or toxic megacolon. Narcotics or nonsteroidal anti-inflammatory drugs are not recommended in the setting of acute severe colitis.
10. PUCAI scores can be used to monitor response and the need for secondary therapy. A score greater than 45 points at day 3 indicates poor response to corticosteroids and a need to prepare for rescue therapy. A score greater than 65 on day 5 indicates a need to a rapid switch to rescue therapy. If PUCAI scores is between 35 and 60 at day 5, steroids can be continued for a further 2–5 days before secondary therapy should be considered. Children with scores of less than 35 points on day 5 are unlikely to require rescue therapy.
11. Plain radiographs of the abdomen should be obtained in any child with clinical signs of toxicity and subsequently as indicated. The diagnostic criteria for toxic megacolon consist of radiological evidence of transverse colonic dilatation (≥56 mm) along with systemic signs. In children less than 10 years old, a radiological evidence of transverse colonic dilatation greater than 40 mm with signs of systemic toxicity is sufficient to diagnose a toxic megacolon. Urgent surgical consultation is required in all children with toxic megacolon. If the child has stable vital signs and there are no signs of sepsis, conservative management may be appropriate. If signs of toxicity worsen or they do not resolve within 48–72 h, immediate colec-

tomy should be performed. Rescue medical therapies are not indicated in the setting of toxic megacolon.
12. Rescue therapies include medical (infliximab or calcineurin inhibitors) and surgical (colectomy) options.
13. Sequential medical rescue therapy is not recommended in children.
14. If colectomy is required in acute severe colitis in children, subtotal colectomy and ileostomy is recommended. Pouch formation can subsequently be considered.
15. Surgical complications can be reduced by avoiding delays in colectomy, improving nutrition, and using perioperative broad-spectrum antibiotic coverage. Preoperative steroid administration is related to an increased risk of anastomotic leak and infectious complications, although surgery should not be delayed to taper steroids.

23.1.6.5 Salvage Therapy

A second-line medical therapy is usually preferred than surgery in children. However, colectomy may be required in several circumstances, such as patients with severe colitis unresponsive to medical therapy, patients with complications (toxic megacolon and/or perforation), and if precancerous lesions are identified. Colectomy could be discouraged in children younger than 5 years old, in whom it could be difficult to distinguish between UC and CD.

The most common medical rescue therapy in steroid-refractory acute severe UC is calcineurin inhibitors (cyclosporine, tacrolimus) and biological agents (infliximab, adalimumab). Several studies reported a high rate of short-term success, though there is a low rate of long-term success of calcineurin inhibitors. Because of its long-term renal toxicity, cyclosporine should only be administered as a "bridge" to thiopurine treatment (azathioprine), which is typically effective after 3–4 months. Although not structurally related to cyclosporine, tacrolimus has a similar mechanism of action and efficacy, though there is a more tolerable side effect profile. Calcineurin inhibitors may also be used as a steroid-sparing "bridge" to surgery. There aren't any comparative prospective trials between cyclosporine and infliximab in children. Infliximab is a monoclonal antibody to tumor necrosis factor-alpha. The recommended dose is 5 mg/kg at 0.2 and 6 weeks, followed by maintenance therapy every 8 weeks. Unlike cyclosporine, infliximab can be continued as long-term maintenance therapy. Infliximab seems to be more effective in obtaining mucosal healing than immunomodulators. Combination therapy with infliximab and azathioprine should be discouraged because of the potential risk or lymphoma, even if combination therapy has reported a good response in many adult studies.

Adalimumab is a fully human monoclonal antibody to tumor necrosis factor-alpha. Extrapolating from the adult literature and pediatric case series, adalimumab should be started at 100 mg/m^2 up to 160 mg, followed by 50 mg/m^2 up to 80 mg after 2 weeks and then 25 mg/m^2 up to 40 mg every other week; dose individualization may be needed. It is generally used in children who either fail to tolerate or become intolerant to infliximab. Adalimumab is an effective and safe treatment that should be considered as the rescue treatment before colectomy in children [1, 4–7].

23.1.7 Surgical Management of UC

Although the primary therapy of ulcerative colitis is medical, surgery may be required in patient who develops severe complications or becomes refractory to medical therapy.

Indications for urgent surgery:

- Massive colorectal bleeding: uncontrolled, life-threatening hemorrhage occurs in a small portion of patient, but it requires immediate surgery.
- Toxic megacolon, which is characterized by systemic toxicity and segmental or total colonic dilatation.
- Perforation: this complication is rare but these patients require colectomy.
- Severe colitis, which has failed to respond to aggressive medical therapy within 2 weeks.

Indications for elective surgery:

- Unresponsive patients: patients who do not respond to medical therapy or cannot be weaned from glucocorticoids or immunomodulatory therapy should be offered a surgical option.
- Side effects: when medical therapy influences the physiologic development (growth failure from steroids), this constitutes an indication to colectomy.
- Cancer risk: bioptic findings at risk for cancer require colectomy [4, 7].

23.1.7.1 Technique

The gold standard technique is *ileal pouch-anal anastomosis* (*IPAA*) firstly described in 1978 by Parks and Nicholls [8]. It consists of colectomy and rectal mucosectomy with an endorectal ileo-anal pull-through, creation of a distal reservoir and ileorectal anastomosis (Fig. 23.2). If urgent surgery is required, the treatment of choice is to perform a colectomy and ileostomy leaving a rectal stump.

IPAA can be performed in one, two, or three stages:

- One-stage IPAA: following the proctocolectomy, an ileal pouch is anastomosed to the anus. Single-stage surgery is feasible, but it seems to be associated to a higher risk of major complication such as anastomotic dehiscence and late pouch failure [9].
- Two-stage IPAA: following the proctocolectomy and the ileal pouch-anal anastomosis, a loop ileostomy is made to protect to lower anastomosis from the fecal stream. The ileostomy is reversed in a second procedure.
- Three-stage IPAA: during the first stage, a colectomy and ileostomy are performed leaving a rectal stump. During the second procedure, the proctectomy is completed, and ileal pouch-anal anastomosis is performed leaving a loop ileostomy which is reversed during a third procedure.

Total *abdominal colectomy with ileorectal anastomosis* is another applicable technique (Fig. 23.3). It consists of colonic removal and ileal anastomosis to the rectum. The rectum serves as native reservoir ensuring continence but local disease persists. Eligible patients for this technique are those who are not suitable for IPAA but refuse a permanent ileostomy, patients with indeterminate colitis in whom Crohn's disease cannot be excluded, and young women who desire preservation of fecundity [10]. In fact some authors reported improved fertility in ileorectal anastomosis, thus avoiding pelvic adhesions. This advantage has to be balanced with the need for endoscopic surveillance and a possible failure of medical control of the residual disease.

Laparoscopic IPAA is increasingly being performed in adults, while the application of this technique to pediatric practice has been slower. Laparoscopic approach offers advantages in terms of wound infection, intra-abdominal abscess, length of stay, and reduced incidence of small bowel obstruction at 1-year follow-up [11, 12].

23.1.7.2 Complications

The major complication of IPAA is inflammation of the pouch (pouchitis). Main symptoms are diarrhea, rectal bleeding, abdominal pain, and malaise. Therapy is based on broad-spectrum antibiotics or glucocorticoid enemas. Other long-term complications are incontinence and a reduction in fertility in females.

23.2 Crohn's Disease

23.2.1 Introduction

The incidence of CD in children is increasing worldwide, ranging from 2.5 to 11.4 per 100,000, with an estimated prevalence of 58/100,000 which is rising in both developed and developing countries. The cause of CD is still poorly understood, but evidence demonstrated that the disease is based on abnormal response to the intestinal microbiota in a genetically susceptible host; in particular in pediatric-onset CD, the genetic component is more dominant, and therefore recurrence within the family is more prevalent than in

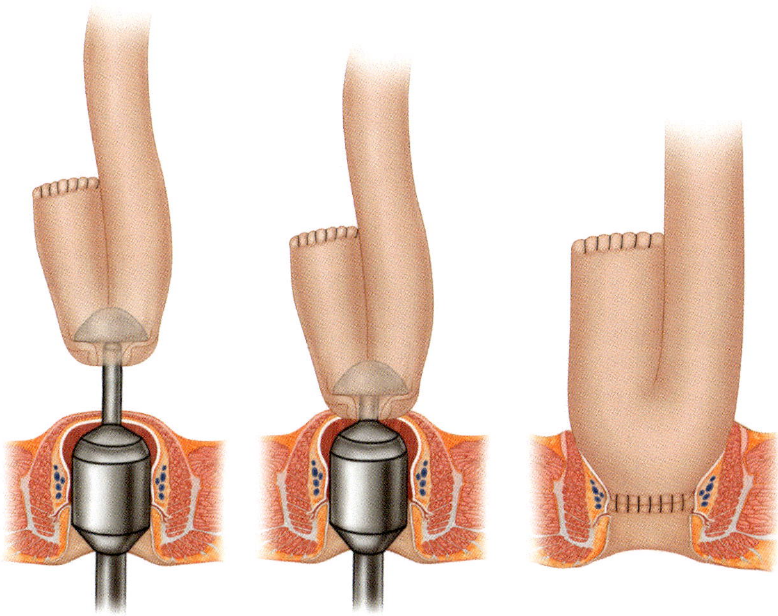

Fig. 23.2 After total colectomy and ileal pouch are performed, circular staple is used to perform ileoanal anastomosis (**a**, **b**). At the end of the procedure, no rectal mucosa should be present (**c**)

adults. Some features are typical of pediatric age; pediatric CD is more often extensive; is associated with a more aggressive disease course, including a greater propensity for disease extension and early use of immunomodulators; presents various phenotypes; and is influenced by nutritional treatment. The cumulative risk of progression to complicated CD (i.e., fistulizing or stricturing disease) is similar to adults, but children are more likely to have undergone surgery by young adulthood [13–15].

23.2.2 Epidemiology

In the last years, CD has shown an increase of incidence, which determinates an increase in the overall mean annual incidence of pediatric IBD. CD highest rates occur in Western and Northern countries, with a decreasing gradient from North to South and from West to East. In Europe data suggest a mean annual incidence rate of 2.6 for pediatric CD. US studies reported a prevalence of 43/100,000. Factors contributing to the increase of CD could be a greater case of diagnosis, the widening case definition, earlier onset, and a greater access to medical care associated to a real increase in the number of affected children. CD is more frequent than UC in childhood with a male predominance. In pediatric CD, most patients have an extensive disease, ileocolonic or colonic, and also an upper gastrointestinal involvement. Pediatric CD usually presents as an inflammatory or nonstricturing, nonpenetrating disease, although complicated disease is fairly unusual at presentation [2].

23.2.3 Etiopathogenesis

In genetically predisposed children, an interaction between luminal contents and the mucosa leads to a dysregulated inflammation, which is the most recognized mechanism of pediatric CD. Different microorganisms are studied to find the pathogen of CD; strains of adherent-invasive *E. coli* have been described both in adults and in children with CD. However no data

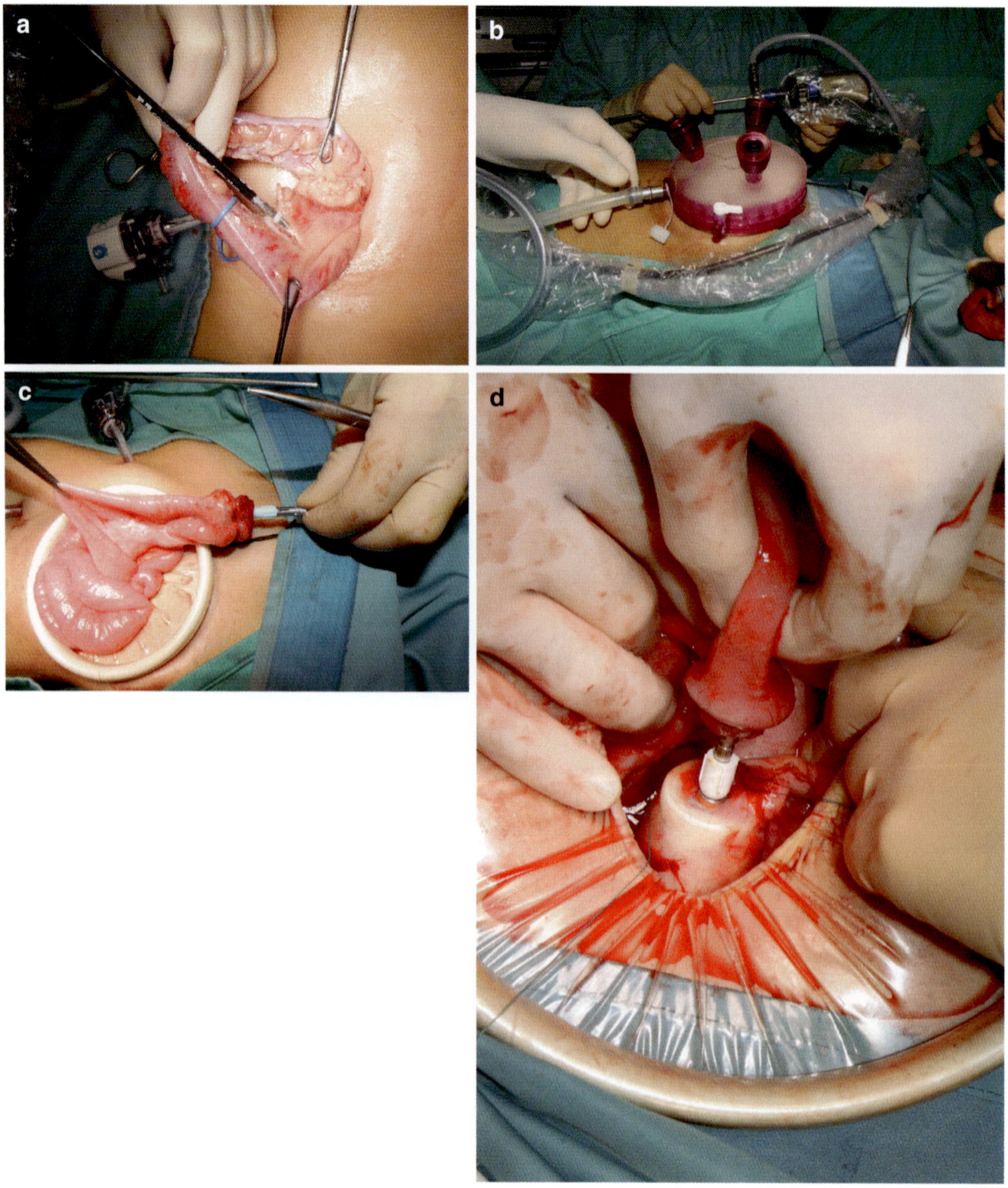

Fig. 23.3 Colectomy can be performed with a video-assisted technique exteriorizing the colon through the umbilical wound during a fist surgical stage (**a**); when intestinal recanalization has to be done, the ileostomy site can be used to free intestinal loop laparoscopically (**b**, **c**) and finally perform an ileorectal anastomosis (**d**)

support the role of any microorganisms as the causative pathogen of CD. Genetics has an important role in CD pathogenesis; monozygotic twins show a phenotype concordance of 50–70 % in CD patients, with an increased risk (800-fold) compared to general population. Several susceptibility genes are discovered: variants of NOD2, IL23 receptor, ATG16L1, and IRGM and mutations of IL10RA, and IL10RB. NOD2 gene defect has an impaired ability to recognize and process bacterial products, a condition which could determinate an abnormal immune response. ATG16L1 and IRGM gene defect have an impaired ability to process cell degradation products and so a disability to eliminate pro-inflammatory factors. Impaired IL10 signaling is associated to a very early-onset CD, an aggressive treatment-resistant CD colitis with perianal involvement.

23.2.4 Clinical Presentation

Crohn's disease is a chronic, relapsing, inflammatory disorder which could develop in any part of the gastrointestinal tract. A percentage of 60 % of children with CD have an extensive ileocolonic involvement and 20–30 % an isolated colonic involvement. Terminal ileum is the most common affected area. Classical symptoms and signs are abdominal pain, diarrhea, weight loss, fever, and failure to thrive. Deficit or delay in sexual development could be present and could be the main presentation of the disease; thus, particular attention should be given to these symptoms. Growth failure has been reported in up to 40 % of children with CD and comes from several factors as malnutrition, increased gastrointestinal loses, malabsorption, and medical effects. Inflammation could have a negative effect upon some linear growth, contributing to growth retardation. Maintaining adequate nutrition, minimizing inflammation, and maximizing corticosteroid-free treatment are goals to achieve in the management of the disease.

23.2.5 Diagnosis

A definite diagnosis is not found by a single specific test, but results from the association of several factors, such as family and personal history, physical examination, laboratory test, imaging, and endoscopic studies. Infectious diseases (*Salmonella*, *Yersinia*, *Shigella*, *E. coli*) and vasculitides such as Henoch-Schonlein purpura and hemolytic-uremic syndrome should be excluded. Several conditions such as intestinal lymphoma could mimic CD, and this entity should be carefully carried out [14].

23.2.5.1 Serologic Test

These tests are the first line in the diagnosis of CD in children. Particular attention should be given to the acute reactants, C-reactive protein, whose levels correlate with clinical, endoscopic, and histologic disease activity. Studies demonstrate the potential role of *Saccharomyces cerevisiae* antibodies (ASCA) and perinuclear antineutrophil cytoplasmic autoantibodies (p-ANCA) as marker of IBD. In particular CD-positive ASCA counts correlated to younger at onset, ileal disease, aggressive behavior, and increased risk of early surgery.

Pseudomonas fluorescens-related protein was related to stenotizing IBD and necessity of surgery, and anti-*E. coli* outer membrane porin C has been associated to penetrating disease. Both the presence and the grade of immune response were correlated with more aggressive disease.

23.2.5.2 Fecal Markers

Calprotectin is a noninvasive test for the diagnosis and monitoring of activity of IBD. Calprotectin is a calcium-binding protein found in the feces, which could be quickly quantified by an enzyme-linked immunosorbent assay (ELISA). On the basis of the stability of the protein in stool specimens, the patient could simply collect a specimen at home without particular precautions. This protein is particularly useful to confirm tissue healing and predict disease relapses. Studies demonstrate a sensitivity of 89–90 % and specificity of 82–83 % for predicting disease relapse.

23.2.5.3 Imaging

Children affected by CD require frequent evaluations during follow-up, so radiation-free imaging test is an important alternative to endoscopy. Magnetic resonance (MR), ultrasound (US), and computed tomography (CT) could be the choice to define activity and complications of the disease. CT exposes the children to a large dose of radiation, so other techniques are preferable. MR with oral contrast (MRE) determinates a luminal distension which permits a better visualization of bowel wall and regularity associated to a detailed assessment of perianal disease. MRE is the imaging study of choice in IBD diagnosis and follow-up in children. Abdominal US presents safety profile and low costs and permits high-resolution images with recent advances. A small intestine contrast ultrasonography (SICUS) is a technique performed after the administration of an oral contrast, which permits to visualize and assess the entire small bowel with higher sensitivity and specificity of standard US [3].

23.2.5.4 Endoscopy

Ileocolonoscopy (IC) and esophagogastroduodenoscopy (EGD) should be recommended as the initial work-up for patients with suspected CD. Endoscopic features in CD are present throughout the entire GI tract. Endoscopic lesions in CD are discontinuous and segmental; frequent are deep serpiginous ulcers (Fig. 23.4) and cobblestoning. These exams are also useful in staging the severity of the disease and monitoring the response to therapies, to evaluate postoperative recurrence and to treat strictures. In selected patients, endoscopic dilation (Fig. 23.5) is a safe and effective alternative to surgery for the management of strictures and should be considered before surgery in short anastomotic strictures (<4 cm). Multiple biopsies should be executed in all areas of gastrointestinal tract, even in the absence of macroscopic lesions. Histologic features in CD are focal crypt distortion, ulcers, mucin depletion, focal cryptitis, focal lymphoplasmacellular infiltration of the lamina propria, granulation tissue-like inflammation, and epithelioid granulomas.

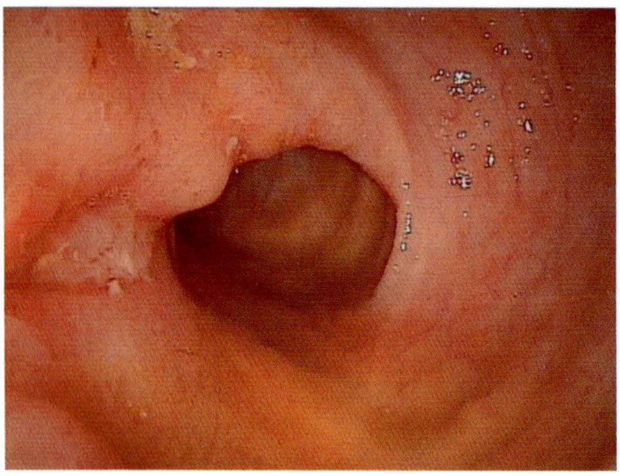

Fig. 23.4 Deep serpiginous ulcer of the terminal ileum

Small bowel capsule endoscopy (CE) permits the study of small bowel lesions without the use of radiation. Advantages of this technique are the capacity to study the entire small bowel, simple preparation, and better tolerance by the children. Disadvantages are the incapacity of performing biopsies, no way to guide the capsule, obscured visualization due to luminal bubbles or debris, or delayed intestinal transit resulting in an inaccurate exam. CE is contraindicated in patients with strictures because of the risk of capsule retention. If stricture is suspected, patency capsule should precede CE. Balloon-assisted enteroscopy (BAE) is indicated in selected cases where biopsies and therapeutic procedures (i.e., stricture dilation) or CE retrieval are needed [1].

23.2.6 Therapy

Treatment of pediatric CD is finalized to achieve and maintain a stable remission with the minimum grade possible of drug toxicity. So the primary aim of CD therapy is to prevent relapses, to preserve growth and pubertal development, and to assure a good quality of life. Conventional therapy is based on the shift from drugs with a better safety profile but lower efficacy (mesalazine, sulfasalazine, antibiotics) to those with

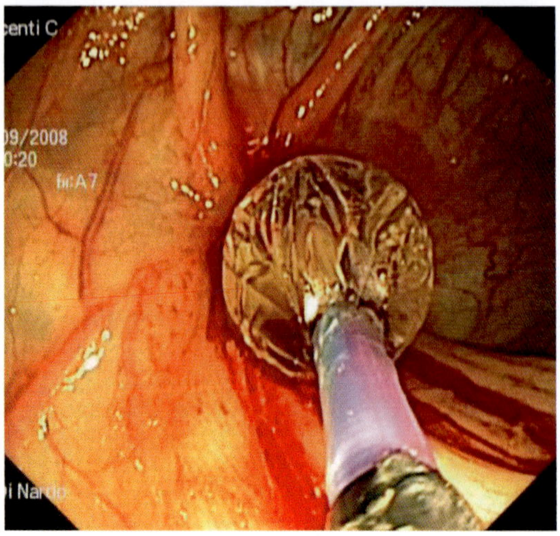

Fig. 23.5 Endoscopic balloon dilation of a short anastomotic stricture

improved efficacy but a greater risk of side effects (steroids, immunomodulators, biologicals, surgery). This "step-up" approach determinates several advantages as reserving more toxic drugs for "particularly resistant" patients [16, 17].

23.2.6.1 Conventional Therapy

Aminosalicylates are frequently used in the management of pediatric CD, although no randomized controlled studies were performed to evaluate the efficacy of these drugs in determining and maintaining the remission in children. No data support the use of this drug in ileal CD.

Corticosteroids are used to induce remission in moderate-to-severe CD. This drug is usually quickly weaned after the induction, on the basis of its understood adverse affects. Particular attention should be given to budesonide, an oral steroid preparation that is released in the distal ileum and proximal colon. This drug should be considered in patients with mild-to-moderate disease of those segments. Budesonide presents less systemic effect than other steroids, but quick withdrawal could determine adrenal insufficiency.

23.2.6.2 Immunomodulators (Azathioprine, 6-Mercaptopurine, Methotrexate)

Thiopurines are usually used in maintenance therapy of pediatric CD. Their efficacy is shown in several studies in maintenance of remission in CD. These drugs are not used for induction of remission on the basis of their slow onset of action (2–3 months). The remission usually can be achieved 1 year after the beginning therapy. Methotrexate is often regarded as a second-line treatment in CD patient not responding or intolerant to thiopurines.

23.2.6.3 Biological Agents

Infliximab, a chimeric monoclonal anti-TNF IgG1 antibody, has been introduced since 15 years ago in the management of pediatric IBD and is given intravenously. This drug has an important role in both inducing and maintaining remission in pediatric CD. The major effects of the use of infliximab are to induce mucosa healing and to reduce the necessity of corticosteroid, the hospitalization, and the surgery. It could also be used in cases with perianal involvement. Induction dose is 5 mg/kg at 0, 2, and 6 weeks, followed by 5 mg/kg maintenance infusion every 8 weeks. This program determinates a remission rate of 60 % at week 30 and of 56 % at week 54. The risk of using this drug is the development of opportunistic infections or a particular type of lymphoma, hepatosplenic T-cell lymphoma (HSTCL), which affects particularly the young male patients.

Adalimumab is a humanized anti-TNF-α drug effective both in induction and maintenance of remission for children with CD. It is useful in particular in patients intolerant or unresponsive to infliximab.

23.2.6.4 Nutrition

Exclusive enteral nutrition (EEN) is used as a treatment to reach remission in children with acute CD. Nutritional therapy is based on the use of several products, such as elemental, semi-elemental, and polymeric formulas, as first treatment to achieve and maintain remission in CD, to improve growth, and to replenish micronutrient deficiency. Evidence of nutritional therapy as the first-line treatment is controversial. The most frequent theory, about its mechanism of action, is that the microbiota of the gut lumen changed under the use of enteral nutrition; the reduction in antigenic load associated to EEN could also contribute to bowel rest. However, the major limitation of EEN is the poor compliance; most parents are reluctant to commit their children to total enteral nutrition for 5–8 weeks as required, and few children are able to consume an adequate volume of formula by mouth, thus requiring the insertion of a nasogastric tube.

23.2.7 Surgical Management of CD

Surgery in Crohn's disease is reserved to those patients who do not respond to medical therapy, have a failure of growth, or develop complications such as fistulas, abscess, strictures, bleeding, obstruction, and perforation. Although surgery cannot cure definitively CD and therapy is primarily medical, approximately 80% of patients will need surgery during their clinical course [18].

The aim of surgery is to restore health and improve quality of life resecting as little bowel as possible since a large part of patients will have recurrence after intestinal resection.

Treatment of left-sided colitis continues to be debated as it has been shown to relapse early following segmental resection or develop complications. Despite this, segmental resection continues to be advocated, citing preservation of anorectal function and decreased postoperative symptoms [19].

Laparoscopy can offer benefits also in pediatric patients with CD. The main advantages include faster postoperative recovery, decreased risk of wound-related complications, formation of fewer intra-abdominal adhesions, and better cosmesis [20].

23.2.7.1 Anastomotic Technique

After segmental resection, anastomosis can be performed with different techniques: end to end or side to side and handsewn or stapled. It's difficult to desume the best choice from the literature data. Simillis et al. concluded that side-to-side anastomosis is associated to a less postoperative complications rate, while an earlier meta-analysis did not show difference between the two techniques. Stapled anastomosis seems to be safer, but familiarity with this technique is mandatory to reduce complications [21, 22].

23.2.7.2 Strictureplasty

Strictureplasty can be performed associated or not to segmental resection. The technique follows the Heineke-Mikulicz principle and involves creation of a longitudinal incision through the narrowed area while closing transversely, which widens the lumen.

Strictureplasty offers good results in chronic stenosis avoiding extensive resections but should not be performed in acutely inflamed bowel.

23.2.7.3 Abdominal Abscess

Abdominal abscess should be treated with systemic antibiotic and percutaneous drainage that promote healing and should be used for >2 cm abscess [23]. The drainage is left in place till the outlet becomes <10 ml/day. Antibiotics against both nosocomial and community-acquired organisms are empirically selected till an antibiogram is obtained and subsequently adapted to the sensitivity of cultured organisms.

Patients with persistent or recurrent abscesses will have benefit from surgical drainage and resection of the affected tract.

23.2.7.4 Intra-abdominal Fistulas

The aim of surgery is to interrupt fistula and resect the affected tract obtaining macroscopically free margins. The resection should be aimed at saving as bowel as possible considering that loss of colonic length is less dire than loss of small bowel.

23.2.7.5 Perianal Disease

Perianal disease is characterized by the onset of perianal abscesses and fistulas. The principles of the management are a prompt identification and drainage of the septic focus, an appropriate medical therapy, and a conservative surgery if necessary. The most recommended surgical approach is the placement of a seton after drainage of purulent collections. Perianal setons promote drainage, prevent abscess recurrence, and provide pain relief but keep the fistula open until seton is removed. On the other hand, the impaired wound healing of patients affected by CD makes extensive perianal surgery quite hazardous. Fistulotomy can be performed in well medical-controlled patients with extra-sphincteric or short low inter-sphincteric fistula tracks.

References

1. Levine A, Koletzko S, Turner D et al (2014) ESPGHAN revised Porto criteria for the diagnosis of inflammatory bowel disease in children and adolescents. J Pediatr Gastroenterol Nutr 58:795–806
2. Benchimol EL et al (2011) Epidemiology of pediatric inflammatory bowel disease: a systemic review of international trends. Inflamm Bowel Dis 17:423–439

3. Kilcoyne A, Kaplan JL, Gee MS (2016) Inflammatory bowel disease imaging: current practice and future directions. World J Gastroenterol 22:917–932
4. Turner D, Levine A, Escher JC (2012) Management of pediatric ulcerative colitis: joint ECCO and ESPGHAN evidence-based consensus guidelines. J Pediatr Gastroenterol Nutr 55:340–361
5. Turner D, Griffiths AM (2011) Acute severe ulcerative colitis in children: a systematic review. Inflamm Bowel Dis 17:440–449
6. Levine A, Griffiths A, Markowitz J et al (2011) Pediatric modification of the Montreal classification for inflammatory bowel disease: the Paris classification. Inflamm Bowel Dis 17:1314–1321
7. Turner D, Travis S, Griffiths AM et al (2011) Consensus for managing acute severe ulcerative colitis in children: a systematic review and joint statement from ECCO, ESPGHAN, and the Porto IBD Working Group of ESPGHAN. Am J Gastroenterol 106:574–588
8. Parks AG, Nicholls RJ (1978) Proctocolectomy without ileostomy for ulcerative colitis. Br Med J 2(6130):85–88
9. Brown J, Meyer F, Klapproth JM (2012) Aspects in the interdisciplinary decision-making for surgical intervention in ulcerative colitis and its complications. Z Gastroenterol 50(5):468–474
10. Mortier PE, Gambiez L, Karoui M et al (2006) Colectomy with ileorectal anastomosis preserves female fertility in ulcerative colitis. Gastroenterol Clin Biol 30(4):594–597
11. Bartels SA, Gardenbroek TJ, Ubbink DT et al (2013) Systematic review and meta-analysis of laparoscopic versus open colectomy with end ileostomy for non-toxic colitis. Br J Surg 100(6):726–733
12. Sheth J, Jaffray B (2014) A comparison of laparoscopic and open restorative proctocolectomy in children. J Pediatr Surg 49(2):262–264; discussion 264
13. Boualit M et al (2013) Long-term outcome after first intestinal resection in pediatric-onset Crohn's disease: a population-based study. Inflamm Bowel Dis 19:7–14
14. Savoye G et al (2012) Clinical predictors at diagnosis of disabling pediatric Crohn's disease. Inflamm Bowel Dis 18:2072–2078
15. Abraham BP et al (2012) Natural history of pediatric-onset inflammatory bowel disease: a systematic review. J Clin Gastroenterol 46:581–589
16. Ruemmele FM et al (2014) Consensus guidelines of ECCO/ESPGHAN on the medical management of pediatric Crohn's disease. J Crohns Colitis 8:1179–1207
17. Schoepfer AM et al (2012) Treatment of fibrostenotic and fistulizing Crohn's disease. Digestion 86:23–27
18. Caprilli R, Gassull MA, Escher JC et al (2006) European evidence based consensus on the diagnosis and management of Crohn's disease: special situations. Gut 55(Suppl 1):i36–i58
19. Andersson P, Olaison G, Hallböök O, Sjödahl R (2002) Segmental resection or subtotal colectomy in Crohn's colitis? Dis Colon Rectum 45(1):47–53
20. Laituri CA, Fraser JD, Garey CL et al (2011) Laparoscopic ileocecectomy in pediatric patients with Crohn's disease. J Laparoendosc Adv Surg Tech 21:193–195
21. Simillis C, Purkayastha S, Yamamoto T, Strong SA, Darzi AW, Tekkis PP (2007) A meta-analysis comparing conventional end-to-end anastomosis vs. other anastomotic configurations after resection in Crohn's disease. Dis Colon Rectum 50:1674–1687
22. McLeod RS, Wolff BG, Ross S, Parkes R, McKenzie M (2009) Recurrence of Crohn's disease after ileocolic resection is not affected by anastomotic type: results of a multicenter, randomized, controlled trial. Dis Colon Rectum 52:919–927
23. Pfefferkorn MD, Marshalleck FE, Saeed SA et al (2013) NASPGHAN clinical report on the evaluation and treatment of pediatric patients with internal penetrating Crohn disease: intraabdominal abscess with and without fistula. J Pediatr Gastroenterol Nutr 57(3):394–400

Anorectal Malformations

24

Tommaso Gargano and Mario Lima

24.1 Introduction

Anorectal malformations (ARMs) are rare birth defects of the digestive system affecting 2–6 per 10.000 births worldwide with an estimated prevalence rate of 3 per 10.000 births in Europe. They are more common among Asians and are somewhat more common in boys (60 %) than in girls. Male patients tend to have more severe malformations than female ones [1]. ARMs are the result of an abnormal development of the distal end of the digestive tract interesting the anus and/or rectum that occur early between the sixth and tenth week of embryonic development. They carry a malformation spectrum of severity depending on the level of disruption of the anorectal canal and of the associated caudal malformations (sacrum and spine). In most ARMs, the anus is not perforated, and the distal enteric component may end blindly (atresia) (Fig. 24.1) or as a fistula into the urinary tract, genital tract, or perineum (Figs. 24.2 and 24.3) [2].

T. Gargano (✉) • M. Lima
Pediatric Surgery, S. Orsola-Malpighi Hospital,
Bologna University, Via Massarenti 11, 40138
Bologna, Italy
e-mail: tommaso.gargano2@unibo.it;
mario.lima@unibo.it

24.2 History

ARM or imperforate anus has been a well-known condition since antiquity. For many centuries, physicians created an orifice in the perineum of children with imperforate anus. Those that survived most likely suffered from a type of defect that would now be recognized as "low." Those with a "high" defect did not survive that treatment. Amussat, in 1835, was the first individual who sutured the rectal wall to the skin edges, which could be considered the first anoplasty. During the first 60 years of the twentieth century, surgeons performed a perineal operation without a colostomy for the so-called low malformations. High imperforate anus was usually treated with a colostomy performed in the newborn period, followed by an abdominoperineal pull-through some time later in life, but surgeons lacked objective anatomic guidelines. Unfortunately this left many patients incontinent and was not an appropriate solution to the spectrum of malformations. The surgical approach to repairing these defects changed dramatically in 1980 with the introduction of the posterior sagittal approach, which allowed surgeons to view the anatomy of these defects clearly, to repair them under direct vision, and to learn about the complex anatomic arrangement of the junction of the rectum and genitourinary tract. It has become the predominant surgical method for anorectal anomalies. In cases when the rectum or the vagina is very high and an

M. Lima (ed.), *Pediatric Digestive Surgery*, DOI 10.1007/978-3-319-40525-4_24

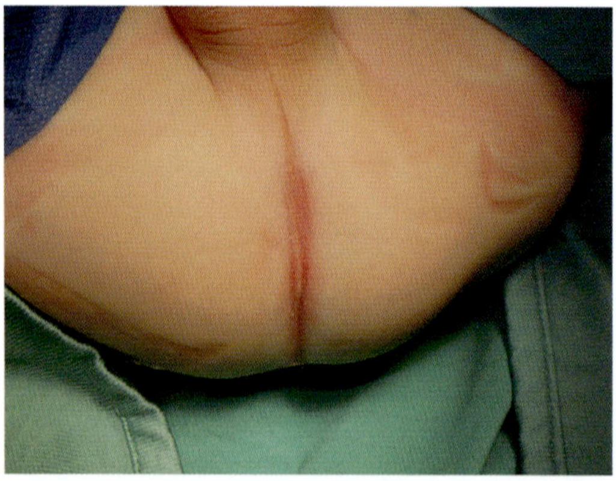

Fig. 24.1 Imperforate anus

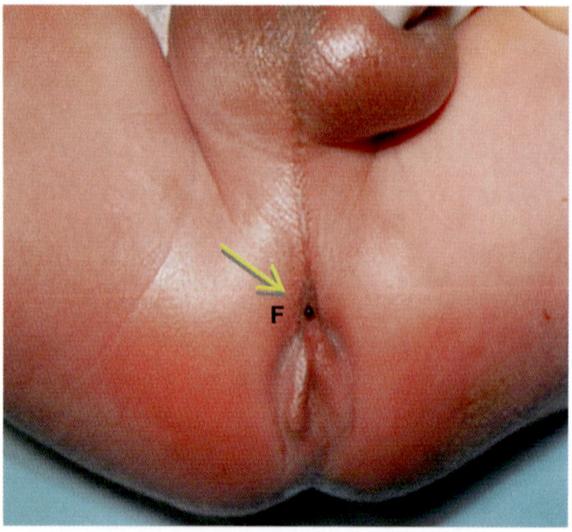

Fig. 24.2 Perineal (cutaneous) fistula in male

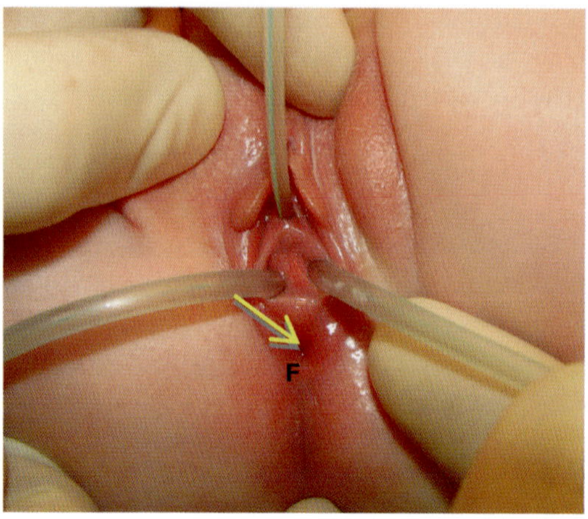

Fig. 24.3 Perineal (cutaneous) fistula in female

abdominal approach as well is needed, laparoscopy can be used in combination with the posterior sagittal approach [3].

24.3 Embryology

The early embryologic development of the anorectum, the primitive urogenital sinus, and the caudal neural tube is closely related, which helps explain the associated malformations of these three systems. In early embryonic life, the distal portion of the hindgut, the primitive cloaca, is divided into dorsal and ventral parts by a coronal sheet of the mesenchyme, the urorectal septum, and separated from the amniotic cavity by the cloacal membrane. Most ARMs result from abnormal development of the urorectal septum. Between weeks 4 and 6 of gestation, both the yolk sac or primitive hindgut and the allantois or primitive urogenital sinus enter into the cloaca. The urorectal septum then develops forklike infoldings (Tourneux and Rathke folds) of the lateral cloacal walls; at the same time, the embryo starts to curve as a result of the longitudinal growth of the developing neural tube and the mesodermal compartment. With these morphologic changes, the distance between the cloacal membrane and the tip of the urorectal septum is progressively reduced. At the end of week 7, the urorectal septum and the cloacal membrane are located at the same level. The cloaca is thus divided into a ventral part (the urogenital sinus) and a dorsal part (the rectum and proximal anal canal). Between them, the tip of the urorectal septum becomes the perineal area. At this time, the cloacal membrane ruptures by apoptosis, thus opening two orifices in the perineum: one ventral or urogenital and one dorsal or anal. Also at the end of week 7, a secondary occlusion of the anorectal canal takes place, initially by adhesion of the walls and later by formation of an epithelial "plug" at the anal level. This secondary closed anal orifice will rupture and recanalize by apoptosis at the end of week 8. Embryologically, ARMs can thus be subdivided into two main groups according to when the disturbances occur: those manifesting as an ectopic anal orifice or fistula are due to early abnormal development of the dorsal part of the cloaca and the cloacal membrane (at weeks 4–7), whereas those manifesting as an abnormal anus in a normal position are due to later defective recanalization of the secondary occluded anal orifice (at weeks 7 and 8) [4].

24.4 General Considerations

ARMs are found as isolated congenital birth defects, as part of a syndrome or associated with other anomalies. Associated anomalies have been reported to occur in approximately 45–65 % of the patients, mostly of the urogenital tract, central nervous system, skeletal system (vertebrae), or the remaining gastrointestinal tract [1]. ARM has been reported to occur in families suggesting that there is a genetic component in its etiology. There appears to be a low rate of association in families, but some appear to have an autosomal dominant inheritance pattern. Consanguinity has been identified as leading to a higher incidence of ARM, particularly in countries in the Gulf and Middle East regions. In addition, familial Currarino associations are well established, and family members have been shown to have sacral anomalies without the full syndrome. In a small number of patients, genetic factors are clearly associated with ARM. Previous studies have suggested the importance of a locus on chromosome 7q39, which includes three genes: SHH, EN2, and HLXB9. These include Towne-Brock syndrome, FG syndrome, Kaufman-McKusick syndrome, and Lowe syndrome. In addition, ARM has been described in association with trisomy 8 mosaicism, as well as Down and fragile X syndromes. Till date, the accurate embryologic defect causing anorectal malformations still remains undetermined. With recent researches in the pathogenesis of anorectal malformations, the previous theories have been discarded. While in the past, defects in lateral fusion were thought to be causative, there is evidence from animal models and from detailed study of human fetuses with major anomalies that a deficiency in the dorsal component of the cloacal membrane and the adjacent dorsal cloaca is causative. A subsequent malfunction of the primitive streak and tail bud in the early development phase around 3–4 weeks has been proposed (yet to be clearly defined) as causation for associated anomalies of the pelvic floor [1, 5].

24.5 Classification

Based on the anatomy, various classifications have been proposed to define the pathology of these anorectal anomalies. The earliest classification dates back to 1953 when Gross proposed a simple differentiation based on the levator muscle, i.e., supralevator, for those above the levator ani, or infralevator anomalies, for those below the levator ani [6].

With advancement in the understanding of the pathology of the malformations, a need was felt to define these lesions more appropriately. During the centenary of the Royal Children's Hospital in Melbourne, a new international classification was proposed in 1970. This classification utilized the concept of levator ani wherein anomalies above the levator were termed as high and those below were termed as low anomalies, but it also introduced intermediate anomalies which were known as translevator anomalies [7].

The best known classification of ARMs is the Wingspread classification of 1984 (Wisconsin). This classification distinguished between high, intermediate, and low anomalies in the male and female, with special groups established for cloacal and rare malformations. High-type anorectal malformations were agenesis without fistula in both sexes. The low-type malformations were classified as anovestibular fistula in the female and, in both sexes, as anocutaneous fistula and anal stenosis. This classification was widely accepted over the years and was based on detailed embryological and anatomic studies performed especially by Stephens et al. and Kelly on anatomic sections and radiographic investigations. They recognized that the pubococcygeal line extending from the upper border of the os pubis to the os coccyx corresponds with the attachment of levator ani muscles to the pelvic wall, separating high-type malformations lying above the levator muscle and intermediate and low forms of anorectal agenesis lying below this anatomic line. Furthermore, in healthy individuals, the lowest point of the ischial tuberosity, the so-called I-point, represents the deepest point of the funnel of the levator ani muscles. Therefore, every blind rectal pouch, lying between the pubococcygeal line and the I-point, was classified as an intermediate anomaly and could be treated by a posterior sagittal anorectoplasty (PSARP). Low lesions below the I-point could be easily managed from a perineal approach. Because of these anatomic relations, the Wingspread classification had a significant impact on the choice of surgical approach. However, some details of the Wingspread classification remained questionable. Therefore, in 1995, Peña proposed a classification based on the type of the fistula present. He distinguished between perineal, vestibular, bulbar, prostatic, and bladder neck fistulas, imperforate anus without fistula, vaginal fistulas, cloacal fistulas, and rectal atresia or stenosis (Table 24.1).

This descriptive and fistula-related grouping became widely accepted over the past decade. The advantage of the classification of Peña is that the type of the fistula provides information not only about localization of the blind pouch but also on the anticipated extent of mobilization of the atretic rectal segment necessary to perform a sacro- or abdominosacroperineal pull-through. It is important to remember that the course of the fistula may vary from one individual to another and can be ascending or descending and of shorter or longer length so that the confluence of the fistula with the urogenital tract or perineum may differ from the lowest point of the blind pouch. This is especially true if the fistula arises from a higher level of the blind-ending rectum and not from its lowermost point. Therefore, the classification of Peña does not distinguish between rectovestibular and anovestibular fistulas. By closely comparing both classifications, that is, the Wingspread classification and the suggestions of Peña, it becomes clear that there is no real contradiction between them. Perineal and vestibular fistulas could be regarded as low malformations, bulbar fistulas, and imperforate anus without a fistula, and most of the vaginal fistulas may be regarded as intermediate-type anomalies, and prostatic and bladder neck fistulas are considered high-type imperforate anus. The same is true for rectal agenesis or stenosis. In addition, rare/regional variants, despite being frequent in certain geographic areas of the world, are not alluded to in either classifications. More recently, the Krickenbeck Conference of 2005 established a new classification, which is based mainly on the presence or absence of fistulas and their type and location, as well as the position of the rectal pouch. It has gained overall popularity in the international community of pediatric surgeons. This classification itself seemed a logical sequel to the Wingspread classification. It distinguishes five types of fistulas: rectoperineal, rectovestibular, rectourethral bulbar, rectourethral prostatic, and rectovesical. Cloacal malformations and the absence of fistulas, anal stenosis, and rare regional variants complete this classification. The extremely rare rectovaginal fistula is considered a variant of cloacal anomaly (Table 24.2) [4, 8].

Table 24.1 Peña classification

Males	Females
Perineal fistula (cutaneous)	Perineal fistula (cutaneous)
Rectourethral fistula	Vestibular fistula
Prostatic	Cloaca
Bulbar	Imperforate anus without fistula
Rectovesical fistula	Rectal atresia
Imperforate anus without fistula	
Rectal atresia	

Table 24.2 Krickenbeck classification

Major clinical groups	Rare/regional variants
Perineal (cutaneous) fistula	Pouch colon
Rectourethral fistula	Rectal atresia/stenosis
Prostatic	Rectovaginal fistula
Bulbar	H fistula
Rectovesical fistula	Others
Vestibular fistula	
Cloaca	
No fistula	
Anal stenosis	

Cloacal anomaly is a complex anatomic disorder that manifests as a unique external perineal opening with a short or long common canal for the genital, urinary, and digestive systems. Isolated rectovaginal fistulas are extremely rare and are considered a variant of cloacal anomaly. The Wingspread and Krickenbeck classifications are very similar. The Wingspread classification allows location of the blind rectal pouch. The Krickenbeck classification is more descriptive and is clinically oriented; its most important advantage is the preoperative identification and anatomic evaluation of not only the rectal pouch but also any fistulas. This information allows the surgeon to anticipate the extent of mobilization of the atretic rectal segment required during surgery and helps determine the most appropriate surgical approach for each case (Tables 24.3 and 24.4) [8].

24.6 Prenatal and Neonatal Management

Prenatal diagnosis of ARM remains rare and occurs in only up to 16% of cases. Currently, the most complex anorectal malformations are the ones that can be most often diagnosed prenatally. The reason for this is the fact that the higher the malformation (recto-bladder neck fistula in males, cloaca in females), the higher is the presence of associated anomalies, and many of these associated defects can be seen in utero. During the prenatal imaging study, one important clue to suspect an anorectal malformation is the finding of multiple systems with abnormalities (digestive, vertebral, genitourinary). The advantages of having a prenatal diagnosis include giving the parents some information about the type of anomaly that the patient will be born with and also giving them the opportunity to make arrangements for the

Table 24.3 Comparison of Wingspread and Krickenbeck classifications in *male patients*

Type of ARM	Wingspread classification (1984)	Krickenbeck classification (2005)
Low	Anal stenosis Anocutaneous fistula	Anal stenosis Imperforate anus without fistula Rectoperineal fistula
Intermediate	Anal agenesis without fistula Anal agenesis with rectourethral bulbar fistula	Anal or anorectal agenesis without fistula Anorectal agenesis with rectourethral bulbar fistula
High	Rectal atresia anorectal agenesis without fistula Anorectal agenesis with rectourethral prostatic fistula	Anorectal agenesis with rectourethral prostatic fistula Anorectal agenesis with rectovesical fistula
	Rare forms	

Table 24.4 Comparison of Wingspread and Krickenbeck Classifications in *female patients*

Type of ARM	Wingspread classification (1984)	Krickenbeck classification (2005)
Low	Anal stenosis Anal agenesis without fistula Anal agenesis with external fistula	Anal stenosis Imperforate anus without fistula Anal agenesis with rectoperineal fistula Anal agenesis with rectovestibular fistula
Intermediate	Anal agenesis without fistula Anal agenesis with rectovestibular fistula Anal agenesis with rectovaginal fistula	Anal or anorectal agenesis without fistula Rectal atresia Cloacal malformations with short (<3 cm) or long (>3 cm) common canal
High	Rectal atresia Anorectal agenesis without fistula Anorectal agenesis with rectovaginal fistula	
	Cloacal malformation Rare forms	

baby to be delivered in a specialized center that is familiar with the neonatal management of patients born with these conditions. Images that can be seen prenatally and should raise suspicions for an anorectal malformation include dilated and or calcified bowel, lack of meconium at the expected rectal level, hydronephrosis, absent kidney, neural tube defects, tethered cord, hydrocolpos, vertebral anomalies, absent radius, and omphalocele in the absence of bladder visualization [9]. During the first 24 h of life, it is important to rule out associated malformations that might be life-threatening. With an echocardiogram, the physician will rule out cardiac conditions, a nasogastric tube should be passed to rule out esophageal atresia, an abdominal x-ray should rule out duodenal atresia, a kidney ultrasound should rule out severe hydronephrosis, and a pelvic ultrasound in females born with a cloaca should rule out a hydrocolpos. A sacral x-ray in anteroposterior and lateral views will allow for the calculation of the sacral ratio, which is an important tool to predict the future prognosis for bowel control. A spinal ultrasound should be ordered to rule out tethered cord. Imaging plays a key role in evaluation of ARM. In the first days of life, clinical and imaging findings facilitate early classification of ARM and allow a decision about whether to perform an immediate colostomy. In children with intermediate and high types of ARM, preoperative pelvic MR imaging after the neonatal period allows accurate evaluation of the morphology and grade of development of the sphincteric muscle complex (Fig. 24.4). This information helps orient the medical and surgical teams as to the postoperative prognosis for continence. During the first 24 h, the surgeon will also have enough information to decide between a primary repair and a descending colostomy. This decision should take into consideration the experience of the surgeon and the condition of the baby. Common indications for a colostomy include flat perineum, meconium in the urine, distal gas on the invertogram taken after 24 h of life above the coccyx, and cloaca (Fig. 24.5). In ARM the ideal colostomy must be completely diverting, leaving enough distal bowel to allow for the future pull-through. Both stomas must be separated enough to accommodate a stoma bag that only covers the proximal stoma.

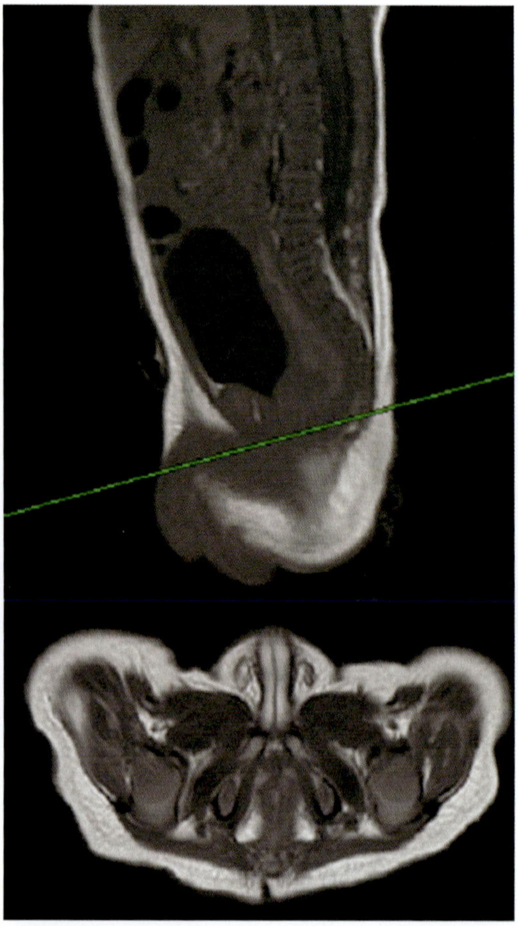

Fig. 24.4 Sphincteric muscle complex

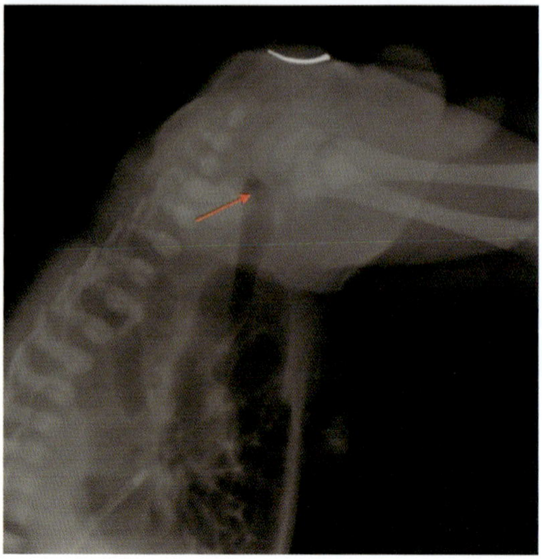

Fig. 24.5 Distal gas on the invertogram above the coccyx

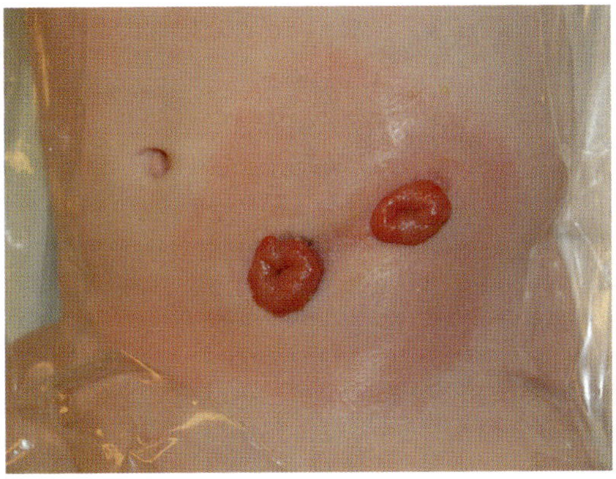

Fig. 24.6 Diverting colostomy in descendent colon

We suggest a descending colostomy taking advantages of the peritoneal attachments of the descending colon to avoid prolapse of the proximal stoma and making the mucous fistula as tiny as possible to avoid prolapse of the distal stoma (Fig. 24.6). During the colostomy opening, the distal bowel should be irrigated with large amounts of saline solution to clear it from any distal meconium. In patients with cloaca, during the first 24 h of life, a pelvic ultrasound should be ordered, specifically looking for a pelvic cystic mass behind the bladder. If a hydrocolpos is diagnosed, it should be drained at the time of colostomy opening with a transabdominal indwelling tube that should be left in place until the time of the main repair (when the patient will have a vaginal opening created). The distal colostogram is the most valuable diagnostic study to determine the specific type of anorectal malformation in male patients (the precise location of the fistula), the length of bowel available for the pull-through, and the relationship between the sacrum, the coccyx, and the rectum (Fig. 24.7). All these informations are important to plan the operation (laparotomy, laparoscopy, or posterior sagittal approach). In addition, it allows for the determination of the future functional prognosis [9].

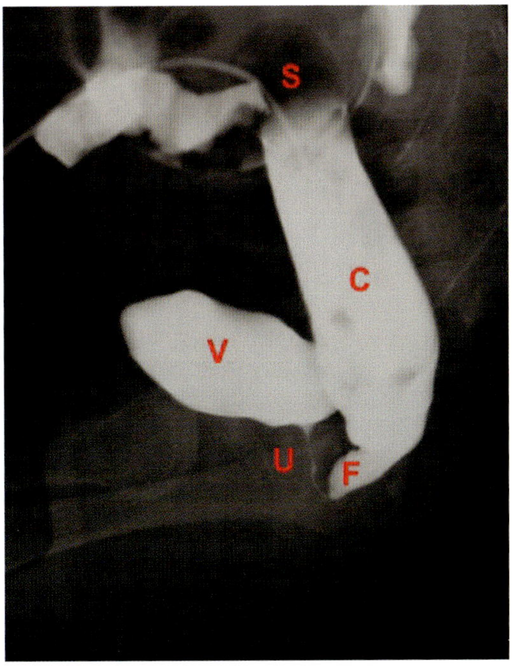

Fig. 24.7 Preoperative distal colostogram

24.7 Surgical Treatment

Almost all ARMs require surgery early in life. The spectrum of malformations sometimes mandates different techniques for different malformations, but the preferred technique is also influenced by the surgeon's preference and surgical education. The most commonly used operative procedures for treatment of ARMs include perineal operations, posterior sagittal anorectoplasty, and laparoscopic abdominoperineal rectoplasty techniques. Cloacal anomaly requires highly specialized reconstructive surgery [1, 2]. ARMs involving a rectal pouch located below the level of the puborectalis muscle, regardless of whether they are associated with a fistula perineal or vestibular, are considered low-type ARM. They may be managed early with a perineal approach involving opening of the rectal pouch and ligature of the fistula, if present. A rectal pouch lying at or above the level of the puborectal sling is considered an intermediate or high type of ARM; it is treated with colostomy in the first days of life and with posterior sagittal anorectoplasty alone or combined with laparoscopic abdominoperineal rectoplasty in a second intervention.

24.7.1 Posterior Sagittal Anorectoplasty (PSARP)

The patient is placed in a prone position with the pelvis elevated (Fig. 24.8).

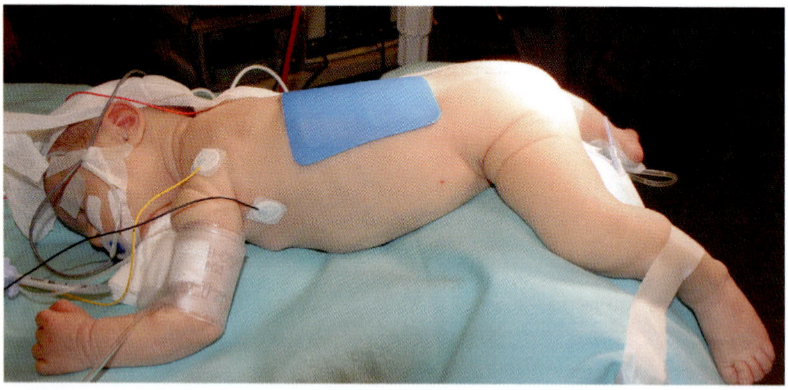

Fig. 24.8 Position of patient in PSARP procedure: prone position with the pelvis elevated

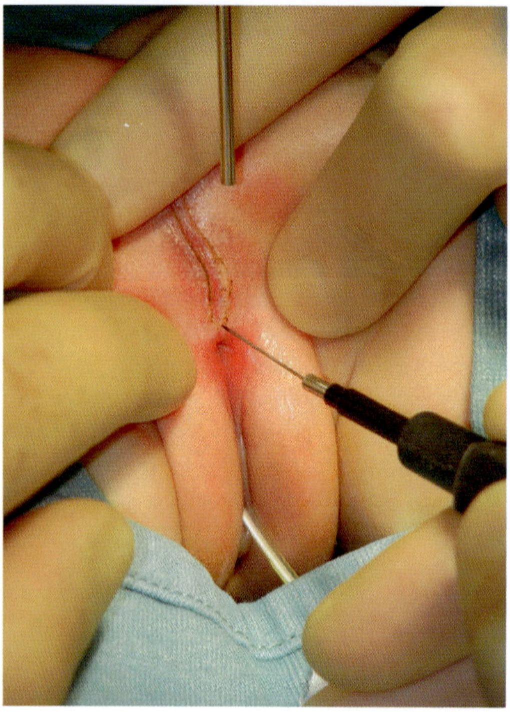

Fig. 24.9 Midline incision from the tip of the coccyx to the perineum

A strictly midline incision is then made from the tip of the coccyx to the perineum. Throughout the procedure, muscles are identified with the help of a muscle stimulator. All muscle groups are separated and opened as if paging through a book, without cutting them, until the rectal pouch is located. The levator ani muscle must then be divided to reach the rectal pouch (Figs. 24.9 and 24.10).

The rectum is then mobilized until a sufficient length is obtained for anal reconstruction.

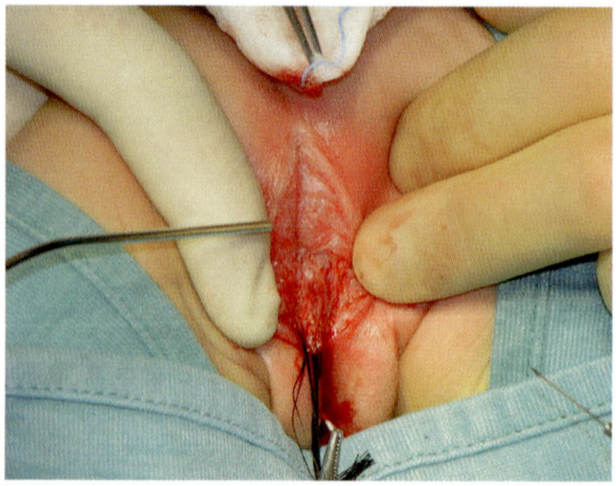

Fig. 24.10 Isolation of rectal pouch

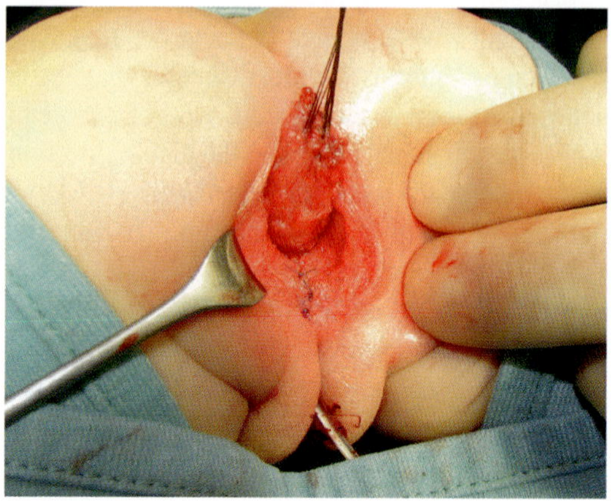

Fig. 24.11 Anterior suturing of the muscular plane

After that, the levator ani muscle is repaired, followed by repair of the muscle complex and external anal sphincter (Figs. 24.11, 24.12, 24.13, and 24.14).

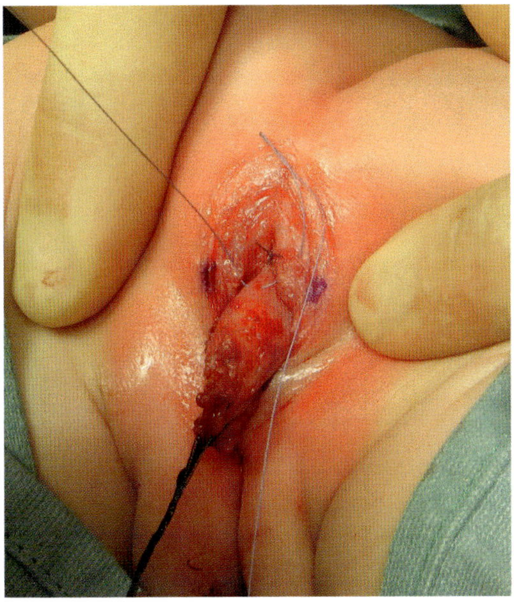

Fig. 24.12 Posterior suturing of the muscular plane

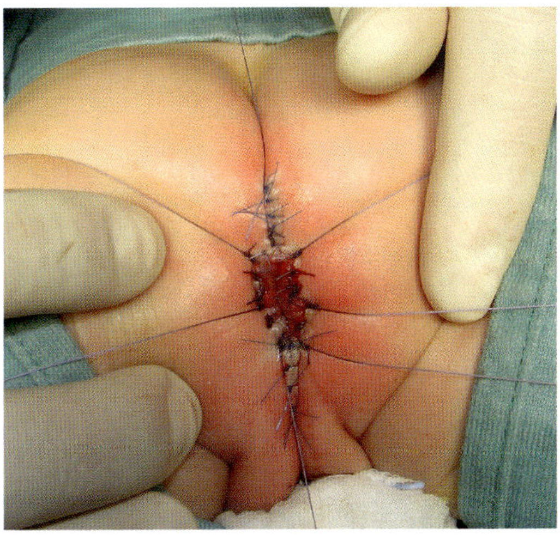

Fig. 24.13 Final step: anoplasty

Very high fistulas, mainly rectourethral prostatic or rectovesical fistulas in boys, are sometimes impossible to visualize exclusively through a perineal sagittal approach, and a laparotomy or laparoscopy (abdominoperineal rectoplasty) is also required. If an abdominal approach is needed, the patient is then positioned faceup, allowing the surgeon to work simultaneously from the abdomen and the perineum.

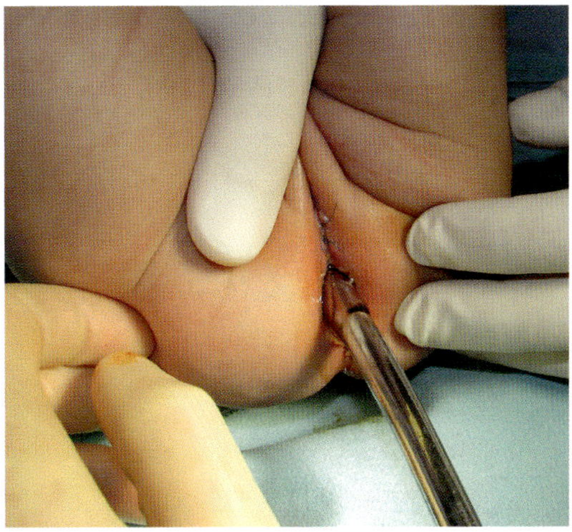

Fig. 24.14 Anal calibration

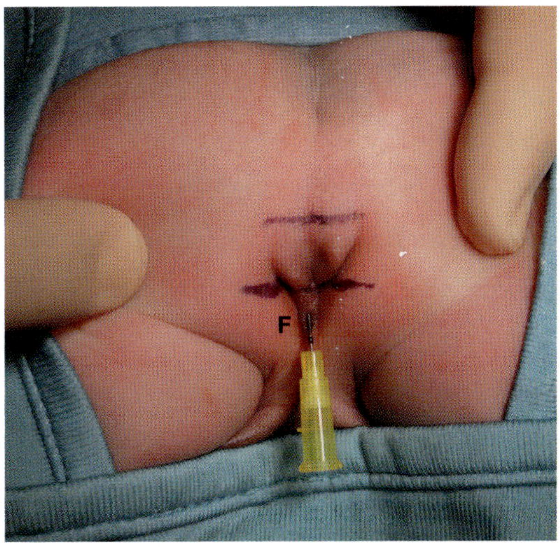

Fig. 24.15 Rectoperineal fistula in male. *F* fistula

24.7.2 Posterior Sagittal Anoplasty for Rectoperineal Fistula

The repair of these defects consists of a small posterior sagittal incision with enough mobilization of the rectum, sufficient to be transposed and placed within the limits of the sphincter (Figs. 24.15, 24.16, 24.17, and 24.18). This is a meticulous operation and can be done during the neonatal period without a colostomy. The most common complication during the repair of this defect in male patients is a urethral injury, which can be avoided by placing a urethral catheter and taking particular care during the dissection of the anterior rectal wall.

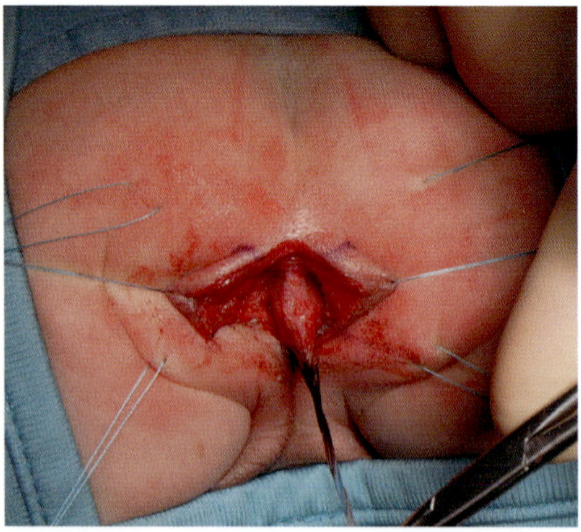

Fig. 24.16 Mobilization of distal pouch

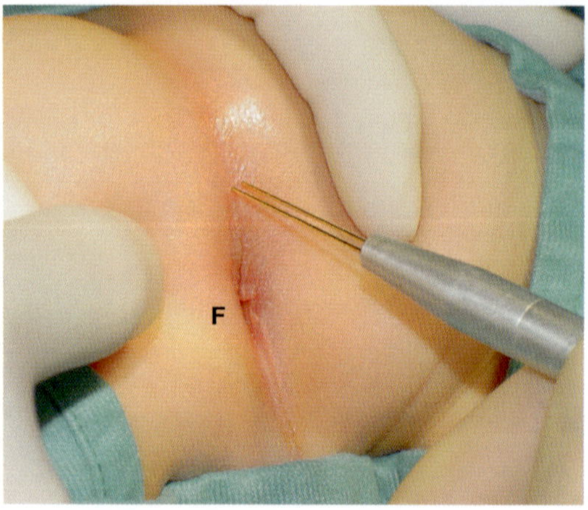

Fig. 24.17 Localization of neoanum with Peña electrostimulator

24.7.3 Posterior Sagittal Anorectoplasty for Rectovestibular Fistula, Rectourethral Bulbar Fistula, Rectourethral Prostatic Fistula, and Imperforate Anus Without Fistula

The key anatomic characteristics that should be kept in mind are that in rectovestibular fistulas the rectum shares a common wall with the vagina, and in rectourethral fistulas and imperforate anus without fistula, the rectum shares a common wall with the urethra. The surgeon has to make two

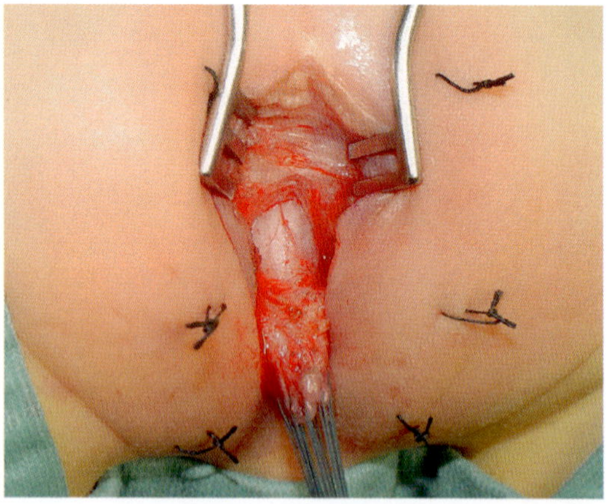

Fig. 24.18 Mobilization of distal pouch

walls out of one with a careful and meticulous separation of these structures. The posterior sagittal incision in these cases should be long enough to allow for adequate rectal mobilization. The posterior rectal wall should be identified, the lateral walls should be dissected, and then the surgeon should concentrate on the most delicate portion of the operation: the separation of the anterior rectal wall, without damaging the urethra in males and the vagina in females.

24.7.4 Laparoscopic-Assisted Posterior Sagittal Anorectoplasty (LAARP)

In 10 % of the male patients, the abdominal cavity has to be entered either through laparoscopy or laparotomy to repair the anorectal malformation. We consider the recto-bladder neck fistulas the ideal indication for laparoscopy as well as some selected rectourethral prostatic fistulas. In 2000, Georgeson proposed a new technique that combines the laparoscopic approach [10]. Yamataka et al. proposed and others confirmed the laparoscopic use of the Peña electrostimulator [11]. The LAARP technique allows treatment of high malformations by pulling down the rectum under direct vision close to the perineal plane. The levator muscles are clearly identified, thanks to intra-abdominal and external electrostimulation, so the surgeon can be sure of the

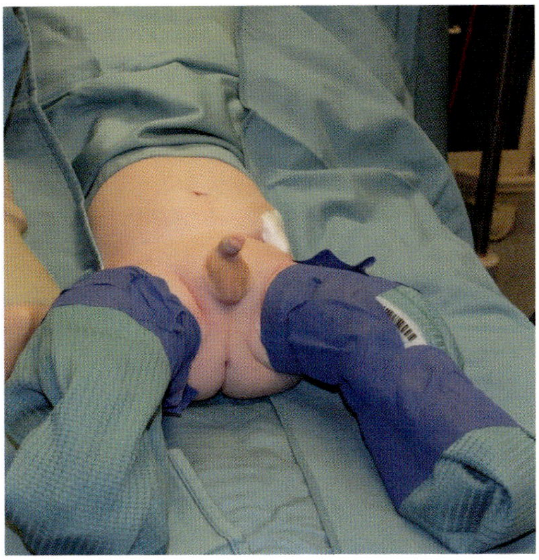

Fig. 24.19 Supine position in LAARP procedure

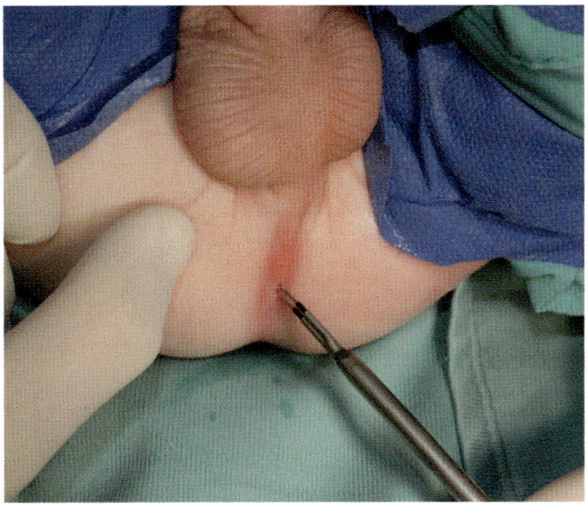

Fig. 24.20 Peña electrostimulation

correct position of the anus, thus avoiding the risks of sagittal dissection. Some studies seem to demonstrate better anorectal manometric findings in patients who underwent LAARP. Although the primary pull-through without colostomy has been described, we prefer to perform the LAARP after a diverting colostomy. We want to emphasize the importance of good positioning of the colostomy in order to avoid problems in mobilizing the rectum. Finally, we want to state the advantage of the intra-abdominal use of the Peña electrostimulator. The bellies of the puborectalis sling are clearly seen, and the contractions indicate the exact site of the pull-through. This can be particularly useful in cases of immature and unclear levator muscles [12] (Figs. 24.19–24.26).

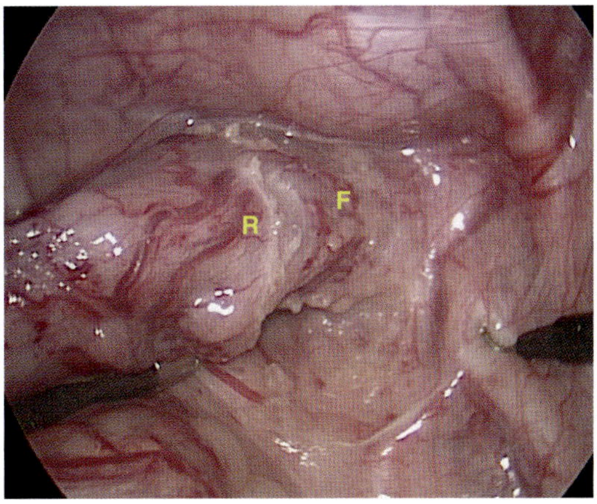

Fig. 24.21 Laparoscopic identification of fistula

24.7.5 Posterior Sagittal Anorectal–Vaginal–Urethral Plasty with Laparotomy for Cloaca with a Common Channel Length of More Than 3 cm

The repair of these complex defects requires the implementation of a rather complicated decision making algorithm. When the total urogenital mobilization (TUM) is not enough for the urethra

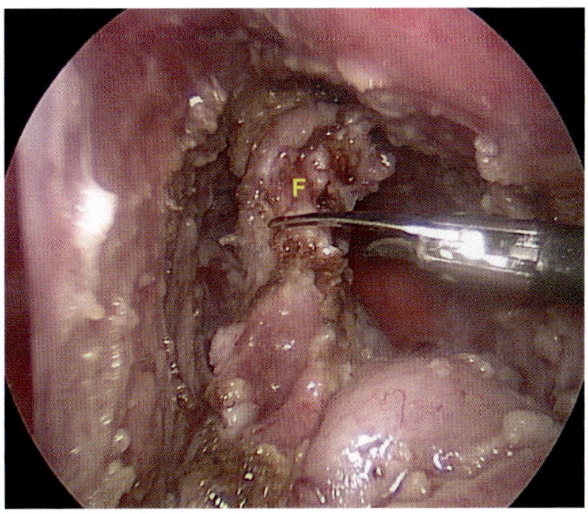

Fig. 24.22 Resection of fistula

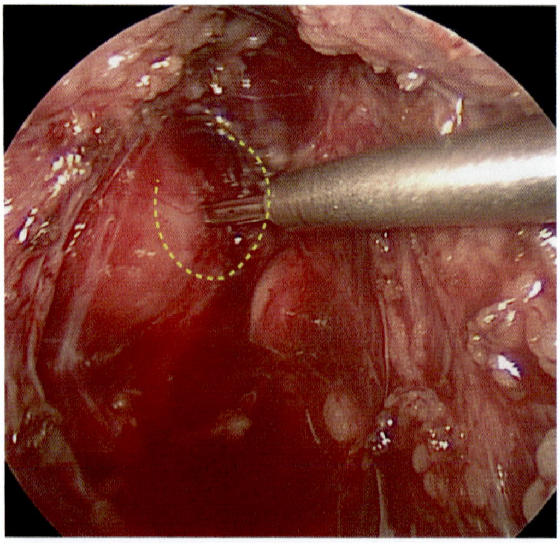

Fig. 24.23 Laparoscopic electrostimulation

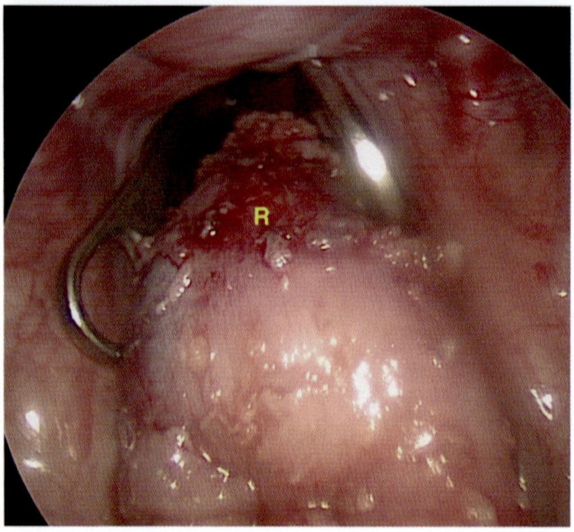

Fig. 24.24 Video-assisted rectal pull-through

and vagina to reach the perineum, carving the pubic cartilage and making a Heineke-Mikulicz maneuver in the vagina may give extra millimeters; when that is not enough, an extended transabdominal total urogenital maneuver is performed. If the structures still do not reach the perineum, the most challenging maneuver should be done, and it consists in the separation of the vagina from the bladder. To do that, the bladder must be open, and catheters have to be inserted into the ureters. At this stage, if the vagina still does not reach, depending on the anatomy, a vaginal switch maneuver can be performed or a partial vaginal replacement using the rectum or colon [6].

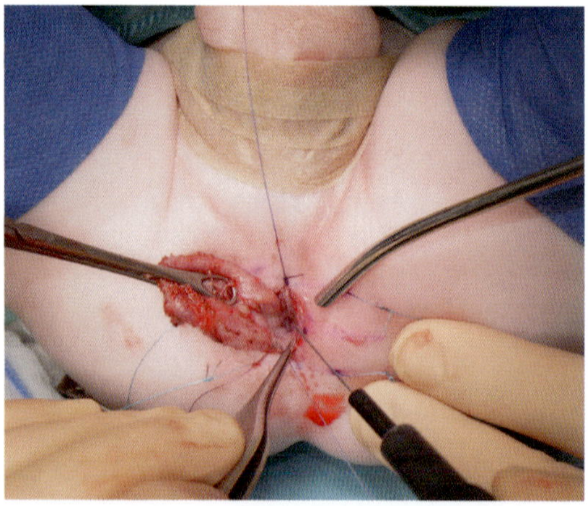

Fig. 24.25 Perineal approach: rectal pull-through

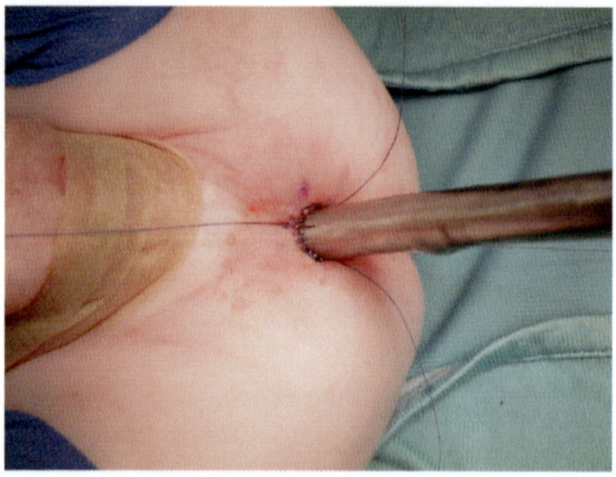

Fig. 24.26 Calibration of neoanum

24.8 Postoperative Management

At 2 weeks postsurgery, anal calibration is performed, followed by a program of anal dilatations to avoid an anoplasty stricture. The anus must be dilated twice daily, and the size of the dilator is increased every week. The final size to be reached depends on the patient's age (Table 24.5).

24.9 Treatment of the Functional Disorders (Constipation and Fecal Incontinence)

Constipation Constipation is the most important problem to avoid after definitive repair. Patients with good prognosis for bowel control

Table 24.5 Postoperative program of anal dilatations

Guidelines for sizing anal dilators	Suggested timing
1–4 months of age: 12	Dilate 2–3 times a day for 1–2 weeks
4–8 months of age: 13	Dilate once daily for 1–2 weeks
8–12 months of age: 14	Dilate once every other day for 1–2 weeks
1–3 years of age: 15	Dilate once every 3–4 days for 2 weeks
3–12 years of age: 16	Dilate once weekly for 4 weeks
>12 years of age: 17–18	

(rectoperineal fistula, rectovestibular fistula, rectourethral bulbar fistula, imperforate anus without fistula, with normal sacrum, and no tethered cord) are the ones that suffer from the most severe type of constipation. These patients usually require laxative dosages much higher than what is conventionally recommended. Patients must be regularly monitored, and laxatives and dietary manipulations are begun at the first sign of constipation. If surgical treatment to restore anatomy as normal as possible is indispensable, postoperative care is essential for these patients whose defecation mechanisms are altered, to reach if not continence, at least a socially acceptable cleanliness.

Fecal incontinence Patients with poor prognosis for bowel control (recto-bladder neck fistulas, cloaca with common channel more than 3 cm in length and tethered cord) should be kept artificially clean with a daily enema. Rectal administration of this daily enema allows the patient to be clean of stool in the underwear for a 24 h period, until the time for the next enema. Patients may complain of soiling. This may represent fecal incontinence in patients with very high ARMs or in those with poor muscles and an abnormal sacrum. These patients require a proper bowel management program. However, in a patient with a good prognosis, soiling may represent overflow incontinence, and constipation must be treated [2].

24.10 Complications

Iatrogenic complications include *dehiscence* and *infection*, which may be avoided with colostomy before the main repair. The *anoplasty stricture* is a possible postoperative complication that may be avoided by a program of dilatations. Posterior *urethral diverticulum* may develop from a fistula remnant.

References

1. De Blaauw I, Wijers CH, Schmiedeke E et al (2013) First results of a European multi-center registry of patients with anorectal malformations. J Pediatr Surg 48(12):2530–2535
2. Cretolle C, Rousseau V, Lottmann H et al (2013) Anorectal malformations. Arch Pediatr 20(Suppl 1):S19–S27
3. Levitt MA, Peña A (2012) Correction: anorectal malformations. Orphanet J Rare Dis 7:98
4. Alamo L, Meyrat BJ, Meuwly JY et al (2013) Anorectal malformations: finding the pathway out of the labyrinth. Radiographics 33(2):491–512
5. Iwai N, Fumino S (2013) Surgical treatment of anorectal malformations. Surg Today 43(9):955–962
6. Gross RE (1953) Malformations of the anus and rectum. The surgery of infancy and childhood. WB Saunders, Philadelphia, pp 348–357
7. Santulli TV, Kiesewetter WB, Bill AH Jr (1970) Anorectal anomalies: a suggested international classification. J Pediatr Surg 5:281–287
8. Holschneider A, Hutson J, Peña A et al (2005) Preliminary report on the International Conference for the Development of Standards for the Treatment of Anorectal Malformations. J Pediatr Surg 40(10): 1521–1526
9. Bischoff A, Levitt MA, Peña A (2013) Update on the management of anorectal malformations. Pediatr Surg Int 29(9):899–904
10. Georgeson KE, Inge TH, Albanese CT (2000) Laparoscopically assisted anorectal pull-through for high imperforate anus: a new technique. J Pediatr Surg 35:927–931
11. Yamataka A, Segawa O, Yoshid R et al (2001) Laparoscopic muscle electrostimulation during laparoscopy-assisted anorectal pull-through for high imperforate anus. J Pediatr Surg 36:1659–1661
12. Lima M, Tursini S, Ruggeri G et al (2006) Laparoscopically assisted anorectal pull-through for high imperforate anus: three years'experience. J Laparoendosc Adv Surg Tech 16:63–66

25 Congenital Hyperinsulinism

Giovanni Boroni, Filippo Parolini, and Daniele Alberti

Transient symptomatic hypoglycemia is the most common metabolic abnormality in newborns, with an incidence of 4 per 1000 term infants and 6 per 1000 premature infants. Up to 1 % of these infants have severe and persistent hypoglycemia, which can cause permanent brain damage. Laidlaw [1] in 1938 coined the term "nesidioblastosis," to indicate diffuse and disseminated proliferation of islet cells budding off from pancreatic ducts. Before the mid-1980s, this increase in β-cell mass was presumed to be responsible of the syndrome of persistent hyperinsulinemic hypoglycemia of infancy, described more than 50 years ago by McQuarrie [2]. However, studies by Rahier et al. [3] and other pathologists had convincingly proven that nesidioblastosis is present not only in hypoglycemic symptomatic infants but also in normoglycemic control patients, and it is just a normal feature of the pancreas in early infancy. Over the past 20 years, remarkable progresses have been made in the understanding of the pathogenesis of the persistent hypoglycemia in infancy; nowadays the inappropriate secretion of insulin by β-cells, which has heterogeneous genetic origins, is recognized as cause of this condition [4]. Therefore, in the recent pediatric literature, the term "nesidioblastosis" has been abandoned in favor of "congenital hyperinsulinism" (CHI), which includes both focal and diffuse pancreatic involvement associated with hyperinsulinism and hypoglycemia.

G. Boroni, MD • F. Parolini, MD
Department of Pediatric Surgery, "Spedali Civili" Children's Hospital, Brescia, Italy

D. Alberti, MD (✉)
Department of Pediatric Surgery, "Spedali Civili" Children's Hospital, University of Brescia, Brescia, Italy
e-mail: daniele.alberti@spedalicivili.brescia.it

25.1 Epidemiology

The estimated incidence of CHI in the general population is 1/30,000 to 1/50,000, but it increases to 1/2500 in communities with high rates of consanguinity. This finding reflects the most common modality of inheritance, that is, autosomal recessive, although dominant mutations have been reported. The male to female ratio is 1.2:1 for diffuse lesions and 1.8:1 for focal lesions [5]. The age at onset is variable: the vast majority of cases occurs early in life, a few hours or days after birth, but occasionally, symptoms can take as long as 5 or 6 months to become apparent. Presentation beyond the age of 2 years is rare. The severity of the disease is quite variable but tends to be greater in the neonatal form.

M. Lima (ed.), *Pediatric Digestive Surgery*, DOI 10.1007/978-3-319-40525-4_25

25.2 Pathogenesis and Molecular Mechanism of CHI

Congenital hyperinsulinism is the result of a dysregulated insulin secretion from pancreatic β-cells. Inappropriate secretion of insulin leads to an increased glucose consumption, suppression of endogenous glucose production by inhibiting glycogenolysis and gluconeogenesis and eventually hypoglycemia. Moreover, insulin inhibits lipolysis, free fatty acid production, and ketogenesis, depriving the brain of both its primary and secondary energy sources (glucose and ketone bodies). Normally insulin secretion is primarily regulated by glucose metabolism. Postprandial glucose is transported into the cytoplasm of pancreatic β-cells by the glucose transporter type 2 (GLUT2) and then phosphorylated by glucokinase. Glucose-6-phosphate is then metabolized via glycolysis, Krebs cycle, and oxidative phosphorylation to generate ATP. An increased ATP/ADP ratio within β-cells leads to the closure of the ATP-sensitive potassium channel (K_{ATP}-channel), which causes depolarization of the cell membrane and opening of the voltage-gated calcium channels. The resulting inflow of calcium ions then causes fusion of the insulin secretory granules with the cell membrane and secretion of insulin outside of the β-cell (Fig. 25.1).

Molecular genetic abnormalities have been identified in nine different genes which cause CHI: these include inactivating mutation of the K_{ATP}-channel genes (ABCC8 and KCNJ11), HNF4A, HNF1A, HADH, and UCP2 or activating mutations of GLUD1, GCK, and SLC16A1 [6, 7]. Mutations in ABCC8 and KCNJ11 genes are estimated to account for 40–45 % of all cases of CHI, while mutations in the remaining genes are identified in approximately 5–10 % of cases. The genetic etiology for the remaining 45–50 % of patients remains unknown.

25.2.1 K_{ATP}-Channel Mutations (ABCC8 and KCNJ11)

Inactivating mutations in the ABCC8 and KCNJ11 genes, which encode the SUR1 and Kir6.2 subunits of the K_{ATP}-channel, are the most frequent cause of CHI. Mutations in these genes impair the ability of MgADP to stimulate channel activity or affect the expression of the K_{ATP}-channels at the surface membrane, resulting in continuous depolarization and inappropriate insulin secretion. Many of these patients show a poor response to diazoxide therapy, which is evident considering the target of the drugs is the K_{ATP}-channel. The mode of inheritance of the K_{ATP}-channel mutations

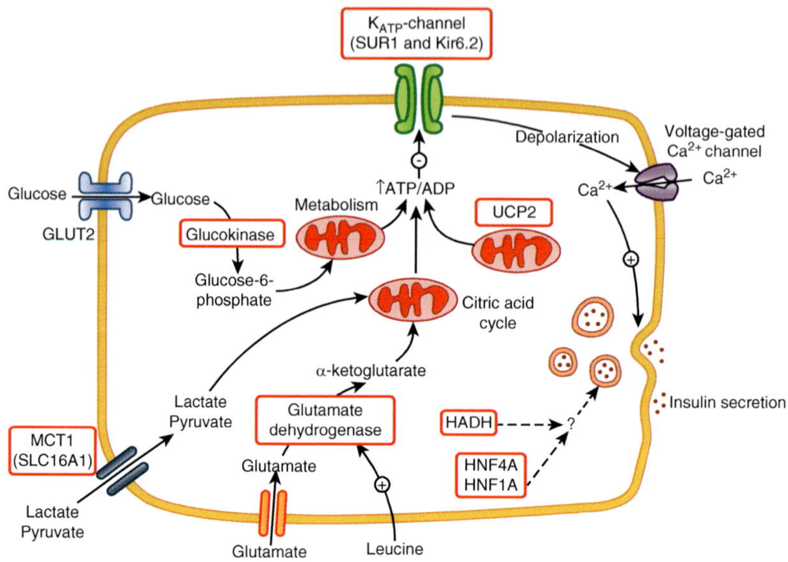

Fig. 25.1 Genetic mechanisms of congenital hyperinsulinism (see text for details)

correlates with the histological type: the identification of two recessive mutations indicates a diffuse disease, whereas, when a single paternally inherited mutation is discovered, a focal lesion is suspected. Indeed focal lesions result from paternal uniparental disomy of chromosome 11p15.5-11p15.1 within a single pancreatic cell. In close proximity with the K_{ATP}-channel genes at chromosome 11p15.1, a region at 11p15.5 harbors maternally expressed tumor suppressors (H19 and CDKN1c) and a paternally expressed growth factor gene (IGF2). When paternal uniparental disomy occurs as a somatic mutation during the development of the pancreas, that β-cell loses K_{ATP}-channel activity. At the same time, the tumor-suppressor activities of H19 and CDKN1C are lost, and the activity of IGF2 is doubled. This leads to a growth advantage for the abnormal β-cells and eventually to a formation of a focal lesion [6, 8]. There are a few reports describing dominant mutations of K_{ATP}-channel genes, in patients with CHI responsive to diazoxide therapy.

25.2.2 Glutamate Dehydrogenase (GLUD1)

Mutations in the GLUD1 gene, which encodes the enzyme glutamate dehydrogenase (GDH), are the most frequent cause of CHI after ABCC8/KCNJ11 mutations. CHI induced by these mutations is also known as the hyperinsulinism/hyperammonemia syndrome. The enzyme GDH, activated by leucine, catalyzes the oxidative deamination of glutamate to α-ketoglutarate and ammonia. Activating mutations in GLUD1 lead to an increased conversion of glutamate to α-ketoglutarate and heightened sensitivity to stimulation by leucine. In β-cells, α-ketoglutarate enters the citric cycle and leads to an increased ATP/ADP ratio, the closure of K_{ATP}-channels and, eventually to an increased insulin secretion [9]. Inheritance is usually autosomal dominant. Patients with GLUD1 mutations usually present a milder form of CHI, with associated hyperammonemia. Hypoglycemia is rapidly precipitated by protein-rich meals. This type of CHI is usually diazoxide responsive, but patients also require a low-protein diet.

25.2.3 Hepatocyte Nuclear Factors (HNF4A and HNF1A)

Hepatocyte nuclear factor 4α (HNF4α), encoded by the HNF4A gene, is a transcription factor critical for liver development and hepatocyte-specific gene expression. In the pancreatic β-cell, HNF4α regulates several genes involved in glucose-stimulated insulin secretion. Heterozygous loss-of-function mutations in this gene have been shown to account for 5 % of cases of diazoxide-responsive hyperinsulinism [10]. The mechanism is currently unknown. Mutations in HNF4A cause also maturity-onset diabetes of the young (MODY1).

Mutations in HNF1A gene have been identified in macrosomic newborns presenting with diazoxide-responsive CHI. However, in later life, patients tend to shift from hypoglycemia to MODY3. The exact mechanism still remains unknown [6].

25.2.4 Glucokinase (GCK)

Congenital hyperinsulinism occurs when a heterozygous-activating mutation (inherited in autosomal dominant manner) in the GCK gene produce an enzyme with an increased affinity for glucose, resulting in the inappropriate insulin secretion at low blood glucose concentration. The age of presentation can vary widely from infancy to adulthood. Patients who require intervention are often responsive to diazoxide therapy, although unresponsive forms have also been described.

25.2.5 Hydroxyacyl-Coenzyme A Dehydrogenase (HADH)

Hydroxyacyl-coenzyme A dehydrogenase (HADH) catalyzes the penultimate step in fatty acid β-oxidation in the mitochondria and is highly expressed in the pancreatic β-cells. Recessively inherited mutations in the HADH gene have been reported, up to now, only in 10 patients, and the mechanism that leads to the unregulated insulin secretion is still unclear [6].

25.2.6 Solute Carrier Family 16, Member 1 (SLC16A1)

Solute carrier family 16, member 1 (SLC16A1) gene encodes a transporter required for the intracellular transport of pyruvate and lactate. The SLC16A1 gene is not usually transcribed in pancreatic β-cells. Mutations that cause inappropriate transcription of this gene in the pancreatic β-cells make these cells sensitive to extracellular levels of lactate and pyruvate and cause exercise-induced hyperinsulinism (EIHI) [11]. In case of EIHI, lactate and pyruvate, produced during anaerobic exercise, enter into the β-cells and are metabolized increasing the ATP/ADP ratio and inducing insulin secretion. Patients are diazoxide responsive, but treatment is not always necessary, as hypoglycemic episodes may be prevented by avoiding strenuous exercise.

25.2.7 Uncoupling Protein 2 (UCP2)

The UCP2 gene encode for the mitochondrial uncoupling protein 2, which uncouples oxidative phosphorylation from ATP synthesis. Under normal condition, UCP2 reduces ATP synthesis and thus suppresses the glucose-stimulated insulin secretion. A loss-of-function mutation in the UCP2 gene was recently suggested as a candidate gene for CHI [12].

25.3 Histopathology

Congenital hyperinsulinism does not correspond to a single pathological entity: many different forms have been reported on the basis of specific genetic defects. Nevertheless, concerning the surgeon's point of view, there are two main pathological subtypes: diffuse (50–70 % of patients) and focal (30–50 % of patients).

In the diffuse type of CHI, the pancreas appears normal both macro- and microscopically. Careful analysis reveals the presence of large β-cells with abnormally large nuclei (as observed in hyperactive endocrine cells). Immunostaining with a specific antibody to proinsulin shows a large Golgi apparatus, reflecting a very high proinsulin synthesis. However, labeling with insulin antibody is very weak, indicating low insulin storage, because of unregulated insulin release.

The focal CHI is a focal adenomatous hyperplasia, characterized by the presence of a small endocrine lesion (3–10 mm in diameter). Histologically this lesion corresponds to the confluence of hyperplastic but normally structured islets, with a large core of β-cells and a peripheral rim of endocrine non-β-cells. Within the focal lesion, the β-cells are hyperactive, with enlarged cytoplasm and a large Golgi apparatus, rich in proinsulin, and with low insulin storage. Outside the focal lesion, the islets are small; their β-cells are resting, with a high storage of insulin and weak production of proinsulin [13].

25.4 Clinical Presentation

The majority of the babies with CHI are macrosomic at birth. Fetal hyperinsulinemia also accounts for the hypertrophic cardiomyopathy and hepatomegaly (increased storage of glucose as glycogen), commonly observed in patients with CHI. The clinical presentation is variable, and patients complain either mild unspecific symptoms of hypoglycemia (poor feeding, lethargy and irritability) or more severe symptoms, as apnea, seizures, or even coma. Seizures are generalized, tonic-clonic, and occur in half of the cases. Other common symptoms are tremors, hypotonia, cyanosis, and hypothermia. Older children and adolescent may present with sweating, confusion, and behavioral changes; in these patients, insulinoma should be considered as alternative diagnosis. Facies is typical with a high forehead, large nose with a short columella, smooth philtrum, and thin upper lip.

In most of cases, symptoms of hypoglycemia appear within 72 h from birth. Hypoglycemia is severe and permanent (both fasting and postprandial). Typically, newborns with CHI have greatly reduced fasting tolerance, and increased intravenous glucose infusion rate is required to maintain adequate blood glucose levels. If not promptly treated, these children are highly susceptible to develop neurological damage, psychomotor retardation, and even death.

25.5 Diagnosis

The main laboratory criteria for the diagnosis of CHI are inappropriately elevated plasma insulin (and/or C-peptide) in the presence of hypoglycemia, low plasma free fatty acids and ketone bodies, and inappropriate response to glucagon.

Some authors suggest that any detectable level of insulin during hypoglycemia is abnormal, whereas others propose different cutoffs; the most frequent value accepted for the diagnosis is serum insulin concentration >3μU/mL in the presence of blood glucose <50 mg/dL.

As insulin inhibits lipolysis, during hypoglycemia, beta-hydroxybutyrate level <1.5–2 mmol/L and free fatty acids <1–1.5 mmol/L are also used as diagnostic adjuncts.

When hypoglycemia is caused by a defect in glycogenolysis or in gluconeogenesis, the patient does not respond to intramuscular/intravenous injection of glucagon. An inappropriate glycemic response to glucagon, with an increase in blood glucose greater than 30 mg/dL at the time of hypoglycemia, is consistent with excess insulin action and is useful in order to confirm the diagnosis [14].

When diagnosis of CHI is confirmed, from a practical point of view, it is important to differentiate focal type from diffuse CHI. When a focal lesion is identified preoperatively, resection of the lesion or partial pancreatectomy can cure the patients without postoperative complications. In case of diffuse type, surgery should be reserved for patients with failure of medical management or poor compliance to therapy, because of the high risk either of persistent hypoglycemia or diabetes, after near-total pancreatectomy [15].

Although focal lesions detected with contrast-enhanced CT scan have been reported [16], they cannot usually be detected using conventional imaging modalities such as ultrasonography, computed tomography (CT), magnetic resonance imaging, and angiography.

Two interventional radiology tests have been used in the past. The arterial stimulation with venous sampling (ASVS) technique involves selective pancreatic angiographic stimulation using intra-arterial calcium and venous sampling. An immediate rise in insulin from stimulation in gastroduodenal artery suggests focal form in pancreatic head; if the test is positive in superior mesenteric artery, the lesion is localized in the uncinate process or in the neck; a rise in insulin from stimulation in splenic artery identifies a lesion in pancreatic body or tail. If the stimulation is effective in all three arteries, a diffuse CHI should be suspected. In transhepatic portal venous catheterization and selective sampling of pancreatic vein (THPVS), the pancreatic venous insulin levels are compared with simultaneous plasma levels of insulin and glucose [17]. Both ASVS and THPVS are technically challenging and have limited specificity and sensitivity, and these techniques have been replaced by 18-Fluorine-L-dihydroxyphenylalanine positron emission tomography (^{18}F-DOPA-PET), usually combined with computed tomography with multiphase contrast media protocols (^{18}F-DOPA-PET/CT). L-DOPA is absorbed by neuroendocrine cells and by pancreas islet cells and metabolized into dopamine. Beta cells of the pancreas have dopamine receptors, and the uptake of ^{18}F-DOPA is very increased in foci with high insulin synthesis rates. ^{18}F-DOPA-PET/CT detects focal lesions as small as 5 mm. This technique, described for the first time in 2003 [18], nowadays represents the most precise method used to differentiate between focal and diffuse form of congenital hyperinsulinism, with a sensitivity of 94 % combined with a specificity of 100 % [19].

25.6 Treatment

In CHI, it is vital to make a prompt diagnosis and to begin early management, as delay in treatment may cause brain damage and permanent neurodevelopmental disorders. Some factors as age, comorbidities, severity, duration, and frequency of hypoglycemic episodes could affect the neurological outcome.

The primary goals of therapy are to achieve normoglycemia and restore production of ketone bodies, inhibiting inappropriate insulin secretion.

The increase in glucose concentration can be achieved either by giving additional glucose or by administration of glycogenolytic and gluconeogenic hormones such as glucagon. Force-feeding must be prevented in order to avoid feeding refusal behavior or severe gastroesophageal reflux. If necessary, intravenous glucose infusion should be used in order to maintain blood glucose >60–70 mg/dL. In neonates with CHI glucose infusion rate necessary to maintain euglycemia is higher than in unaffected newborns (>6–8 mg/kg/min compared to a normal of 4–6 mg/kg/min).

On the other hand, for decreasing serum insulin, medications that inhibit insulin secretion (diazoxide, octreotide) and/or pancreatic resection will be required.

25.7 Medical Therapy

Diazoxide is a potent inhibitor of insulin secretion that binds the SUR1 subunit of the K_{ATP}-channel, activating it. This drug is considered the first-line drug for treatment of CHI but requires an intact K_{ATP}-channel. Therefore, children with diffuse disease due to inactivating mutations in ABCC8 and KCNJ11 and most patients with focal lesions are unresponsive to diazoxide. Diazoxide is daily administered orally in three divided doses, at 5–15 mg/kg/day. Most common side effects include hypertrichosis and salt and fluid retention, which could lead to severe complications, such as congestive hearth failure and reopening of the ductus arteriosus [20]. Other frequent side effects of the therapy with diazoxide are nausea, vomiting, and loss of appetite. When diazoxide is used in higher dose (20 mg/kg/day), it could lead to paradoxical hypoglycemia. In addiction to diazoxide, administration of a thiazide diuretic (chlorotiazide 7–10 mg/kg/day in two divided doses) is advised to prevent fluid retention and for its synergistic effect on the suppression of insulin secretion.

Octreotide is a long-acting analogue of somatostatin that inhibits the secretion of a variety of hormones (including insulin) and is the second line of treatment for patients unresponsive to diazoxide. Octreotide inhibits insulin secretion by inducing hyperpolarization of β-cells by direct inhibition of voltage-dependent calcium channels. Moreover, octreotide activation of somatostatin receptor 5 (STTR 5) decreases insulin gene promoter activity, resulting in reduced insulin biosynthesis. Octreotide is administered as multiple daily subcutaneous injection (3–4 times/day) or by continuous subcutaneous infusion using an insulin pump, at a dose of 5–35 μg/kg/day [14, 21]. After the first 2–3 doses, a tolerance to its effects may be observed, and increased doses could be necessary. Adverse effects include anorexia, nausea, abdominal discomfort, and diarrhea; rarely, serious side effects are drug-induced hepatitis, necrotizing enterocolitis, and long QT syndrome.

Lanreotide, a long-acting somatostatin analogue, has been successfully used in the treatment of CHI patients as a four weekly intramuscular injection or deep subcutaneous injection [22].

The calcium channel blocker nifedipine (0.25–2.5 mg/kg/day in 2–3 divided doses) inhibits insulin secretion, inactivating voltage-gated calcium channels. Some authors reported few cases of nifedipine-responsive forms of CHI [23]. A large, multicentric, randomized clinical trial would be desirable to elucidate the effectiveness and safety of nifedipine in this setting [24].

Glucagon stimulates glycogenolysis and gluconeogenesis; in emergency situation, intramuscular administration increases blood glucose within a few minutes. Administered also by intravenous and subcutaneous routes, glucagon is used mainly for short-term control of diazoxide-unresponsive patients. Nevertheless, successful long-term therapy with subcutaneous infusion has been reported [25].

Recently, novel medications for diazoxide-unresponsive CHI have been proposed. An antagonist of glucagon-like peptide 1 (GLP1) receptor, exendin, has been shown to be effective for the treatment of CHI in randomized clinical trial [26]. Sirolimus, one of the mammalian target of rapamycin (mTOR) inhibitors, usually used as immunosuppressant to prevent rejection in organ transplantation and to treat neoplasm, was successfully used to treat patients with diazoxide unresponsive CHI [27].

25.8 Surgical Management

Medical therapy represents currently the first line of treatment for CHI. However, when patient does not respond to medical therapy and cannot be weaned off treatment with intravenous glucose infusion, pancreatectomy should be considered. In this eventuality, the differentiation between focal and diffuse type is crucial. Indeed focal lesion can be cured with a limited pancreatic resection, reducing the risk of diabetes and exocrine pancreatic deficiency. Differently, diffuse disease usually requires a near-total (95–98 %) pancreatectomy, with a high risk of postsurgical endocrine and/or exocrine pancreatic insufficiency. Genetic mutation analysis may predict focal and diffuse disease: focal CHI is associated with loss of heterozygosity for paternally inherited mutations in K_{ATP}-channel genes, whereas homozygous-recessive or compound heterozygote mutations cause a diffuse disease. ^{18}F-DOPA-PET/CT is also required for the differentiation between focal and diffuse CHI and for a precise preoperative localization of the focal lesions within the pancreas. Almost 35–45 % of patients with CHI are unresponsive to medical therapy and eventually require surgery [7].

25.8.1 Surgery for Diffuse CHI

In diffuse congenital hyperinsulinism, the optimal extent of resection has been largely debated. Gross in 1953 reported on 65 % pancreatic resection (lateral to the superior mesenteric vessels). In the following years, there was a gradual shift in opinion toward 80–90 % resection, which involved removal of all pancreas distal to the right side of the superior mesenteric vessels. This procedure was associated with a 25–50 % incidence of recurrent hypoglycemia [5]. Nowadays most authors agree that a "near-total" pancreatectomy is required to prevent unacceptable high incidence of recurrent hyperinsulinemia. The procedure involves removal of 95 % of pancreatic tissue (tail, body, uncinate process, and part of pancreatic head), leaving behind an amount of pancreatic tissue around the common bile duct and along the medial border of the duodenum. Some authors suggested that up to a 98 % pancreatectomy, in which only small islands of tissue are left along the pancreaticoduodenal arcade bordering the duodenum, may be required in refractory cases [28]. Other authors adopt a conservative approach and recommend only a 50–75 % resection as first step, associated with subsequent medical therapy; if necessary, they reexplore the patient and do a further resection [29] (Fig. 25.2).

25.8.1.1 Open Procedure

Laparotomy is performed via supraumbilical transverse incision. The anterior surface of the pancreas is exposed by entering the lesser peritoneal sac through the gastrocolic omentum. The duodenum is Kocherized to expose the head of the pancreas. Three biopsies from the head, corpus, and tail (and, if present, biopsy of any

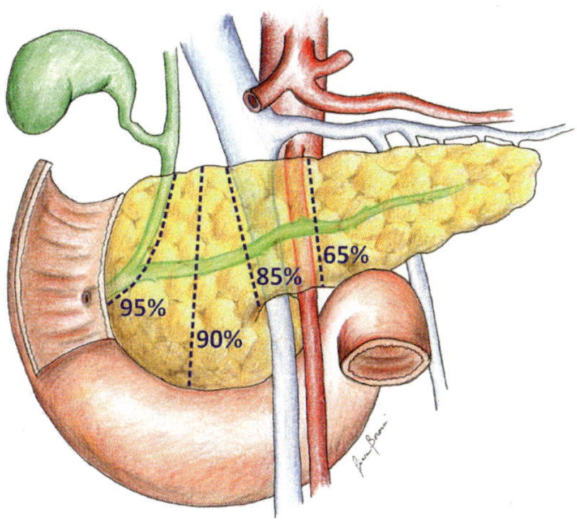

Fig. 25.2 Schematic representation of various degrees of pancreatectomy

suspicious nodule) are sent for frozen section histologic examination. If, unexpectedly, they show resting or suppressed islet cells, a focal lesion has to be searched. If frozen section analysis confirms diffuse CHI, a near-total pancreatectomy can be performed. A stay suture is placed in the tail of the pancreas to allow traction; the tail is carefully dissected out of the splenic hilum, and the short pancreatic vessels are coagulated or tied and divided. The dissection proceeds medially toward the corpus and neck; short pancreatic arteries and veins passing from splenic vessels to the pancreas are meticulously dissected, coagulated using bipolar diathermy, or ligated and divided. Once the dissection has arrived to the right of superior mesenteric vessels, attention is directed to the uncinate process and to the pancreatic head. The uncinate process, which may represent up to 30 % of the pancreatic weight, lies behind the superior mesenteric vessels. A sling may be passed around these vessels, retracting them to the left and facilitating the dissection of uncinate process. As the head of the pancreas is approached, it is essential to define accurately the course of the common bile duct. This is achieved by identifying the common bile duct above the first part of duodenum and passing a sling around the duct. A blunt forceps is passed, within the concavity of the C-loop of the duodenum, behind the duodenum; the sling is then grasped and brought out above the head of the pancreas. This becomes the guide to the position of the common bile duct during subsequent dissection. The head can now be mobilized safely. The superior and inferior pancreaticoduodenal vessels are ligated and divided; the pancreatic duct is identified, ligated with non-adsorbable ligature, and divided and pancreatic resection completed [30, 31] (Fig. 25.3).

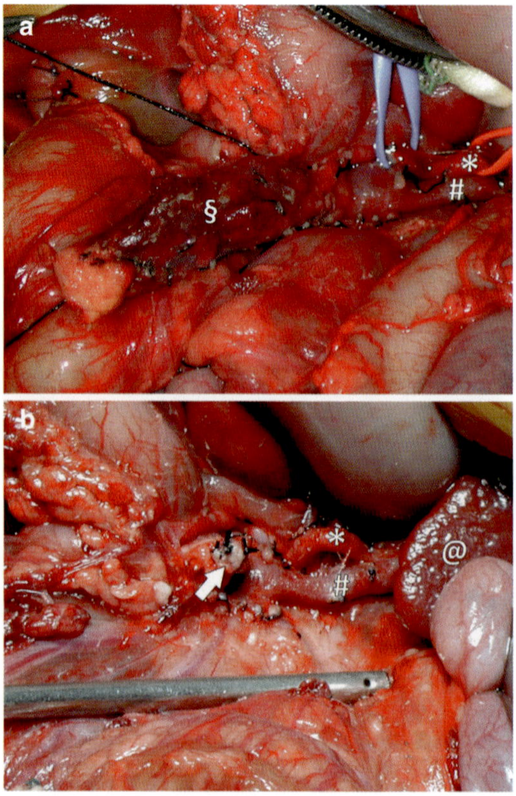

Fig. 25.3 Open near-total pancreatectomy, during the dissection (*A*) and at the end of the procedure (*B*) (* splenic artery; # splenic vein; § pancreas; @ spleen; *arrow* ligated Wirsung)

25.8.1.2 Laparoscopic Procedure

A 10-mm Hasson port is inserted at the umbilicus through an open technique for a 30° scope (this large port allows the retrieval of the pancreas after resection). The following ports are inserted under direct vision: a 5-mm port in the left lower quadrant, a Nathanson retractor in the epigastrium (to retract the stomach), and a further working port (3 or 5 mm) in the right flank. The gastrocolic ligament is divided and the lesser sac entered. The Nathanson retractor is used to retract upward the stomach. A stay suture is placed into the pancreatic tail and used to retract the gland. Dissection proceeds from the tail toward the head; the short pancreatic vessels are divided using a 3-mm hook diathermy at very high coagulation settings. The pancreatic tail is resected using harmonic scalpel and removed through the umbilical port. The tail is sent for frozen section analysis to confirm the diagnosis. Further dissection is facilitated by the insertion of a stay suture at the cut surface of remaining pancreas. The pancreas is resected in segments of about 2 cm. To facilitate excision of the head, a stay suture is placed in the uncinate process and a second one in the head of the pancreas, which is retracted superiorly. Near-total pancreatectomy is performed by leaving a small rim of pancreas along the medial border of the duodenum, where the common bile duct is expected [30, 31]. As in the open procedure, the pancreatic duct is ligated with non-adsorbable suture.

25.8.2 Surgery for Focal CHI

In patients with focal CHI, the goal of surgery is the resection of the lesion, sparing healthy pancreatic tissue, and eventually the cure of the disease without complications.

As in diffuse CHI, three intraoperative biopsies are performed for frozen section. Histology may reveal the presence of the focal lesion or a normal pancreas with resting or suppressed islet cells, excluding a diffuse CHI. The pancreas is then inspected and palpated for a nodular area, which can indicate the site of the focal lesion. These lesions differ from insulinoma: their size usually varies between 3 and 7 mm in diameter, they are not provided with capsule, and their architecture and structure are preserved. In the rare cases of superficial lesions, they may be simply enucleated, remembering that lesions often have small branches extending in the surrounding tissue. In case of lesions located deep in the parenchyma, the surgical access differs according to the location of the lesion. If the focal lesion is deep in the head or neck of the pancreas, open resection of the lesion with a rim of surrounding normal pancreatic tissue is recommended. A pancreaticojejunostomy is then performed to allow drainage of distal pancreas. For the lesion in the tail or body, a distal pancreatectomy may be done, by laparotomy or laparoscopy, as in the diffuse form. In any case, an adequate resection margin has to be confirmed by frozen section analysis [29, 30].

25.8.3 Complications and Outcomes

The most serious surgical complication in near-total pancreatectomy, or in partial resection for focal lesions in the head of the pancreas, is biliary tree injury, with an incidence of 2–15 %.

Moreover, if more than 90 % of focal CHI cases were proven to be cured after surgery [15], in diffuse CHI, reported complications include recurrent hyperinsulinemic hypoglycemia (sometimes requiring further pancreatic resection) and pancreatic endocrine and exocrine insufficiency.

In large series, only 25 % of patients with diffuse CHI were well controlled postoperatively with no medications, while up to 58 % of cases required medical treatment for persistent hypoglycemia and up to 33 % needed further pancreatic resection.

The need for pancreatic enzyme replacement ranged from 4 to 37 %, and postoperative diabetes mellitus was reported in 12–56 % of patients [30]. The long-term metabolic outcome of these patients is even worse. Beltrand reported that hyperglycemia was found in 53 % of 58 patients after surgery, but this incidence increased regularly with age, reaching 100 % at the age of 13 years. Similarly, the incidence of insulin therapy increased from 19 % postoperatively to 42 % at 8 years and 91 % during adolescence [32].

References

1. Laidlaw GF (1938) Nesidioblastoma: the islet cell tumor of the pancreas. Am J Pathol 14:125–134
2. McQuarrie I (1954) Idiopathic spontaneously occurring hypoglycemia in infants: clinical significance of problem and treatment. Am J Dis Child 87:399–428
3. Rahier J, Guiot Y, Sempoux C (2000) Persistent hyperinsulinaemic hypoglycaemia of infancy: a heterogeneous syndrome unrelated to nesidioblastosis. Arch Dis Child Fetal Neonatal 82:F108–F112
4. Palladino AA, Stanley CA (2011) Nesidioblastosis no longer! It's all about genetics. J Clin Endocrinol Metab 96(3):617–619
5. Goel P, Choudhury SR (2012) Persistent hyperinsulinemic hypoglycemia of infancy: an overview of current concepts. J Indian Assoc Pediatr Surg 17(3): 99–103
6. Rahman SA, Nessa A, Hussain K (2015) Molecular mechanisms of congenital hyperinsulinism. J Mol Endocrinol 54(2):R119–R129
7. Flanagan SE, Kapoor RR, Hussain K (2011) Genetics of congenital hyperinsulinemic hypoglycemia. Semin Pediatr Surg 20(1):13–17
8. Saint-Martin C, Arnoux JB, de Lonlay P et al (2011) KATP channel mutations in congenital hyperinsulinism. Semin Pediatr Surg 20(1):18–22

9. Marquard J, Palladino AA, Stanley CA et al (2011) Rare forms of congenital hyperinsulinism. Semin Pediatr Surg 20(1):38–44
10. Flanagan SE, Kapoor RR, Mali G et al (2010) Diazoxide-responsive hyperinsulinemic hypoglycemia caused by HNF4A gene mutations. Eur J Endocrinol 162:987–992
11. Otonkoski T, Jiao H, Kaminen-Ahola N et al (2007) Physical exercise-induced hypoglycemia caused by failed silencing of monocarboxylate transporter 1 in pancreatic beta cells. Am J Hum Genet 81:467–474
12. González-Barroso MM, Giurgea I, Bouillaud F et al (2008) Mutations in UCP2 in congenital hyperinsulinism reveal a role for regulation of insulin secretion. PLoS One 3, e3850
13. Rahier J, Guiot Y, Sempoux C (2011) Morphologic analysis of focal and diffuse forms of congenital hyperinsulinism. Semin Pediatr Surg 20(1):3–12
14. Yorifuji T (2014) Congenital hyperinsulinism: current status and future perspectives. Ann Pediatr Endocrinol Metab 19(2):57–68
15. Palladino AA, Stanley CA (2011) A specialized team approach to diagnosis and medical versus surgical treatment of infants with congenital hyperinsulinism. Semin Pediatr Surg 20(1):32–37
16. Hashimoto Y, Sakakibara A, Kawakita R et al (2015) Focal form of congenital hyperinsulinism clearly detectable by contrast-enhanced computed tomography imaging. Int J Pediatr Endocrinol 2015(1):20
17. Adzick NS (2012) The pancreas. In: Coran AG, Caldamone A, Scott Adzick N et al (eds) Pediatric surgery, 7th edn. Elsevier, Philadelphia , pp 1371–1384
18. Otonkoski T, Veijola R, Huopio H et al (2003) Diagnosis of focal persistent hyperinsulinism of infancy with 18F-fluoro-L-dopa PET. Horm Res 60:2
19. Mohnike W, Barthlen W, Mohnike K et al (2011) Positron emission tomography/computed tomography diagnostics by means of fluorine-18-L-dihydroxyphenylalanine in congenital hyperinsulinism. Semin Pediatr Surg 20(1):23–27
20. Shah P, Demirbilek H, Hussain K (2014) Persistent hyperinsulinaemic hypoglycaemia in infancy. Semin Pediatr Surg 23(2):76–82
21. Thornton PS, Alter CA, Katz LE et al (1993) Short- and long-term use of octreotide in the treatment of congenital hyperinsulinism. J Pediatr 123(4): 637–643
22. Le Quan Sang KH, Arnoux JB, Mamoune A et al (2012) Successful treatment of congenital hyperinsulinism with long-acting release octreotide. Eur J Endocrinol 166(2):333–339
23. Baş F, Darendeliler F, Demirkol D et al (1999) Successful therapy with calcium channel blocker (nifedipine) in persistent neonatal hyperinsulinemic hypoglycemia of infancy. J Pediatr Endocrinol Metab 12(6):873–878
24. Müller D, Zimmering M, Roehr CC (2004) Should nifedipine be used to counter low blood sugar levels in children with persistent hyperinsulinaemic hypoglycaemia? Arch Dis Child 89(1):83–85
25. Neylon OM, Moran MM, Pellicano A et al (2013) Successful subcutaneous glucagon use for persistent hypoglycaemia in congenital hyperinsulinism. J Pediatr Endocrinol Metab 26(11–12):1157–1161
26. Calabria AC, Li C, Gallagher PR et al (2012) GLP-1 receptor antagonist exendin-(9–39) elevates fasting blood glucose levels in congenital hyperinsulinism owing to inactivating mutations in the ATP-sensitive K+ channel. Diabetes 61(10):2585–2591
27. Senniappan S, Alexandrescu S, Tatevian N et al (2014) Sirolimus therapy in infants with severe hyperinsulinemic hypoglycemia. N Engl J Med 370(12): 1131–1137
28. Spitz L (2006) Surgery for hyperinsulinemic hypoglycaemia. In: Spitz L, Coran AG (eds) Operative pediatric surgery, 6th edn. Hodder Arnold, London, pp 733–738
29. Barthlen W (2011) Surgery in congenital hyperinsulinism-tips and tricks not only for surgeons. A practical guide. Semin Pediatr Surg 20(1):56–59
30. Pierro A, Nah SA (2011) Surgical management of congenital hyperinsulinism of infancy. Semin Pediatr Surg 20(1):50–53
31. Spitz L, Pierro A (2013) Pancreatic resection. In: Spitz L, Coran AG (eds) Operative pediatric surgery, 7th edn. CRC Press, Boca Raton, pp 740–749
32. Beltrand J, Caquard M, Arnoux JB et al (2012) Glucose metabolism in 105 children and adolescents after pancreatectomy for congenital hyperinsulinism. Diabetes Care 35(2):198–203

Hepatobiliary Pediatric Surgery

26

Arnaud Bonnard, Florent Guerin, and
Pascal de Lagausie

26.1 Introduction

Hepatobiliary pediatric surgery remains rare and should be, for some pathologies such as biliary atresia and hepatic transplantation, performed in very specialized pediatric centers.

On the other hand, other pathologies are common, and most of the pediatric surgeons must be able to take care of these children. Firstly, we will establish some considerations about biliary stones, either in the gallbladder or in the common bile duct, about some congenital abnormalities (choledochal cyst, biliary atresia) and a quick overview on how to manage hepatobiliary trauma. Then, we will talk about some pancreatic conditions, which can sometimes require a surgical approach.

26.2 Biliary Stones

Even though biliary stones can be found at any age, from fetal life to adolescence, this pathology remains quite rare in children. Cholelithiasis occurs in 1 % of children, mainly due to hemolytic disorders and distal ileum pathology in infancy and dyslipidemia in adolescents [1]. Sex ratio is about 4 to 1 with a female preponderance at the age of adolescence.

26.2.1 Etiologies

In about 30 % of cholelithiasis, no cause is identified. This means that an etiology is determined in 70 % of the cases. Hemolytic disorders (spherocytosis, sickle cell disease, thalassemia) are probably the most frequent causes. A congenital abnormality of the bile duct can also be found (stenosis, choledochal cyst). During fetal life, cholelithiasis can occur at any time. The appearance of cholelithiasis after 30 weeks of gestation, without any risk factors, is associated with a satisfying prenatal and neonatal clinical course [2]. Ceftriaxone has been reported as a possible cause for pseudolithiasis formation, with associated risk factors being fasting and bed rest [3].

An increase in the frequency of cholecystectomy in children has been described during the last decades, mainly explained by the fact that more and more cholecystectomies are performed in children, not only for gallstone disease but also for dyskinesia of the gallbladder [4]. In this population, obesity is predominant. However, the risk of developing gallstones for obese children and adolescents during a lifestyle intervention is

A. Bonnard, MD, PhD (✉)
Department of Pediatric surgery, Robert Debré Children University hospital, APHP, Paris, France
e-mail: arnaud.bonnard@rdb.aphp.fr

F. Guerin, MD, PhD
Department of Pediatric Surgery, Kremlin Bicetre Children University Hospital, APHP, Paris, France

P. de Lagausie, MD PhD
Department of Pediatric Surgery, Hôpital Timone-Enfant, Marseille, France

M. Lima (ed.), *Pediatric Digestive Surgery*, DOI 10.1007/978-3-319-40525-4_26

reported to be limited and mainly related to weight loss. Patients who lost more than 10 % of their initial body weight were exposed to develop more lithiasis, with an even higher prevalence in those who had lost more than 25 % of their initial weight [5].

26.2.2 Clinical Signs and Complications

Abdominal pain in the right upper quadrant is the most frequent sign, sometimes associated to a positive Murphy sign. If the patient is febrile, a cholecystitis should be suspected. Jaundice is highly associated with lithiasis in the common bile duct (CBD).

Prenatal diagnosis can be done, usually during the third trimester. Cholelithiasis at this age has been reported to be associated with some fetal and maternal conditions such as hydramnios, congenital anomalies (gastrointestinal, cardiac), or Down syndrome [6].

Complications are possible: migration of cholelithiasis in the CBD is responsible of jaundice, hepatic cytolysis, and sometimes pancreatitis. If the patient is febrile, cholecystitis or angiocholitis must be suspected. In this last case, pain in the right upper quadrant associated with fever and jaundice is typical.

26.2.3 Preoperative Workout

A blood workout should be done to determine a cause for cholelithiasis (dyslipidemia, hemolytic disorders). Hepatic enzyme and lipase should also be done to rule out any complication.

26.2.4 Treatment

26.2.4.1 Elective Cholecystectomy

For a child with a short bowel syndrome on whom the surgery should be discussed because sometimes very difficult to perform regarding the previous surgery, ursodeoxycholic acid (Ursofalk®, Vifor Fribourg, Switzerland) could be a treatment of choice to prevent cholelithiasis occurrence. This treatment seems effective in prevention, but also as a postoperative treatment after obesity surgery [7].

In patients with hematologic disorders, cholecystectomy should be performed even if the patient is asymptomatic, in order to prevent the potential complications of biliary colics, acute cholecystitis, and choledocholithiasis, which leads to major risks in this population. Laparoscopic cholecystectomy is the procedure of choice, as it has become the gold standard over the last year. Recently, an interest for a single-port surgery has been published. Although this needs confirmation, it does not seem to offer more advantages than classic laparoscopic cholecystectomy [8, 9]. Robotic surgery in this indication has also been reported, but it remains reserved to a few pediatric centers [10]. At last, it seems that performing this surgery with a same-day discharge does not generate an increase in complication rate in children [11].

On the other hand, asymptomatic cholelithiasis in patients without any associated comorbidity should be simply monitored with an ultrasound exam every year. Although the natural history of this lithiasis remains misunderstood, an elective cholecystectomy can be indicated if the child has to spend time away from health-care access.

Cholelithiasis which has been diagnosed prenatally usually presents a good prognosis without surgery. It sometimes disappears spontaneously; in case of migration, a transhepatic washout of the common bile duct can be performed.

26.2.4.2 Treatment of Complications

- *Acute cholecystitis*: The main debate in literature is on the optimal moment to perform the laparoscopic cholecystectomy, whether it should be early (ELC) or delayed (DLC). A paper from the Cochrane database published in 2013 [12] found no significant difference between early (within 7 days) and late laparoscopic (after 6 weeks) cholecystectomy on the primary outcomes (bilious complications). However, trials with high-bias risk indicate that early laparoscopic cholecystectomy during acute cholecystitis seems safe and may shorten the total hospital stay. More recently, ELC appears as safe and effective as DLC. ELC might be associated with lower hospital costs, fewer workdays lost, and greater patient satisfaction [13]. In children, there are no randomized control trials. A retrospective study reports an identical rate of complications and conversion for early and delayed cholecystectomy [14]. Most of the time, such complications occur on patients with hematologic disorders, and preoperative conditions can be poor. Thus, time to improve the clinical condition before surgery is necessary, making the ELC rarely feasible within the 3 days. The bilious complications reported to be less than 1 % in this indication [15], and precise guidelines for appropriate patient selection, adequate experience, and proper laparoscopic technique are absolutely necessary.

- *Common bile duct (CBD) stones*: A sequential approach with endoscopic retrograde cholangiopancreatography (ERCP) and endoscopic sphincterotomy (ES) followed by a laparoscopic cholecystectomy is an effective and standardized treatment of CBD stones in adults.

In children, this treatment remains controversial. Although experience with diagnostic and therapeutic ERCP with ES in children has grown during the past few years [16–18], the data concerning safety and technical outcomes is poor in comparison with ERCP in adults [19]. Moreover, performing an ERCP requires almost systematically general anesthesia (GA) in children [18]. At last, long-term consequences of ERCP with ES on the papilla and cancer risk in children have yet to be evaluated. For these reasons, a one-stage total laparoscopic treatment of CBD stones in children has been demonstrated to be as effective as the others options allowing to clear the CBD in 72 % of the cases with a simple washout of the duct in majority of the cases [20].

26.2.4.3 A Few Words About Technique

Different positions are possible for laparoscopic surgery, but the best remains the "French position" with the operator between the patient's legs, the assistant on the patient's left, the scrub nurse on the patient's right side, and the monitor close to the patient's right shoulder.

A three-port technique (two operative ports and one port to present the gallbladder) is the most common. It can also be done using a single transumbilical port and a special instrument dedicated to or even two ports with a transabdominal stitch to expose the gallbladder. The dissection of the Calot triangle is most of the time the first step of the surgery with the left hand holding onto the gallbladder and the right hand performing the dissection. In children, the cystic artery rarely requires a clip or a knot; the monopolar hook is effective in most of the cases. At this point, we prefer to control the cystic duct by an intracorporeal knot instead of clip since complications have been reported with clips. The second step usually consists of a retrograde cholecystectomy. In case of cholecystitis, anterograde cholecystectomy is sometimes more accessible, the pedicle being difficult to dissect because of inflammation and edema. Cholecystectomy should begin once the cystic duct has been completely isolated.

If the preop medical history and ultrasound are highly in favor of a CBD stone, the catheterization of the cystic duct and a transcystic washout should be performed. A Fogarty or a Dormia catheter can be used. In case of failure to clear the CBD, postoperative ERCP can be useful.

26.3 Congenital Malformations

26.3.1 Choledochal Cyst (CC)

26.3.1.1 Introduction and Etiology

A choledochal cyst is a cystic dilatation of the common bile duct, which occurs in approximately 1 to 10.000–13.000 live births, more commonly in girls (3–4:1) and is more frequent in Asia (up to 1:1000), especially in Japan. There are two principal hypotheses: the pancreatic reflux hypothesis and the obstructing segment hypothesis. The main anatomical disorder seems to be an abnormality of the pancreaticobiliary junction with the terminal bile duct and pancreatic bile duct having a long common channel (more than 1 cm from the sphincter). This could explain the reflux of the pancreatic secretion and enzyme in the common bile duct and the chronic inflammation induced [21, 22]. The weakness of the bile duct wall or an obstruction of the distal choledochus or both can be also incriminated [23]. More recently, it has been suggested that there were finally two major entities explaining the CC malformation. One entity consists of a high pressure in the bile duct, usually diagnosed prenatally and in relation with a congenital obstruction leading to the dilatation. In this case, amylase dosage in the cyst, used as a marker of reflux, is low. The second entity is in relation with a pancreatic secretion reflux into the bile duct, with a high amylase level in the cyst, and pancreatitis instead of jaundice is the most important clinical sign [24].

26.3.1.2 Clinical Signs and Complications

Prenatal diagnosis can be made by showing a cyst in the hepatic area. Differential diagnostics include a duplication cyst, biliary atresia, or even ovary cyst in a female. A fetal MRI can be performed. At birth, stool color should be closely monitored in order to avoid a late diagnosis of biliary atresia.

Otherwise, jaundice, cholangitis, and pancreatitis are frequent complications if the cyst is not diagnosed until later, usually within the first decade of life. It can also be diagnosed through a palpable mass in the right upper quadrant, sometimes associated with pain and jaundice, forming the classic triad, only present in less than one third of the patient.

26.3.1.3 Preoperative Workout

MRI is the most useful tool to confirm the diagnosis and plan the surgery. It allows the surgeon to determine the anatomy of the common channel and the presence of an accessory bile duct. It also has the advantage of replacing the ERCP which used to be done before surgical treatment of CC. A classification has been established in five types: type I (cystic or fusiform dilatation) is the most common type. Type IV involving the hepatic duct convergence is the second most frequent type. The others remain rare. A special type V also called Caroli disease involving the entire biliary tract has been described. Recently another classification from the King's College of London has been reported, establishing a difference between the cystic and the fusiform dilatation of the type I in relation with either a stenosis or a reflux [24]. Contrast study of the biliary tract should be performed during the surgery in order to appreciate perfectly the anatomy before any resection and sometimes dose the amylase in bile. Additionally, a preoperative hepatic biopsy to evaluate the hepatic fibrosis must be done.

26.3.1.4 Treatment

Surgery is the only treatment. It can be performed either with an open approach or laparoscopically or even with a robot. Numerous papers have already been published on the laparoscopic approach of the CC. Concern on the type of biliary intestinal anastomosis that should be done remains controversial. Liem NT in an extensive series of 400 patients and comparing biliary-digestive continuity reestablished by hepatico-duodenostomy (HD) or hepaticojejunostomy (HJ) showed no difference in term of postoperative cholangitis (1.6 % vs 0.5 %) [25]. Timing of surgery remains also discussed for prenatally diagnosed CC. A randomized control trial has been carried out, comparing a group of patients operated on before 1 month with another group operated on after the age of 1 month [26]. During the first month of life, 32 infants out of the 68 fetuses diagnosed with CC became symptomatic (e.g., developed jaundice) and were excluded from the trial. Grades III and IV hepatic fibroses were significantly more common in the late operation group and in patients who were diagnosed during early pregnancy, which pleads in favor of early surgery for neonates with a prenatal diagnosis of CC.

26.3.1.5 A Few Words About Technic

Patient's installation is the French position. Trocar placement is the same used for a cholecystectomy. Technically, laparoscopic approach is making the resection and the anastomosis, while the Roux-en-Y loop is usually done through an umbilical approach which is quicker than a total intracorporeal reconstruction [27]. The minimal handling of the bowel when it's done intracorporealy appears to minimize postoperative ileus and allows for early postoperative feeding and discharge between 4 and 8 days. Starting with the gallbladder dissection and ligation of the cystic, and hanging it to put it down, allows visualizing easily the top of the cyst, the biliary convergence, and eventually an accessory bile duct. Also, a contrast study can be done through the cystic duct. Make the dissection of the cyst; opening it or not is depending on the surgeon's preferences. We could say that, in case of inflammation and difficulties, for a better security, avoiding to injure the portal vein, opening the cyst, and making the dissection as close as possible from the cyst are safer. Not ligating the distal stump is a feasible approach for managing CC with stenotic distal choledochus. It simplifies the operative procedure and may minimize pancreatic duct injury [28].

Attention should be paid to late complications, other than cholangitis that has been published with intrahepatic gallstones formation. This is commonly attributed to the remaining intrahepatic bile duct dilatation and the stenosis located between the intrahepatic bile duct dilatation and the common hepatic duct. Accordingly, these results support the total excisional procedure for this condition. However, regarding the cases associated with cystic dilatation of intrahepatic bile ducts, completely free bile drainage from the dilated intrahepatic biliary system should be performed at the radical operation [29].

26.3.2 Biliary Atresia

26.3.2.1 Definition

Biliary atresia is a neonatal obliterative cholangiopathy affecting both intra- and extrahepatic parts of the biliary system.

26.3.2.2 Pathogenesis

The histological appearance of the liver is characterized by portal tract edema, bile duct plugging and proliferation, and a small cell and variably giant cell infiltrate with an inflammatory process. Progression of the condition results in cholestasis, hepatic fibrosis, and ultimately cirrhosis. Experimental, genetic, and epidemiologic studies have not yet reach an agreement on the origin of the disease. The main hypothesis is a combination of toxic, immunologic, and genetic origin [30, 31].

26.3.2.3 Epidemiology

Biliary atresia is a rare disease with an incidence in North America and Europe varying from 1 in 15,000 to 1 in 20,000 live births. There is a western to eastern increase with the highest reported incidence from Taiwan and French Polynesia with about 1 in 5,000 live births [32, 33].

26.3.2.4 Classification

- *The Japanese pediatric surgical* classification is based on the level of obliteration of the extrahepatic duct, of which Type 3 (obliteration at the level of the porta hepatis) is the commonest, occurring in about 85 % of cases. Obstruction at the level of the common hepatic duct (Type 2) or common bile duct (Type 1) is much less common but carries a better prognosis (Fig. 26.1a).
- *Other surgical classifications* are based on the on the patency of both the gallbladder and the common bile duct in order to perform rather a Kasai portocholecystostomy (KPC) than a Kasai portoenterostomy (KPE) (Fig. 26.1b) [34].
- *The UK group developed a clinical classification* based on the outcome:
  1. *Cystic BA* is that variant characterized by cystic change within otherwise obliterated ducts. The cyst communicates poorly with intrahepatic ducts, with a cloudy appearance on cholangiogram (Fig. 26.2). It should not be confused with true choledochal cysts. They usually have a better outcome than the isolated complete BA [35].
  2. *Biliary atresia splenic malformation (BASM)* is a peculiar constellation of anomalies and occurs in ~10 % of Caucasian series; Table 26.1 illustrates the associated anomalies. There is a marked detrimental effect of age at Kasai in this subtype than the isolated type of BA [36].

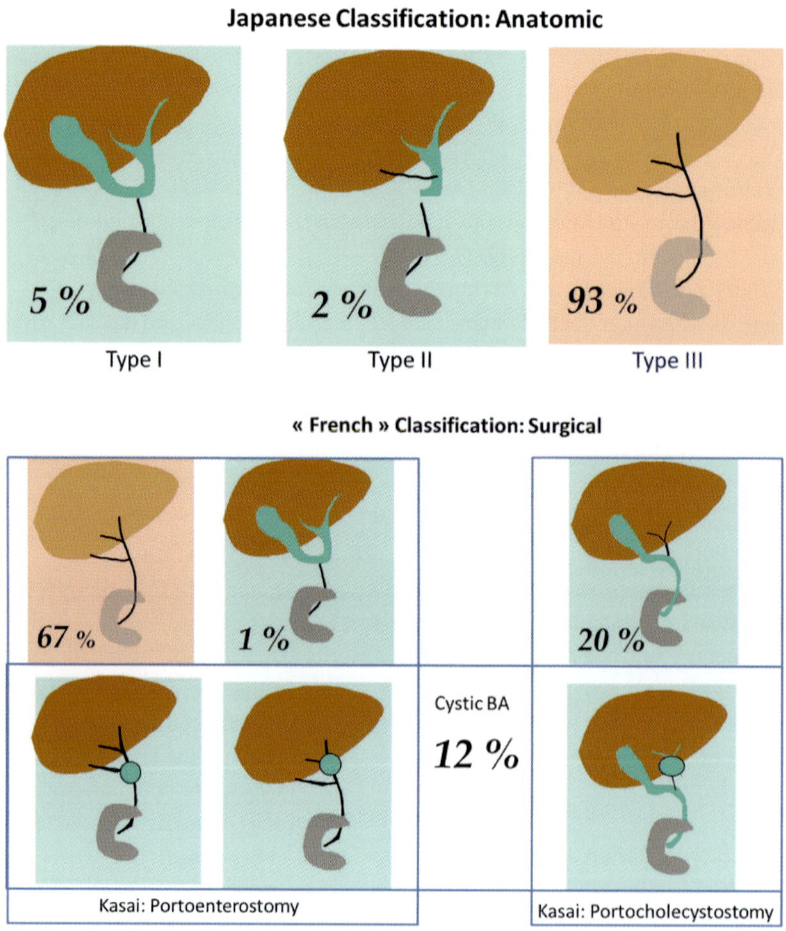

Fig. 26.1 Japanese classification (**a**) and the "French" classification (**b**) depending on the patency of both the gallbladder and common bile duct. Cystic BA is also included in this classification

3. *CMV IgM positive associated biliary atresia* is a recent entity with a poorer outcome than isolated BA [37].

26.3.2.5 Diagnosis

Prenatal Diagnosis

Prenatal detection of BA is a rare situation, found on 20 patients over 15 years in our center (with about 20 pts/year referred for BA). Prenatal signs on ultrasound performed at the second trimester of gestation include:

1. Absence of the gallbladder: 35 % (although most of the prenatal absence of the gallbladder is benign and not related to BA)
2. Cyst located on the liver hilum: 50 % (differentials include choledochal cyst or duplication)
3. Elements of the splenic malformation syndrome: 15 % (situs inversus, polysplenia, etc.)

Great care should be deserved for the prenatal counseling regarding the likelihood of BA, although a complete and early postnatal assessment should be performed before the second week of life.

Neonatal Diagnosis

Infants with BA present with a conjugated jaundice, dark urine, and pale stools. These signs are usually present from birth. Initially the infants

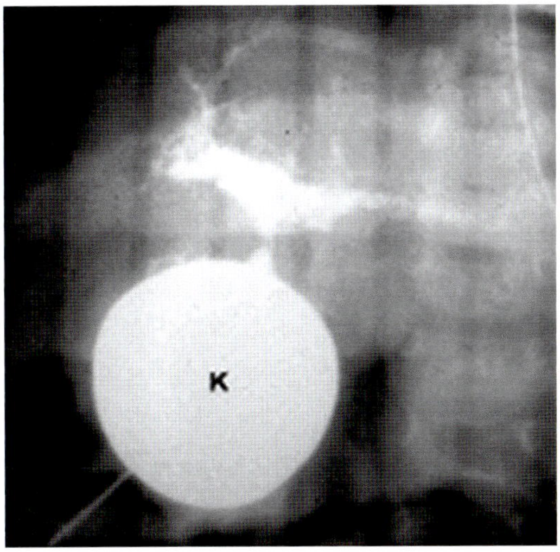

Fig. 26.2 Cholangiogram of a cystic BA showing that the cyst (K) communicates with the intrahepatic bile ducts, although these latest have a cloudy appearance. This is rather the feature of BA than choledochal malformation

Table 26.1 Recognized anomalies in the biliary atresia splenic malformation syndrome

Abnormality	Frequency (%)
Polysplenia/double spleen	98–95
Situs inversus	50
Preduodenal portal vein	45
Malrotation	30
Cardiac anomalies	25
Absent IVC	50–70
Annular pancreas	10
Asplenia	2–5
Immotile cilia syndrome	1

feed normally though their weight gain is subnormal due to their inability to digest fat and soluble vitamins. The liver is usually enlarged and firm in older infants (e.g., more than 10 weeks), and there may be ascites and or splenomegaly indicating the onset of portal hypertension along with cirrhosis.

Diagnosis Work-Up

The diagnosis of BA is an operative diagnosis, but is accurate when performed preoperatively in more than 90 % of cases. In our institution, this is achieved by exclusion of various medical causes of conjugated jaundice (Fig. 26.3). Ultrasonography is equivocal of BA if it excludes intrahepatic bile duct dilatation (found in choledochal malformation) and the absence, irregular, or very small gallbladder after a 4 hours long fasting, and the specific triangular cord sign (which corresponds to the fibrotic remnant at the hilum) is found in about 80 % of cases [38] (Fig. 26.4). In our center, ERCP is indicated if there is any doubt regarding the color of stools or the presence of a gallbladder without the triangular cord sign on US. ERCP showing stained bile at the papilla or intrahepatic bile ducts excludes BA [39].

26.3.2.6 Surgery: The Kasai Operation

The first step is to formerly establish the operative diagnosis of BA, by either the mean of a limited incision or by laparoscopy. The gallbladder patency is checked to see whether it is atretic or normal. If normal the cholangiogram is performed and the steps are detailed in Fig. 26.5. Once the diagnosis of BA is confirmed (no opacification of the intrahepatic bile ducts), the scar is enlarged, the liver is exteriorized through the wound avoiding transection of the triangular ligaments, and the dissection is performed but only above the level of the portal and arterial bifurcation in order not to compromise both the arterial vascularization of the liver and a further transplantation. The remnant is excised leaving the liver capsule intact (Fig. 26.5). The third step is the reconstruction: mainly by a Roux-en-Y loop (Kasai portoenterostomy) performed at the level of the second jejunal limb, in an antegrade fashion, and should be long enough (45 cm), both to prevent ascending cholangitis especially when the child is transplanted, as the extremity is chopped out (Fig. 26.5). Elements of the splenic malformation syndrome are checked for, and a Meckel's diverticulum should be resected during the surgery, anti-adhesive barriers could be used to facilitate a hypothetic liver transplantation. In case of a patent gallbladder and main bile duct, we would rather perform the less common Kasai portocholecystostomy (Fig. 26.5).

Referring the patient to a primary transplantation should probably only be considered when clinical imaging and biologic features of cirrhosis and portal hypertension are present (e.g., obvious ascites, widening of the small omentum, high figures of elastometry, parenchymal heterogeneity) especially when associated with signs of liver failure (raised INR and low albumin).

The role of the laparoscopy for BA is still controversial. Although laparoscopy for the diagnosis steps is not challenged, many high-volume centers, including those which have tried this technique, do not advocate using laparoscopy for the Kasai since the results have been proven to be worse compared to the open approach [40, 41]. However worldwide, in Japan and Brazil, some centers still use it with fair results, not comparative, though, and difficult to recommend for this rare disease, with a likely long learning curve [42].

26.3.2.7 Postoperative Complications

Ascending Bacterial Cholangitis

Cholangitis occurs most commonly in the days following primary surgery but can be delayed. It is recorded in about 40–50 % of cases in most

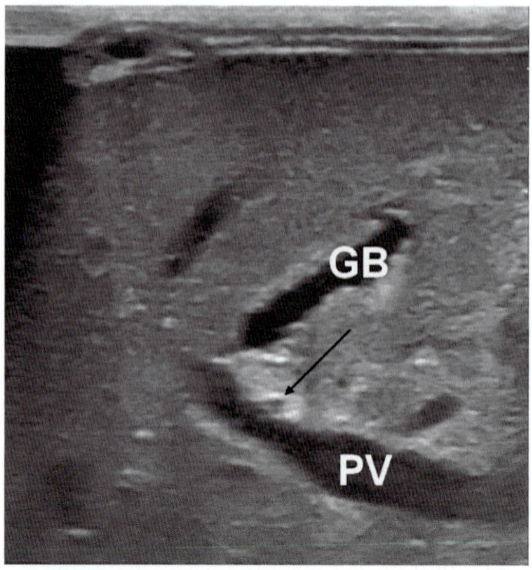

Fig. 26.4 Sagittal view of a hepatic ultrasonography, the triangular cord sign (*white arrow*) is located above the portal vein; this sign corresponds to the biliary fibrous remnant

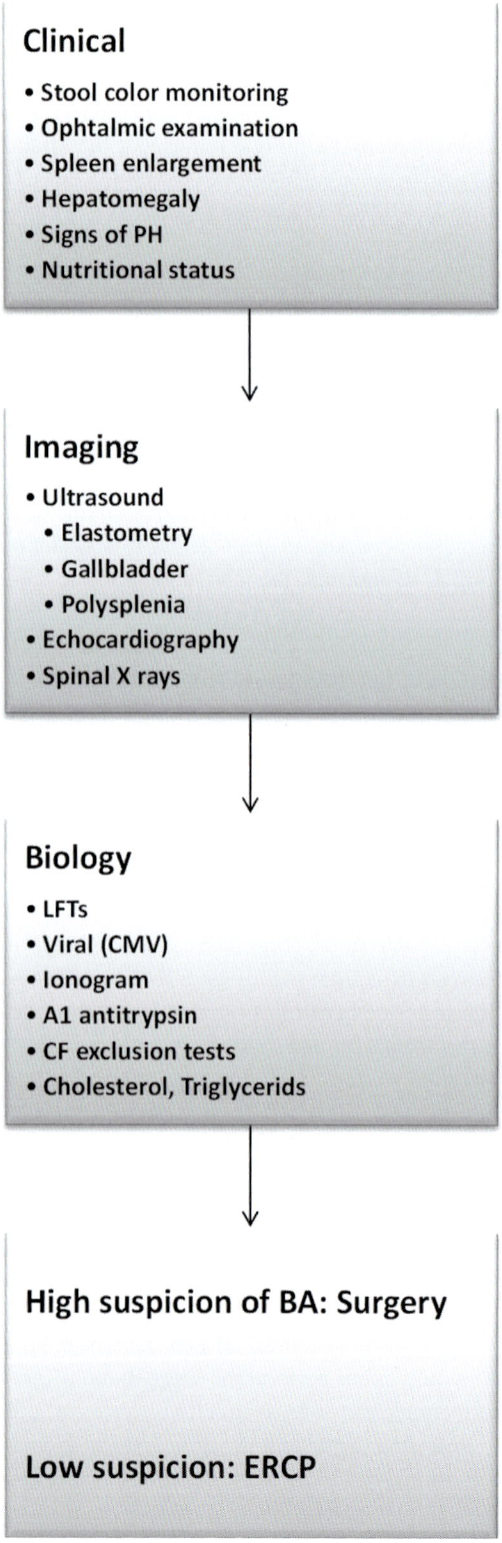

Fig. 26.3 Algorithm to achieve an accurate diagnosis of BA in our center. *Abbreviations*: *PH* portal hypertension, *LFT* liver function tests, *CMV Cytomegalovirus*, *CF* cystic fibrosis, *ERCP* endoscopic retrograde cholangiopancreatography

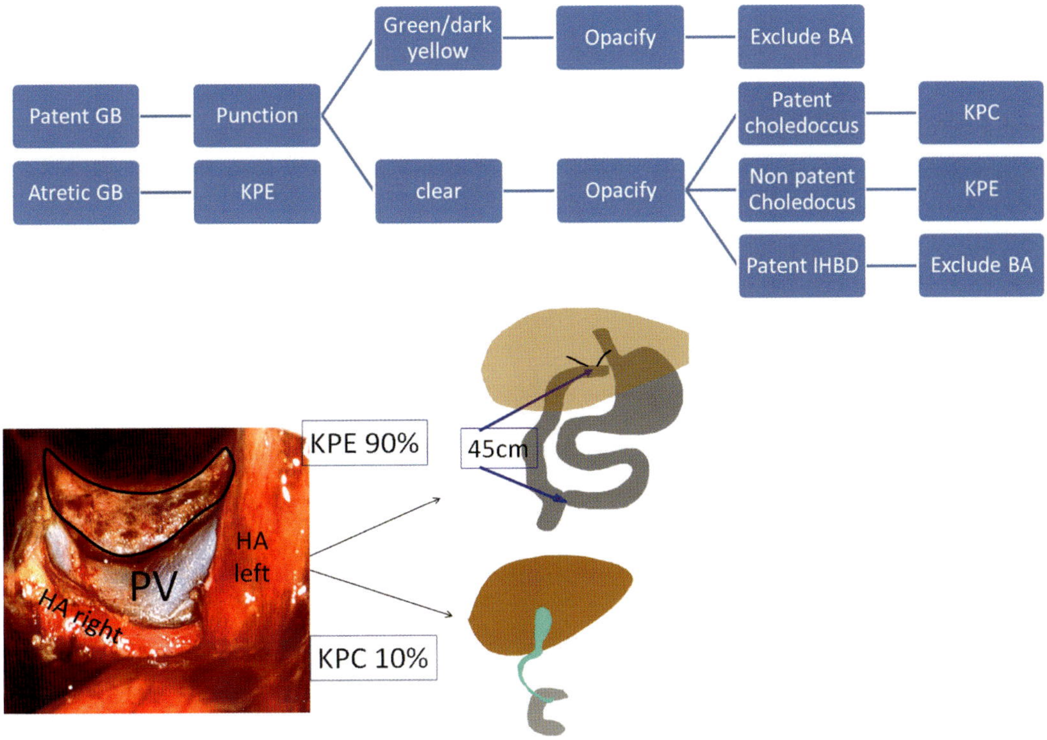

Fig. 26.5 Operative algorithm for biliary atresia. *GB* gallbladder, *KPE* Kasai portoenterostomy, *KPC* Kasai portocholecystostomy, *BA* biliary atresia, *HBD* intrahepatic bile ducts, *HA* hepatic artery, *PV* portal vein

series and almost always occurs in children with at least some degree of bile flow, not those with early failure. Clinically, it is characterized by worsening jaundice, fever, and acholic stools. The diagnosis may be confirmed by blood culture, but it is important to treat suspected cases early with broad-spectrum antibiotics effective against gram-negative organisms.

Bowel obstruction: It is difficult to diagnose as these infants do not have stained vomiting postoperatively. Pain, uncomfort, clear or bilious vomits, as well as high temperature (obstruction after the Roux-en-Y limb) should raise the diagnosis. Adherence-related bowel obstruction has become rare since the use of anti-adhesive barriers in our center; however, postoperative ileo-ileal intussusception is a rare cause of mechanic bowel obstruction and compromises both the bile flow and the Roux-en-Y sutures. Peritonitis by anastomotic leak at the bottom limb of the Roux-en-Y is very rare, but the diagnosis and the adequate treatment are delayed as it is confused with an ascending cholangitis.

Inguinal hernia, usually occurring in about 10 % of these infants, should be checked before discharge and repaired especially if the child has a successful Kasai [43].

Biliary leakage does not occur after Kasai portoenterostomy, but in Kasai portocholecystomy. This technique is given up by most of the teams, even though the risk of leakage should be balanced with the risk of cholangitis.

26.3.2.8 Results of the Kasai Operation

The earliest measurable outcome is clearance of jaundice to normal bilirubin values within 6 months in large; typically multicenter series have varied from 27 to 57 %, translation into a 5- (or 4)-year native liver survival of 37–52 % for the most recent cohorts [30, 44–46]. Uncorrected biliary occlusion causes progressive intrahepatic disease, and the longer this is allowed to persist, the more irreversible it becomes, explaining why age at surgery (especially before 6–8 weeks of age), although without obvious cutoff, has become the main prognosis factor. Series from France, *the USA*, and the UK suggest that about 30–45 % of the children may survive to reach 10 years of age with their native liver intact [33, 45, 46].

26.3.2.9 Indication for Liver Transplantation

Biliary atresia is still the commonest indication for liver transplantation during childhood and is indicated in case of:

Failure of Kasai (persistence or recurrence of jaundice) with any of the following:

Failure to thrive, liver failure which can be precipitated by infection, portal hypertension with uncontrolled esophageal varices, portopulmonary syndrome, onset of pulmonary hypertension, and recurrent cholangitis

In patients who have a sustainable successful Kasai, portal hypertension may benefit from either surgical or transjugular intrahepatic portosystemic shunts. Recurrent ascending cholangitis can be treated by the revision of Roux-en-Y which may be too short or having a mechanic chronic obstruction (role of a HIDA scan) [47].

The 5- and 10-year actuarial survival rates of patients that underwent liver transplantation for biliary atresia in France and the USA are 82–87 % and 82–86 %, and the 5- and 10-year graft actuarial survival rates are 73–76 % and 71–72 %, respectively [48, 49].

26.3.3 Hepatic Trauma

The spleen and the liver are the most frequent solid organs involved in traumatology. Their damage is present in 5 % of pediatric blunt abdominal trauma with 52 % hepatic injury and 43 % splenic injury, and in 5 % both organs are injured [50]. The most frequent mechanism is motorized vehicle accident, the child being either a pedestrian hit by car or a car passenger. Penetrating trauma is rare. Apparent benign blunt abdominal trauma occurring in a backyard or during sport activities can also lead to liver injury.

26.3.3.1 Assessment

As for all patients presenting with abdominal trauma, ABC should be performed at the arrival in the trauma room [51]. Two intravenous accesses is the rule. At the end of this first assessment, you should be able to know what exam to perform, either a FAST evaluation or a total body CT scan. Based on 136 papers accepted among 900 on pediatric abdominal trauma, Sang-Woo Pak speculated in 2013 that if the clinical exam shows abdominal wall or lower chest bruising, abdominal pain or tenderness, and/or low blood pressure without shock, a FAST scan and a blood work should be performed searching for liver enzyme increase. In case of anomalies, a CT scan can be discussed. If not, the patient can be admitted to the ward for monitoring [52].

26.3.3.2 Treatment

The liver has a tremendous capacity of healing, and the success rate has been reported to be between 82 and 100 % [53]. The treatment is mainly guided by the patient's hemodynamic status more than by the liver injury scale [54]. The initial management should follow the Advanced Trauma Life Support (ATLS) principles of aggressive fluid resuscitation, guided by monitoring of central venous pressure and urinary output [51]. Actually, the only indication of surgery is the need for blood transfusion above 40 ml/kg (half body mass index). Nonoperative management involves admission to a unit and the monitoring of vital signs, with strict bed rest, frequent monitoring of hemoglobin concentration, and repeated abdominal examinations [55]. In case of failure, angio-embolization can be an interesting option. A perfect collaboration between the anesthesiologist, the interventional radiologist, and the surgeon is therefore crucial. Angio-embolization can be necessary either in a high-grade liver injury (grade IV and V) associated to unstable hemodynamic or after a first surgical procedure such as a packing when the patient remains unstable [56]. Success has been reported to be between 68 and 87 % [56]. Complications can be related to the nonoperative management (liver hematoma, false aneurysm, biloma, or biliary ascites) or to angioembolization (hepatic necrosis, liver abscess). Incidence increases accordingly with the grade of injury. In a series of 337 patients with liver injury grades III–V treated nonoperatively, those with grade III had a complication rate of 1 %, grade IV 21 %, and grade V 63 % [57]. Patients with grades IV and V injuries are more likely to require surgery and to develop complications of nonoperative treatment.

If the patient requires surgery because of instability, laparoscopic approach has no place. Through a midline incision, after a complete exploration of the abdominal cavity, the surgeon should be able to see the liver fracture and starts by packing with surgical dress. Indeed, severe coagulopathy, acidosis, and hypothermia can occur in case of important hemorrhage and make the resuscitation challenging to save the patient. Initial control of hemorrhage and contamination followed by packing and temporary abdominal closure, ICU restoration of normal physiology, and delayed definitive repair is also well known as “the damage control” technic. The group at the University of Pennsylvania has popularized this technic in 1993 [58]. If the patient remains unstable, an attempt to see where the bleeding comes from should be done carefully, especially in case of hepatic vein rupture. Indeed, if the surgeon tries to bring down the liver with his hand, the risk of aggravating the hepatic vein lesion is major. The next step would be the Pringle maneuver, which consists in clamping the whole hepatic pedicle. This maneuver is controversial, but it can be maintained up to 1 h without compromising the blood supply to the liver. Despite this, if the patient continues to be unstable, the next step is to clamp the inferior vena cava. After this, surgeon should consider performing a hepatic resection in case of continuous bleeding or repair a hepatic vein or vena cava injury.

The treatment of a bile leakage is most of the time a conservative treatment. A simple drainage of the ascites or a cholecystostomy can be done if the leak is heavy with a considerable amount of ascites. Stenting the bile duct through radiologist intervention is another interesting and valid option [59].

26.3.3.3 Posttrauma Care

For isolated liver injury, a guideline with the number of hospitalization days has been published depending on the grade of the injury from 2 to 5 days for grade I to grade IV [60]. An even shorter hospital stay has been also reported with a discharge at day 1 or 2 after the trauma [61, 63]. Considering the risk of secondary bleeding, it could be safer to keep the patient to the hospital longer especially in case of high-grade liver injury.

26.3.4 Hepatoblastoma

26.3.4.1 Epidemiology

Hepatoblastoma (HBL) is the most common malignant hepatic tumor in children typically seen in the first 3 years of life. Incidence is about 1.2–1.5 cases per million [62]. Those that occur after 5 years of age, formerly called transitional hepatocellular carcinoma (HCC), tend to have a worse prognosis, probably because their behavior is similar to a HCC [63]. Most HBLs do not have an abnormal genetic background, but predisposing factors include trisomy 18, Beckwith-Wiedemann syndrome, familial adenomatous polyposis, and prematurity [64].

26.3.4.2 Clinical Presentation

The most common presentation is an isolated abdominal mass. As some HBL found to have an HCG excretion, mild signs of virilization should be looked for. They rarely present signs of rupture, i.e., acute abdominal pain with guarding or contracture.

Investigations

α-fetoprotein (α-FP) is the key marker in HBL and its level has a prognostic value. An abnormal level of α-FP (below 100 IU/l or higher than 1 million IU/l) predicts a poor outcome whether it correlates with tumor pathology or not. α-FP is excreted by the fetal liver and is increased at birth but should decrease to a normal level (i.e., 5 IU/l or ng/ml) after 1 year of age. In infants

Table 26.2 Elevation of α-fetoprotein (α-FP)

Physiological	Newborn until 1 year Liver regeneration Pregnancy
Nonneoplastic conditions	*Congenital persistence of AFP* Acute/chronic hepatitis Hemochromatosis Tyrosinemia Ataxia-telangiectasia Cirrhosis
Neoplasia	
Benign	Mesenchymal hamartoma Hemangioendothelioma
Malign	Hepatoblastoma Hepatocellular carcinoma Mixed fibrolamellar carcinoma Yolk sac tumors Pancreatoblastoma Acinar cell carcinoma of the pancreas

with a malignant liver tumor and a normal AFP, the diagnosis of a rhabdoid tumor of the liver should be evoked. α-FP may be increased in various other malignant or benign conditions (Table 26.2).

Human chorionic gonadotropin (HCG) hormone is a marker, which might be raised in some HBL, although its prognosis value has not yet been determined.

Liver ultrasound with Doppler is used to assess the intrahepatic extent of the tumor and patency of the portal and hepatic veins.

Thoracoabdominal CT scan (with arterial and mixed portal and venous phases) is used to assess the input and output blood vessels of the liver and is sent for review in national referral centers in the SIOPEL or COG studies to set up the *pretreatment extent (PRETEXT)* of disease [64]. The PRETEXT is used for locoregional involvement only. The PRETEXT relies on the Brisbane classification with sections (right posterior, right anterior, left anterior, and left lobe) outlined by the right, median hepatic veins and the umbilical fossa (Fig. 26.6). The PRETEXT formula is for numbers of adjacent tumor-free sections. Pulmonary lesions documented on the chest CT scan are considered as unequivocally metastatic if there is one nodule > 10 mm or several nodules with at least one > 5 mm. In the other cases, the metastases will be considered as doubtful, and a surgical biopsy of one of the nodules should be discussed. Patient with a PRETEXT equal or superior to III or/and with either P2 or V3 should be, before chemotherapy, referred for a possible liver transplant, which may happen promptly according to the extent of disease, after neoadjuvant chemotherapy.

Pretreatment biopsies are strongly recommended in European protocols and may exclude other differential diagnoses such as liver metastases of a yolk sac tumor, benign liver tumors, and HCC in older children. Biopsies are carried out with a minimum of 5 and preferably 10 cores and should also include a biopsy of the adjacent non-tumoral liver whenever possible.

Different pathologic subtypes consist of epithelial, fetal, or mixed fetal and epithelial hepatoblastoma. Small cell undifferentiated carcinoma (SCUD) is a special subtype with a worse prognosis [65]. Transitional hepatoblastoma/carcinoma is defined by the age rather than by the pathology [66]. Children are then classified into three risk groups according to outcomes identified in previous SIOPEL studies. This is based on clinical data, tumor biology, imaging, and pathology (Table 26.3).

26.3.4.3 Chemotherapy: The European Experience

The chemotherapy of hepatoblastoma is based on *platin family* and *anthracyclines*. Neoadjuvant chemotherapy has been administered to all patients in SIOPEL protocols as compared to the North American protocol, although this may change in the future. The type and frequency of drug administration are reported in Fig. 26.7, as well as the timing of surgery.

26.3.4.4 Surgery

Careful preoperative assessment is mandatory before surgery. Patients should be referred to a radiologist and a surgeon with expertise in liver resection and imaging. Early referral after diagnosis improves surgery planning. After the chemotherapy, preoperative assessment includes CT scan and post-neoadjuvant chemotherapy (POSTEXT) evaluation coupled with operative or preoperative Doppler ultrasound to carefully identify the limits of the tumor with the main

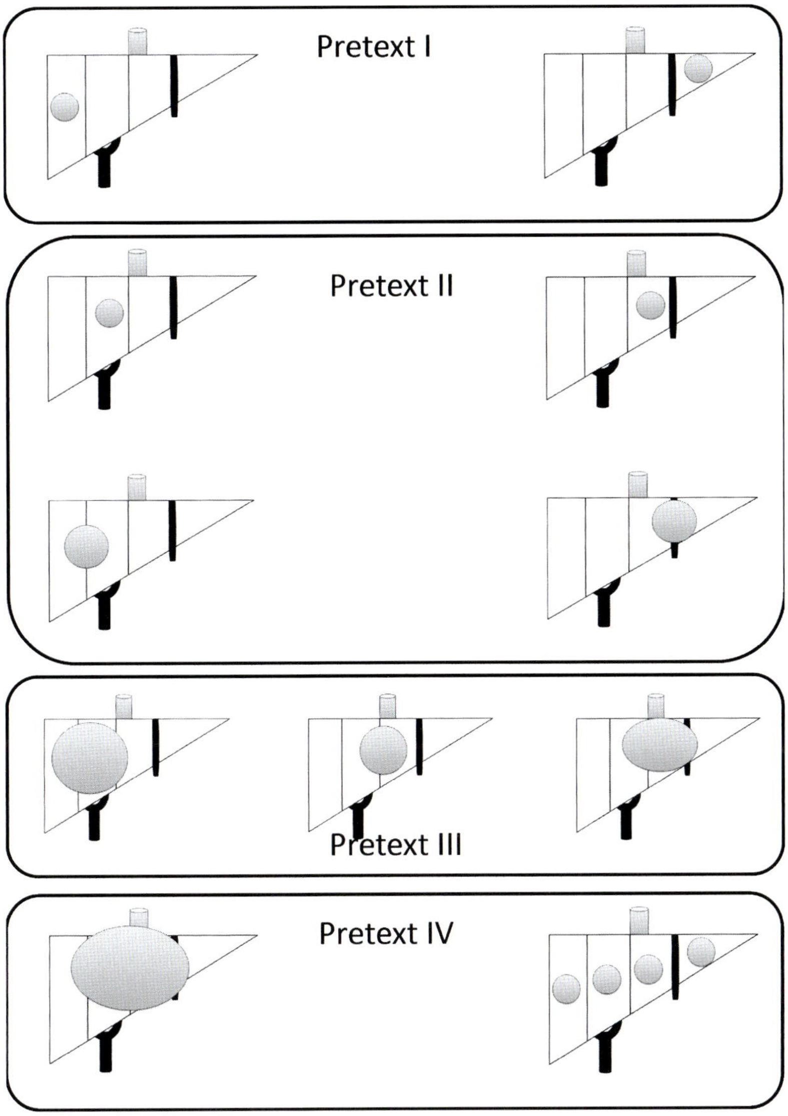

Fig 26.6 The PRETEXT classification in the liver

hepatic vessels. α-FP decrease should be monitored and documented. Echocardiography is mandatory in order to assess both anthracycline-related toxicity and the tolerance to a potential hepatic vascular exclusion. For these large tumors with a poor prognosis in case of local relapse, both minimally invasive surgery and wedged surgical excision are not recommended. Transverse or subcostal laparotomy is performed. The abdominal cavity is inspected. The hepatic pedicle is encircled by a tape in prevision of a Pringle maneuver, triangular ligaments are sectioned, and total vascular exclusion of the liver is prepared. Anatomic resection of the liver is performed via vascular ligature of the inflow to the involved part of the liver. Transection is done with the help of either thermic or ultrasound sealing devices. The aim is complete microscopic resection of the tumor with minimum blood loss and avoiding air embolism via the main hepatic veins. This is why, in our experience, we perform a brief total vascular exclusion of the liver (i.e., less than 30 min)

Table 26.3 Risk stratification in current SIOPEL studies

Risk group	Criteria	Recommended protocol	Expected CR, EFS, OS
Standard risk	*PRETEXT I–III* M0 P and V in involved sectors, E0, N0 100<AFP No SCUD	*SIOPEL 6*	3y CR=99 % 3y EFS=83 % 3y OS=95 % [66]
High risk	None of criteria of standard and very high risk groups or *PRETEXT IV* M0 or P2 or V3 or E+	*SIOPEL 3 HR*	3y CR=89 % 3y EFS=75 % 3y OS=86 % [67]
Very high risk	Metastatic or AFP<100 IU/L (apart from very small tumors)	*SIOPEL 4 HR*	3y CR=70 % 3y EFS=77 % 3y OS=79 % [68] Supportive care

when the tumor borders are in the vicinity of the hepatic veins. Morbidity of this procedure is low given that the remaining liver parenchyma is healthy.

26.3.4.5 Liver Transplantation

In current protocols LT is recommended for PRETEXT IV or sometimes PRETEXT III patients with uncertainty on surgical margins prior to liver resection, providing that the children are cleared of their lung metastases either by chemotherapy or surgery. Liver transplantation is not currently considered as a treatment of local relapses [67].

26.3.4.6 Relapses

Treatment strategy for recurrent HBL has not been standardized, but either local or distant (the lungs, peritoneal, and brain) relapses can be managed with platin, doxorubicin, irinotecan, and high doses of cyclophosphamide. Surgical removal or radiofrequency ablation (RFA) of detectable tumor foci is recommended whenever feasible either at diagnosis of relapse or following chemotherapy for patients with non-resectable disease. A recent paper from the SIOPEL group, compiling SIOPEL 1–3 studies, showed that relapse was local in 36 %, metastatic in 55 %, and combined in 9 % of children. Fifty-two percent of children achieved a second complete remission, 58 % of them were alive after a median of 84 (range 3–175) months, and 32 % were alive in complete remission after a second relapse, which proves that treatment of relapse combining surgery, RFA, and chemotherapy is efficient [68, 70, 71].

26.4 Pancreatic Pathology

26.4.1 Solid Pseudopapillary Pancreatic Tumor (Frantz Tumor)

26.4.1.1 Introduction

Solid pseudopapillary tumor (SPPT) of the pancreas is a rare tumor representing 1–2 % of all pancreatic tumors. Its incidence in infant has been reported between 8 and 16 % [69]. The tumor is predominant in Asian and African American women [72, 73]. Usually it is described as a low-grade malignant potential, but in older men it appears more aggressive [74]. In 2003, a review of the pediatric literature reported 92 cases in children with an average age of 10.5 years (range 8–16 years) and a male/female ratio of 1:4 [75].

26.4.1.2 Clinical Presentation

Clinic is poor and patients are asymptomatic most of the time. Sometimes, a mass is palpable and is the main purpose for visiting a physician. Rarely, the tumor is painful and can mimic an acute abdomen related probably to an internal tumor bleeding [76]. Thus, diagnosis is often delayed, which explains the predominance of huge tumors, mostly in the upper part of the abdomen.

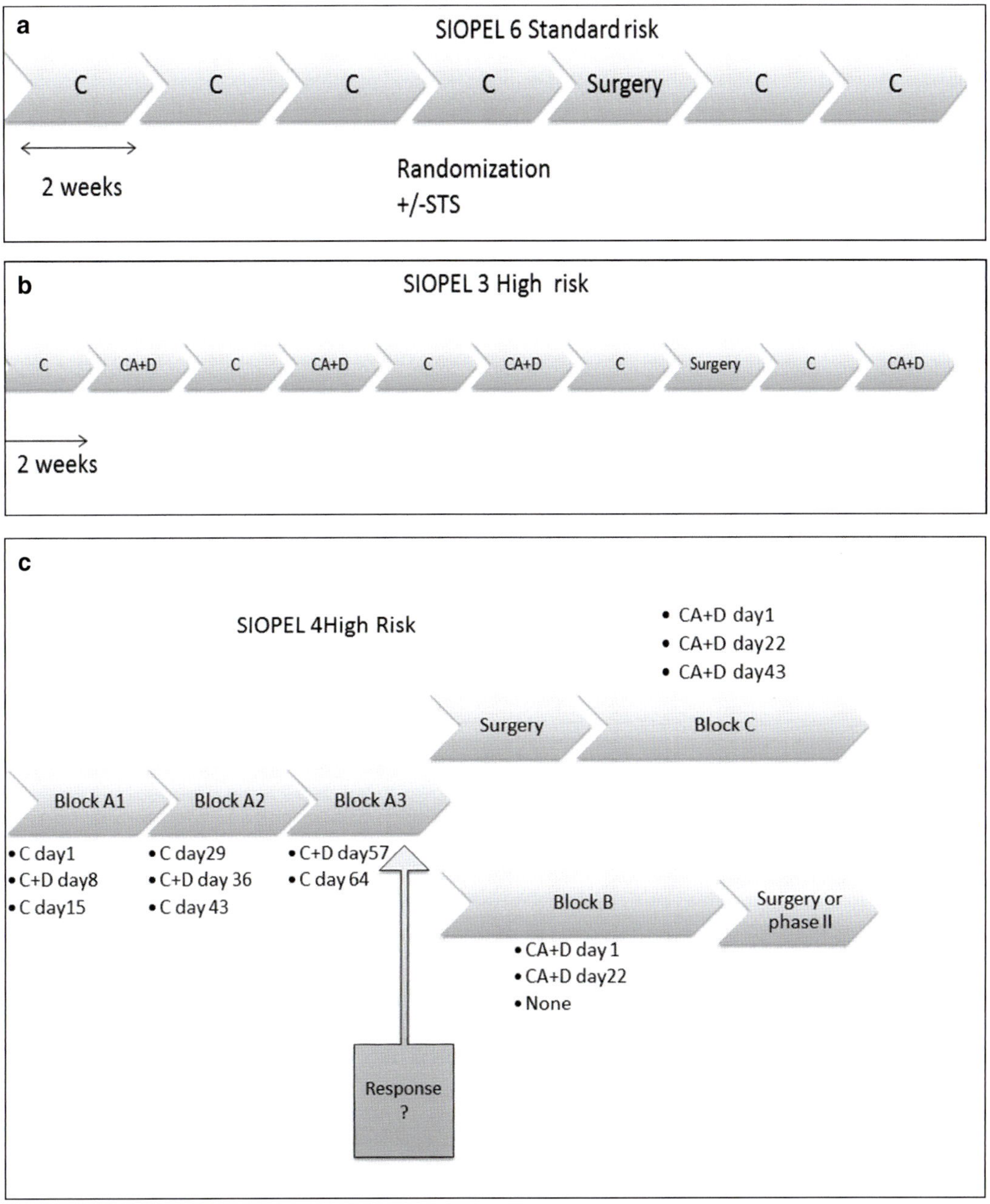

Fig. 26.7 Current SIOPEL protocols: SIOPEL 6 protocol for standard risk: CDDP, cisplatin; STS, sodium thiosulfate (ear protection). SuperPlado protocol in SIOPEL 3: C=cisplatin, D=doxorubicin, CA=carboplatin, 1 arrow=2 weeks. High-risk protocol in SIOPEL 4: C=cisplatin, D=doxorubicin, CA=carboplatin

26.4.1.3 Diagnosis

Usually, an ultrasound sonography and a CT scan make the diagnosis, showing an association of solid and cystic component. It is crucial to determine preoperatively if the tumor is malignant or benign. Yin has compared CT scan and MRI's efficiency in determining this [77]. In this paper, firstly, malignancy was more frequent in a group of patients aged from 11 to 19 years old, followed by a group aged from 50 to 65 years old. Secondly, the authors found that when the tumor was located in the tail and the size was equal or larger than

6.0 cm, the positive and negative predictive value, sensitivity, and specificity for a malignant SPN were 61.5 %, 100 %, 100 %, and 78.6 %, respectively. Complete encapsulation was more frequent in benign tumors. Amorphous or scattered calcifications, all near-solid tumors, and the presence of upstream pancreatic ductal dilatation were associated with benignity. A well-marginated, large, encapsulated, solid, and cystic mass with areas of hemorrhagic degeneration, as revealed by high-signal intensity on T1-weighted imaging, should be considered as a benign tumor [78].

26.4.1.4 Pathology and Immunohistochemistry

Immunohistochemistry is recommended in order to establish the diagnosis. Antivementine antibodies are positive in 90 % of the cases [79]. Anti-*neuron-specific enolase* (NSE) and anti-alpha1-antitrypsine antibodies are positive in around 50 % of the cases [80]. Interestingly, hormonal receptor antibodies for progesterone and estrogenic hormone are positive in some tumors, raising the highly suspicious hypothesis of hormono-dependency and even more when it occurs on young female.

26.4.1.5 Treatment

The only treatment is surgical. Radical resection with negative margins should be performed. Thus a pancreatectomy should be done if the tumor is either in the tail, the body, or the head [81]. Although the splenectomy associated with the resection has been already published, everything should be done to preserve it, keeping in mind that the margins should be negative. Pancreatic tissue sparing is the rule to limit the potential postoperative endocrine and exocrine insufficiency.

Sometimes, because this tumor is surrounded by a dense fibrous capsule, an enucleation has been purposed as a possible surgical option [82], but appropriate surgical treatment is still controversial in children.

The laparoscopic approach seems to be feasible and reported in 2003 by Carricaburu et al. [83] but quickly abandoned because of peritoneal metastasis recurrence several months after [84]. Recurrences after laparoscopic management may have been due to diffusion of tumor cells caused by gas insufflation especially during the biopsy.

Since this, Namgoong JM has published a large series of laparoscopic resection of SPPT in 2014 [85]. Fourteen patients were operated on for a SPPT with distal pancreatectomy and spleen-sparing surgery for 70 % of the cases. Indeed, laparoscopic distal pancreatectomy seems to be a good alternative over the open approach [86]. The median tumor size on pathology was 4.4 (range 2.0–8.4) cm in the LDP group and 10.0 (range 1.8–15.0) cm in the ODP group ($p = 0.060$) meaning that this approach should be reserved to a tumor size under approximately 10 cm, assuming that larger tumor is more likely to present malignancy. In this series, there was only one case of recurrence at 82 months after surgery. This was a localized recurrence without peritoneal dispersion. In conclusion, a biopsy should not be done during a laparoscopic approach in case of SPPT, but complete resection should be attempted instead.

26.4.2 Pancreatic Traumatism

26.4.2.1 Background

Pediatric pancreatic injury is quite rare in children and can be associated with surrounding organ injuries such as the duodenum, spleen, and liver. In adults, it can be potentially dangerous due to the location of the pancreas near the aorta, the superior mesenteric artery, and the vena cava. Diagnosis can be challenging due to his position as a retroperitoneal organ and eventually associated lesions on other organs. For this reason, lipasemia is often requested in the blood work for abdominal blunt trauma. In Europe, penetrating trauma is even more rare, and the pancreas injury is easier to diagnose since most of these patients would undergo a laparotomy. Blunt pancreatic trauma is the most common type of trauma mechanism in children, and it is typically seen after crashes involving a bicycle handlebar and road traffic crashes.

The main question is if a patient with pancreatic injury should have a laparotomy and what could be the optimal management between conservative treatment and surgery. In case of surgery, different techniques can be discussed: resection, drainage, or, ideally, repair. None of these procedures have shown a real advantage over another.

26.4.2.2 Diagnosis and Classification

According to the pancreas injury scaling [87], 5 grades have been described from the stage 1 with a hematoma or contusion to the complete head avulsion in the stage 5. A complete distal section is graded as stage 3. Diagnosis is correctly made with a CT scan showing edema, disruption, or even ascites, which can be very extensive in case of unknown injury. Endoscopic retrograde cholangiopancreatography (ERCP) has been evaluated in a retrospective study to assess the pancreatic duct injury. ERCP is helpful when pancreatic duct injury is suspected, in order to exclude ductal leakage, localize it, and eventually treat it. It can accelerate diagnosis of higher grade of pancreatic injuries if the CT scanning is not accurate [88]. ERCP can also safely provide definitive treatment for some patients, which could be an argument for a more frequent indication of ERCP [89].

26.4.2.3 Management

The only remaining question is if the treatment at the acute phase should be conservative and nonoperative or surgical. Up to now, there has not been any randomized control trial published in literature to answer this question [90]. The rate of pancreatic trauma complications, such as pancreatic pseudocyst formation, pancreatitis, and pancreatic fistula formation, is reported as being between 19 % and 55 % [91].

The treatment is clear and should be conservative for the low-grade injuries (grade 1 and 2). It may involve a parenteral nutrition, painkillers, and bed rest for a short or longer time in case of associated lesions and organ injuries. Attitude remains unclear in grade 3 and 4 injuries. There might be a trend toward nonoperative treatment of blunt severe pediatric pancreatic lesions [92]. In this series, de Blaauw et al. reported only 10 % of the patients treated conservatively requiring secondary surgery. Pseudocysts develop in 50 %, and half of these are managed nonoperatively. Mean duration of hospital stay was 29 days in the operative group and 24 days in the nonoperative group.

If surgery is indicated, distal pancreatectomy with attempt at preserving the spleen, drainage, ideal repair of the pancreatic duct, and rarely, duodenopancreatectomy or Roux-en-Y loop and anastomosis have all been published. This shows how the choice of procedure is highly dependent of the surgeon, the team habit, and the type of the lesions. Even in case of complete pancreatic transaction, the conservative management is effective with 44 % patients developing pseudocyst and requiring drainage [91]. Median hospital stay was 24 days with a maximum of 60 days. The authors made the hypothesis that anatomically the distal body and tail usually atrophies; however, occasionally, the gland can heal and appear to recanalize.

Laparoscopy in this indication is feasible. It has been reported for a simple drainage of a pseudocyst [93] or for a distal pancreatectomy [94]. Most of the papers published are case reports. Rutkoski JD et al. reported three cases. In this indication, hospital stay was short, less than 15 days, without complications. Laparoscopy could be ideally indicated in patients with isolated pancreatic injury, grades 3 and 4, and hemodynamically stable. Surgery should be performed in the first days after trauma in order to have minor adhesions.

References

Biliary Stone

1. Debray D, Franchi-Abella S, Irtan S, Girard M (2012) Cholelithiasis in infants, children and adolescents. Presse Med 41:466–473
2. Troyano-Luque J, Padilla-Pérez A, Martínez-Wallin I, Alvarez de la Rosa M, Mastrolia SA, Trujillo JL, Pérez-Medina T (2014) Short and long term outcomes associated with fetal cholelithiasis: a report of two cases with antenatal diagnosis and postnatal follow-up. Case Rep Obstet Gynecol 71:42–71
3. Murata S, Aomatsu T, Yoden A, Tamai H (2015) Fasting and bed rest, even for a relatively short period, are risk factors for ceftriaxone-associated pseudolithiasis. Pediatr Int 57:942–946
4. Langballe KO, Bardram L (2014) Cholecystectomy in Danish children – a nationwide study. J Pediatr Surg 49:626–630

5. Heida A, Koot BG, vd Baan-Slootweg OH, Pels Rijcken TH, Seidell JC, Makkes S, Jansen PL, Benninga MA (2014) Gallstone disease in severely obese children participating in a lifestyle intervention program: incidence and risk factors. Int J Obes (Lond) 38:950–953
6. Triunfo S, Rosati P, Ferrara P, Gatto A, Scambia G (2013) Fetal cholelithiasis: a diagnostic update and a literature review. Clin Med Insights Case Rep 15: 153–158
7. Adams LB, Chang C, Pope J, Kim Y, Liu P, Yates A (2015) Randomized, prospective comparison of ursodeoxycholic acid for the prevention of gallstones after sleeve gastrectomy. Obes Surg. doi:10.1007/s11695-015-1858-5
8. Ostlie DJ, Juang OO, Iqbal CW, Sharp SW, Snyder CL, Andrews WS, Sharp RJ, Holcomb GW 3rd, St Peter SD (2013) Single incision versus standard 4-port laparoscopic cholecystectomy: a prospective randomized trial. J Pediatr Surg 48:209–214
9. Chandler NM, Danielson PD (2011) Single -incision laparoscopic cholecystectomy in children: a retrospective comparison with traditional laparoscopic cholecystectomy. J Pediatr Surg 46:1695–1699
10. Jones VS (2015) Robotic-assisted single-site cholecystectomy in children. J Pediatr Surg 50:1842–1845
11. Dalton BG, Gonzalez KW, Knott EM, St Peter SD, Aguayo P (2015) Same day discharge after laparoscopic cholecystectomy in children. J Surg Res 195:418–421
12. Gurusamy KS, Davidson C, Gluud C, Davidson BR (2013) Early versus delayed laparoscopic cholecystectomy for people with acute cholecystitis. Cochrane Database Syst Rev. (6):CD005440
13. Cao AM, Eslick GD, Cox MR (2015) Early laparoscopic cholecystectomy is superior to delayed acute cholecystitis: a meta-analysis of case–control studies. Surg Endosc. doi:10.1007/s00464-015-4325-4
14. Avrutis O, Friedman SJ, Meshoulm J, Haskel L, Adler S (2000) Safety and success of early laparoscopic cholecystectomy for acute cholecystitis. Surg Laparosc Endosc Percutan Tech 10:200–207
15. Zeidan MM, Pandian TK, Ibrahim KA, Moir CR, Ishitani MB, Zarroug AE (2014) Laparoscopic cholecystectomy in the pediatric population: a single-center experience. Surg Laparosc Endosc Percutan Tech 24:248–250
16. Paris C, Bejjani J, Beaunoyer M, Ouimet A (2010) Endoscopic retrograde cholangiopancreatography is useful and safe in children. J Pediatr Surg 45:938–942
17. Rocca R, Castellino F, Daperno M, Masoero G, Sostegni R, Ercole E, Lavagna A, Barbera C, Canavese F, Pera A (2005) Therapeutic ERCP in paediatric patients. Dig Liver Dis 37:357–362
18. Varadarajulu S, Wilcox CM, Hawes RH, Cotton PB (2004) Technical outcomes and complications of ERCP in children. Gastrointest Endosc 60:367–371
19. Otto AK, Neal MD, Slivka AN, Kane TD (2011) An appraisal of endoscopic retrograde cholangiopancreatography (ERCP) for pancreaticobiliary disease in children: our institutional experience in 231 cases. Surg Endosc 25:2536–2540
20. Muller CO, Boimond MB, Rega A, Michelet D, El Ghoneimi A, Bonnard A (2015) Safety and efficacy of one-stage total laparoscopic treatment of common bile duct stones in children. Surg Endosc 29: 1831–1836

Choledochal Cyst

21. Todani T, Watanabe Y, Fujii T, Uemura S (1984) Anomalous arrangement of the pancreatobiliary ductal system in patients with a choledochal cyst. Am J Surg 147:672–676
22. Yamashiro Y, Miyano T, Suruga K, Shimomura H, Suda K, Matsumoto M, Nittono H (1984) Experimental study of the pathogenesis of choledochal cyst and pancreatitis, with special reference to the role of bile acids and pancreatic enzymes in the anomalous choledocho-pancreatico ductal junction. J Pediatr Gastroenterol Nutr 3:721–727
23. Kato T, Asakura Y, Kasai M (1974) An attempt to produce choledochal cyst in puppies. J Pediatr Surg 9: 509–513
24. Makin E, Davenport M (2012) Understanding choledochal malformation. Arch Dis Child 97:69–72
25. Liem NT, Pham HD, le Dung A, Son TN, Vu HM (2012) Early and intermediate outcomes of laparoscopic surgery for choledochal cysts with 400 patients. J Laparoendosc Adv Surg Tech A 22:599–603
26. Diao M, Li L, Cheng W (2012) Timing of surgery for prenatally diagnosed asymptomatic choledochal cysts: a prospective randomized study. J Pediatr Surg 47:506–512
27. Gander JW, Cowles RA, Gross ER, Reichstein AR, Chin A, Zitsman JL, Middlesworth W, Rothenberg SS (2010) Laparoscopic excision of choledochal cysts with total intracorporeal reconstruction. J Laparoendosc Adv Surg Tech A 20:877–881
28. Diao M, Li L, Cheng W (2011) Is it necessary to ligate distal common bile duct stumps after excising choledochal cysts? Pediatr Surg Int 27:829–832
29. Ohi R, Yaoita S, Kamiyama T, Ibrahim M, Hayashi Y, Chiba T (1990) Surgical treatment of congenital dilatation of the bile duct with special reference to late complications after total excisional operation. J Pediatr Surg 25:613–617

Biliary Atresia

30. Davenport M (2015) Biliary atresia: clinical aspects. Semin Pediatr Surg 21(3):175–184
31. Lorent K, Gong W, Koo KA, Waisbourd-Zinman O, Karjoo S, Zhao X et al (2015) Identification of a plant

isoflavonoid that causes biliary atresia. Sci Transl Med 7:28ra667
32. Chardot C, Carton M, Spire-Bendelac N, Le Pommelet C, Golmard JL, Auvert B (1999) Epidemiology of biliary atresia in France: a national study 1986–96. J Hepatol 31:1006–1013
33. Livesey E, Cortina Borja M, Sharif K, Alizai N, McClean P, Kelly D et al (2009) Epidemiology of biliary atresia in England and Wales (1999–2006). Arch Dis Child Fetal Neonatal Ed 94:F451–F455
34. Lefkowitch JH (1998) Biliary atresia. Mayo Clin Proc 73:90–95
35. Caponcelli E, Knisely AS, Davenport M (2008) Cystic biliary atresia: an etiologic and prognostic subgroup. J Pediatr Surg 43:1619–1624
36. Davenport M, Caponcelli E, Livesey E, Hadzic N, Howard E (2008) Surgical outcome in biliary atresia: etiology affects the influence of age at surgery. Ann Surg 247:694–698
37. Zani A, Quaglia A, Hadzić N, Zuckerman M, Davenport M (2015) Cytomegalovirus-associated biliary atresia: an aetiological and prognostic subgroup. J Pediatr Surg 50:1739–1745
38. Lee H-J, Lee S-M, Park W-H, Choi S-O (2003) Objective criteria of triangular cord sign in biliary atresia on US scans. Radiology 229:395–400
39. Shanmugam NP, Harrison PM, Devlin J, Peddu P, Knisely AS, Davenport M et al (2009) Selective use of endoscopic retrograde cholangiopancreatography in the diagnosis of biliary atresia in infants younger than 100 days. J Pediatr Gastroenterol Nutr 49:435–441
40. Lishuang M, Zhen C, Guoliang Q, Zhen Z, Chen W, Long L et al (2015) Laparoscopic portoenterostomy versus open portoenterostomy for the treatment of biliary atresia: a systematic review and meta-analysis of comparative studies. Pediatr Surg Int 31:261–269
41. Ure BM, Kuebler JF, Schukfeh N, Engelmann C, Dingemann J, Petersen C (2011) Survival with the native liver after laparoscopic versus conventional kasai portoenterostomy in infants with biliary atresia: a prospective trial. Ann Surg 253:826–830
42. Yamataka A (2013) Laparoscopic Kasai portoenterostomy for biliary atresia. J Hepato-Biliary-Pancreat Sci 20:481–486
43. Zani A, Davenport M (2012) Inguinal hernias associated with biliary atresia. Eur J Pediatr Surg Off J Austrian Assoc Pediatr Surg Al Z Für Kinderchir 22:117–120
44. Davenport M, De Ville de Goyet J, Stringer MD, Mieli-Vergani G, Kelly DA, McClean P et al (2004) Seamless management of biliary atresia in England and Wales (1999–2002). Lancet Lond Engl 363:1354–1357
45. Nio M, Ohi R, Miyano T, Saeki M, Shiraki K, Tanaka K et al (2003) Five- and 10-year survival rates after surgery for biliary atresia: a report from the Japanese Biliary Atresia Registry. J Pediatr Surg 38:997–1000
46. Chardot C, Buet C, Serinet M-O, Golmard J-L, Lachaux A, Roquelaure B et al (2013) Improving outcomes of biliary atresia: French national series 1986–2009. J Hepatol 58:1209–1217
47. Bondoc AJ, Taylor JA, Alonso MH, Nathan JD, Wang Y, Balistreri WF et al (2012) The beneficial impact of revision of Kasai portoenterostomy for biliary atresia: an institutional study. Ann Surg 255:570–576
48. Fouquet V, Alves A, Branchereau S, Grabar S, Debray D, Jacquemin E et al (2005) Long-term outcome of pediatric liver transplantation for biliary atresia: a 10-year follow-up in a single center. Liver Transpl 11:152–160
49. Barshes NR, Lee TC, Balkrishnan R, Karpen SJ, Carter BA, Goss JA (2005) Orthotopic liver transplantation for biliary atresia: The U.S. experience. Liver Transpl 11:1193–1200

Hepatic Trauma

50. Bond SJ, Eichelberger MR, Gotschall CS, Sivit CJ, Randolph JG (1996) Nonoperative management of blunt hepatic and splenic injury in children. Ann Surg 223:286–289
51. Advance For Trauma Life Support (ATLS), student course manual, 7th edition (2004)
52. Sang-Woo Pak (2013) The evaluation of pediatric blunt abdominal trauma. Eastern Association for the Surgery of Trauma
53. Ein SH, Shandling B, Simpson JS, Stephens CA (1978) Nonoperative management of traumatized spleen in children: how and why. J Pediatr Surg 13(2):117–119
54. Moore EE et al (1989) Organ injury scaling: spleen, liver, and kidney. J Trauma 29:1664–1666
55. Pachter HL, Guth AA, Hofstetter SR, Spencer FC (1998) Changing pat- terns in the management of splenic trauma: the impact of nonoperative management. Ann Surg 227:708–717
56. Lin BC, Wong YC, Lim KE, Fang JF, Hsu YP, Kang SC (2010) Management of ongoing arterial haemorrhage after damage control laparotomy: optimal timing and efficacy of transarterial embolisation. Injury 41:44–49
57. Kozar RA, Moore JB, Niles SE et al (2005) Complications of non-operative management of high-grade blunt hepatic injuries. J Trauma 59:1066–1071
58. Asensio JA, Roldan G, Petrone P et al (2003) Operative management and out- comes in 103 AAST-OIS grades IV and V complex hepatic injuries: trauma surgeons still need to operate, but angioembolization helps. J Trauma 54:647–654
59. Almaramhi H, Al-Qahtani AR (2006) Traumatic pediatric bile duct injury: nonoperative intervention as an alternative to surgical intervention. J Pediatr Surg 41:943–945
60. Stylianos S (2000) Evidence-based guidelines for resource utilization in children with isolated spleen or liver injury. The APSA Trauma Committee. J Pediatr Surg 35:164–167; discussion 167–9

61. St Peter SD, Sharp SW, Snyder CL, Sharp RJ, Andrews WS, Murphy JP, Islam S, Holcomb GW 3rd, Ostlie DJ (2011) Prospective validation of an abbreviated bedrest protocol in the management of blunt spleen and liver injury in children. J Pediatr Surg 46:173–177

Hepatoblastoma

62. von Schweinitz D (2012) Hepatoblastoma: recent developments in research and treatment. Semin Pediatr Surg 21:21–30
63. Maibach R, Roebuck D, Brugieres L, Capra M, Brock P, Dall'Igna P et al (2012) Prognostic stratification for children with hepatoblastoma: The SIOPEL experience. Eur J Cancer 48:1543–1549
64. Birch JM (2011) Epidemiology of pediatric liver tumors. In: Zimmermann A, Perilongo G, Malogolowkin M, von Schweinitz D (eds) Pediatric liver tumors. Springer, Heidelberg, pp 15–26
65. Perilongo G, Malogolowkin M, Feusner J (2012) Hepatoblastoma clinical research: lessons learned and future challenges. Pediatr Blood Cancer 59:818–821
66. López-Terrada D, Alaggio R, de Dávila MT, Czauderna P, Hiyama E, Katzenstein H et al (2014) Towards an international pediatric liver tumor consensus classification: proceedings of the Los Angeles COG liver tumors symposium. Mod Pathol 27: 472–491
67. Czauderna P, Otte JB, Aronson DC, Gauthier F, Mackinlay G, Roebuck D et al (2005) Guidelines for surgical treatment of hepatoblastoma in the modern era–recommendations from the Childhood Liver Tumour Strategy Group of the International Society of Paediatric Oncology (SIOPEL). Eur J Cancer 41:1031–1036
68. Semeraro M, Branchereau S, Maibach R, Zsiros J, Casanova M, Brock P et al (2013) Relapses in hepatoblastoma patients: Clinical characteristics and outcome – Experience of the International Childhood Liver Tumour Strategy Group (SIOPEL). Eur J Cancer 49:915–922
69. Perilongo G, Maibach R, Shafford E, Brugieres L et al (2009) Cisplatin versus cisplatin plus doxorubicin for standard-risk hepatoblastoma. N Engl J Med 361:1662–1670
70. Zsiros J, Maibach R, Shafford E, Brugieres L et al (2010) Successful treatment of childhood high-risk hepatoblastoma with dose-intensive multiagent chemotherapy and surgery: final results of the SIOPEL-3HR Study. J Clin Oncol 28:2584–2590
71. Zsiros J, Brugieres L, Brock P, Roebuck D et al (2013) Dose-dense cisplatin-based chemotherapy and surgery for children with high-risk hepatoblastoma (SIOPEL-4): a prospective, single-arm, feasibility study. Lancet Oncol 14:834–842

Solid Pseudopapillary Tumor of the Pancreas

72. Das PC (2007) Solid pseudo papillary tumor of the pancreas in a child. J Indian Assoc Pediatr Surg 12:148–150
73. Sun CD, Lee WJ, Choi JS, Oh JT, Choi SH (2005) Solid-pseudo papillary tumours of the pancreas: 14 years experience. ANZ J Surg 75:684–689
74. Persson M, Bisgaard C, Nielsen BB, Christiansen T, Kroustrup JP (1986) Solid and papillary epithelial neoplasm of the pancreas presenting as a traumatic cyst. Case report. Acta Chir Scand 152:223–226
75. Coleman KM, Doherty MC, Bigler SA (2003) Solid-pseudo papillary tumor of the pancreas. Radiographics 23:1644–1648
76. Pattanshetti VM, Vinchurkar K, Pattanshetti SV (2014) Solid pseudo papillary tumor of pancreas: presenting as acute abdomen in a female child. Indian J Med Paediatr Oncol 35:184–186
77. Yin Q, Wang M, Wang C, Wu Z, Yuan F, Chen K, Tang Y, Zhao X, Miao F (2012) Differentiation between benign and malignant solid pseudopapillary tumor of the pancreas by MDCT. Eur J Radiol 81:3010–3018
78. Cantisani V, Mortele KJ, Levy A, Glickman JN, Ricci P, Passariello R et al (2003) MR imaging features of solid pseudo papillarytumor of the pancreas in adult and pediatric patients. AJR Am J Roentgenol 181:395–401
79. Shaoquin C, Shengquan Z, Qibao D, Peisheng H, Weihua C (2007) The clinicopathological and immunohistochemical analysis of solid pseudopapillary tumor of the pancreas: report of nine cases. J Nanj Med Univ 21:398–401
80. Guedira M, Hrora A, Raïss M, El Alaoui M, Kettani F, Tounsi A (2006) Tumeurs pseudopapillaires et solides du pancréas. J Chir 143:271–273
81. Morita K, Urushihara N, Fukumoto K, Miyano G, Yamoto M, Nouso H, Miyake H, Kaneshiro M (2014) Solid pseudopapillary tumor of the pancreas in children: surgical intervention strategies based on pathological findings. Pediatr Surg Int 30:253–257
82. Raffel A, Cupisti K, Krausch M, Braunstein S, Tröbs B, Goretzki PE, Willnow U (2004) Therapeutic strategy of papillary cystic and solid neoplasm (PCSN): a rare non-endocrine tumor of the pancreas in children. Surg Oncol 13:1–6
83. Carricaburu E, Enezian G, Bonnard A, Berrebi D, Belarbi N, Huot O, Aigrain Y, de Lagausie P (2003) Laparoscopic distal pancreatectomy for Frantz's tumor in a child. Surg Endosc 17:2028–2031
84. Fais PO, Carricaburu E, Sarnacki S, Berrebi D, Orbach D, Baudoin V, de Lagausie P (2009) Is laparoscopic management suitable for solid pseudo-papillary tumors of the pancreas? Pediatr Surg Int 25:617–621
85. Namgoong JM, Kim DY, Kim SC, Kim SC, Hwang JH, Song KB (2014) Laparoscopic distal pancreatec-

tomy to treat solid pseudopapillary tumors in children: transition from open to laparoscopic approaches in suitable cases. Pediatr Surg Int 30:259–266
86. Abu Hilal M, Hamdan M, Di Fabio F, Pearce NW, Johnson CD (2012) Laparoscopic versus open distal pancreatectomy: a clinical and cost-effectiveness study. Surg Endosc 26:1670–1674

Pancreatic Injury

87. Moore EE, Moore FA (2010) American Association for the Surgery of Trauma Organ Injury Scaling: 50th anniversary review article of the Journal of Trauma. J Trauma 69:1600–1601
88. Keil R, Drabek J, Lochmannova J, Stovicek J, Rygl M, Snajdauf J, Hlava S (2016) What is the role of endoscopic retrograde cholangiopancreatography in assessing traumatic rupture of the pancreatic in children? Scand J Gastroenterol 51:218–224
89. Garvey EM, Haakinson DJ, McOmber M, Notrica DM (2015) Role of ERCP in pediatric blunt abdominal trauma: a case series at a level one pediatric trauma center. J Pediatr Surg 50:335–338
90. Haugaard MV, Wettergren A, Hillingsø JG, Gluud C, Penninga L (2014) Non-operative versus operative treatment for blunt pancreatic trauma in children. Cochrane Database Syst Rev 12:1–19
91. Wales PW, Shuckett B, Kim PC (2001) Long-term outcome after nonoperative management of complete traumatic pancreatic transection in children. J Pediatr Surg 36:823–827
92. de Blaauw I, Winkelhorst JT, Rieu PN, van der Staak FH, Wijnen MH, Severijnen RS et al (2008) Pancreatic injury in children: good outcome of nonoperative treatment. J Pediatr Surg 43:1640–1643
93. Bonnard A, Lagausie P, Malbezin S, Sauvat E, Lemaitre AI, Aigrain Y (2001) Mediastinal pancreatic pseudocyst in a child. A thoracoscopic approach. Surg Endosc 15:760
94. Rutkoski JD, Segura BJ, Kane TD (2011) Experience with totally laparoscopic distal pancreatectomy with splenic preservation for pediatric trauma – 2 techniques. J Pediatr Surg 46:588–593

Portal Hypertension in Children 27

Neil Di Salvo, Michela Maffi, and Mario Lima

27.1 Definition

Portal hypertension is defined as an increase of blood pressure in the portal venous bed beyond the physiological values of 5–10 cm H_2O or as an increase of pressure gradient of more than 5 cm H_2O between the hepatic veins and the portal circulation (hepatic venous pressure gradient or HVPG) [1–5].

27.2 Classification and Etiology

It is caused by either:

- An increase of resistance to the blood flow from the mesenteric venous circulation through or to the liver (which is way more frequent in childhood)
- An increase of the blood flow to the portal circulation

The increase of resistance is the consequence of an obstruction in the portal system. Depending on the site of this obstruction, we can divide all causes of portal hypertension into three main categories:

- *Prehepatic portal hypertension*, also known as extrahepatic portal vein obstruction (EHPVO). Unlike in adulthood, this represents the most frequent type of portal hypertension in children (60–75 %).
- *Intrahepatic portal hypertension*, secondary to hepatocellular injury leading to cirrhosis. This is the second most frequent type of portal hypertension in childhood. Among all hepatocellular diseases leading to portal hypertension (Table 27.1), biliary atresia is the most common.
- *Post-hepatic portal hypertension*. It is caused by thrombosis of large or small veins draining blood from the liver into the inferior vena cava (Budd-Chiari syndrome, rare in children).

Extrahepatic portal vein obstruction can be caused by:

- Thrombosis of the portal vein (Fig. 27.1): instrumentation and cannulation of the umbilical vein at birth including umbilical vein catheters for intravenous access in the first days of life, omphalitis, sepsis, hypovolemic shock and hereditary hypercoagulable states represent risk factors for this condition. Regarding the umbilical cannulation, some authors report a 40 % risk of thrombosis after

N. Di Salvo (✉) • M. Maffi • M. Lima
Pediatric Surgery, S. Orsola-Malpighi Hospital, Bologna University, Via Massarenti 11, 40138 Bologna, Italy
e-mail: neildisalvo@hotmail.com; michela.maffi@libero.it; mario.lima@unibo.it

M. Lima (ed.), *Pediatric Digestive Surgery*, DOI 10.1007/978-3-319-40525-4_27

the catheter is left in place for 48 hours; 100 % if more than 72 hours. Some others believe this risk has been nowadays reduced by the improvement of catheters' materials. However the principle is that this kind of venous line must be taken into consideration only if extremely needed.

- Portal vein congenital stenosis/atresia (Fig. 27.2a) or postnatal fibrotic stenosis (Fig. 27.2b). The latter is due to abnormal spreading of the normal process, obliterating the umbilical vein or ductus venosus of Aranzio, to the trunk of the portal vein.

Occlusion of the main trunk of the portal vein may lead to recanalization of the vein and its transformation into a series of smaller collateral

Table 27.1 Hepatocellular diseases leading to portal hypertension

Biliary atresia
Postinfectious cirrhosis
Congenital hepatic fibrosis
Congenital disorders of bile acid metabolism
Sclerosing cholangitis
Autoimmune hepatitis
Drug toxicity
Metabolic diseases (e.g., alpha-1 antitrypsin deficiency)

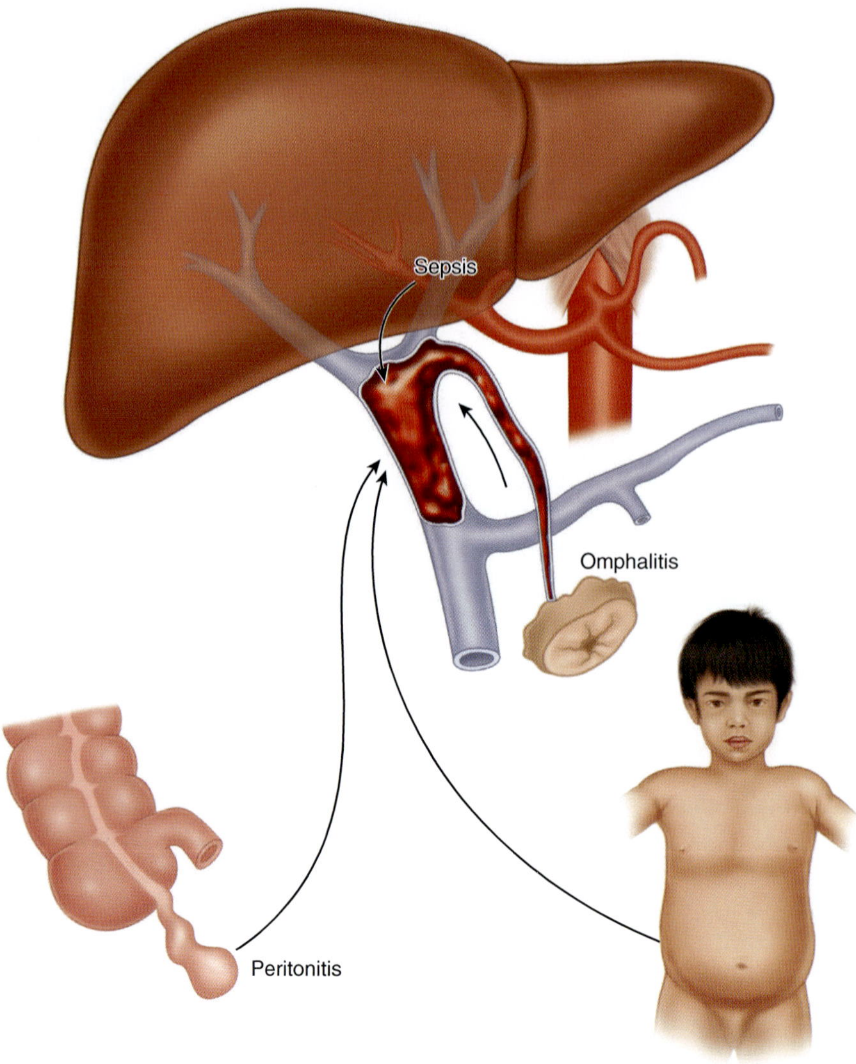

Fig. 27.1 Causes of prehepatic portal hypertension: portal vein thrombosis

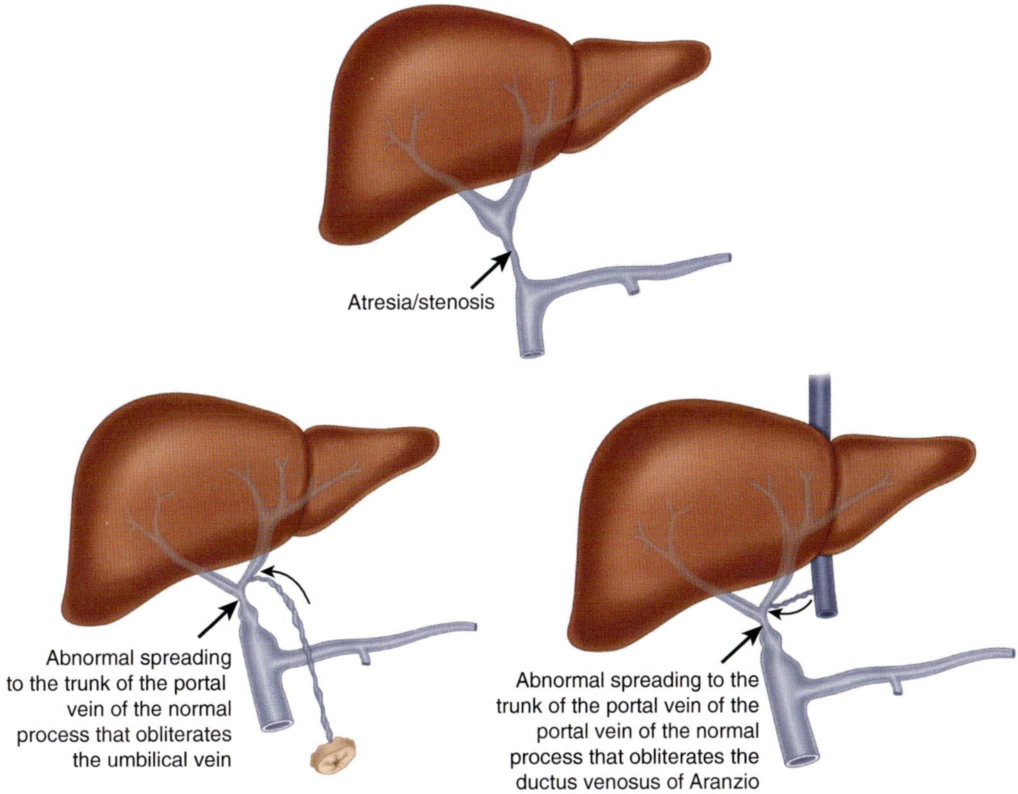

Fig. 27.2 Causes of prehepatic portal hypertension. (**a**) Atresia/stenosis of the portal vein. (**b**) Postnatal fibrotic stenosis

veins that assume the appearance of a venous cavernoma. It is a network of small collaterals that supply the liver with a small amount of mesenteric blood and keep the intrahepatic portal circulation patent, even though hypoplastic (Fig. 27.3). Even though the role of all these risk factors is established, in daily practice the etiology remains unknown in about 50 % of cavernomas [2–6].

27.3 Pathophysiology and Collateral Circulation

The main areas where the abnormal shunts between the systemic and portal venous system occur are:

- Gastroesophageal area: left gastric (coronary) vein and short gastric veins to oesophageal veins (forming submucosal oesophageal varices) thence to azygous/hemiazygous veins in the thorax
- Hemorrhoidal plexus in the rectum: superior hemorrhoidal veins to the middle and inferior hemorrhoidal veins and ultimately to the inferior vena cava
- Paraumbilical network: paraumbilical and umbilical veins to superficial veins of the abdominal wall and the superior/inferior epigastric veins (forming the "caput medusae")
- Intestinal veins to the branches of the inferior vena cava in the retroperitoneum (veins of Retzius)

Depending on the type of Portal obstruction, every "shunting" area will be more or less developed. For instance, in the EXPVO, the paraumbilical plexus will be little represented since the umbilical veins drain beyond the obstruction (Figs. 27.4 and 27.5) [5].

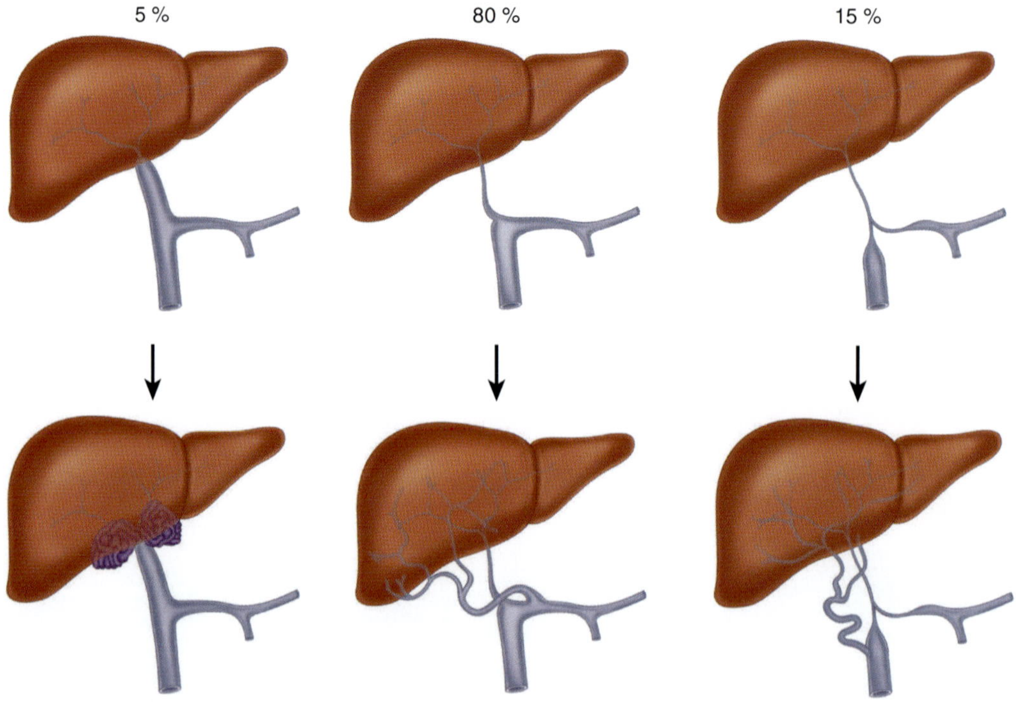

Fig. 27.3 Anatomic variants of cavernomas

27.4 Clinical Presentation

Unlike children with preexisting liver disease (mainly the ones affected from cirrhosis secondary to biliary atresia), children with extrahepatic portal vein obstruction are usually completely well before the sudden onset of symptoms. The significant manifestation of portal hypertension in childhood is massive upper gastrointestinal bleeding. Oesophagogastric varices have been noted in very young infants and 70 % of patients experience their first bleeding episode before the age of 7. Almost 90 % of patients with bleeding varices secondary to extrahepatic obstruction of the portal vein hemorrhage before the age of 10 (Fig. 27.6).

The second most common finding is splenomegaly and progressive fibrosis of the organ (fibro-congestive splenomegaly) together with a certain degree of functional hyperactivity (hypersplenism). By the term hypersplenism, we mean an excessive splenic sequestration of red and white blood cells and platelets, therefore resulting in anemia, thrombocytopenia and leukopenia.

Encephalopathy, ascites, and pulmonary disorders are associated to an advanced liver disease (cirrhosis), therefore extremely unusual in childhood [1–5, 9].

27.5 Diagnosis

Routine lab parameters of liver function (transaminases, bilirubin, albumin, alkaline phosphatase, gamma-GT, PT) and splenic sequestration of cells (blood cells count) are essential. A coagulation work-up is often required if no risk factors (like an umbilical catheter) are present in order to rule out a hereditary hypercoagulable state (C and S protein, AT –III, etc.).

This could sometimes be hard to interpret because anomalies in both the pro- and anticoagulant pathway may be secondary to the hepatic deprivation of portal blood and are reversible after the successful restoration of portal flow.

The presence of a cavernoma and portal vein thrombosis are usually first diagnosed by ultrasonography with Doppler interrogation.

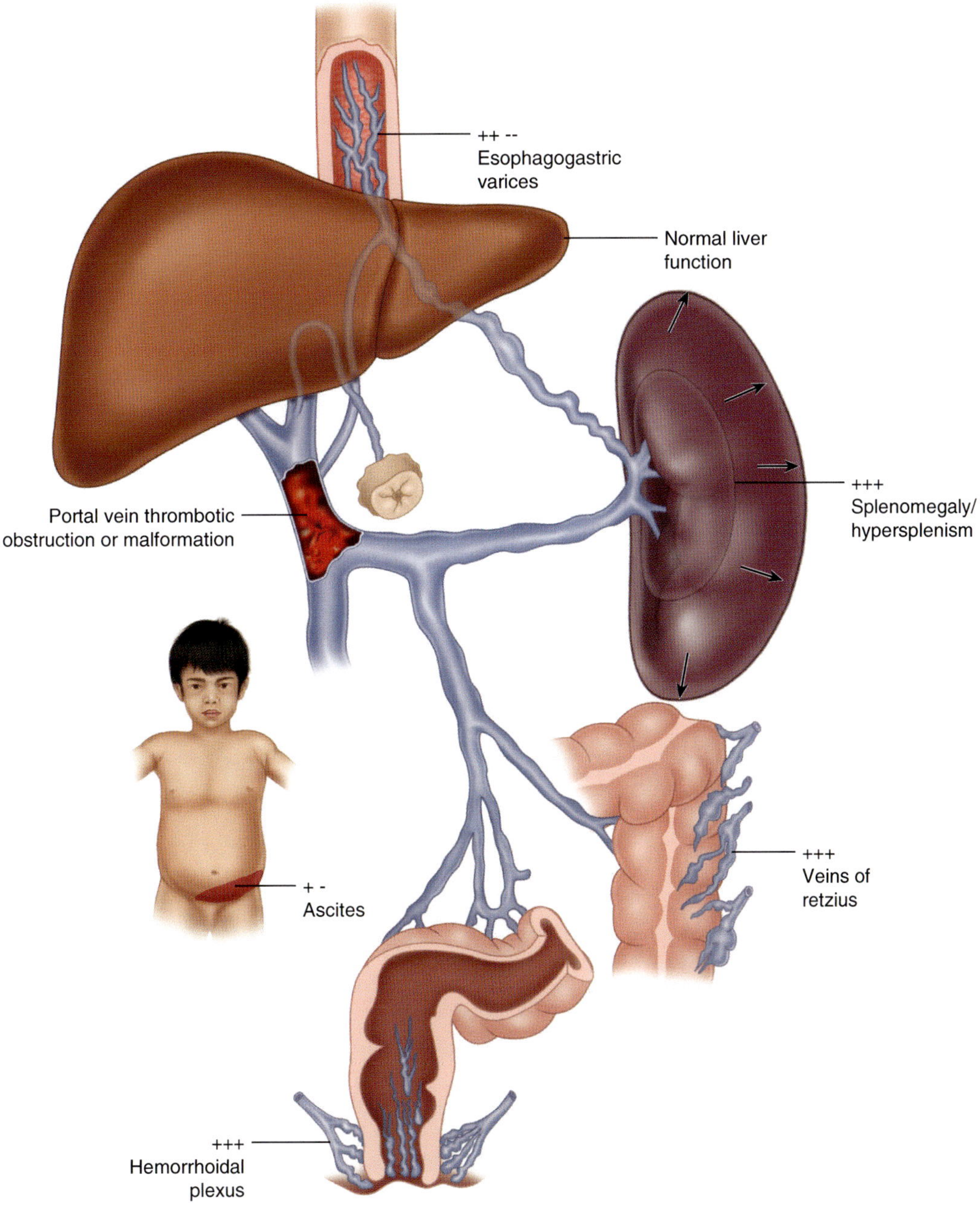

Fig. 27.4 Development of portosystemic shunts in prehepatic portal hypertension

The precise portal venous anatomy must be assessed, first by Doppler ultrasound which is suitable to demonstrate patency and flow (Fig. 27.7).

Afterward patients being considered for shunting should also be evaluated by CT or MR angiography (each with its own advantages) that has replaced traditional invasive angiography except for retrograde trans-jugular portal venogram which can still be a useful tool, especially when evaluating Rex process patency (Fig. 27.8) [1–4].

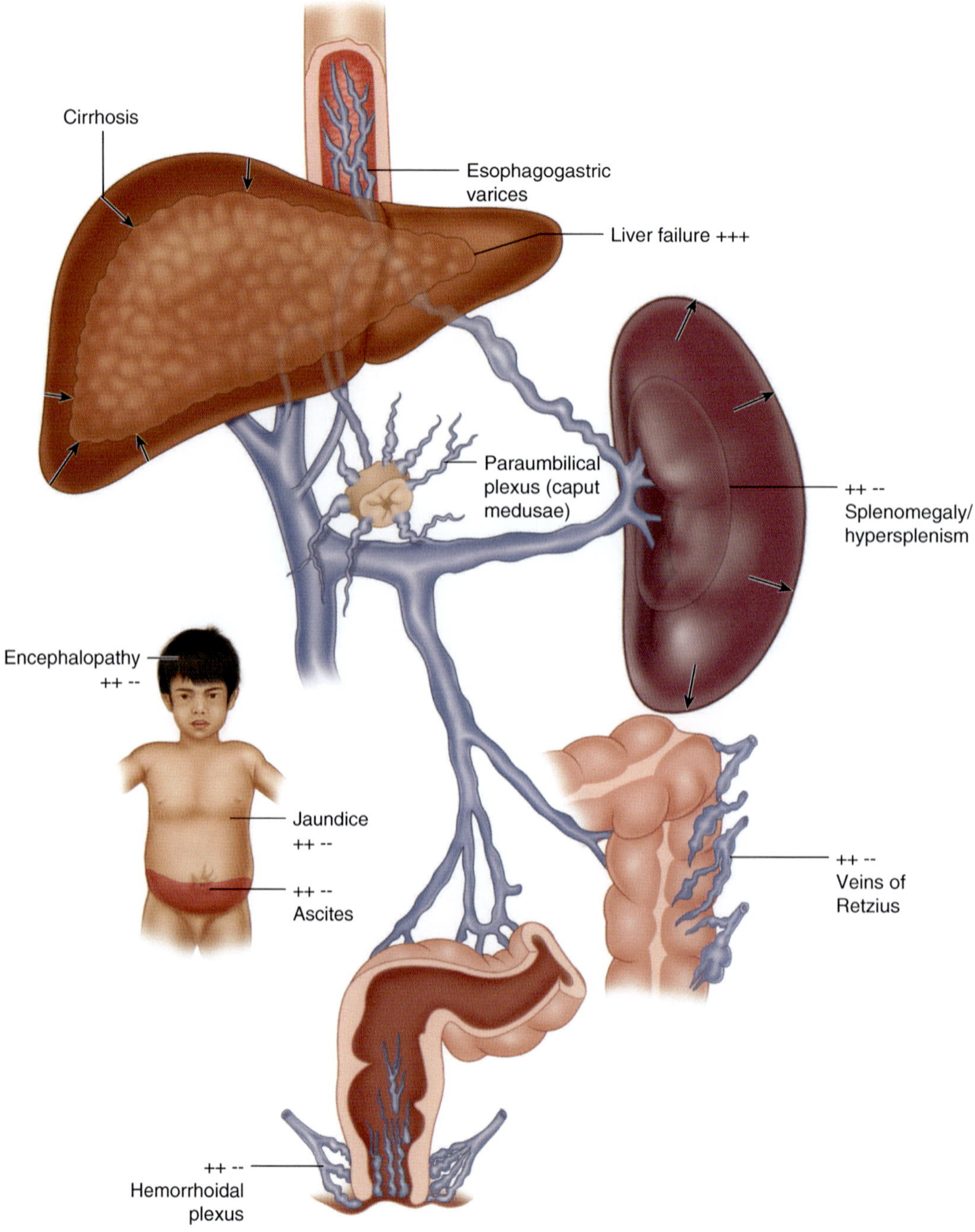

Fig. 27.5 Development of portosystemic shunt in intrahepatic portal hypertension

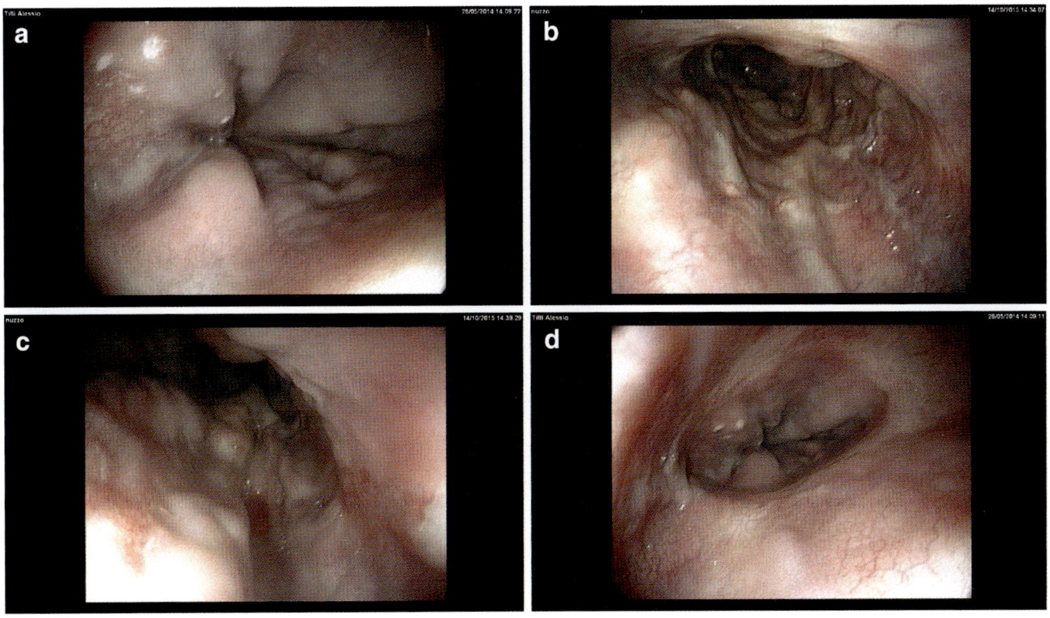

Fig. 27.6 (**a–d**) Endoscopic diagnosis of oesophageal varices

27.6 Treatment

27.6.1 Prevention

Prevention of variceal bleeding, both in children and adults, is obtained by administering nonselective beta-blockers such as propranolol which reduces portal pressure by vasoconstriction of splanchnic circulation and decreased cardiac output. If there are no contraindications to therapy such as asthma, cardiac failure, diabetes, etc., propranolol is used in the pediatric population with a dose ranging between 0.5 mg and 1.5 mg/kg/day (divided into two to four doses). During treatment basal heart rate should not decrease more than 25 %. Treatment is usually started after the first bleeding episode that is to say, in childhood, at the time of diagnosis after the infant has overcome the acute event. Certainly an effective prophylaxis is represented by the endoscopic treatment of varices which is also an emergency treatment [9–11].

27.6.2 Emergency Variceal Bleeding Treatment

Being upper gastrointestinal bleeding often the first significant manifestation of portal hypertension in childhood, as we said before, when a child is presenting hematemesis, we do not often know the cause of it. As a matter of fact, the first-line treatment of acute bleeding from ruptured oesophageal varices does not differ from that used for secondary hematemesis from other causes such as oesophagitis, hemorrhagic gastritis, etc. In the first place, we need to cope with the prevention or treatment of the subsequent hypovolemic shock (placement of at least two peripheral venous line if not a central venous access, IV fluid infusion, vital signs and diuresis monitoring, preparation for a possible transfusion). Nasogastric tube placement is safe and may be an essential part of the management of these patients. It allows documentation of the rate of ongoing bleeding and removal of blood, a

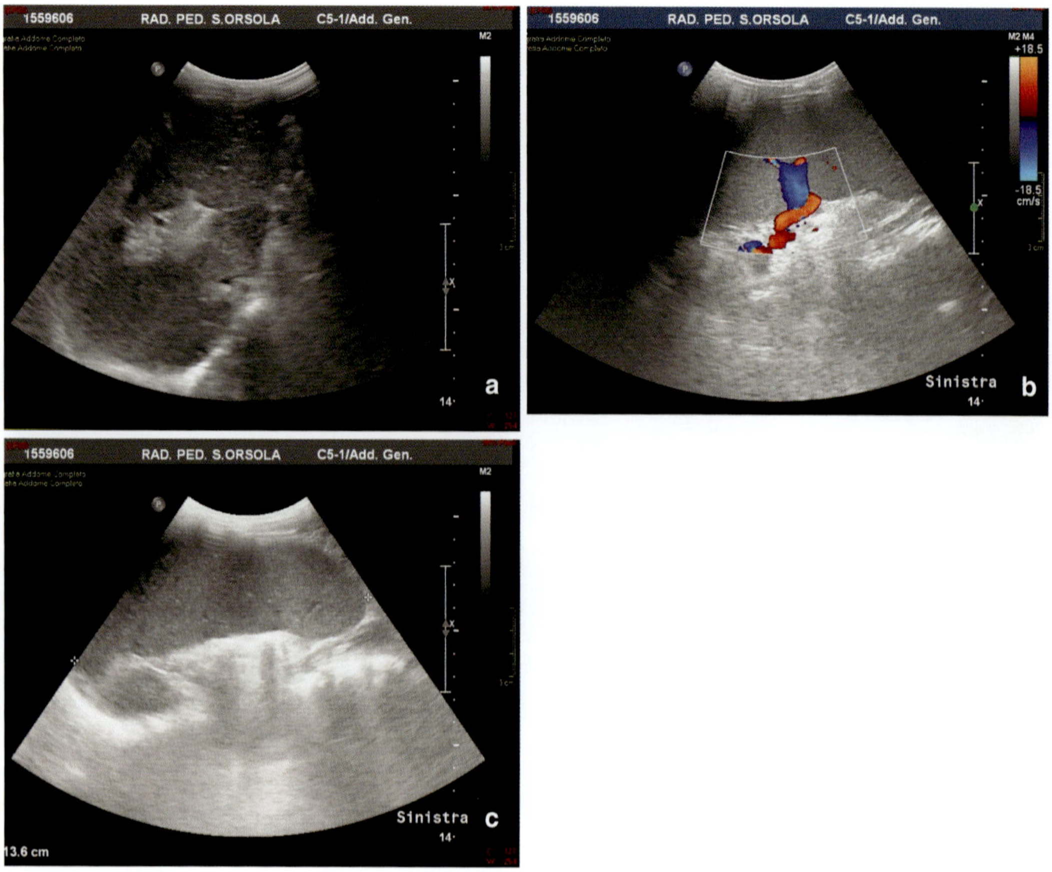

Fig. 27.7 Ultrasound with Doppler interrogation for the study of portal venous anatomy and flow

protein source that may precipitate encephalopathy. In addition, the blood in the stomach increases splanchnic blood flow and could aggravate portal hypertension and ongoing bleeding. Secondly, the administration of certain drugs like somatostatin analogs such as octreotide is very effective in stopping the acute bleeding through vasoconstriction of the splanchnic circulation and thereby reducing the portal blood flow. Octreotide is administered by continuous infusion at a rate of 1–2 μg/pro kilo/h to a maximum dose of 100 μg/h even though it may need to be initiated by the administration of a bolus. It is also recommended giving proton pump inhibitors and antibiotics. In particularly serious cases (severe uncontrollable hemorrhage), a Sengstaken-Blakemore tube can be used. It is a tube designed to stop hemorrhage by mechanically compressing oesophageal and gastric varices (Fig. 27.9). The patient requires significant sedation for its use and the airway is often secured by endotracheal intubation. This therapy is very effective in controlling acute bleeding; unfortunately it is associated with significant number of complications (for instance, aspiration pneumonia if not intubated, mucosal necrosis, balloon displacement) and high incidence of re-bleeding when the tube is removed. The balloon is deflated after 12–24 h at the time of endoscopy. Endoscopy plays an essential role in the diagnosis and emergency treatment of oesophageal varices. There is no unanimous consensus about the proper timing of emergency endoscopy, but there is general agreement in saying that endoscopy should be performed as soon as possible, once the bleeding has been

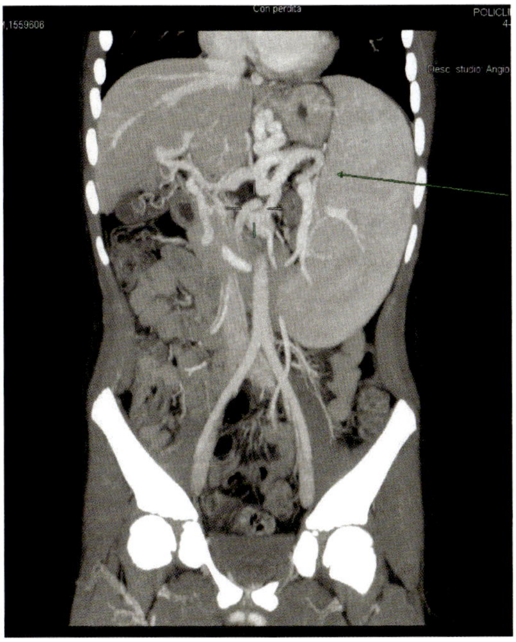

Fig. 27.8 CT angiography for portal anatomy assessment in a patient considered for a shunting procedure

stopped with the above mentioned means and after appropriate stabilization of the patient. It is carried out after approximately 24–72 h from the event's onset [3, 9–11].

27.6.3 Endoscopic Treatment: Endosclerosis and Banding of Varices

Injecting sclerosing solutions into the tissue around a varix or directly into a varix to obliterate the vessel was the earliest attempt to control variceal bleeding. Endoscopic variceal band ligation utilizes mechanical ligation and strangulation of varices with elastic O-rings (Fig. 27.10). Banding was found to be a more effective, more rapid, and safer method of reducing the chance of bleeding from varices. Oesophageal banding together with pharmacologic control has become the procedure of choice in the early therapy of bleeding oesophageal varices. Subsequent sessions are aimed at ligating residual varices or varices that arise after the larger ones are tied off. Ligation is effective in most children and is less associated with many of the adverse side effects of sclerotherapy such as oesophageal ulceration, perforation and stricture. This is why endoscopic sclerotherapy has been largely abandoned in favor of endoscopic variceal ligation. The only indication for sclerotherapy still remains the very small infant (approximately less than 12–15 kg body weight) for whom currently available equipment for variceal banding (addition of the band ligation device to the endoscope) is too large to introduce into the oesophagus [2, 9–11].

27.6.4 Shunt Surgical Procedures

The treatment of choice for symptomatic portal hypertension from extrahepatic portal obstruction is a surgical shunt. Surgical shunts are of two kinds: portosystemic shunts and the mesentericoportal shunt. The first one is inspired on the principle of artificially improving the portosystemic derivation that the organism puts into action spontaneously, but often in an insufficient degree, through the collateral circles both superficial and deep. Portosystemic shunts are usually divided into two categories: nonselective and selective (Table 27.2). Selective shunts preserve the majority of portal or mesenteric blood flow to the liver while shunting blood from high-pressure gastroesophageal varices into the low-pressure systemic venous circulation. Whenever possible, all forms of nonselective shunting should be avoided in order to diminish the following encephalopathy thus preserving neurocognitive function. The second one, unlike portosystemic shunting, restores portal flow to the liver, thus acting as a physiologic bypass (see description below).

Portal hypertension accompanied by advanced liver dysfunction from either venous outflow obstruction or intrinsic liver disease is ultimately treated by transplantation [1–8, 10, 11].

27.6.4.1 Mesocaval Shunt

One of the first mesocaval shunts was described by Clatworthy. It consisted of a side-to-side anastomosis between the superior mesenteric vein and the inferior vena cava. Since this procedure

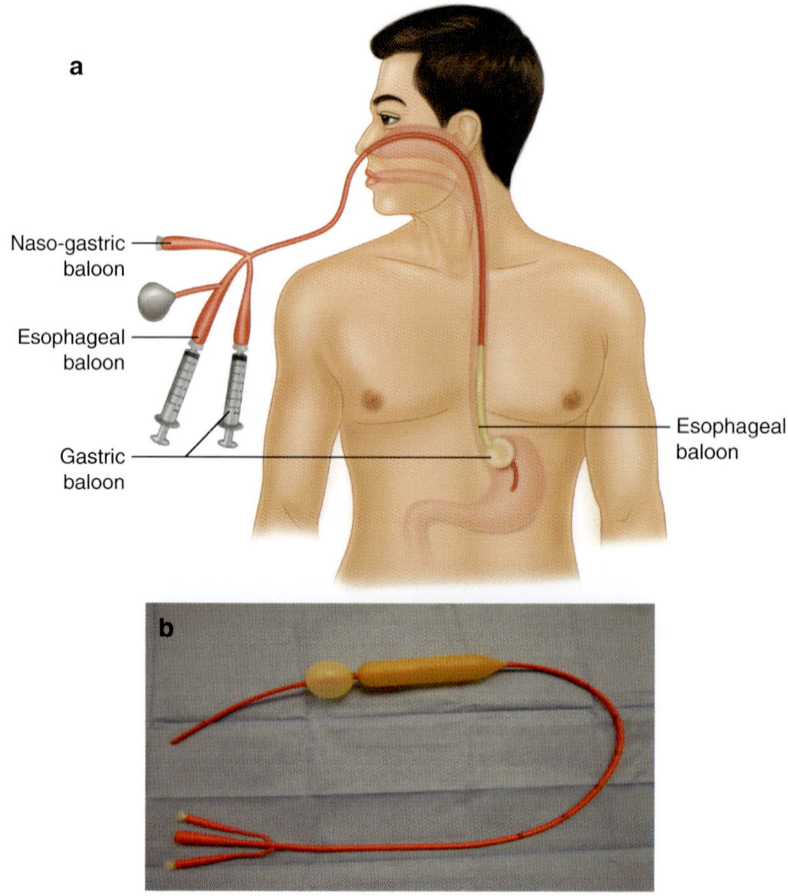

Fig. 27.9 Sengstaken-Blakemore probe: the device consists of a rubber tube with at least two balloons: it is passed into the stomach, where the first balloon is inflated and pulled up snug against the gastroesophageal junction. Once the tube is secured in place, the second balloon is inflated in the esophagus at a pressure that compresses the varices without necrosing the oesophagus. A channel in the rubber tube allows gastric contents to be sampled for evidence of bleeding. Correct positioning must be verified by x-rays

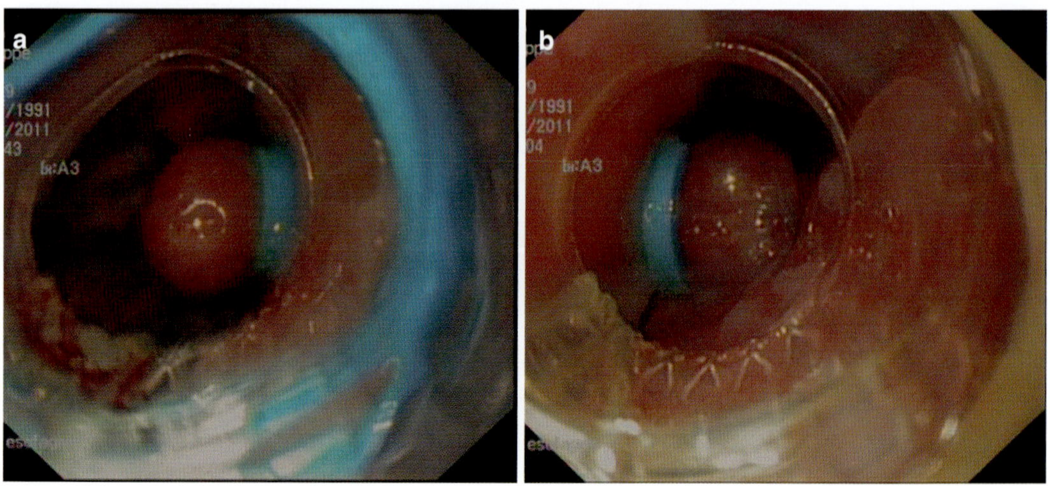

Fig. 27.10 Banding of oesophageal varices

required division of the inferior vena cava (IVC), it could frequently result in swelling of the lower extremities. This is why a mesocaval shunt using an interposition graft between the superior mesenteric vein (SMV) and IVC, without interrupting it, has been developed (H-mesocaval shunt) (Fig. 27.11). The graft can be a short autologous vein (usually the internal jugular vein) or a prosthetic graft (goretex).

Obviously an autologous graft offers the best chance of long-term patency. As a matter of fact, a synthetic vascular graft is only used in cases when the distance between the two major veins is too much to be filled by an autologous graft. It is easier to perform than some other shunts in children because the veins used are larger. The indications for this type of shunt are the impossibility to perform a splenorenal shunt as in the following cases:

- Children in whom the splenic vein is thrombosed
- Left renal agenesia/nephrectomy
- Small diameter of vessels like in very young patients [1, 4, 5]

Table 27.2 Classification of the most common portosystemic shunts

Nonselective shunts
Proximal splenorenal shunt
Mesocaval shunt: H-mesocaval shunt (with autologous or prosthetic graft)
Selective shunts
Distal splenorenal shunt (Warren)

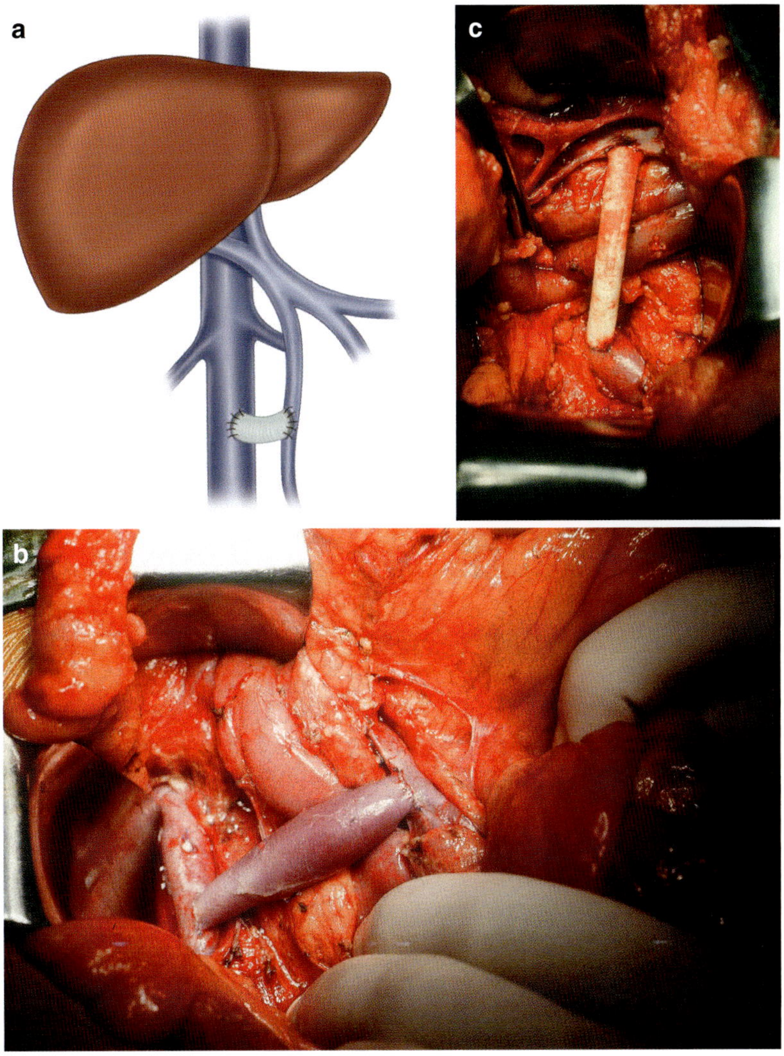

Fig. 27.11 H-mesocaval shunt. (**a**) Schematic representation. (**b**) With interposition of an autologous graft, intraoperative image. (**c**) With interposition of a prosthetic graft, intraoperative image

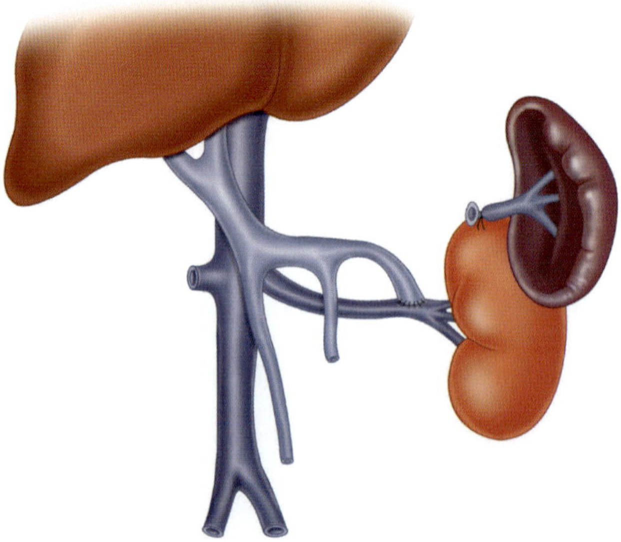

Fig. 27.12 Schematic representation of proximal splenorenal shunt

27.6.4.2 Proximal Splenorenal Shunt

The splenic vein is divided close (proximal) to the spleen and then sewn to the side of the left renal vein so that all the blood from the superior and inferior mesenteric veins is shunted into the systemic venous circulation through the left renal vein. The spleen is removed (Figs. 27.12 and 27.13) [1, 4, 5].

27.6.4.3 Distal Splenorenal Shunt

The distal splenorenal shunt was described by Warren in order to diminish the encephalopathy that followed portacaval shunting and to preserve the spleen. The portal circulation is divided into two components: one maintains anterograde portal flow toward the liver via the SMV, and the other flows away from the oesophageal varices to the short gastrics then through the splenic vein (ligated distally from the spleen) into the renal vein. After ligation of the coronary vein, the varices are therefore both decompressed by allowing them to drain via the short gastric vessels and splenic vein into the left renal vein and by decreasing blood flow to the varices by tying off the blood that reaches them through reverse flow in the coronary vein (Fig. 27.14) [1, 4, 5, 12–14].

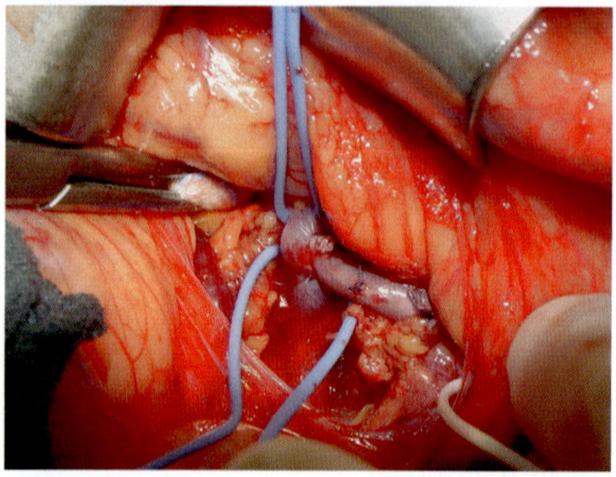

Fig. 27.13 Proximal splenorenal shunt. Termino-lateral anastomosis between the splenic and renal vein (intraoperative image)

27.6.4.4 Mesentericoportal Shunt (Rex Shunt)

The mesenteric-to-left portal vein bypass (Rex shunt) was originally developed for the treatment of portal vein blockage following liver transplant. The procedure allows relief of portal hypertension by redirecting blood from the obstructed mesenteric system to the still patent intrahepatic portal vein. It is the only shunt that is able to restore flow from the portal circuit back to the liver via the intrahepatic left

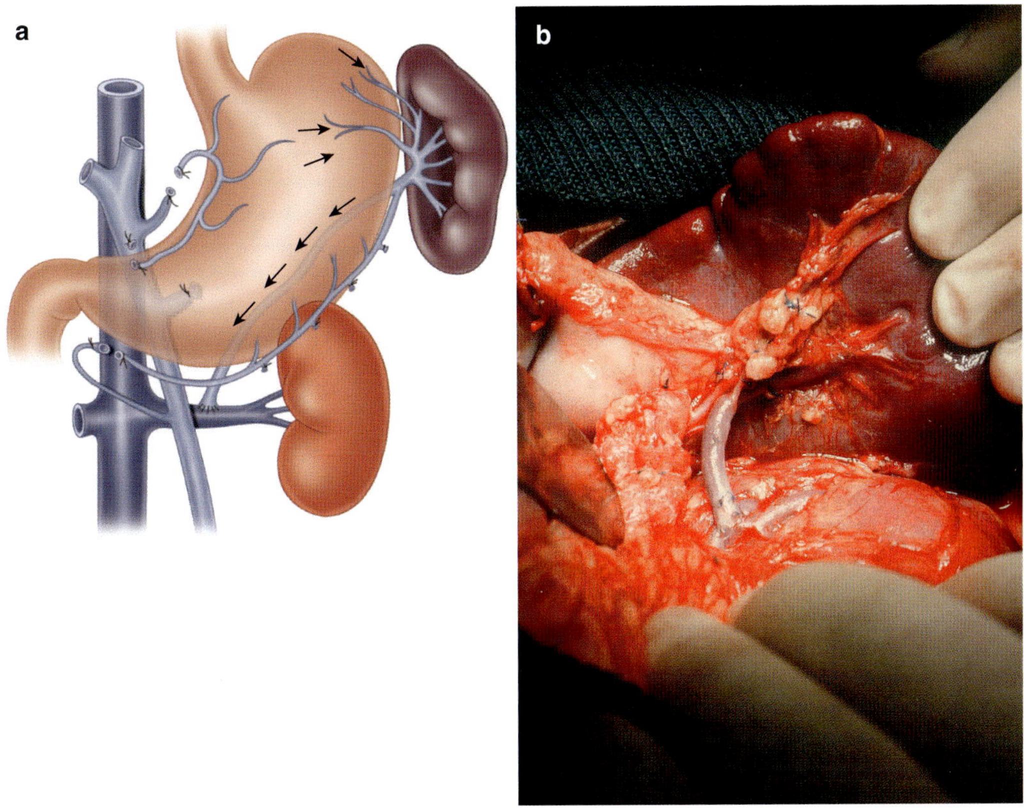

Fig. 27.14 Distal splenorenal shunt by Warren. (**a**) Schematic representation. (**b**) Termino-lateral anastomosis between the splenic and renal vein

portal vein. For this reason, it has been defined as a "physiologic shunt." This vein remains patent in about two-thirds of patients with cavernous transformation of the portal vein. Thus it is essential to preoperatively establish the patency of such vein (which is a prerequisite) by noninvasive angiography. The intrahepatic portal vein may be difficult to visualize by preoperative imaging and a final assessment may be possible only at the time of surgery. Once the intrahepatic left portal vein has been isolated, the jugular vein (either right or left) is removed and sewn first to the intrahepatic portal vein and then to the superior mesenteric vein. Enthusiasm for the utilization of the meso-Rex shunt is increasing because of the physiologic nature of the procedure to the point that many surgeons consider it the procedure of choice when feasible (Fig. 27.15) [2–4, 10, 11, 15].

27.7 Postoperative Outcome

Shunt thrombosis is a potential complication after surgery as in any other vascular procedures. This risk is particularly consistent since we are dealing with low-flow vessels. This is the reason why anticoagulants such as heparin and antiplatelet drugs like low-dose aspirin are often used. The latter is also useful as a systemic antithrombotic agent after splenectomy if platelets count exceeds 1,500,000/ mm^3. Literature suggests that shunts should remain patent in the long run in more than 90% of cases, thanks to a good operative technique and the postoperative antithrombotic prophylaxis. Prognosis depends on shunt patency and on the severity of liver disease. Those with cirrhosis eventually require liver transplantation before the development of end-stage disease. With complimentary medical therapy, endoscopic intervention and shunt surgery, the ultimate prognosis is excellent [2–4, 10, 11].

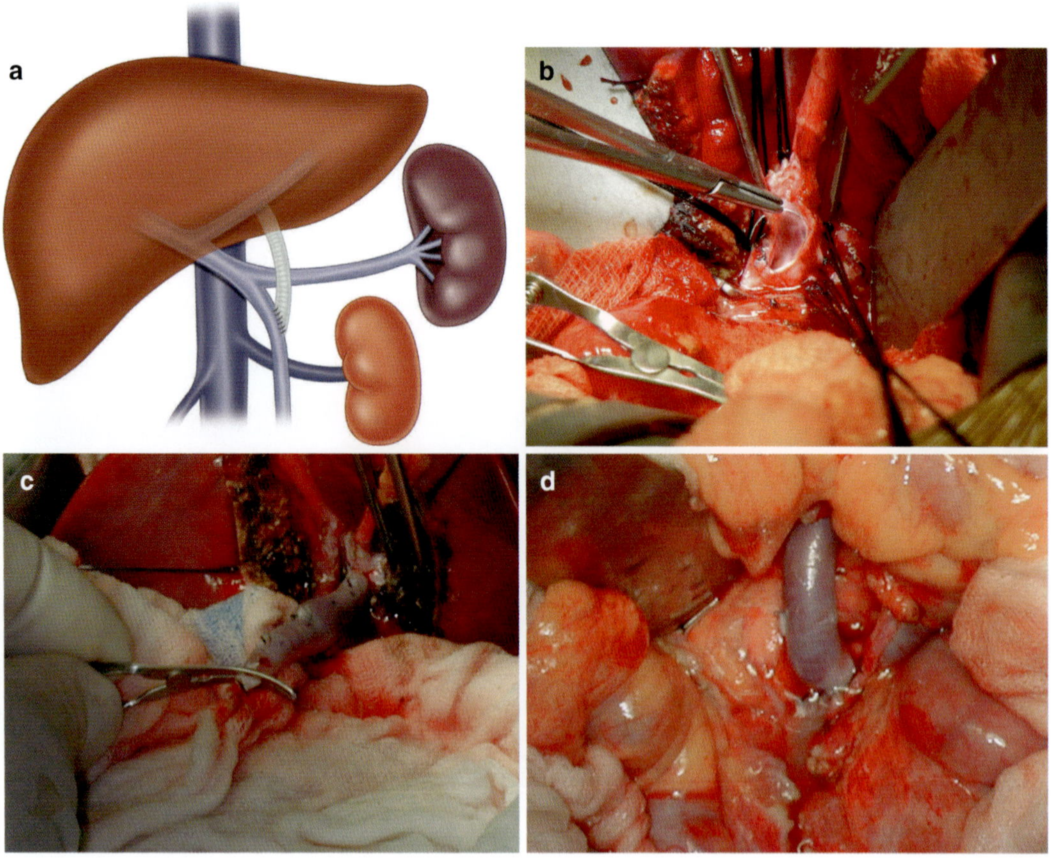

Fig. 27.15 Meso-Rex shunt. (**a**) Schematic representation. (**b**) The intrahepatic left portal vein is isolated in the Rex process. (**c**) Anastomosis between the graft and the left portal vein. (**d**) Completed anastomosis between the superior mesenteric vein and the left portal vein

References

1. Dòmini R, Lima M (2003) Lezioni di Chirurgia Pediatrica. Clueb editore
2. Spitz L, Coran A (2013) Operative pediatric surgery. Taylor 5 Francis Group
3. Coran A (2012) Pediatric surgery. Elsevier
4. Lima M, Ruggeri G (2015) Chirurgia Pediatrica. Edises editore
5. Appignani A, Lima M, Ceccarelli PL, Ricci S (1982) Endoscopia dell'esofago varicoso. Rass It Chir Ped 24(4):155–158
6. Appignani A, Lima M (1984) Recent advances in the treatment of portal hypertension in paediatric age. "Centro Studi Humana". Editore, Milano
7. Cacciari A, Ricci S, Appignani A, Lima M et al (1983) Vantaggi dello shunt di Warren nella chirurgia dell'ipertensione portale infantile con particolare riferimento alla correzione dell'ipersplenismo. Rass It Chir Ped 25(2):117–120
8. Domini R (1968) L'Ipertensione Portale dell'Infanzia. Piccin Editore
9. Domini R, Appignani A, Lima M (1985) L'ipertensione portale nell'infanzia. Aggiornamento Medico 7(3):189–194
10. Domini R, Appignani A, Lima M (1986) Ipertensione portale nell'infanzia. Progressi clinici: Chirurgia. L'ipertensione portale. Piccin Editore, Padova. N. 5, vol. 1, cap. 11, p. 291
11. Gugig R, Rosenthal P (2012) Management of portal hypertension in children. World J Gastroenterol 8:1176–1184
12. Lima M, Appignani A (1985) L'anastomosi splenorenale secondo Warren nel ratto: studio sperimentale preliminare. Rass It Chir Ped 27(4):302–306
13. Ricci S, Lima M, Cacciari A, Appignani A et al (1983) Utilizzazione dei mezzi ottici di ingrandimento nelle

derivazioni porto-sistemiche. Rass It Chir Ped 25(1): 23–28
14. Lautz TB, Keys LA, Melvin JC, Ito J, Superina RA (2013) Advantages of Meso-Rex bypass compared to porto-systemic shunt in the management of extra-hepatic portal vein obstruction in children. J Am Coll Surg 216(1):83–89
15. Ling SC (2012) Advances in the evaluation and management of children with portal hypertension. Semin Liver Dis 32(4):288–297

28 The Pediatric Short Bowel State: Practical Concepts Toward Enteral Autonomy

Adrian Bianchi

28.1 Introduction

Unlike adults where the short bowel state is most often due to bowel disease (Crohn's disease) or vascular causes (cardiac disease, superior mesenteric artery embolus), the pediatric short bowel state (PSBS) is commonly secondary to congenital anomalies, specifically midgut volvulus complicating malrotation (Fig. 28.1) or gastroschisis (Fig. 28.2), and long-segment aganglionosis (Hirschsprung's disease).

Postnatal necrotizing enterocolitis (NEC) and its attendant surgery account for the greater proportion of the remainder (Fig. 28.3). Whereas it is not presently possible to prevent intrauterine bowel loss, a high index of suspicion will reduce postnatal midgut volvulus, while cautious feeding in premature babies and earlier pre-necrosis bowel-preserving surgery for NEC will salvage greater lengths of functional bowel.

Intestinal failure (IF) can be regarded as the inability to sustain survival and growth because of inadequate absorption from the available autologous bowel. Most children with PSBS who suffer from IF have a residual mucosa that is healthy, but is of insufficient amount and of inappropriate configuration. Survival following major loss of absorbing bowel depends on the natural adaptation response [1, 2] that includes bowel elongation and dilatation with a major increase in absorptive brush border surface area consequent on mucosal hypertrophy (increase in villus height) and villus cellular hyperplasia (increased numbers of cells per villus). It is noteworthy that the ileum develops a greater adaptation response and is preferable to the jejunum also because of its specific absorption sites for vit B_{12} and bile salts. The ileocecal valve (IC valve) is helpful in delaying transit, thereby increasing mucosal contact time for absorption. Greater lengths of the colon are relevant to fluid and electrolyte absorption, with particular advantage for the right colon as the site of production of glucagon-like peptide 2 (GLP-2), an intestinotrophic mediator that is the most potent stimulator of small bowel mucosal adaptation.

Prior to total parenteral nutrition (TPN) and bowel reconstruction, minimum lengths of 40–60 cm of small bowel with an IC valve and the colon were considered necessary for survival. However the length of small bowel compatible with independent survival is markedly influenced by the type, configuration, and health of the residual bowel. TPN, a better understanding of PSBS, and improved techniques for bowel management have increasingly offered hope of enteral autonomy with acceptable quality long-term life, even to patients with extreme short bowel. Patients who have no functional bowel, who have failed autologous bowel management, who have poor quality life, and those who have lost venous

A. Bianchi, MD, FRCS, FRCSEd
Neonatal and Paediatric Reconstructive Surgeon,
The Cabin, 1 Elleray Road, Alkrington, Middleton,
M24 1NY Manchester, UK
e-mail: bianchi54@gmail.com

M. Lima (ed.), *Pediatric Digestive Surgery*, DOI 10.1007/978-3-319-40525-4_28

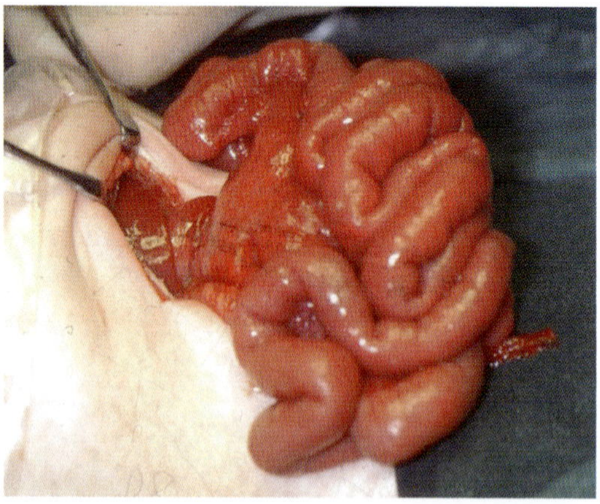

Fig. 28.1 Midgut volvulus complicating malrotation and mesenteric non-fixation

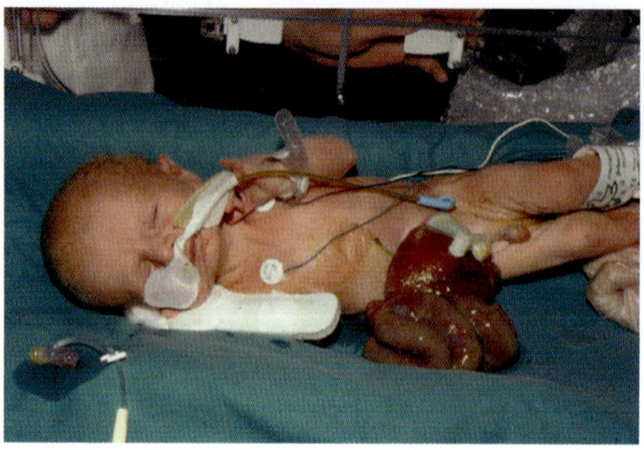

Fig. 28.2 Gastroschisis with extruded bowel on a narrow-based mesentery

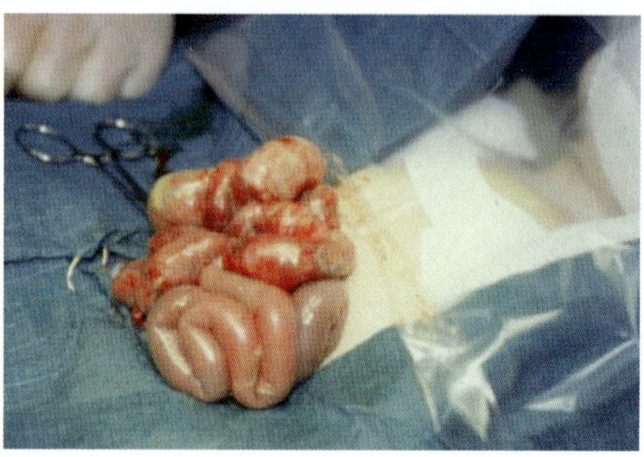

Fig. 28.3 Neonatal necrotizing enterocolitis

access or suffer irreversible liver failure have the option of small bowel-colon or liver-bowel transplantation, with improving long-term outcomes. However, graft rejection and the infective and neoplastic risks associated with immunosuppression remain significant. Furthermore, the constant need for monitoring for acute rejection and the insidious onset of chronic rejection with loss of graft function impacts on quality of life, such that transplantation should not be the first choice but a welcome final resort.

28.2 The Pediatric Short Bowel State

Antenatal midgut volvulus with loss of the superior mesenteric vascular territory presents as a high jejunal atresia (Fig. 28.4) with an occluded dilated loop of the jejunum commonly of 20–40 cm (<10 % of normal) measured from the ligament of Treitz along the antimesenteric border, and an atrophic left transverse colon through to the anus. This residual bowel is usually peristaltic and absorptive with adaptive potential.

Postnatal midgut volvulus and NEC present as life-threatening peritonitis from ischemic and inflamed bowel and bacterial sepsis. The length and variety of the residual bowel will depend on the *extent of the disease*, the *timing of surgery*, and the degree of *bowel conservation* practiced by the surgeon. The residual proximal and distal bowel are not dilated and are of similar caliber. Significantly, surviving bowel after NEC may not be functionally normal, also having a reduced adaptive potential.

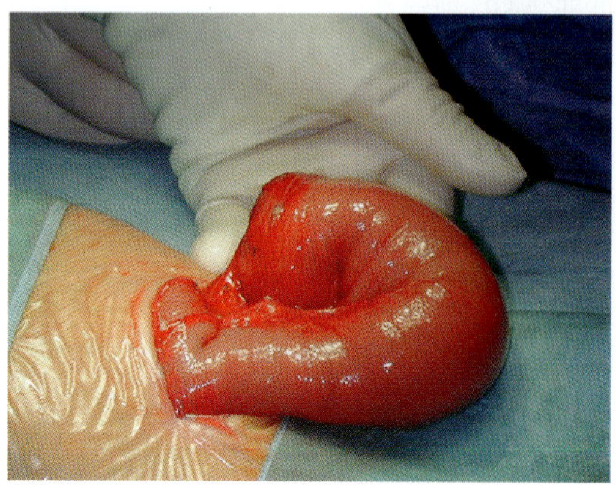

Fig. 28.4 30 cm residual jejunum following antenatal midgut loss

The "lucky" patient with long-segment jejunal aganglionosis (Hirschsprung's disease) may have a variable length of ganglionic jejunum that is usually of normal function and adaptive potential. All aganglionic bowel distal to the transition zone is aperistaltic and nonabsorptive but should not be removed unless it is the source of infection, since it serves to retain abdominal cavity volume that is relevant to an eventual bowel transplant.

Conventional atresia management with a high jejunal stoma on the abdominal wall or by similar caliber jejunocolic anastomosis is followed by rapid transit and severe loss of fluid, electrolytes, and nutrients. Anastomosis of the *markedly dilated* proximal jejunum in intestinal atresia, to the smaller diameter distal bowel, is contraindicated since it leads to a "functional obstruction," with failure of propulsion across a patent anastomosis despite active peristalsis (Fig. 28.5). Stasis within the dilated loop generates bacterial overgrowth with D-lactic acidosis, mucosal inflammation, and bacterial translocation causing liver injury and septicemia. If left untreated, the short bowel state is rapidly fatal from dehydration, malnutrition, and sepsis. TPN offers hope of long-term patient survival with reasonable quality of life and opens the way to autologous bowel rehabilitation and reconstruction and, when all else fails, to transplantation.

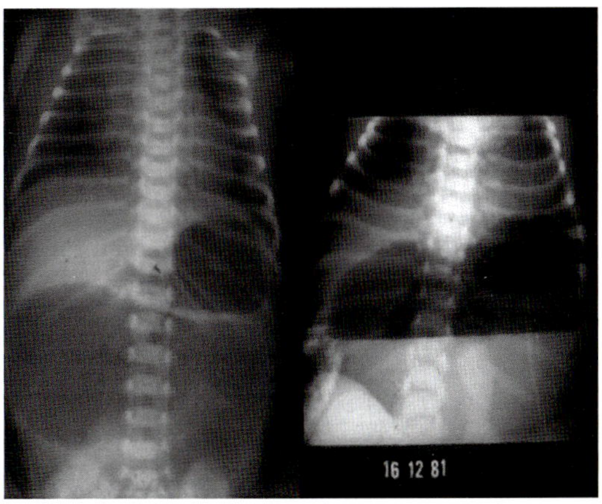

Fig. 28.5 Functional obstruction following a "big-to-small" anastomosis

28.3 The "Hub and Spoke" Model

At an annual incidence of around 1:15,000, the short bowel state in children is of significant impact. Survivors on TPN require intermittent specialist hospital care and long-term home support that places a major burden for dedicated and expensive management on patient's families and on health service providers. It is essential for long-term care to be delivered close to the family home and local community, allowing easier access to the child for better integration within family and social life and for keeping the family unit within their established work, school, and social environment. Management is best guided from a dedicated specialist pediatric IF and PSBS center (Table 28.1), that is preferably also close to adult services. Its role is to provide advice, training, and support to local carers, to offer specialist surgical and other clinical services and to generate a reference database and research. The specialist center will cover a wide area and will act as a "hub" offering support to less experienced referring hospitals and local services ("spokes").

Ongoing care is delivered through the local services and the referring hospital, with patients transferring to the center only at the request of local clinicians for specific surgical episodes and planned review. The basic mandate of the central team (Table 28.2) at the hub is *to help the parents to manage their child's problem*. The team coordinator and nurse specialists are essential for implementing an agreed patient-specific management plan and for the training and transfer of care to the family and the local carers, thereby retaining a "functional family unit within their local community."

28.4 The Patient-Specific PSBS Management Plan

A high level of cooperation between the different medical specialities and the parents is essential at every stage. Survival is followed by implementation of a patient-specific management plan (Table 28.3) that is agreed between the specialist

Table 28.1 "Hub and Spoke" model for PSBS care

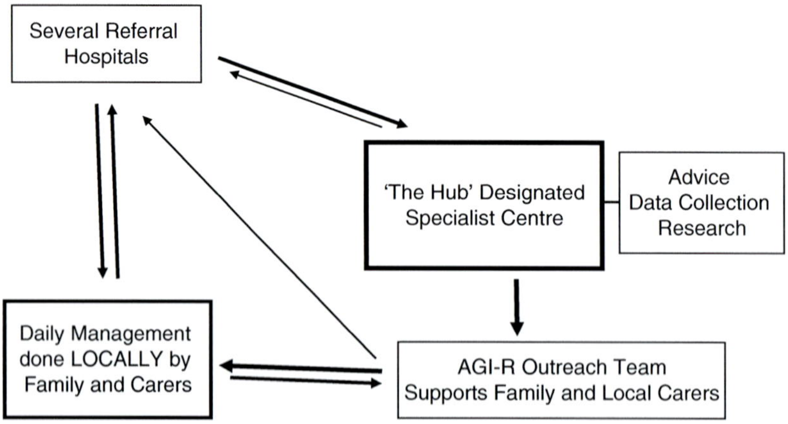

Table 28.2 Multidisciplinary Team essential to appropriate PSBS management

Team coordinator	The referring hospital
Gastroenterologist	Specialist outreach team
Neonatal-Pediatric Surgeon	HPN team
Psychologist	Social services support
Nutritionist	Family doctor
Pharmacist	Others – radiology, anesthesia
Play workers	
Transplant team	

team at the hub, the local clinical services, and the family. As the child stabilizes, the family rapidly takes on the responsibility for delivery of *in-hospital* care, including cyclical TPN and enteral feeding, also taking the child home during the daytime. Hospitalization is kept to a minimum, and home parenteral nutrition (HPN) completes the transfer of care to the home.

28.5 The "Dedicated" Central Venous Feeding Catheter

A secure central venous catheter is conveniently placed, to be used solely for long-term cyclical parenteral nutrition. The cuffed single-lumen catheter (Broviac), of narrowest gauge consistent with the child's size and TPN requirement (4.2–6 F), is passed by open or percutaneous access preferably through the neck veins, verifying by intraoperative ultrasound or radiology the tip position at the junction of the superior vena cava with the right atrium. The catheter should be handled only by nominated carers under strict sterile conditions to minimize the risk of infection, occlusion, and central vein thrombosis. Experience has confirmed the much reduced incidence of catheter complications and sepsis associated with nominated catheter care and HPN. At each use the hub should be thoroughly cleansed with a Hibiscrub (Chlorhexidine) soap solution (or similar) and then immersed in absolute alcohol to ensure sterility. After each use it should be flushed with 0.9% IV saline solution and locked during injection of 1–2 ml of a urokinase solution (1000 units/ml) to avoid intra-catheter backflow and thrombosis and to keep the lumen free of deposits.

It is important to differentiate between catheter-related sepsis with skin organisms (*Staphylococcus albus*, *Staphylococcus aureus*) and septicemia from gram-negative intestinal bacteria (*Escherichia coli*, *Klebsiella*) that requires appropriate bowel management. Catheter change should be kept to a minimum and only if through-catheter antibiotic therapy and urokinase lock have not been successful at eliminating catheter sepsis. Prolonged broad-spectrum or multiple antibiotic therapy is inadvisable and likely to lead to fungal (*Candida*) catheter infection, cardiac colonization, and sepsis. Persistent significant infection, irreparable catheter damage, and catheter occlusion will require a change of central line that should be

Table 28.3 Structured plan for management of pediatric short bowel state

The Child: Survival & Growth

Intact Liver	**Oral Enteral Feeds**	**Normal Psychology**
No/Low Soya TPN - ↓ Sepsis	Habit - Mucosal Stimulus	Family - Social & Community

Preserve Venous Access

- **Dedicated Catheter Care**
- **Urokinase Lock**
- Antibiotics prn
- Reuse of Venous Access Sites

The Bowel

- **Conserve All viable bowel**
- **Minimal Early Surgery** – Tube-stomas
- **Patient-specific A G I R** – Expansion & 'Housekeeping'
  - Tailoring and lengthening
  - Reversed Segments & Other
  - Pharmacology
  - **Transplantation**

undertaken through the same venous access site as often as possible. Loss of venous access sites for essential TPN seriously compromises long-term survival, limits opportunity for autologous bowel reconstruction, and forces earlier referral for "rescue" bowel transplantation.

Extensive central vein thrombosis is difficult to treat, eventually forcing complex catheter placement transhepatically or by open access to the right atrium. Highly specialist interventional radiological techniques are being developed for canalizing and stenting thrombosed central veins, thereby relieving cardiac strain and establishing the high venous flow that is necessary for a central feeding catheter.

28.6 Total Parenteral Nutrition and Home Parenteral Nutrition

The child with extensive bowel loss and intestinal failure will require a long period of parenteral nutrition to ensure survival and growth. Present-day regimens, although still not perfect, will provide sufficient fluid, electrolytes, and nutrients for normal physical and mental development and for supporting long-term life. Fat- and water-soluble vitamin and trace element supplements (zinc, copper, selenium, manganese) attempt to replace normal intake and reduce deficiencies. It is not the scope of this dissertation to detail the composition of the parenteral solutions and supplements that is available from the manufacturers and appropriate texts. As absorption improves with increasing bowel adaptation, the volume and composition of IV fluid and nutrients and the ratio of parenteral to enteral nutrition will alter with reduction of the parenteral component. It is relevant to track daily calorific intake and to avoid hyperalimentation. Whereas parenteral protein and carbohydrate solutions are now largely standardized, there is still difficulty over the lipid component. Following the work of Clayton [3] and Iyer [4] demonstrating the cholestatic effect of contaminant plant phytosterols, it is now well accepted that plant phytosterols within soya-based lipid solutions induce a rapidly progressive hepatitis and end-stage liver failure. A new less toxic intravenous lipid solution derived from fish oils containing omega-3 fatty acids is preferable for long-term parenteral nutrition; however on its own, it does not provide a full range of essential fatty acids. A combination of small amounts of soya-based lipid, medium-chain triglycerides, olive oil, and fish oil (SMOF) provides a more complete lipid profile.

Once TPN is established and the family is familiar with its cyclical nighttime delivery, appropriate funding and practical arrangements are made for home parenteral nutrition. This is an involved process that requires the provision of sufficient home storage space for equipment and refrigeration facilities for the TPN solutions that are often delivered on a weekly basis by a specialist company. The family home may need spatial adjustment to provide a dedicated "clean area" for central vein catheter care that is so crucial to long-term survival.

28.7 Enteral Nutrition and Brain Learning

Neonatal physiology dictates that the newborn child must learn feeding (bolus formation, swallowing) and food recognition (taste, texture) through the stimulus of normal oral feeding that commences immediately at birth. It is not uncommon in order to maximize absorption that the PSBS child with rapid transit and large enteral losses, is often continuously drip fed by nasogastric or gastrostomy tube and is denied the cyclical oral bolus feeding with normal foods at normal rate and volume that is crucial to brain learning. Food intake and enjoyment is a key element of long-term good quality life, and failure to develop a basic feeding pattern in physiological time will persist as serious "food aversion and denial," becoming an intractable problem even after enteral autonomy is established.

In striving to maximize absorption, predigested and elemental diets can sometimes prove helpful. However there is little evidence that predigested and elemental diets, even given continuously or cyclically, are better than normal foods at stimulating the mucosal adaptation response and increasing absorption. Additives in the form of starches (rice) and proteins are better absorbed and serve also to thicken the food, whereas fats in the form of medium-chain triglycerides (MCT) are more easily absorbed. It is particularly relevant to remember that food needs to be palatable if it is to be acceptable to the PSBS child, and it cannot be overemphasized that it is normal food given orally and following a normal feeding pattern that are most acceptable and by far the best stimulus for natural mucosal adaptation. It is important to recognize the diverse beneficial effects, in supplementing TPN, of even small amounts of normal foods locally within the bowel and generally following absorption in reducing deficits, protecting the liver and sustaining the intricate enzyme systems relevant to cellular functions.

28.8 Family and Social Life

Long-term survival accentuates the need for a home and social life of quality for both the child and the family. During the initial admission, the delivery of *in-hospital* care is taken up by the family who learns to set up cyclical parenteral nutrition over the night hours and who takes the child home during the day. HPN allows complete transfer of care to the home and has the advantage of a much reduced rate of central venous feeding catheter sepsis. Home care is supported by local carers and specialist nurses from the "hub" so that the family is kept as a "unit within its local environment" where the child finds opportunity for acceptance and bonding and interaction with siblings and friends.

28.9 Autologous Gastrointestinal Rehabilitation (AGI-R)

The surgical management of the short bowel state is a multistage program working with the natural intestinal adaptation response to increase absorption and to develop new functional bowel suitable for reconstruction [5]. It spans a prolonged period and requires determination and a strong commitment from the patient, the family, and the carers.

28.10 Acute Surgery

Of equal importance to child survival is "bowel salvage" which will determine the quality of long-term life. Thus earlier surgical intervention before bowel necrosis provides an opportunity for minimal resection and maximal conservation of potentially viable bowel. Conventional management with a high proximal jejunostomy on the abdomen or a jejunocolic anastomosis with bowel of similar caliber leads to uncontrollable large volume losses. A large-to-small caliber anastomosis causes "functional obstruction" (Fig. 28.5) with failure of propulsion across a patent anastomosis despite active peristalsis.

It is preferable to establish *controllable* intraluminal drainage through a tube jejunostomy brought out onto the abdominal wall, with a wide-bore catheter (Malecot, de Pezzer, Foley) that is passed into the distal end of the proximal jejunal loop (Fig. 28.6a, b), also closing off any pre-existing stoma. The child is immediately able to feed orally (Fig. 28.7), providing the crucial natural stimulus for brain learning and a lifelong feeding pattern and delivering the essential nutrient stimulus for mucosal adaptation. A second smaller gauge catheter is passed into the proximal end of any functional distal bowel (commonly the left colon) and brought out onto the abdominal wall. The jejunostomy effluent is stored at 4 °C to limit bacterial overgrowth [6] and is sieved and warmed for recycle through the distal catheter by slow

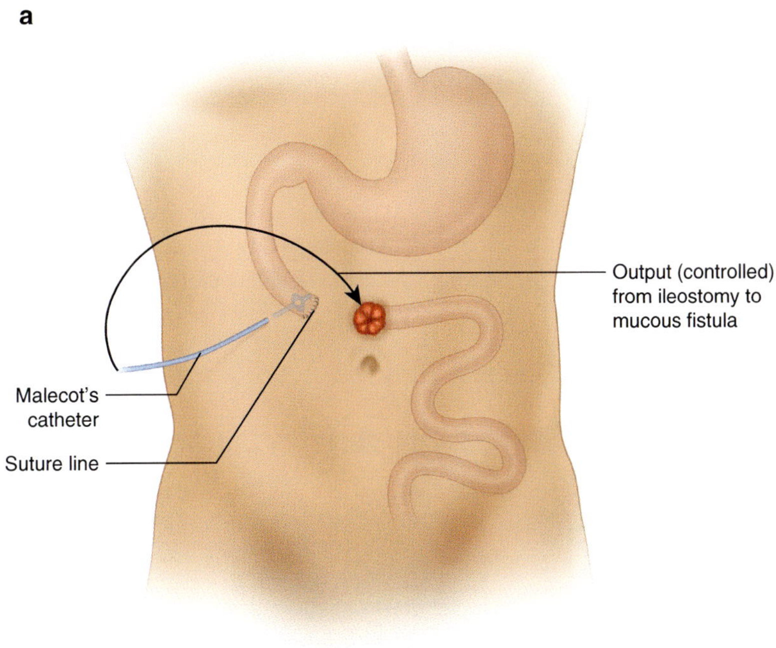

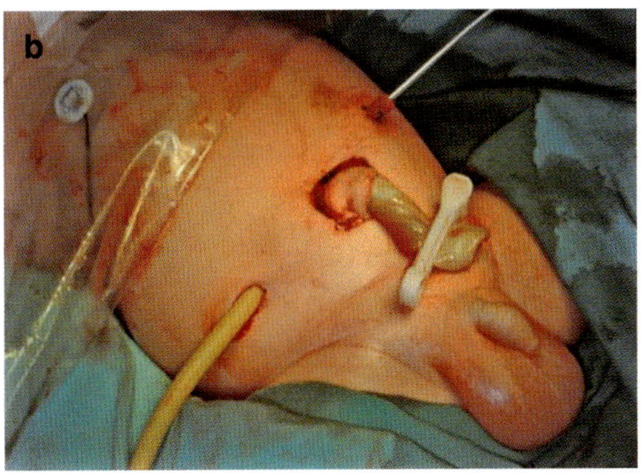

Fig. 28.6 Tube jejunostomy: (**a**) diagram, (**b**) tube jejunostomy only (no functional bowel distally)

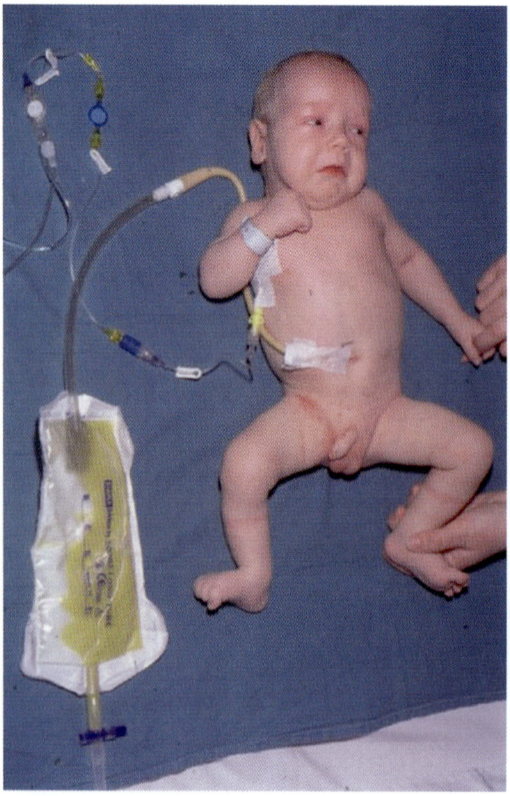

Fig. 28.7 Tube jejunostomy – child able to feed orally and effluent collected for recycle as in (Fig. 28.8)

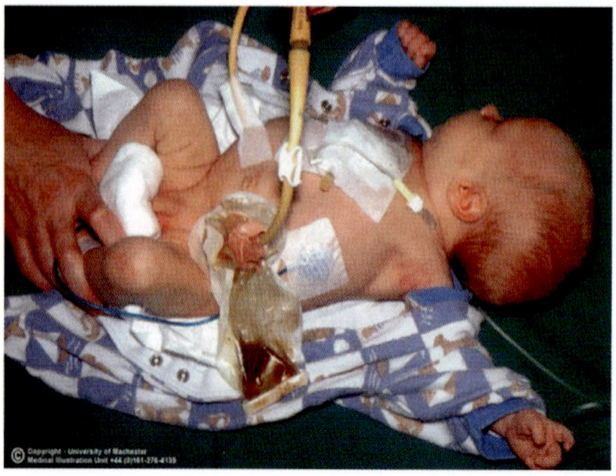

Fig. 28.8 Double-tube stomas for jejunal drainage and bowel expansion. Distal tube stoma for colonic recycle

Table 28.4 Advantages of "controllable" tube stomas

Proximal tube stoma	Distal tube-stoma
Minimal bowel surgery and no loss of bowel	Recycle of proximal collected nutrients
Overcomes jejunal obstruction and allows free drainage	Stimulation and adaptation of distal bowel
Access to the jejunal lumen for washout, bacteriology, etc.	Increased absorption of fluid, electrolytes and nutrients
Allows immediate full oral feeding	Allows physiological cortico-anal learning for continence
Gives control of proximal jejunal losses and longer nutrient contact with the absorptive mucosa	Develops normal perianal skin toleration of feces
Timed occlusion forces bowel elongation and dilatation with generation of new full-thickness functional tissue	Easily replaceable

gavage or syringe pump infusion during the night hours, to stimulate adaptation and absorption particularly of fluids and electrolytes from the distal bowel (Fig. 28.8 and Table 28.4).

The recycle of jejunostomy effluent into the distal bowel has other major advantages in simulating normality with improvement of colonic function and the passage of stools and flatus transanally that allows for the development of cortico-anal neural pathways relevant to continence and avoids severe perianal excoriation by habituation of the perianal skin to fecal flow.

28.11 "Controlled" Bowel Expansion and "Housekeeping"

Intermittent clamping of the proximal tube jejunostomy allows effective control of jejunostomy losses that is not possible with a conventional stoma on the abdominal wall, and prolongs contact of nutrients with the mucosa to promote absorption. The periods of tube jejunostomy occlusion are gradually increased from an initial 10 min to 2–3 hours and alternate with "jejunal housekeeping" that consists of brief periods of complete loop drainage and an occasional washout to avoid intraluminal stasis and bacterial overgrowth. Over a 6-month period, such controlled obstruction forces a gradual natural bowel elongation and dilatation that generates new full-thickness functional autologous tissue for reconstruction [7]. Mucosal adaptation and greater absorption become manifest as an increasing tolerance of enteral feeding and a steady weight gain, with a welcome reduction in parenteral nutrition.

28.12 Autologous Gastrointestinal Reconstruction (AGIR)

Dilatation is a valuable asset for autologous reconstruction [8]. The dilated bowel is tailored to a normal propulsive diameter with the excess vascularized tissue being used to increase bowel length. Isoperistaltic bowel continuity through the anus can be established at the same time, or another tube jejunostomy can be placed at the distal end of the lengthened jejunum for a second phase of expansion and lengthening.

28.13 Bowel Tailoring and Lengthening Techniques

Following the original publication by Bianchi in 1980 [9] on longitudinal intestinal lengthening and tailoring (LILT) and its first successful clinical application to a 4-year-old boy by Boeckman and Traylor [10], there are presently three techniques available for tailoring and lengthening the small bowel and the colon that can be applied separately, in combination, or sequentially.

28.14 Longitudinal Intestinal Lengthening and Tailoring (LILT)

This procedure divides the dilated bowel longitudinally along its antimesenteric and mesenteric borders (Fig. 28.9), passing along an ample natural intra-mesenteric plane which easily develops by blunt dissection between the mesenteric vessels that enter the bowel one-third of the way up each sidewall.

Bowel division with the cutting wave of the bipolar diathermy (Fig. 28.10) is relatively

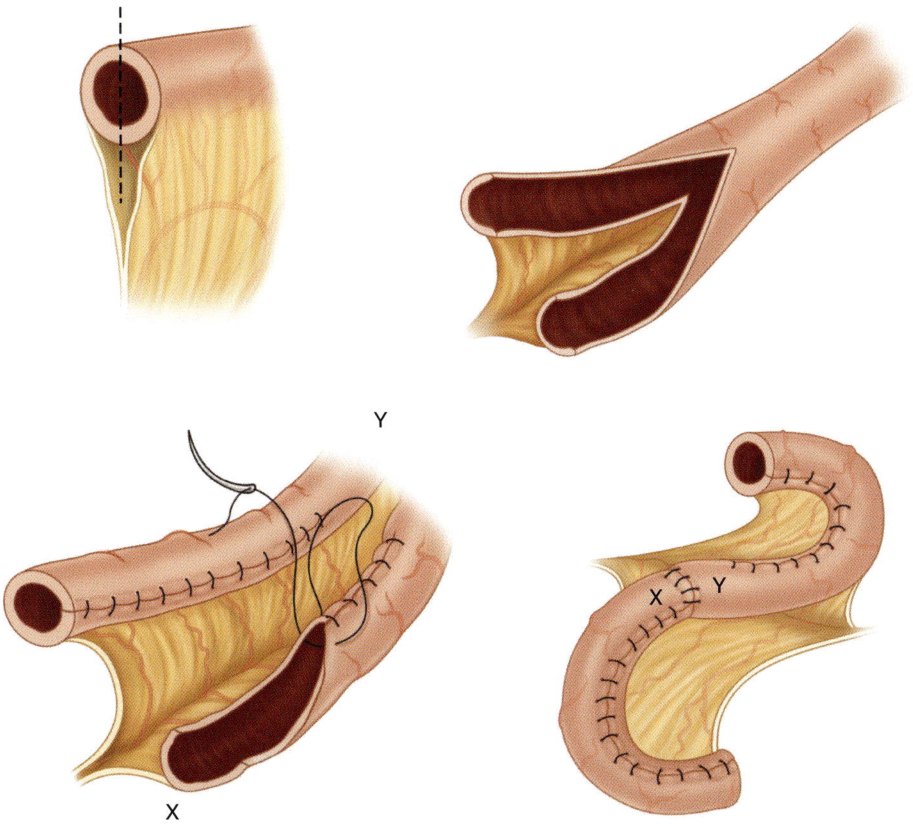

Fig. 28.9 Longitudinal intestinal lengthening and tailoring – LILT diagram

bloodless and is safer than stapling for avoiding injury to the mesenteric vessels. The vascularized hemisegments (Fig. 28.11) are sutured manually under clear vision, turning the cut margins inward toward the lumen, to form two tubes of equal length (Fig. 28.12) that are anastomosed *isoperistaltically* and to the distal bowel to establish bowel continuity (Fig. 28.13).

LILT converts the dysfunctional dilated loop, to a peristaltic propulsive bowel of half the diameter and double the length of the original dilated segment, retaining all absorptive tissue and without significant disturbance to peristalsis. It is applicable to dilated small bowel and colon, but is not suitable for the dilated duodenum. LILT cannot be repeated, but can be applied to the bowel that has been previously tailored and lengthened by other methods.

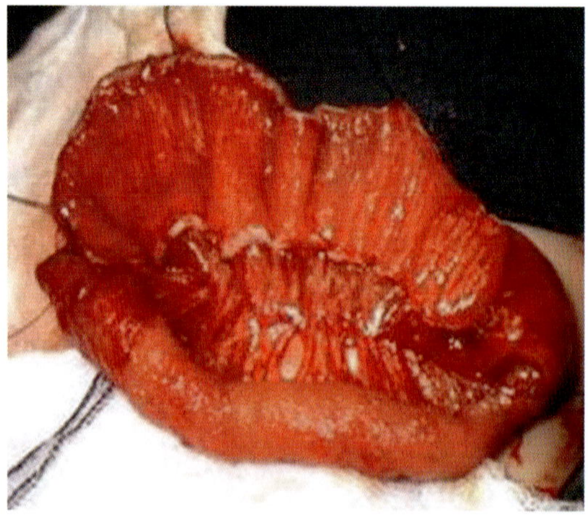

Fig. 28.12 LILT – tubularized hemisegments of half diameter

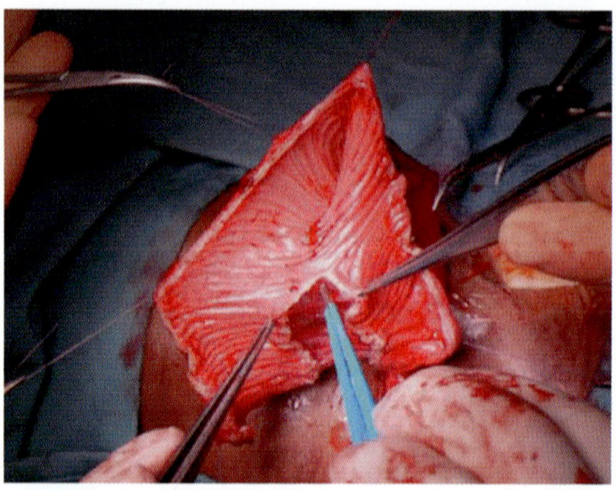

Fig. 28.10 LILT – Bowel division with bipolar cutting wave for bloodless bowel surgery

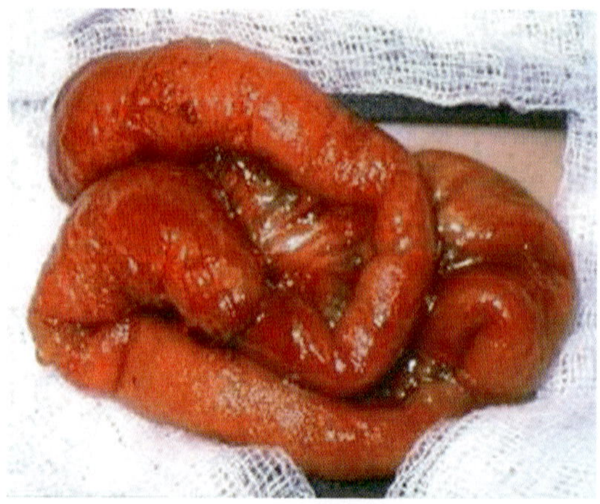

Fig. 28.13 Longitudinally tailored jejunum anastomosed isoperistaltically to double the original length, and anastomosed to the colon

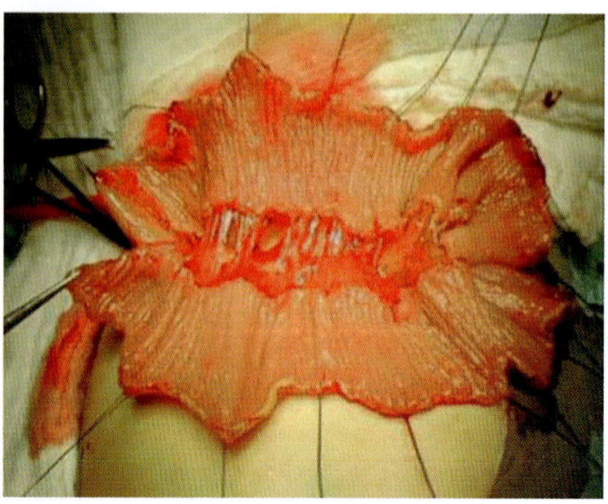

Fig. 28.11 LILT – vascularized hemisegments after longitudinal division

28.15 Serial Transverse Enteroplasty (STEP)

The technique was introduced in 2003 by Kim et al. [11, 12] as an alternative to LILT, but has found application also in combination with, or after LILT for additional tailoring and lengthening. The Endo-GIA autostapler (Covidien (UK) Commercial Ltd.) is applied alternately to either side along the length of the dilated loop (Fig. 28.14), passing parallel to the mesenteric vessels and without dissection within the mesentery.

To avoid stenosis the residual bowel diameter should be of at least 2 cm, and it is preferable to oversew the tip of each staple line to ensure that there is no leakage. The technique is also suitable for tailoring the dilated duodenum. Recurrent bowel dilatation can be managed by a second STEP; however further STEPs beyond this may severely disrupt peristalsis and propulsion.

28.16 Spiral Intestinal Lengthening and Tailoring (SILT)

Spiral tailoring and lengthening was introduced in 2010 by Cserni et al. [13] and is a welcome addition to LILT [9] and STEP [11, 12]. This technique cuts the dilated bowel at a 60° angle, spiraling along its length (Fig. 28.15). The bowel is incised with the cutting wave of the bipolar diathermy with minimal blood loss and under clear vision, passing between the mesenteric vessels. Release incisions are made at the mesenteric border extending longitudinally in the avascular mesentery toward the mesenteric base, to allow free rotation during elongation and suturing.

The opened-out bowel is stretched and draped over a large guide catheter, allowing tissue rotation, and is sutured to form a well-vascularized

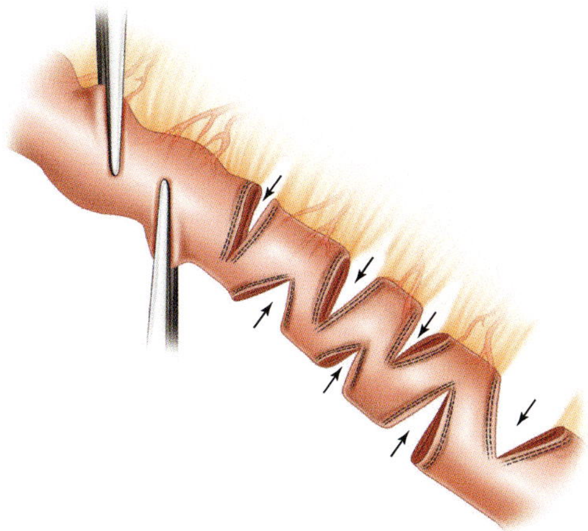

Fig. 28.14 Serial transverse enteroplasty (STEP) according to Kim et al.

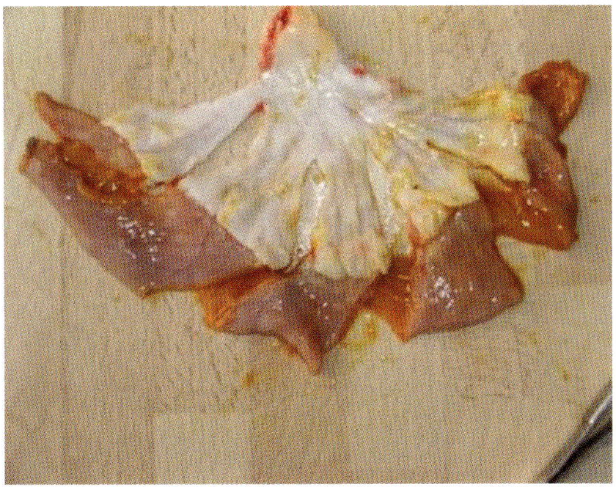

Fig. 28.15 Spiral intestinal lengthening and tailoring (SILT) according to Cserni et al. showing 60° spiral incision

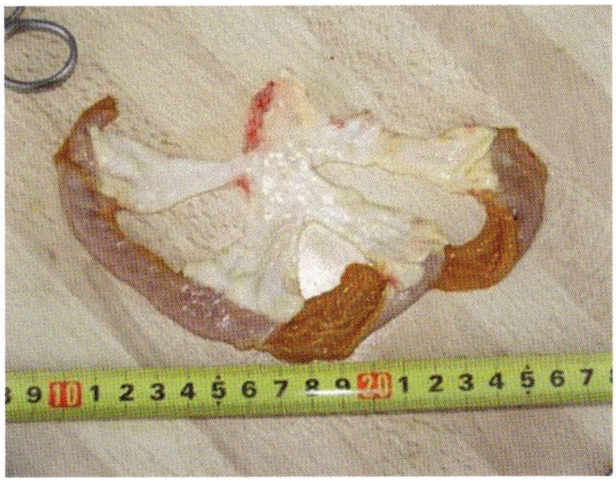

Fig. 28.16 SILT demonstrating elongation and diameter reduction and longitudinal incisions in the avascular mesentery to allow free rotation during suture

elongated bowel of 2 cm propulsive diameter (Fig. 28.16) that can be placed in immediate bowel continuity with the distal colon or can be catheter intubated for further bowel expansion. SILT does not disrupt peristalsis, can be repeated in the event of recurrent dilatation, and can be used in combination or subsequent to LILT and STEP.

28.17 The Post-tailoring and Lengthening Phase

Following the three lengthening procedures, routine post-laparotomy healing should be expected with a rapid return of bowel function within a few days. There is no operative mortality, and morbidity is minimal. Vascular problems are rare, but loss of a hemisegment following LILT has been reported [14]. Suture line dehiscence is unusual, and rarely, cutaneous and interloop fistulae or anastomotic stenoses may develop. It is usual for lengthening procedures to be followed by a reduction in bowel-related sepsis, a steady increase in absorption and enteral feeding, and a reduction in parenteral nutrition with possible enteral autonomy within 4–12 months. However bowel adaptation is known to continue for several years so that persistence is required, and "cutoff points" [15] are inappropriate. A healthier bowel and increasing adaptation and enteral nutrition are also associated with improvement in liver function and general health [16]. Recurrence of bowel-related septicemia and D-lactic acidosis suggest stenosis, stasis within a diverticulum, or excessive recurrent dilatation that can be a welcome opportunity for additional tailoring and lengthening and are best dealt with surgically. Failure to progress toward enteral autonomy is an indication for further reconstruction that may take the form of a repeat bowel expansion and lengthening and/or the addition of supplementary procedures.

28.18 Supplementary Procedures

Few of the previously published procedures designed to delay transit and to increase mucosal contact have come to regular application because, on their own, the outcome has been inconsistent.

Colonic interposition (Fig. 28.17) transposes a segment of iso- or antiperistaltic colon proximal to the jejunum [17] or between the jejunum and the ileum [18] and uses the slower motility of the colon to pass nutrients over the small bowel absorptive surface [19]. Antiperistaltic or reversed small bowel segments (Fig. 28.18) are simple to construct; however the length of the segment is critical to success. Publications by Pigot et al. [20] and Panis et al. [21] have reported good outcomes with lengths of 15 cm in young adults. All of their patients returned to functional social lives, with half dispensing with parenteral nutrition within 36 months and others taking significantly longer (>4 years) to reach

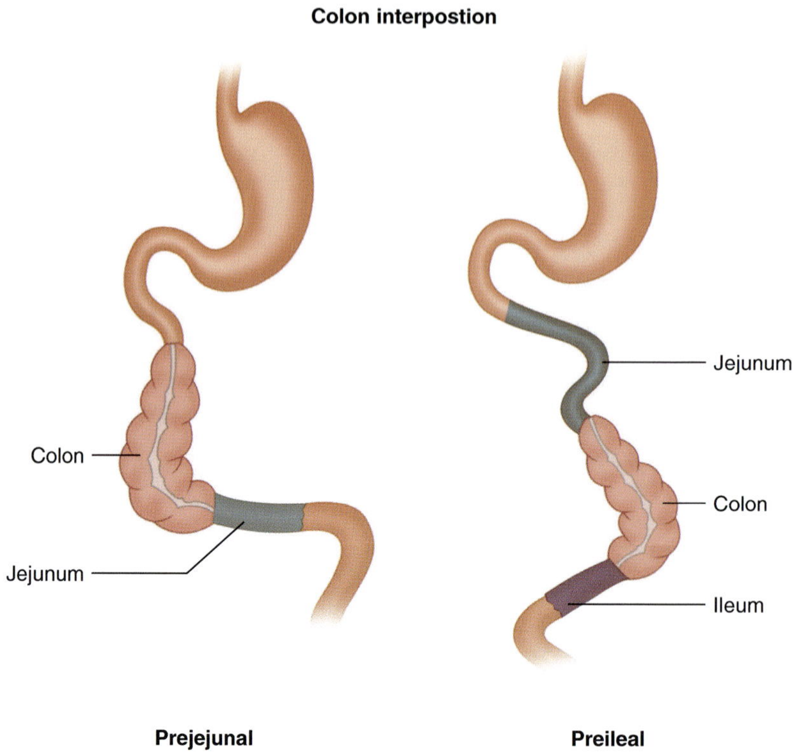

Fig. 28.17 Prejejunal and preileal colon interposition

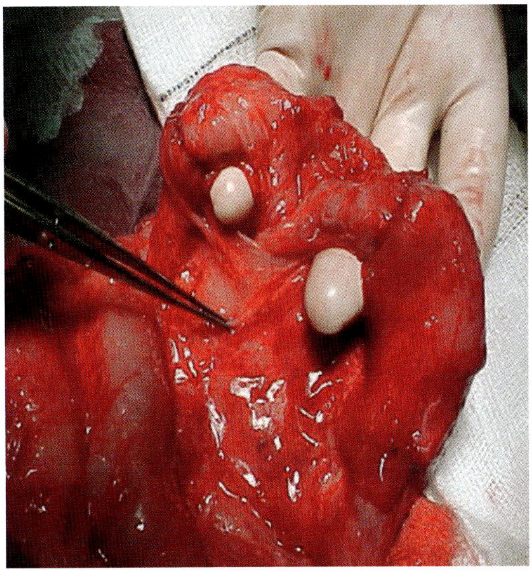

Fig. 28.18 Reversed (antiperistaltic) small bowel segment of 12 cm length

enteral autonomy. Children require a length of 5–15 cm (depending on age) to effectively slow transit without causing functional obstruction and stasis. Multiple reversed segments can be placed along the small bowel, but the position and length for maximal effect are as yet undetermined.

28.19 Combined or Sequential Reconstruction

Bowel reconstruction for the short bowel state is a patient-specific structured program of timely interventions designed to enhance natural bowel adaptation (Table 28.5). There has been greater success when procedures have been combined or added sequentially rather than when used alone. Thus controllable catheter bowel expansion is followed by tailoring and lengthening on one or several occasions, with constant pharmacological enhancement of absorption, and supplementary surgery (reversed segments or colon interposition) as relevant. As experience increases it may be appropriate to combine two or more procedures at the same session e.g. lengthening with reversed segments, for better absorption and a more rapid conversion to enteral autonomy

Table 28.5 Autologous gastrointestinal reconstructive techniques for management of the short bowel state

Bowel tailoring	Antimesenteric tailoring
	Plication
Bowel expansion	*Controlled jejunal occlusion* and *recycle* (Bianchi)
	Uncontrollable semiobstructive valve (Georgeson)
Tailoring and lengthening	*LILT* and combined LILT (Bianchi)
	STEP and second STEP (Kim et al.)
	SILT and combined SILT (Cserni et al.)
	Colonic lengthening by LILT (Devesa et al) by SILT (Alberti et al, Bianchi)
Delaying Transit	Single/Multiple Reversed (antiperistaltic) Segments
	Prejejunal/preileal colonic Interposition (iso-/antiperistaltic)
	IC valve substitutes
Pharmacology	Loperamide, *oral clonidine*, GLP-2 (teduglutide)
	Proton pump inhibitors
	Antibiotics
	Probiotics
	Manipulation of Multibionta
Transplantation	Isolated small bowel, small bowel + colon
	Liver + bowel, multivisceral

28.20 Pharmacology

Pharmacological management is invaluable in reducing potential complications and increasing absorption. Antacids and proton pump inhibitors are relevant to counteract the hyperchlorhydria from the hypergastrinemia that is associated with SBS and that induces gastritis and duodenal ulceration. High-dose loperamide and codeine help to increase mucosal contact time by slowing small bowel transit. Clonidine, an alpha-2-adrenergic blocker, when given in low oral dose [22] or transdermally [23] as a skin patch, significantly increases the absorption of fluids and electrolytes. It is thought to act preferentially on sodium uptake from the colon, but clinical experience has demonstrated its value in increasing fluid, electrolyte, and nutrient absorption also from the small bowel when the colon has been totally absent. The low oral dose has no effect on blood pressure; however as adaptation occurs, increased clonidine absorption may induce sedation and drowsiness.

Glucagon-like peptide 2 (GLP-2) is a powerful intestinotrophic mediator that is naturally produced in the ascending colon and induces small bowel hyperplasia [24]. Effort should therefore be made to preserve the ascending colon during surgery. Early trials suggest that GLP-2 can be of great value in driving intestinal adaptation [25], but it is as yet uncertain whether the mucosal hyperplasia is sustained once it is withdrawn. Concerns have been expressed over its long-term use because of possible induction of gut neoplasia.

Children with PSBS who have lost their ileal vit B_{12} absorption sites will require lifelong replacement. Water-soluble and fat-soluble vitamin supplements are routinely given enterally and parenterally, but requirements will alter as enteral absorption increases. Similarly iron and trace element (zinc, copper, selenium, magnesium) supplements are necessary to avoid deficiencies and to sustain metabolism and growth. The loss of ileal bile salt binding sites interferes with the enterohepatic bile salt circulation and leads to the excretion of an abnormal bile with a high risk of cholelithiasis. Free bile acids passing into the colon have a laxative effect and are unavailable for combining with fats, which then bind dietary calcium leaving free oxalates that are absorbed from the colon and excreted in the urine, with a higher risk of urinary calculi. Cholestyramine given orally binds bile salts and counteracts these colonic effects, but long-term use has been associated with neoplasia.

Continuous administration of broad-spectrum antibiotics and attempts at "bowel sterilization" are largely contraindicated. Repeated gut-related infection is often due to stenosis, sepsis within diverticulae, or to recurrent bowel dilatation with stasis and should be managed surgically. Some children will continue to present with recurrent symptomatic D-lactic acidosis that is an indicator of intraluminal bacterial overgrowth and that may then require long-term oral chemotherapeutic (metronidazole) or antibiotic (erythromycin, vancomycin, gentamicin) therapy.

Probiotics can sometimes prove useful in colonizing the gut with helpful organisms that may actively suppress pathogens. There is increasing interest in the normal beneficial symbiotic microbiota (bacterial flora) [26] in the gut, which may be relevant to absorption, immunological function, and general good health. Manipulation of gut flora may play a useful role in the overall management of the short bowel state and is a serious consideration for limiting the use of broad-spectrum antibiotics.

28.21 Experimental Developments

Experimental work with stem cells has been successful at generating "human intestinal organoids" from human pluripotent stem cells [27], possessing all of the neuromuscular elements and the diverse mucosal cells and enzymes appropriate to human small bowel. Such specimens, of only 1 cm size and without a mesentery, are grown as grafts on the kidney of specific nonreactive mice, but are vascularized only by recipient mouse vessels. Although presently limited to the laboratory and far from clinical application, such research provides understanding and additional promise for the future.

28.22 Long-Term Life

TPN, the move away from hepatotoxic soya-based lipids, and preservation of venous access have given a long-term lifeline to the PSBS patient. Thus 10-year survival on total parenteral nutrition alone is now over 92 %, and the longest survivor has had TPN for >40 years. However serious psychological issues may arise, and patients will occasionally reach a point of resenting their TPN dependence and refuse essential TPN support. The psychologist is a major member of the management team supporting the family from an early stage, offering an ongoing care commitment, and taking the child and family through adolescence and into adulthood.

AGIR with a structured combination of procedures has made significant inroads toward total enteral autonomy. The degree of enteral absorption determines the quantity and quality of intravenous supplements so that some patients may absorb sufficient nutrients but will still require partial fluid and electrolyte support and/or the occasional TPN boost. Several patients still manage a social and work life of acceptable quality, which is reduced by the nighttime obligatory intravenous supplements and other bowel-related factors, e.g. stoma, frequency of motions, and fecal soiling.

Many of the long-term survivors, largely managed by the LILT technique, are now approaching 20–35 years of enteral autonomy and have appreciably normal social lives. The majority have bowel continuity without a stoma and are continent, passing some 4–6 semisolid or liquid motions daily. They have shown good physical and mental growth through puberty achieving a reasonable, if not always normal, physique. Some have had uncomplicated pregnancies without additional parenteral feeding [28] and have delivered normal children. Long-term complications have not been marked; however there is an increased incidence of gallstones and renal oxalate stones and a tendency to osteoporosis. Colicky abdominal pain has sometimes been a feature, which should be investigated for possible bowel stenosis that is amenable to surgery. Similarly D-lactic acidosis, diarrhea, ulceration, and bleeding may be a consequence of bacterial overgrowth within dilated or obstructed loops or diverticulae that although manageable by a reduced carbohydrate diet and cyclical oral nonabsorbable antibiotics, may better respond to surgical intervention. Recurrent dilatation is not always unwelcome and, when complicated by stasis and sepsis, is amenable to further bowel tailoring and possibly lengthening.

Common to patients undergoing AGIR and transplant is the not infrequent recalcitrant problem of food aversion that is particularly marked in children who have not been fed orally during the neonatal period. These patients remain gastrostomy or feeding-tube dependent despite having achieved enteral autonomy, highlighting the need to recognize the importance of brain learning for food recognition during the early weeks of postnatal life. Older patients may present with food refusal or aversion as a symptom of more severe psychological illness and merit ongoing skilled psychological care.

It is not the intention, in this discourse, to list every complication but rather to highlight the commoner long-term concerns. Suffice to say that the majority of patients undergoing bowel reconstruction have achieved enteral autonomy and are physically and mentally stable, with a minority who still require a much reduced level of parenteral support, often only fluid and electrolyte supplements, and still able to lead lives of acceptable quality.

28.23 Transplantation

Transplantation should be regarded as a very definite and significant option for those suffering from intestinal failure. Patients with no residual small bowel, those with a poor quality of life despite autologous reconstruction, and those with precarious venous access or severe hepatic disease will be candidates for isolated bowel, liver-bowel, or multivisceral transplant. Better understanding and more refined immunosuppression have increased graft and patient survival to >95 % at 1 year with most patients on enteral nutrition alone. However despite the more recent inclusion of the colon with the graft, posttransplant bowel function is not normal with an increased frequency of motions. The need for constant monitoring detracts from the quality of life, and acute graft rejection, sepsis, and an increased incidence of posttransplant lymphoproliferative disease reduce the 5-year survival to 55–65 %. Chronic graft rejection with loss of graft function and graft-versus-host rejection further reduces survival to 50 % at 10 years. Despite reasonable survival rates, transplantation should not be the first choice but remains a final and most welcome option for those SBS patients who have exhausted autologous bowel alternatives.

Conclusions

The introduction of total parenteral nutrition has been vital for the long-term survival of patients with the short bowel state. The shift away from hepatotoxic soya-based lipids has markedly reduced the liver injury and end-stage liver failure that was a major cause of death or referral for transplantation. Better venous feeding catheter management and HPN have preserved central venous access and have reduced catheter-related sepsis and central vein thrombosis. Long-term survival on TPN opened the way to the development of autologous bowel reconstruction within an intestinal failure rehabilitation program. There is now a better-structured care pathway with improving outcomes so that patients unfortunate enough to suffer disastrous loss of their midgut can genuinely hope for enteral autonomy and good quality life of relatively normal longevity.

References

1. Williamson RC (1978) Intestinal adaptation: structural, functional and cytogenetic changes. N Engl J Med 298(25):1393–1402
2. Williamson RC (1978) Intestinal adaptation: mechanisms of control. N Engl J Med 298(26):1444–1450
3. Clayton PT, Whitfield P, Iyer K (1998) The role of phytosterols in the pathogenesis of liver complications of pediatric parenteral nutrition. Nutrition 14(1):158–164
4. Iyer KR, Spitz L, Clayton P (1998) BAPS prize lecture: new insight into mechanisms of parenteral nutrition-associated cholestasis: role of plant sterols. J Pediatr Surg 33(1):1–6
5. Bianchi A (2006) From the cradle to enteral autonomy: the role of autologous gastrointestinal reconstruction. Gastroenterology 130(2 Suppl 1):S138–S146
6. Pataki I, Szabo J, Varga P, Berkes A, Nagy A, Murphy F, Morabito A, Rakoczy G, Cserni T (2013) Recycling of bowel content: the importance of the right timing. J Pediatr Surg 48(3):579–584
7. Collins J 3rd, Vincente Y, Georgeson K, Kelly D (1996) Partial intestinal obstruction induces substantial mucosal proliferation in the pig. J Pediatr Surg 31(3):415–419
8. Bianchi A, Morabito A (2009) The dilated bowel: a liability and an asset. Semin Pediatr Surg 18(4):249–257
9. Bianchi A (1980) Intestinal loop lengthening – a technique for increasing small intestinal length. J Pediatr Surg 15(2):145–151
10. Boeckman CR, Traylor R (1981) Bowel lengthening for short gut syndrome. J Pediatr Surg 16(6):996–997
11. Kim HB, Fauza D, Garza J, Oh JT, Nurko S, Jaksic T (2003) Serial transverse enteroplasty (STEP): a novel bowel lengthening procedure. J Pediatr Surg 38(3): 425–429
12. Kim HB, Lee PW, Garza J, Duggan C, Fauza D, Jaksic T (2003) Serial transverse enteroplasty for short bowel syndrome: a case report. J Pediatr Surg 38(6):881–885
13. Cserni T, Varga G, Erces D, Kaszaki J, Boros M, Laszio A, Murphy F, Foldvari A, Morabito A, Bianchi A, Rakoczy G (2013) Spiral Intestinal lengthening and Tailoring – first in vivo study. J Pediatr Surg 48(9):1907–1913
14. Thompson JS, Rikkers LF (1987) Surgical alternatives for the short bowel syndrome. Am J Gastroenterol 82(2):97–106
15. Sondheimer JM, Cadnapaphornchai M, Sontag M, Zerbe GO (1998) Predicting the duration of dependence on parenteral nutrition after intestinal resection. J Pediatr 132(1):80–84
16. Iyer KR, Horslen S, Torres C, Vanderhoof JA, Langnas AN (2004) Functional liver recovery parallels autologous gut salvage in short bowel syndrome. J Pediatr Surg 39(3):340–344
17. Hutcher NE, Mendez-Picon G, Salzberg AM (1973) Prejejunal transposition of colon to prevent the development of short bowel syndrome in puppies with 90% small intestine resection. J Pediatr Surg 8(5):771–777
18. Lloyd DA (1978) Colonic interposition between the jejunum and ileum after massive small bowel resection in rats. Prog Pediatr Surg 12:51–106
19. Glick PL, de Lorimier AA, Adzick NS, Harrison MR (1984) Colon Interposition: an adjuvant operation for short gut syndrome. J Pediatr Surg 19(6):719–725
20. Pigot F, Messing B, Chaussade S, Pfeiffer A, Pouliquen X, Jian R (1990) Severe short bowel syndrome with a surgically reversed small bowel segment. Dig Dis Sci 35(1):137–144
21. Panis Y, Messing B, Rivet P, Coffin B, Hautefeuille P, Matuchansky C, Rambaud JC, Valleur P (1997) Segmental reversal of the small bowel as an alternative to intestinal transplantation in patients with short bowel syndrome. Ann Surg 225(4):401–407
22. McDoniel K, Taylor B, Huey W, Eiden K, Everett S, Fleshman J, Buchman TG, Alpers D, Klein S (2004) Use of clonidine to decrease intestinal fluid losses in patients with high-output short-bowel syndrome. J Parenter Enteral Nutr 28(4):265–268
23. Buchman AL, Fryer J, Wallin A, Ahn CW, Polensky S, Zaremba K (2006) Clonidine reduces diarrhea and sodium loss in patients with proximal jejunostomy: a controlled study. J Parenter Enteral Nutr 30(6):487–491
24. Jeppesen PB, Pertkiewicz M, Messing B, Iyer K, Seidner DL, O'keefe SLD, Forbes A, Heinze H, Joelsson B (2012) Teduglutide reduces need for parenteral support among patients with short bowel syndrome with intestinal failure. Gastroenterology 143(6):1473–1481
25. Compher C, Gilroy R, Pertkiewicz M, Ziegler TR, Ratcliffe SJ, Joly F, Rochling F, Messing B (2011) Maintenance of parenteral nutrition volume reduction, without weight loss, after stopping teduglutide in a subset of patients with short bowel syndrome. J Parenter Enteral Nutr 35(5):603–609
26. Goulet O (2015) Potential role of the intestinal microbiota in programming health and disease. Nutr Rev 73(Suppl 1):32–40
27. Watson CL, Mahe MM, Múnera J, Howell JC, Sundaram N, Poling HM, Schweitzer JI, Vallance JE, Mayhew CN, Sun Y, Grabowski G, Finkbeiner SR, Spence JR, Noah F, Shroyer NF, Wells JM, Helmrath MA (2014) An *in vivo* model of human small intestine using pluripotent stem cells. Nat Med 20(11):1310–1314
28. Byrd LM, Johnston TA, Bianchi A (2006) Successful pregnancy following maternal small bowel reconstruction for congenital short bowel syndrome. BJOG 113(1):117–119

Intestinal Polyposis 29

Luca Pio, Alessio Pini Prato, and Girolamo Mattioli

29.1 Introduction

A polyp is any growth or mass protruding from a mucous membrane into the gastrointestinal (GI) tract. Isolated/single polyps usually occur in children with an overall incidence of 2% without an increased risk of gastrointestinal cancer [1]. Multiple polyps (juvenile polyposis syndrome) are relatively rare, with an incidence ranging between 0.625 and 1 into 100,000 children [2] and a predisposition toward malignancy [3].

Histologically, polyposis is classified as hamartomatous or adenomatous polyposis.

29.1.1 Hamartomatous Polyposis

29.1.1.1 Juvenile Polyposis

As defined by the WHO classification, juvenile polyposis (JP) is a familial cancer syndrome with an autosomal dominant trait [4]. Initially reported by McColl in 1964 [5], the diagnosis is based on the following major diagnostic criteria reported by the World Health Organization (WHO) [6]:

- More than five juvenile polyps in the colon or rectum
- Juvenile polyps throughout the gastrointestinal tract
- Any number of juvenile polyps in a person with a family history of juvenile polyposis

JP has an incidence ranging between 0.625 and 1 into 100,000 children without gender preponderance. In the vast majority of cases, JP is diagnosed before the second decade of life, usually between 6 months and 5 years of age [7, 8]. JP can involve the entire GI tract without a specific site preponderance. Though, in majority of cases, they occur in the hindgut.

Presenting symptoms include abdominal pain, prolapse, intussusception, anemia, melena, and protein-losing enteropathy. The most severe form presents in infancy with severe diarrhea, hypoalbuminemia, macrocephaly, and a worse prognosis. The severity of manifestation is directly related to the number of polyps.

Congenital associated malformations can occur in 11–15% of patients, involving the genitourinary tract, central nervous system, heart and soft tissues with hemorrhagic telangiectasia, and arteriovenous malformations reported in several papers [4].

The macroscopic aspect of polyps is characterized by the sessile aspect in the stomach and pedunculated polyps in the other GI tract with a maximum diameter approaching 5 cm. Multilobulated polyps represent 20% of the overall JP. The histopathology reveals edematous stroma, dilated glands, and inflammatory cells.

L. Pio • A. Pini Prato • G. Mattioli (✉)
Pediatric Surgery Unit, Istituto Giannina Gaslini, DINOGMI University of Genoa, Via Getolamo Gaslini 5, 16147 Genoa, Italy
e-mail: girolamomattioli@ospedale-gaslini.ge.it

M. Lima (ed.), *Pediatric Digestive Surgery*, DOI 10.1007/978-3-319-40525-4_29

Molecular genetics demonstrated germline mutations of BMPR1A and SMAD4 genes in up to 20–30 % of patients, with incomplete penetrance. These genes are involved in the TGF-B/BMP pathway, essential for a correct intestinal development. Around 20–50 % of patients have a family history of JP [9].

A malignant transformation can involve up to 20 % of JP located in the upper GI and 34 % for those in the colon and rectum, with an overall cumulative risk of malignant transformation of 39 % [10]. No risk analysis was ever performed with regard to the development of upper GI cancer [3]. Nonetheless, prevention and surveillance is based on genotype as SMAD4 mutations seem to be associated to a further increased risk of developing malignancy [11].

No international guideline provides a suggestion of prophylactic surgery as endoscopic polypectomies should be considered the treatment of choice, whenever feasible. Total proctocolectomy is suggested only in case of massive polyps that cannot be dealt with endoscopically or in case of malignant transformation. Regular endoscopic surveillance is recommended [12, 13]. Prevention and endoscopic surveillance should be scheduled yearly, starting at 12 years of age or earlier if symptoms occur (depending on polyp characteristics) [13].

29.1.1.2 Cowden Syndrome

Cowden syndrome (CS) was firstly reported by Lloyd and Dennis in 1963 [14]. It is also known as multiple hamartoma syndrome. The WHO classification defined CS as an autosomal dominant disease with multiple hamartomas localized in organs derived from all the germ cell layers.

CS is due to a germline mutation of the PTEN gene with an age-related penetrance and variable expression: several extra-gastrointestinal diseases were reported as uterine leiomyoma, macrocephaly, breast carcinoma, melanoma, thyroid abnormalities, and gangliocytoma of the cerebellum (Lhermitte-Duclos disease) [4]. About 44 % of PTEN mutations occurred de novo; however, a genetic testing is indicated in at-risk relatives.

The reported incidence of CS is among 1:200,000 [9]. Hamartomatous polyps were reported in 35–85 % of CS patients, but also colonic lipomas, adenomas, inflammatory polyps, and ganglioneuromatous and hyperplastic polyps may be present, and among 70 % of patients have more than one polyp [15].

CS polyps typically presented as juvenile polyps are characterized, with the same surgical management and a low risk of malignancies. Prophylactic colectomy is not advocated, though some papers reported an increased risk of developing colorectal cancer (16 %, 95 % CI 8 %, 24 %). Of note, endoscopic surveillance is recommended starting before 40 years of age with a follow-up interval depending by the type and number of polyps [16]. Surveillance of patients with CS should include thyroid, breast, skin, kidney, and uterine cancer screening [13].

29.1.1.3 Peutz-Jeghers Syndrome

Peutz in 1921 and Jeghers in 1944 reported the first cases of the association of mucocutaneous pigmentation and intestinal polyps [17, 18].

Peutz-Jeghers syndrome (PJS) is described by the WHO as a cancer syndrome with mucocutaneous melanin pigmentation and polyposis mainly localized in the small intestine. Other extra-gastrointestinal localizations were described with uterine, breast, pancreatic, testis, and ovarian tumors. The pigments may appear on the buccal mucosa, lips, hand, and face; gastrointestinal polyps occur in 88 % of patients with the vast majority in the small bowel (96 %) [13].

Diagnosis requires the concomitant presence of two of the following three diagnostic criteria: (1) family history of PJS, (2) mucocutaneous lesions with hyperpigmentation, and (3) hamartomatous polyps in the GI tract.

PJ polyps have a central core of smooth muscle and are covered by the native mucosa, and in case of intussusception, the pathological examination can be complicated by a secondary ischemic necrosis (Fig. 29.1). Polyps may appear multilobulated, with a heterogeneous size (small sessile nodules or pedunculated large polyps).

Mutations of STK11 (previously known as LKB1) were described in 80–94 % of tested individuals with PJS. The frequency of pathogenetic variants in familial cases can be as high as 100 % [13].

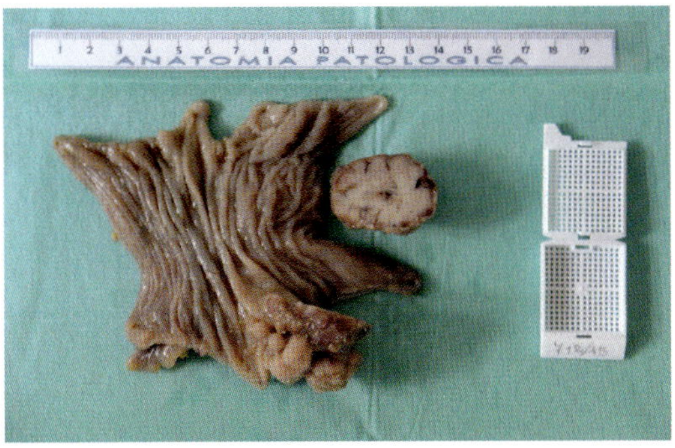

Fig. 29.1 Macroscopic findings of an isolated polyp in Peutz-Jeghers syndrome: polyp is characterized by a central core of smooth muscle and is covered by the native mucosa

PJS has a prevalence of 1:50,000 to 1:200,000 without ethnic or gender preponderance [9].

PJ polyps may cause intussusception, bleeding, anemia, intestinal obstruction, and abdominal pain. One third of PJS polyps are symptomatic at 10 years of age. Diagnostic imaging can include conventional endoscopy, upper gastrointestinal and small bowel contrast study, computed tomography, and capsule endoscopy that was recently adopted in children [19].

Surgical resection by enterotomy with intraoperative endoscopy is recommended in the case of all polyps larger than 15 mm of diameter, and extensive intestinal resection is not warranted. Surveillance of PJS patients should be started with capsule endoscopy at age 8 years and repeated every 3 years, and a second baseline examination should be started at age 18 years and repeated every 3 years [13].

29.1.2 Adenomatous Polyposis

29.1.2.1 Familial Adenomatous Polyposis (FAP)

The definition of familial adenomatous polyposis was firstly provided by Chargelaigue in 1859 [20]: an inherited condition in which numerous adenomatous polyps arise mainly from the epithelial lining of the large bowel. The WHO defined FAP as an autosomal dominant disease characterized by more than 100 adenomatous polyps [4].

The incidence of FAP is between 1:10,000 and 1:15,000 live births [13]. Familial history can be negative in over 20 % of patients given the possible misdiagnosis of relatives affected by the disease or the presence of a de novo APC gene mutation. The disease is caused by a germline mutation of the APC gene with a 100 % of penetrance. Another gene called MUTYH accounts for the so-called autosomal recessive FAP which is milder and definitely less frequent.

FAP is mostly present in the second and third decade of life, and polyps increase in size and number with age. Cancer develops among 40–50 years of age [21] with a cumulative risk of colorectal cancer development higher than 90 % after the age of 50.

Aspecific symptoms include diarrhea, abdominal pain, rectal bleeding, palpable masses, and constipation.

FAP polyps occur throughout the colon, but fundic gland polyps have also been described in the stomach in 90 % of patients, though without increased cancer risk development. Duodenum can also be involved with adenomatous polyps carrying a 5 % of progression to cancer [21].

Extraintestinal manifestations were described including dental anomalies, lipomas, desmoid tumors, epidermoid cysts, osteomas, congenital hypertrophy of the retinal pigment epithelium (CHRPE), and brain tumors.

Diagnosis is based on clinical presentation and familial history. Usually a sigmoidoscopy or a full colonoscopy with biopsies provides diagnosis of FAP. Nonetheless, genetic testing provides the ultimate diagnosis in 95 % of cases.

Prophylactic laparoscopic total colectomy is advocated with rectal mucosectomy and ileal J-pouch anastomosis. Post-colectomy surveillance should include physical examination with examination of the pouch and the transitional anal zone.

A careful attention must be done also to the upper gastrointestinal surveillance, for the screening of gastric and proximal small bowel tumors with a gastroduodenoscopy starting at age 25–30 years and repeated every 0.5–4 years according to the Spigelman stage of polyposis [14].

29.1.2.2 Gardner Syndrome

Gardner syndrome (also known as familial colorectal polyposis) was firstly described by Eldon J. Gardner in 1951 [22] as a variant of FAP associated to epidermoid cysts, dental anomalies, desmoid tumors, and multiple osteomas that can be localized in the skull (mostly in the mandibular angle), the paranasal sinuses, and in the long bones. GS is an autosomal dominant disorder caused by a mutation of the APC gene, with an estimated incidence of 1:14,025 live births [23] and no gender preponderance.

GS may also have a gastric localization with multiple polyps [24].

Colorectal cancer develops in 100% of GS patients with colonic polyps. On the ground of these considerations, surgical strategies are similar than FAP, with restorative proctocolectomy and ileal pouch-anal anastomosis [25].

29.1.2.3 Turcot Syndrome

Turcot syndrome (TS) was originally described by Turcot and colleagues in 1959 and represents a variant of FAP, with an association with brain tumors (medulloblastoma and glioblastoma) [26].

29.2 Surgical Treatment

Usually a staged procedure is preferred and includes total proctocolectomy with J-pouch ileoanal anastomosis and diverting ileostomy in order to avoid anastomotic leakage and prevent pouchitis [27, 28]. Reported surgical outcomes are good in terms of quality of life, patient satisfaction, and intestinal function, with satisfactory continence reported in nearly 90% of patients. The most common surgical complications include pouchitis, anastomotic strictures, anastomotic leakage, and fistula and have been reported in 10–30% of cases [29, 30].

29.2.1 Laparoscopic Proctocolectomy and J-Pouch Ileoanal Anastomosis

A 12-mmHg CO_2 pneumoperitoneum is created after insertion of a 12-mm port in the umbilicus. Two operative 5-mm ports are inserted in the flanks, and a third 12-mm operative port is inserted in the right iliac region.

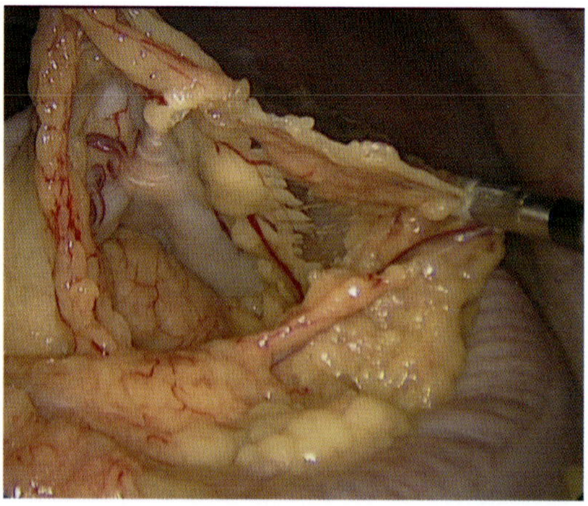

Fig. 29.2 Transverse colon dissection and omentectomy with preservation of gastric vessels

Dissection of the colon is started at the recto-sigmoid junction using vessel-sealing devices for the sigmoid arteries and inferior mesenteric artery, which is spared, thanks to the marginal dissection of the large bowel (provided malignant transformation did not occur). Colectomy is then carried out in an anticlockwise direction up to the last ileal loop. Bundles for a correct and safe laparoscopic colectomy are (1) ureter identification, (2) transverse colon dissection with gastric vessel preservation (Fig. 29.2), (3) careful identification and preservation of the Treitz ligament at the splenic flexure, and (4) careful identification and preservation of the duodenum at the hepatic flexure during Kocher maneuver. The rectum is then dissected down to the peritoneal reflection and interrupted with a mechanical linear stapling device (Fig. 29.3). Under laparoscopic view, the colon is then extracted extending slightly the incision of the right iliac trocar where the terminal ileostomy will be fashioned.

29.2.2 Ileal Pouch-Anal Anastomosis, Proctectomy, and Rectal Mucosectomy

A 3-cm J-pouch ileal reservoir with vascular supply control is created using the right iliac incision used to extract the colon (Fig. 29.4). The J-pouch

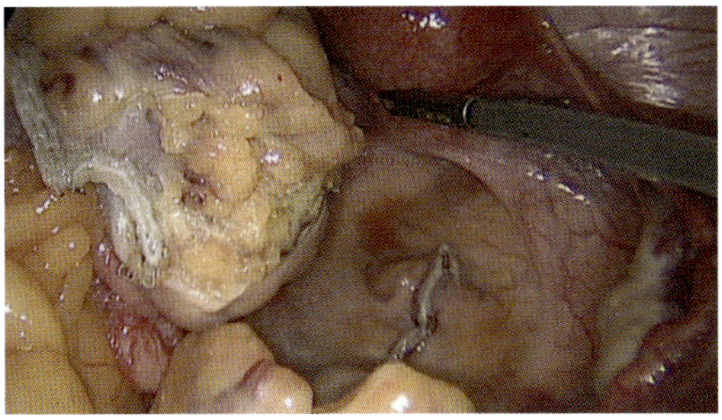

Fig. 29.3 Residual rectal stump with identification of pelvic organs

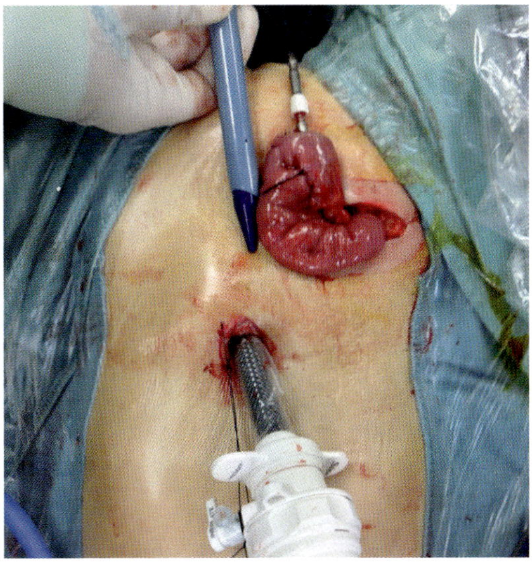

Fig. 29.4 Creation of a 3-cm J-pouch ileal reservoir

is returned in the peritoneal cavity and a multichannel-access flexible SILS® Port (Covidien plc, Cherrywood Business Park, Loughlinstown Co., Dublin, Ireland) is inserted in the ileostomy site and used for further two 5-mm service instruments (Fig. 29.5).

Again a 12-mmHg CO_2 pneumoperitoneum is created and the rectal stump is identified. Radicalization of proctectomy is performed either close to the rectum or inside the muscular rectal wall (robotic surgery, personal unpublished experience) to preserve the innervation and integrity of pelvic organs (ureters, vagina, or seminal vesicles). Mesorectal vessels are well identified, coagulated close to the rectum, and dissection is performed down to the levator ani muscle.

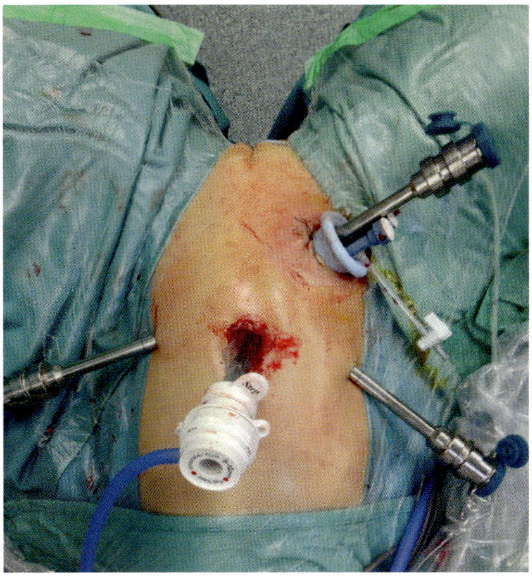

Fig. 29.5 Port position during ileal pouch-anal anastomosis and proctectomy

Endorectal mucosectomy is then performed after identification and careful preservation of the dentate line, paying great attention not to retain mucosal islands during endorectal dissection. The rectal stump is then everted through the anus and removed.

A careful control avoiding any J-pouch torsion is performed, and a hand-sewn J-pouch ileoanal anastomosis is performed. At the end of the procedure, a terminal ileostomy is created in the site of colon extraction (right iliac fossa) in order to avoid anastomotic leak as stated above.

References

1. Nugent KP, Talbot IC, Hodgson SV, Phillips RK (1993) Solitary juvenile polyps: not a marker for subsequent malignancy. Gastroenterology 105:698–700
2. Burt RW, Bishop DT, Lynch HT, Rozen P, Winawer SJ (1990) Risk and surveillance of individuals with heritable factors for colorectal cancer. WHO Collaborating Centre for the Prevention of Colorectal Cancer. Bull World Health Organ 68:655–665
3. Aytac E, Sulu B, Heald B, O'Malley M, LaGuardia L, Remzi FH, Kalady MF, Burke CA, Church JM (2015) Genotype-defined cancer risk in juvenile syndrome. Br J Surg 102(1):114–118
4. Bosman T, Carneiro F, Hruban RH, et al. WHO classification of tumours of the digestive system. 4th ed. WHO Press; 2010.

5. McColl I, Busxwy HJ, Vaele AM, Morson BC (1964) Juvenile polyposis coli. Proc R Soc Med 57:896–897
6. Stoler MA, Mills SE, Carter D, Greenson JK, Reuter VE (2009) Sternberg's diagnostic surgical pathology. Lippincott Williams & Wilkins, Hagerstwon
7. Brosens LA, Langeveld D, van Hattem WA, Giardiello FM, Offerhaus GJ (2011) Juvenile polyposis syndrome. World J Gastroenterol 17(44):4839–4844
8. Jelsig AM, Qvist N, Brusgaard K, Nielsen CB, Hansen TP, Ousager LB (2014) Hamartomatous polyposis syndromes: a review. Orphanet J Rare Dis 9:101
9. Brosens LA, van Hattem A, Hylind LM, Iacobuzio-Donahue C, Romans KE, Axilbund J, Cruz-Correa M, Tersmette AC, Offerhaus GJ, Giardiello FM (2007) Risk of colorectal cancer in juvenile polyposis. Gut 56(7):965–967
10. Howe JR, Mitros FA, Summers RW (1998) The risk of gastrointestinal carcinoma in familial juvenile polyposis. Ann Surg Oncol 5(8):751–756
11. Cairns SR, Scholefield JH, Steele RJ, Dunlop MG, Thomas HJ, Evans GD, Eaden JA, Rutter MD, Atkin WP, Saunders BP, Lucassen A, Jenkins P, Fairclough PD, Woodhouse CR; British Society of Gastroenterology; Association of Coloproctology for Great Britain and Ireland (2010) Guidelines for colorectal cancer screening and surveillance in moderate and high risk groups (update from 2002). Gut 59(5):666–689.
12. Latchford AR, Neale K, Phillips RK, Clark SK (2012) Juvenile polyposis syndrome: a study of genotype, phenotype, and long-term outcome. Dis Colon Rectum 55(10):1038–1043
13. Syngal S, Brand RE, Church JM, Giardiello FM, Hampel HL, Burt RW, American College of Gastroenterology (2015) ACG clinical guideline: Genetic testing and management of hereditary gastrointestinal cancer syndromes. Am J Gastroenterol 110(2):223–262
14. Lloyd KM 2nd, Dennis M (1963) Cowden's disease. A possible new symptom complex with multiple system involvement. Ann Intern Med 58:136–142
15. Stanich PP, Owens VL, Sweetser S, Khambatta S, Smyrk TC, Richardson RL, Goetz MP, Patnaik MM (2011) Colonic polyposis and neoplasia in Cowden syndrome. Mayo Clin Proc 86(6):489–492
16. Mester J, Eng C (2015) Cowden syndrome: recognizing and managing a not-so-rare hereditary cancer syndrome. J Surg Oncol 111(1):125–130
17. Peutz JLA (1921) Over een zeer merkwaardige, gecombineerde familiaire polyposis van de slijmliezen van den tractus intestinalis met die van de neuskeelholte en gepaard met eigenaardige pigmentaties van huid-en slijmvliezen. Ned Maandschr v Gen 10:134–146
18. Jeghers H, McKusick VA, Katz KH (1949) Generalized intestinal polyposis and melanin spots of the oral mucosa, lips and digits; a syndrome of diagnostic significance. N Engl J Med 241:993–1005, 1031–1036
19. Gastineau S, Viala J, Caldari D, Mas E, Darviot E, Le Gall C, Maurage C, Michaud L, Dabadie A (2012) Contribution of capsule endoscopy to Peutz-Jeghers syndrome management in children. Dig Liver Dis 44(10):839–843
20. Spigelman AD (2004) Extracolonic polyposis in familial adenomatous polyposis: so near and yet so far. Gut 53(3):322
21. Half E, Bercovich D, Rozen P (2009) Familial adenomatous polyposis. Orphanet J Rare Dis 4:22
22. Gardner EJ (1951) A genetic and clinical study of intestinal polyposis, a predisposing factor for carcinoma of the colon and rectum. Am J Hum Genet 3(2):167–176
23. Panjwani S, Bagewadi A, Keluskar V, Arora S (2011) Gardner's syndrome. J Clin Imaging Sci 1:65
24. Gu GL, Wang SL, Wei XM, Bai L (2008) Diagnosis and treatment of Gardner syndrome with gastric polyposis: a case report and review of the literature. World J Gastroenterol 14(13):2121–2123
25. Sebastián-Domingo JJ, Charro-Calvillo M, Navarro-Dourdi M, Cabrera-Chaves T, Ceña-Lázaro G, Ortiz-Lucas M (2011) Refractory ulcerative chronic pouchitis in a patient with Gardner syndrome following restorative proctocolectomy with ileal pouch-anal anastomosis. Rev Esp Enferm Dig 103(11):600–601
26. Turcot J, Despres JP, St Pierre F (1959) Malignant tumors of the central nervous system associated with familial polyposis of the colon: report of two cases. Dis Colon Rectum 2:465–468
27. Kartheuser A, Stangherlin P, Brandt D, Remue C, Sempoux C (2006) Restorative proctocolectomy and ileal pouch-anal anastomosis for familial adenomatous polyposis revisited. Fam Cancer 5(3):241–260; discussion 261–262
28. Kennedy RD, Zarroug AE, Moir CR, Mao SA, El-Youssef M, Potter DD (2014) Ileal pouch anal anastomosis in pediatric familial adenomatous polyposis: a 24-year review of operative technique and patient outcomes. J Pediatr Surg 49(9):1409–1412
29. Ozdemir Y, Kiran RP, Erem HH, Aytac E, Gorgun E, Magnuson D, Remzi FH (2014) Functional outcomes and complications after restorative proctocolectomy and ileal pouch anal anastomosis in the pediatric population. J Am Coll Surg 218(3):328–335
30. Zmora O, Natanson M, Dotan I, Vinograd I, Nagar H, Rabau M, Tulchinsky H (2013) Long-term functional and quality-of-life outcomes after IPAA in children. Dis Colon Rectum 56(2):198–204

30 Gastrointestinal Tumors in Children and Adolescents

Andrea Pession

30.1 Introduction and Epidemiology

Primary gastrointestinal (GI) tumors are rare entities in children, accounting for only 1 % of neoplasms, with estimated prevalence of 9–12 per 100,000 [1]. Therefore, the majority of information available is derived from small case series or single case reports, and clinical management often mirrors experience in adults. Due to the rarity of these conditions, patients should be referred to specialized hospitals. Lymphoma represents the most common GI tumor, followed by colorectal carcinoma, neurogenic tumors, and polyps [1].

30.2 Clinical Features

As opposed to adult, clinical onset is often abrupt in children, with diagnosis occasionally made during urgent abdominal exploration due to acute presentation, usually intestinal obstruction caused by an irreducible intussusceptions, appendicitis, or bleeding. Other times, vague symptoms such as nonspecific abdominal pain, nausea, vomiting, changes in bowel habits, and weight loss last a long time before the correct diagnosis is suspected [2]. Physical examination may reveal a palpable abdominal mass or blood during digital rectal examination. It is important to know that, albeit the majority of GI tumors are sporadic, they can occur in the setting of inheritable predisposing syndromes. In this case it is particularly crucial to early recognize specific warning signs through accurate inspection of the patient and family history. When possible, establishing a genetic diagnosis is the first step for starting a proactive cancer screening program both for the patient herself who often has increased risk of other extra GI neoplasms, and for her family [3].

30.3 Diagnosis

Diagnosis usually is based on a combined approach of imaging technique, such as CT, MRI, ultrasound, and PET, but definitive diagnosis is made based on histological examination. In some cases specific blood or urine test is useful for characterizing and monitoring the disease; that is the case of specific hormones for NETs [4].

30.4 Management

As previously said, due to the rarity of GI tumors in children, comprehensive guidelines for clinical management are often lacking; hence, there is uncertainty about the optimal treatment strategies.

A. Pession
Pediatrics Units, S. Orsola-Malpighi Hospital, University of Bologna, Via Massarenti 11, 40138 Bologna, Italy
e-mail: andrea.pession@unibo.it

M. Lima (ed.), *Pediatric Digestive Surgery*, DOI 10.1007/978-3-319-40525-4_30

The mainstay of treatment for the majority of tumors is surgical radical resection although specific approach combining surgical to radio-/chemotherapy depends on the histological type. In the same way, follow-up of the patient depends on the type and the stage of lesion. For inherited syndromes conferring an augmented risk of cancer, a rigid screening for other neoplasms is mandatory, following specific guidelines [3, 5].

30.5 Primary GI Lymphoma

Lymphoma accounts for the majority of GI malignancies. In a recent review of the SEER cancer registry [6], the annual incidence of primary GI lymphoma was approximately 0.199 cases per 100,000 with a striking majority of cases occurring in males. The most common type is non-Hodgkin lymphoma (NHL) and specifically Burkitt lymphoma (BL). Most frequently GI lymphoma involves the terminal ileum and cecum, as opposed to the stomach in adults, but can involve all portions of the GI tract. Symptoms depend on the location and usually include a history of nonspecific abdominal pain, nausea, vomiting, or weight loss followed by an acute exacerbation due to intussusception or GI perforation. The diagnosis of primary GI lymphoma follows the Dawson's criteria: absence of peripheral lymphadenopathy and enlarged mediastinal lymph nodes, normal white blood cell count, and predominance of bowel lesion at the time of laparotomy with only lymph nodes affected in the immediate vicinity and no involvement of liver and spleen [7]. Appropriate diagnosis and staging is based on endoscopic ultrasound (EUS) with biopsies when possible, computed tomography (CT), magnetic resonance imaging (MRI), and 18F-fluorodeoxyglucose positron emission tomography (FDG–PET). Bone marrow biopsy is needed for complete staging. While surgery has been considered for long the standard of care for treatment of GI lymphoma, its role to date is debated except for the case of acute complications, and management is often based on combination with chemo-/radiotherapy depending on the stage at presentation [6, 8, 9]. 5- and 10-year DSS (disease-specific survival) for all patients is 85 % and 81 %, respectively, but tumor location is an independent predictor of survival, with better outcome for small and large bowel tumors compared with gastric tumors [6].

BL is the most common GI lymphoma in children. It is an aggressive mature B-cell neoplasm with three clinical variants: the endemic form associated to EBV infection in Africa, where BL represents the most common malignancy in children, the sporadic variant which is associated with EBV only in 30% of the cases, and immunodeficiency-associated BL, associated with HIV infection. All three subtypes characteristically harbor one of the pathogenetic rearrangements of c-Myc oncogene causing cell cycle deregulation and tumor formation [10]. While the endemic form typically presents as a jaw or facial bone tumor, clinical presentation of GI BL is usually marked by the rapid growth of an intra-abdominal mass, causing symptoms of bowel obstruction or intussusceptions. Rarely it could masquerade as appendicitis; therefore, it should be considered a differential diagnosis especially in children from endemic areas presenting with atypical and long-lasting right iliac fossa pain. In this case histological examination of appendicectomy specimen is warranted [11]. In the setting of an acute abdomen, imaging techniques such as US and CT are useful in detecting a mass, but this should be distinguished from other common pediatric malignancies such as neuroblastoma and Wilms' tumor and other forms of lymphoma. Therefore, careful histopathologic analysis is needed. Gallium 67 scintigraphy and PET are also needed to evaluate stage and treatment response [12]. Even if untreated cases rapidly progress to widespread metastases and death, BL is chemosensitive and the introduction of multiagent high-intensity chemotherapeutic regimens has led to an optimal remission rate [10].

30.6 Polyps and Polypoid Diseases

Colorectal polyps in children are usually benign and could be easily resected via endoscopic polypectomy, but a small fraction of cases hides risk for cancer and should be carefully evaluated.

Typical clinical signs at presentation include rectal bleeding with anemia, abdominal pain, diarrhea, passage of tissue per rectum, and intussusception. Based on microscopic appearance, colorectal polyps can be divided into two different types: hamartomas and adenomas. The former are generally benign, but infrequently could show dysplastic changes and have neoplastic potential, while the latter are properly dysplastic, precancerous lesions.

Hamartomas The majority of polyps found in children are isolated juvenile polyps, more frequently involving the colon and the rectum, with minimal risk of malignant transformation. In this case, the hamartoma could be removed endoscopically with no need for additional follow-up. However, a family history of juvenile polyps or germline mutations should prompt the evaluation for a premalignant condition, such as juvenile polyposis syndrome (JPS) or Peutz–Jeghers syndrome (PJS) even in the presence of a single polyp [13]. JPS is a rare (incidence of 1 in 100,000) autosomal dominant condition with variable penetrance, characterized by multiple gastric, small intestinal, and colonic polyps. The majority of them, usually 50–100, are found in the colon [14]. A family history is reported in 75 % of patients. Only half of patients clinically diagnosed with JPS carry a germline mutation in the SMAD4 or BMPR1A gene; therefore, more often diagnosis cannot rely on genetic screening and is based on the following clinical criteria: (i) at least five juvenile polyps in the colorectum, (ii) juvenile polyps in other parts of the GI tract, or (iii) any number of juvenile polyps in a person with a known family history of juvenile polyps [3]. Patients usually develop symptoms in the first two decades of life. JPS patients carry a cumulative lifetime risk of colorectal cancer of 39 % [13] and increased risk for gastric, duodenal, and pancreatic cancers. For these reasons, surveillance colonoscopy and upper endoscopy every 1–3 years are recommended from the age of 12. Limited number of polyps could be treated with endoscopic polypectomy, but colectomy with IRA (ileal–rectal anastomosis) is indicated in the case of cancer or high-grade dysplasia followed by surveillance of the remaining rectum or pouch [3].

Peutz–Jeghers syndrome (PJS) is a rare (1 in 120,000 births) autosomal dominant syndrome with variable penetrance characterized by mucocutaneous pigmentation, that is present in more than 95 % of patients, and increases the risk of GI, breast, testicular, pancreatic, ovarian, and uterine cancers. Mucocutaneous pigmentation is 1–5 mm spots of the perioral area and buccal mucosa which appear in childhood and may fade with age (Fig. 30.1). They could also involve the forearms, palms, digits, soles, perianal area, and, rarely, intestinal mucosa. A common primary presentation is intussusception of small bowel polyps requiring urgent surgical procedure. Histological features of polyps are unique (nondysplastic, with normal overlying epithelium and muscularis mucosae extending into branching fronds of the polyp). Genetic testing is based on LKB1/STK11 mutation screening, which can be found in 94 % of cases. Once identified, the mutation should be searched for in other family members [3]. Screening recommendations include colonos-

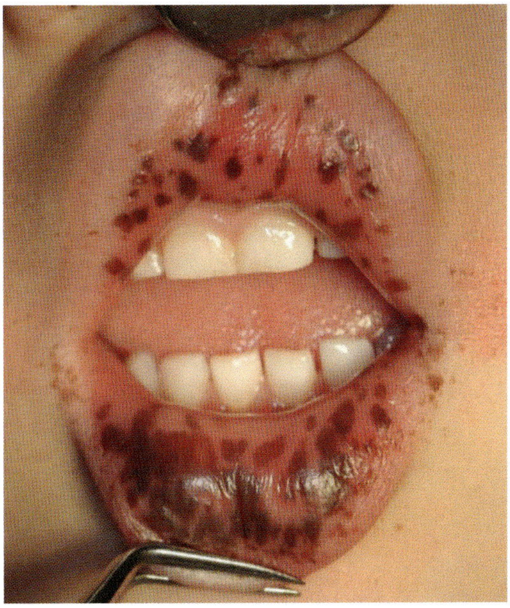

Fig. 30.1 Mucocutaneous pigmentation representative of Peutz–Jeghers syndrome (PJS) (Reproduced from Alawi 2013 [15])

copy, upper GI endoscopy, and small bowel video capsule endoscopy starting from the age of 8 with removal of polyps up to 1 cm in diameter. Colectomy should be considered further in the clinical management.

Adenomas This type of polyps is usually associated with polyposis syndromes such as familial adenomatous polyposis (FAP), attenuated familial adenomatous polyposis (AFAP), and MYH-associated polyposis (MAP). FAP is the most common, while the other two conditions rarely present with intestinal lesions during childhood or adolescence and are no further described in this chapter. FAP is an inherited condition characterized by early onset of multiple adenomas (>100) throughout the large bowel. Its estimated frequency is 1 in 13,000–18,000 live births [16]. It is caused by a mutation of the adenomatous polyposis coli (APC) gene, usually inherited in an autosomal dominant manner, but in 20–30 % of cases represents a *de novo* condition. Even if the most common alteration is a truncating mutation, many other causative mutations have been reported to date. Genotype–phenotype correlations have been observed and should be taken into consideration in decision making [17]. Adenomas first appear at an average age of 16, and progression to colorectal cancer is almost inevitable by the age of 50 [14]. Usually patients present to physicians' attention either because of symptoms of multiple and large adenomas, e.g., rectal bleeding or anemia or other nonspecific complaints such as change in bowel habits, constipation, diarrhea, and abdominal pains, or for evaluation after a family member has been diagnosed. In the first setting, the finding of multiple adenomas (>10) should address the patient to comprehensive genetic testing for one of the various polyposes, including APC and MUTYH gene mutation analysis [3]. In more than 90 % of cases, it is possible to identify the causative mutation by commercially available gene sequencing on a routine blood sample [14]. Nevertheless, the absence of a mutation does not definitively rule out a clinical diagnosis if the phenotype is striking. On the contrary, a negative test in a relative of a patient with known pathogenetic mutation allows the physicians to exclude the diagnosis. The main goal in managing these patients is cancer prevention. For colorectal cancer screening, a sigmoidoscopy is recommended every 1–2 years starting at 10–12 years of age and should include registration of polyp number, size, and distribution and multiple biopsies [3]. Colectomy remains the cornerstone of cancer prevention and is usually recommended between 15 and 25 years of age [13]. Early surgery is mandatory in the case of documented or suspected cancer and should be taken into consideration in case of large polyps (>10 mm), high-grade dysplasia polyps, and marked increase in number of polyps and symptoms. Surgical procedures of choice are colectomy with IRA (ileal–rectal anastomosis) or proctocolectomy with IPAA (ileal pouch–anal anastomosis). Number and localization of polyps and type of APC mutation are to be considered in determining the optimal procedure. Of note, adenomas and cancer may still develop in the remaining rectal epithelium or in the anal transition zone; therefore, postsurgical surveillance should include yearly endoscopy of the rectum or ileal pouch and examination of the ileostomy every 2 years [3]. In individuals with FAP, there is also an increased risk for upper GI adenomas and cancer, even if mean age of duodenal cancer diagnosis is later in the course of the disease (usually between 47 and 51) [16]. Upper GI screening should therefore be performed starting at the age of 25–30 [3]. Another important cause of morbidity and the second cause of death in these patients are desmoid tumors, occurring in 15 % of them. The usual sites are small bowel mesentery and abdominal wall, with few arising in the trunk or limbs, ranging from 1 to 10 per individual. They could remain asymptomatic or cause bowel or ureteric obstruction, perforation, fistula, or hemorrhage, and their treatment still remains a challenge for the risk of bleeding, recurrence, or consequent short bowel syndrome [16]. Other malignancies associated with FAP are thyroid cancer, for which annual thyroid ultrasound is also recommended; hepatoblastoma, for which the need of screening with α-fetoprotein monitoring and liver ultrasound is still debated [3]. Congenital hypertrophy of the retinal pigment epithelium (CHRPE) is another typical feature of FAP, present in roughly 70–80 % of patients. It refers to the presence of characteristic pigmented fundus lesions that are usually present at birth, asymptomatic, and with no malignant potential, but ophthalmological examination could be a useful early diagnostic test for at-risk family members, combined with genetic analysis [16].

30.7 Colorectal Carcinoma

Colorectal carcinoma (CRC) is the most common neoplasm arising from the colon. Although it is a very common cancer in adults, it is extremely rare in people aged less than 20, with an annual incidence of only about 1 case per million in this population [18]. Due to the rarity of this disease, it is difficult to understand the underlying causes, but it seems unlikely that risk factors associated with an increase incidence in adults, such as obesity, excess alcohol or red meat consumption, and smoking, play an important role in the pathogenesis of the disease in younger patients. In the same way, the stepwise malignant transformation from adenomas to invasive carcinoma, validated for adult CRC, appears to be less clear. In fact, the early age of presentation, the different histology, and the paucity of premalignant adenomas do not support this hypothesis except in the case of FAP [19]. The majority of cases of CRC are sporadic, but 10–20 % of patients present a predisposing condition such as FAP or other polyposis syndromes. These conditions are rare but, when present, greatly increase the risk of future development. Another important predisposing condition is hereditary nonpolyposis colon cancer (HNPCC) syndrome (Lynch syndrome) due to germline mutation of DNA mismatch repair genes. Criteria to identify patients affected are clinical (Revised Amsterdam Criteria) and require a diagnosis of CRC in at least three individuals spanning two generations, at least one of whom is a first-degree relative of the other two. These families also carry a higher risk of other tumors, such as gastric, small bowel, hepatobiliary, gynecologic, and urinary cancers [20]. Inflammatory bowel diseases such as ulcerative colitis and Crohn disease are also associated with the development of CRC. The earlier the age of diagnosis of this disease, the earlier and the higher is the risk of cancer [20]. Hallmarks of CRC in children are the advanced stage and aggressive biology, as revealed by a considerably higher rate of mucinous histology (62 %) than in adults (11–13 %) which globally confer a poorer outcome [21]. Diagnosis in children is often delayed, due to underestimation of vague symptoms of early CRC resembling those of benign common pediatric illnesses. Anemia, abdominal or rectal pain, bleeding, weight loss, and bowel habit modifications are the most reported complaints, with a median duration of symptoms of 3 months [21]. Due to the rarity of the disease in children, experience in clinical management is limited, with recommendations deriving mostly from adult patients. Thus, complete evaluation of a patient with suspected CRC should include chest X-ray; CT of the chest, abdomen, and pelvis; and a bone scan. But definitive diagnosis is obtained only with histopathologic examination. Total colonoscopy is also recommended in order to identify other lesions or polyps. The role of FDG–PET scans and carcinoembryonic antigen (CEA) assay is unclear in children, since they appear to be less helpful in these patients [19]. Recommended staging system is the same adopted for adults, with the American Joint Committee on Cancer (AJCC) Staging System being the most widely used. The mainstay therapy is surgical complete resection, following principles established in adults. That consist of en bloc resection of the tumor and any other structures attached to it and removal of vascular and lymphatic vessels. At least 5 cm of margin of normal bowel and 12 negative lymph nodes should be obtained in order to consider the resection adequate [19]. In cases with advanced disease, combination therapy with fluorouracil, folinic acid, oxaliplatin, irinotecan, and bevacizumab should be attempted [20].

30.8 Gastroenteropancreatic Neuroendocrine Tumors

Neuroendocrine tumors (NETs) are rare entities arising from cells of the neuroendocrine system. They can occur in many organs including the lungs, bronchial tree, thymus, testis, and thyroid, but over 50% involves the gastrointestinal tract and the pancreas (gastroenteropancreatic NETS or GEP-NETs). The term "carcinoids" previously used referring to the presumed benign behavior is now considered inappropriate, since it is well established that all NETs can become fully malignant, and it is no longer included in the 2010 WHO classification [22]. Histological features of this particular type of neoplasms are peculiar and consist of small blue cells positive to markers of neuroendocrine tissue, including neuron-specific enolase, synaptophysin, and chromogranin. In addition, specific histological features vary according to the site of origin [4]. While the majority of GEP-NETs are sporadic, it is well worth to point out that they can occur in the setting of specific inherited familial syndromes including multiple endocrine neoplasia type 1 (MEN1) and type 2 (MEN2), von Hippel–Lindau disease, neurofibromatosis type 1, and tuberous sclerosis. For this reason it is necessary to ask the patient about family and personal history of other neoplasms linked to one of these syndromes (medullary thyroid carcinoma, pheochromocytoma, adrenocortical tumors, thymic and/or bronchial tube endocrine tumors, clear cell renal carcinoma) and look for peculiar signs during physical examination such as neuromas, café au lait macules of the skin, or signs of hyperparathyroidism [5]. In case of suspect, it is mandatory to address the patient to a specialist center, both for genetic diagnosis and counseling and for proactive screening and, if necessary, surgical procedures. Clinical presentation of NET is quite variable, depending on whether the tumor is functioning or not. Functioning tumors secrete hormones, such as serotonin, insulin, and gastrin, responsible for specific clinical syndromes. The most common symptoms related to the predominant form of hormone secreted by specific type of NET are listed in Table 30.1. A peculiar clinical presentation is the so-called carcinoid syndrome which refers to facial flushing, diarrhea, wheezing, colicky abdominal pain, and edema caused by the release of serotonin directly in the systemic circulation, therefore bypassing its metabolization into inactive products within the liver. This is a rare condition, occurring in only 20% of well-differentiated NETs of the midgut, when the disease has metastasized to the liver, has invaded the retroperitoneum, or, rarely, involves the rectum, and therefore the venous drainage bypasses the liver. On the other hand of the spectrum, nonfunctioning tumors can be asymptomatic or only manifest with local compression or the discovery of a mass [4].

Table 30.1 Clinical features of functioning NETs

Tumor	Symptoms
Insulinoma	Confusion, sweating, weakness, unconsciousness, and relief of symptoms with eating
Gastrinoma	Peptic ulceration and diarrhea (Zollinger–Ellison syndrome) or diarrhea alone
Glucagonoma	Weight loss, diabetes mellitus, diarrhea, and necrolytic migratory erythema
VIPoma	Profuse diarrhea and marked hypokalemia (Verner– Morrison syndrome)
Somatostatinoma	Weight loss, diarrhea, steatorrhea, and diabetes mellitus

Reproduced from [4]

The most common type of GEP-NETs in children is appendiceal NETs, which are usually nonfunctioning. Pancreatic NETs account for almost a third of all GEP-NETs and are also usually nonfunctioning. Among the functioning ones, insulinoma is the most common, as opposed to gastrinoma in adults. Gastric and colonic/rectal NETs are very rare. Diagnosis can be made with a combination of clinical, biochemical, and imaging techniques. In case of functioning NETs, measuring the specific hormone secreted is useful both for primary diagnosis and for monitoring tumor progression/response to treatment. A combined approach based on CT, MRI, endoscopic ultrasound, MIBG scintigraphy, and gallium 68 PET/CT is used with the aim of detecting the primary tumor and especially the possible presence of multifocal disease, while definitive diagnosis is confirmed only by histopathology. As a general approach, complete surgical resection is considered the only curative treatment. Surgery can be useful even in the case of advanced disease with the aim of reducing the tumor burden and improving quality of life. In the last years, novel therapeutic options are developed for nonresectable NETs, including transhepatic embolization of liver metastasis, image-guided radiofrequency ablation, targeted radionuclide therapy (MIBG and radiolabeled peptide therapy), the use of somatostatin analogues, and chemotherapy [4]. Overall 5-year survival for children and adolescents with NETs (all site) is 78 %, with particularly favorable outcome for appendix and colon/rectum location (>95 % 5-year survival) [23].

Appendiceal carcinoid tumors are the most common GEP-NET in children. Usually they are detected incidentally during specimen examination after emergency appendicectomy, representing approximately 0.2 % of patients with acute appendicitis [24]. As for many other rare cancers, there are no specific guidelines on management in pediatric population and recommendations for treatment and surveillance are based on the North American Neuroendocrine Tumor Society consensus guidelines for adults. According to them, it is accepted that tumors <1.0 cm that are completely excised with appendicectomy are considered cured and do not warrant additional follow-up, whereas for tumors >2 cm, incompletely resected tumor, lymphovascular invasion, invasion of the mesoappendix, or high-grade or mixed histology, it is indicated to perform secondary right hemicolectomy and follow-up with clinical evaluation, serum chromogranin A and 24-h urine 5-HIAA monitoring, CT scan or MRI, plus somatostatin receptor scintigraphy (octreotide scan) if metastatic disease is suspected [25]. These indications are derived from the observation that tumor size correlates with metastatic potential, usually involving the regional lymph nodes rather than the liver [26]. Luckily, the majority of cases in children are <1 cm, and the risk of invasive disease is decreased compared to adults; moreover, there are reports of long disease-free survival in children with tumors >2 cm treated with appendicectomy alone; thus, it is in doubt whether the need for additional surgery and follow-up should be based solely on tumor size [27].

30.9 Gastrointestinal Stromal Tumors (GISTs)

GISTs are rare tumors in pediatric population, with an expected incidence in patients 18 years or younger of 0.08 per million [28]. Nevertheless, they deserve mentioning because of the unique features that distinct pediatric GIST from the adult counterpart. The main difference from adult GIST is that KIT and PDGFRA mutations are very rare, accounting for only 15 % of cases, and consequently response to kinase inhibitors is poor. GIST can occur sporadically or in association with genetic syndromes (Carney triad and Carney–Stratakis syndrome in case of pediatric GIST). Median age at presentation is 13, with a female predominance. Most cases are located in the stomach with a nodular growth pattern (Fig. 30.2) often ulcerated in the surface, causing acute or chronic bleeding. In fact, typical signs at presentation are gastrointestinal bleeding and anemia. Multitumor foci and lymph node or liver metastasis are extremely common. Small intestine GISTs are rare and usually show a more aggressive behavior [29].

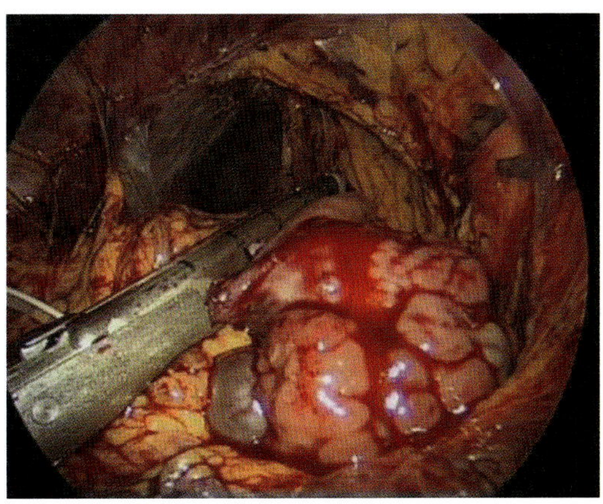

Fig. 30.2 Nodular growth pattern characteristic of GIST (Reproduced from Lima et al. 2015 [31])

In addition to upper GI imaging, revealing single or multiple solid nodular masses with well-circumscribed round margins, histological examination is necessary to confirm the diagnosis. Tissue samples can be obtained by endoscopic (with the help of ultrasound endoscopy in order to identify intramural tumors) or percutaneous approach, but, when localized, resection is preferable [30]. Chemotherapy plays no role in GIST treatment, while it is recommended to evaluate all cases for KIT/PDGRFA mutations that, although rare, predict a good response to the use of imatinib or sunitinib. The mainstay of therapy is surgical removal, but relapse occurs in more than 70 % of cases, often due to peritoneal seeding. Given the high recurrence rate, despite the radicality of resection, but at the same time the indolent course of this tumor in pediatric population, surgical procedure should take into consideration a conservative approach [28]. Laparoscopy is gaining increasingly important role to evaluate the extension of the lesion and confirm the diagnosis and, when possible, to immediately proceed to tumor resection [31].

References

1. Ladd AP, Grosfeld JL (2006) Gastrointestinal tumors in children and adolescents. Semin Pediatr Surg 15(1):37–47
2. Bethel C, Bhattacharyya N, Hutchinson C, Ruymann F, Cooney DR (1997) Alimentary tract malignancies in children. J Pediatr Surg 32(7):1004–1009
3. Syngal S, Brand RE, Church JM, Giardiello FM, Hampel HL, Burt RW (2015) ACG clinical guideline: genetic testing and management of hereditary gastrointestinal cancer syndromes. Am J Gastroenterol 110(2):223–262, Nature Publishing Group
4. Johnson PRV (2014) Gastroenteropancreatic neuroendocrine (carcinoid) tumors in children. Semin Pediatr Surg 23:91–95, Elsevier
5. Gut P, Komarowska H, Czarnywojtek A, Waligórska-Stachura J, Bączyk M, Ziemnicka K et al (2015) Familial syndromes associated with neuroendocrine tumours. Contemp Oncol 19(3):176–183
6. Kassira N, Pedroso FE, Cheung MC, Koniaris LG, Sola JE (2011) Primary gastrointestinal tract lymphoma in the pediatric patient: review of 265 patients from the SEER registry. J Pediatr Surg 46:1956–1964, Elsevier Inc
7. Ghimire P, Wu GY, Zhu L (2011) Primary gastrointestinal lymphoma. World J Gastroenterol 17(6):697–707
8. Bandyopadhyay R, Sinha SK, Chatterjee U, Mukhopadhyay S, Chowdhury SR, Biswas PK (2011) Primary pediatric gastrointestinal lymphoma. Indian J Med Paediatr Oncol 32(2):92
9. Cirocchi R, Farinella E, Trastulli S, Cavaliere D, Covarelli P, Listorti C et al (2011) Surgical treatment of primitive gastro-intestinal lymphomas: a systematic review. World J Surg Oncol 9:145
10. Bautista-Quach MA, Ake CD, Chen M, Wang J (2012) Gastrointestinal lymphomas: morphology, immunophenotype and molecular features. J Gastrointest Oncol 3(3):209–225
11. Weledji EP, Ngowe MN, Abba JS (2014) Burkitt's lymphoma masquerading as appendicitis – two case reports and review of the literature. World J Surg Oncol 12:187
12. Grajo JR, Kayton ML, Steffensen TS, Dragicevic N, Guidi CB (2012) Presentation of ileal Burkitt lymphoma in children. J Radiol Case Rep 6(8):27–38
13. Thakkar K, Fishman DS, Gilger MA (2012) Colorectal polyps in childhood. Curr Opin Pediatr 24(5):632–637
14. Barnard J (2009) Screening and surveillance recommendations for pediatric gastrointestinal polyposis syndromes. J Pediatr Gastroenterol Nutr 48(Suppl 2):S75–S78
15. Alawi F (2013) Pigmented lesions of the oral cavity: an update. Dent Clin North Am 57(4):699–710
16. Galiatsatos P, Foulkes WD (2006) Familial adenomatous polyposis. Am J Gastroenterol 101(2):385–398
17. Half E, Bercovich D, Rozen P (2009) Familial adenomatous polyposis. Orphanet J Rare Dis 4(1):22
18. Ferrari A, Rognone A, Casanova M, Zaffignani E, Piva L, Collini P et al (2008) Colorectal carcinoma in children and adolescents: the experience of the Istituto Nazionale Tumori of Milan, Italy. Pediatr Blood Cancer 50:588–593
19. Goldberg J, Furman WL (2012) Management of colorectal carcinoma in children and young adults. J Pediatr Hematol Oncol 34(May):10–12
20. Saab R, Furman WL (2008) Epidemiology and management options for colorectal cancer in children. Paediatr Drugs 10(3):177–192
21. Hill DA, Furman WL, Billups CA, Riedley SE, Cain AM, Rao BN et al (2007) Colorectal carcinoma in childhood and adolescence: a clinicopathologic review. J Clin Oncol 25(36):5808–5814
22. Bosman F, Carneiro F, Hruban R, Al E (2010) WHO classification of tumours of the digestive system. IARC, Lyon
23. Allan B, Davis J, Perez E, Lew J, Sola J (2013) Malignant neuroendocrine tumors: incidence and outcomes in pediatric patients. Eur J Pediatr Surg 23:394–399
24. Fallon SC, Hicks MJ, Carpenter JL, Vasudevan SA, Nuchtern JG, Cass DL (2015) Management of appen-

diceal carcinoid tumors in children. J Surg Res 198:384–387, Elsevier Inc
25. Kim SS, Kays DW, Larson SD, Islam S (2014) Appendiceal carcinoids in children—management and outcomes. J Surg Res 192:250–253, Elsevier Inc
26. Tchana-Sato V, Detry O, Polus M, Thiry A, Detroz B, Maweja S et al (2006) Carcinoid tumor of the appendix: a consecutive series from 1237 appendectomies. World J Gastroenterol 12(41):6699–6701
27. Assadi M, Kubiak R, Kaiser G (2002) Appendiceal carcinoid tumors in children: does size matter? Med Pediatr Oncol 38:65–66
28. Pappo AS, Janeway K, Laquaglia M, Kim SY (2011) Special considerations in pediatric gastrointestinal tumors. J Surg Oncol 104(8):928–932
29. Shimomura M, Ikeda S, Takakura Y, Kawaguchi Y, Tokunaga M, Takeda H et al (2010) Gastrointestinal stromal tumors of the small intestine in pediatric populations: a case report and literature review. Pediatr Surg Int 26(6):649–654
30. Benesch M, Wardelmann E, Ferrari A, Brennan B, Verschuur A (2009) Gastrointestinal stromal tumors (GIST) in children and adolescents: a comprehensive review of the current literature. Pediatr Blood Cancer 53:1171–1179
31. Lima M, Gargano T, Ruggeri G, Pession A, Mariotto A, Maffi M (2015) Laparoscopic resection of a rare gastrointestinal stromal tumor in children. Springerplus 4:73

Augmented Reality in Minimally Invasive Digestive Surgery

31

Luc Soler, Stéphane Nicolau, Patrick Pessaux,
Didier Mutter, and Jacques Marescaux

31.1 Introduction

The introduction of an optical device into the abdomen of a patient in order to carry out a surgical procedure via a miniaturized camera represented a major evolution in the surgical world of the twentieth century: the "minimally invasive" surgery era was born. Although the benefits for patients of laparoscopic surgery have been clearly demonstrated, it brings up new difficulties for surgeons by greatly reducing their maneuvering capabilities. The first difficulty is the loss of several senses such as the sense of touch, along with a modification in the force feedback. This lack of force feedback is also exemplified by current robotic systems such as the da Vinci from Intuitive Surgical, currently the most used surgical robot worldwide. However, the use of stereoscopic vision allowed to lessen that perception limit with a 3D view of the operative field filmed by two cameras. Another solution applicable to both monoscopic and stereoscopic systems consists in using virtual reality and augmented reality.

Indeed, from a patient's medical image (CT scan or MRI), the virtual reality software provides a 3D model and visualization of the patient. With an improved preoperative knowledge of each patient's internal anatomy, practitioners can establish an improved diagnosis and plan for the best suited therapy in a given case. Therefore, 3D patient modelling is generally used as a diagnosis support or for surgical planning. By combining this preoperative 3D modelling with intraoperative information, two major computer-assisted surgical procedures have been developed: computer-assisted guiding systems, using real information to control the virtual environment, and augmented reality (AR) systems that superimpose virtual information onto real images [1]. These make up for the lack of touch by improved surgical images augmented by virtual information. Computer assistance will therefore avoid having to locate tumors or vessels using the sense of touch, providing visualization through virtual transparency instead.

AR is based on two main components. The first one is the 3D visualization of anatomical or pathological structures that appear on the medical image. The second one is the registration of this visualization on the patient's real images and the tracking of surgical instruments, thus allowing to create virtual transparency. We will present such AR systems by describing existing techniques and expected clinical benefits.

L. Soler (✉)
Luc Soler, IRCAD, 1 place de l'hôpital,
67091 Strasbourg, France
e-mail: luc.soler@ircad.fr

S. Nicolau
IRCAD, 1 place de l'hôpital, 67091 Strasbourg,
France

P. Pessaux • D. Mutter • J. Marescaux
IHU Strasbourg, IRCAD, 1 place de l'hôpital,
67091 Strasbourg, France

M. Lima (ed.), *Pediatric Digestive Surgery*, DOI 10.1007/978-3-319-40525-4_31

31.2 Visualization of Anatomical and Pathological Structures

The first expected benefit of an AR system is to provide a fast, efficient, and easy way to implement a view of the patient's anatomy. Any software meeting these needs will therefore allow for the reading of images recorded during the clinical routine in DICOM, the international standard format. Moreover, this software will have to allow for at least two types of immediate rendering: a 2D view of image slices and a 3D view. Several types of 3D volume rendering are being used in routine: direct volume rendering, MIP (maximum intensity projection) rendering, and ray casting rendering for virtual navigations, such as a colonoscopy or fibroscopy. Currently, many of the available software applications for the visualization consoles of radiology departments must be paid for, or can be freely downloaded from the Internet. OsiriX [2] is the most notorious and used software among radiologists. Although it is very complete, it presents two drawbacks: it only works on Mac OS and its user interface is not particularly intuitive for surgeons as it is too similar to the software of postprocessing consoles used in radiology. Whether it is free or must be paid for, we have noticed that these software applications are scarcely used by surgeons due to their complexity: the user interface is submerged with complicated options and lengthy training is sometimes required to use the software.

To overcome this recurring drawback, we have developed a software, VR-Render (©IRCAD 2010), that has the advantage of being very easy to use and requires little training time. This software has been transferred to the Visible Patient Company that has optimized it, renamed it Visible Patient Planning™, and obtained its certification as a medical device (CE Mark, 510 k FDA, Canadian Health). Visible Patient Planning is today freely available and can be downloaded on Mac OS and Windows (https://www.visiblepatient.com/en/products/software). For surgeons, the first advantage is its direct volume rendering which is automatically computed by the software from the CT or MRI slices of the DICOM image (Fig. 31.1).

This technique, available on all current imaging systems (MRI or CT scan), can be sufficient for a good 3D visualization of anatomical and pathological structures and can thus be a useful tool for preoperative planning [3, 4]. It consists in replacing the standard slice view by the visualization of all slices simultaneously and in 3D. In order to see internal structures, the initial voxel gray level is replaced by an associated voxel color and transparency. This transparency allows to view the organ borders as they are not delineated in reality. With VR-Render, the user simply selects automatically computed 3D renderings from a very explicit list. That volume can also be cut along the three main axes (axial, frontal, or sagittal) or with an oblique mouse-controlled plane. In clinical routine, direct volume rendering can be of great preoperative interest. This is the case for all malformation pathologies, in particular vascular or bone malformation, but also for thoracic and digestive pathologies.

Direct volume rendering is a very useful tool as it is accessible without any preprocessing; however, it does have some limitations. It can provide neither the volume of organs nor the dimensions since these organs are not delineated. For the same reason, it is not possible to provide a volume after resection or to cut a section of these structures without cutting neighboring structures. To overcome this limit, each anatomical and pathological structure in the medical image has to be delineated. To do it, several software are available on the market essentially for liver (Myrian© from Intrasense, Ziostation© from Ziosoft, Iqqa® Liver from Edda Technology, ScoutTM Liver from Pathfinder) and more rarely for all digestive areas (Synapse© Vincent from Fujinon). Another solution consists in using 3D modelling distant services (MeVis Distant Service, Visible Patient Service from Visible Patient) that do not

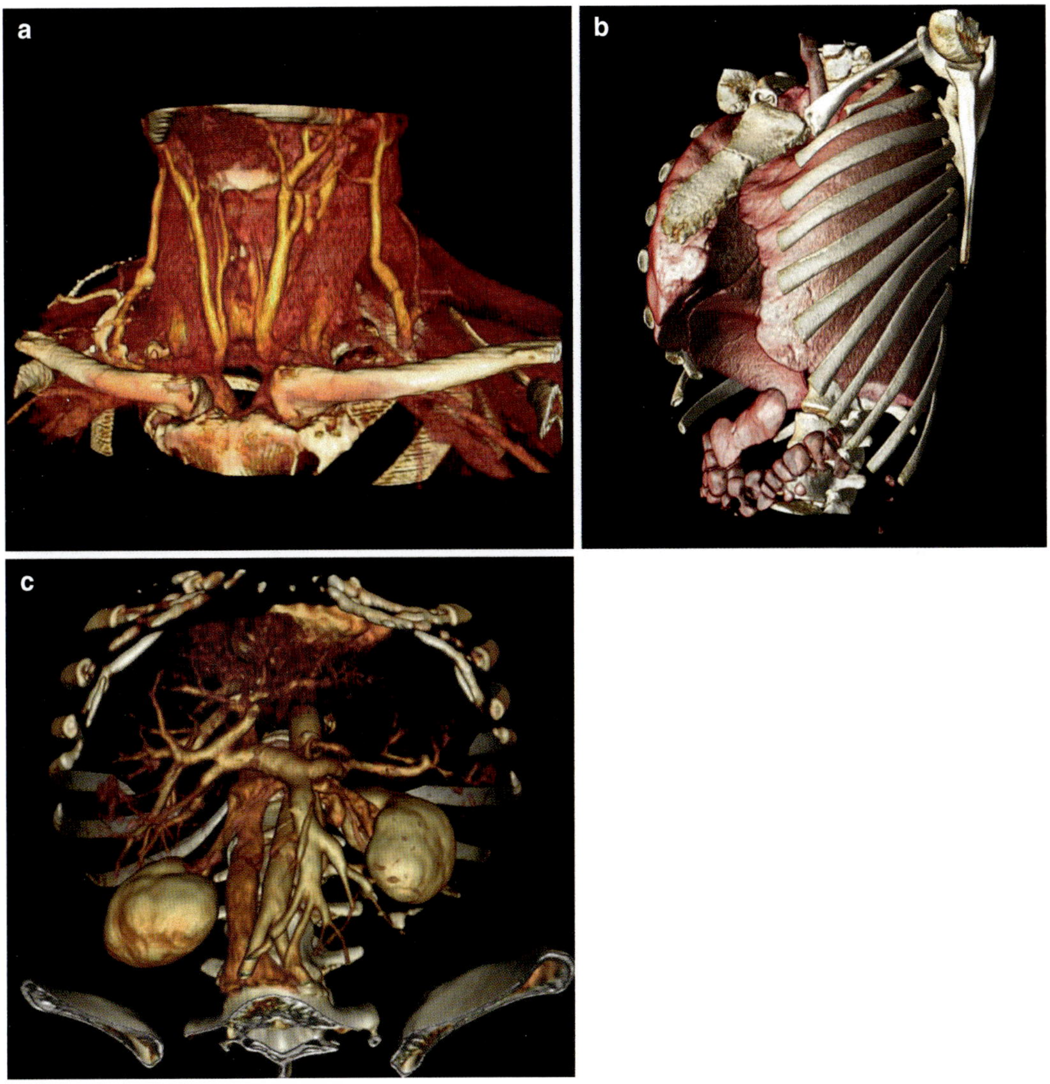

Fig. 31.1 Direct volume rendering of three different clinical cases from their DICOM image, here CT scan of the neck (**a**), thorax (**b**), and abdomen (**c**)

request the purchase and use of expensive modelling workstations, the modelling being realized at distance by experts in image processing. If MeVis Distant Service is limited to the liver, Visible Patient Service is today the only service available for any part of the body, from baby to adult. Results of the 3D modelling process can be visualized from Visible Patient Planning software through surface rendering or fusion between surface and volume rendering (Fig. 31.2).

Beside the 3D visualization of delineated and modelled structures, Visible Patient Planning also allows to interactively change transparency of any structure, to interact on them, to navigate anywhere, and therefore to simulate any kind of endoscopy such as laparoscopy, fibroscopy, gastroscopy, or colonoscopy (Fig. 31.3).

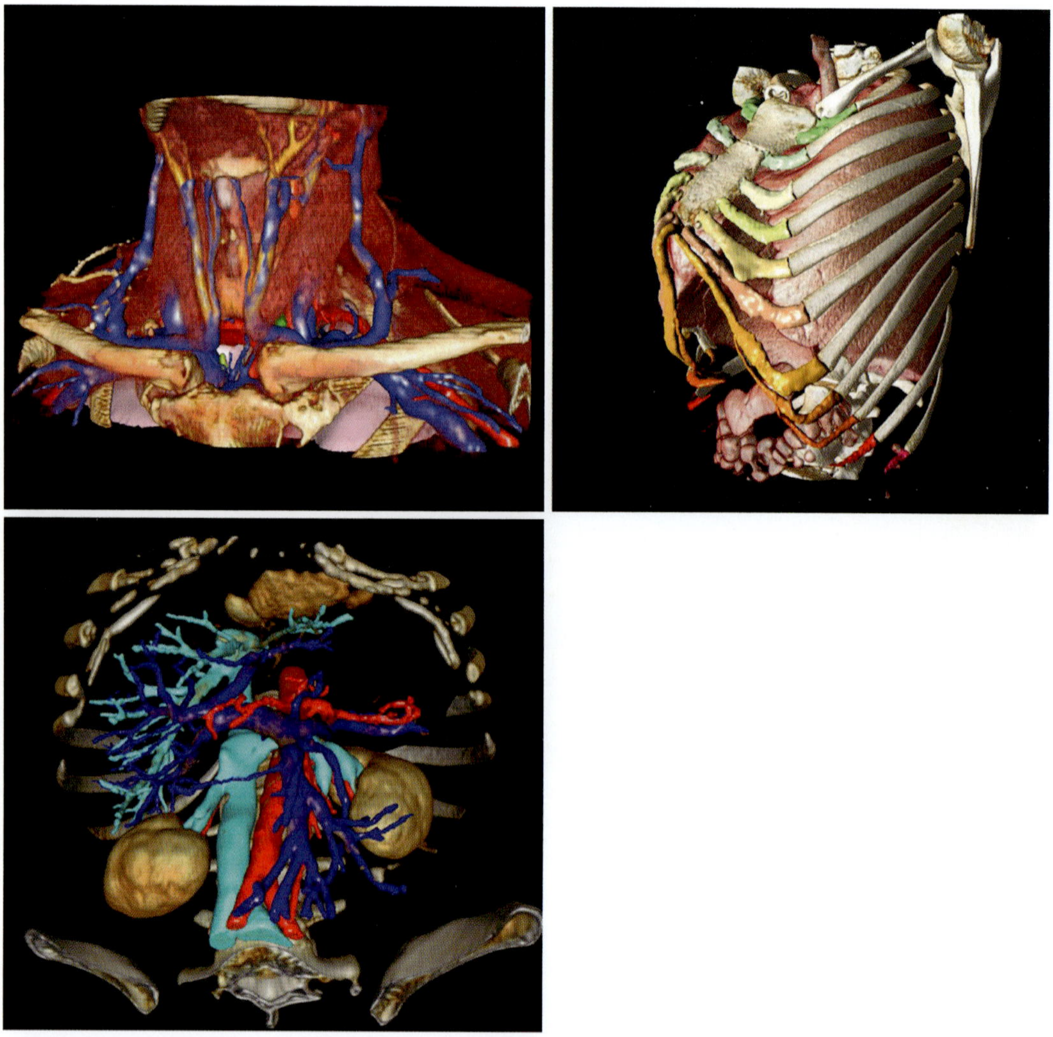

Fig. 31.2 Visible patient 3D modelling of patients of Fig. 31.1 with a fusion of direct volume rendering and surface rendering provided by Visible Patient Planning software

In liver surgery, a simple 3D visualization is frequently not sufficient to efficiently plan surgery. Virtual resection and volume computation after resection are then usually mandatory and requested by surgeons. Visible Patient Planning software gives such possibility through virtual clip applying that provides in real time the vascular territory of the clipped portal subtree defining the anatomical segment. It allows for multi-segmentectomy and automatically computes the future liver remain rate (see Fig. 31.4). Such computation allows for the improvement of preoperative surgical planning [5–7] and sometimes also of surgical eligibility in liver surgery, thanks to better patient-specific anatomical knowledge and better postoperative volume definition.

31.3 Interactive Augmented Reality

Preoperative surgical planning and simulation can significantly improve the efficiency of a surgical procedure, thanks to better preoperative knowledge of the patient's anatomy. However, the preoperative use of such systems is not suffi-

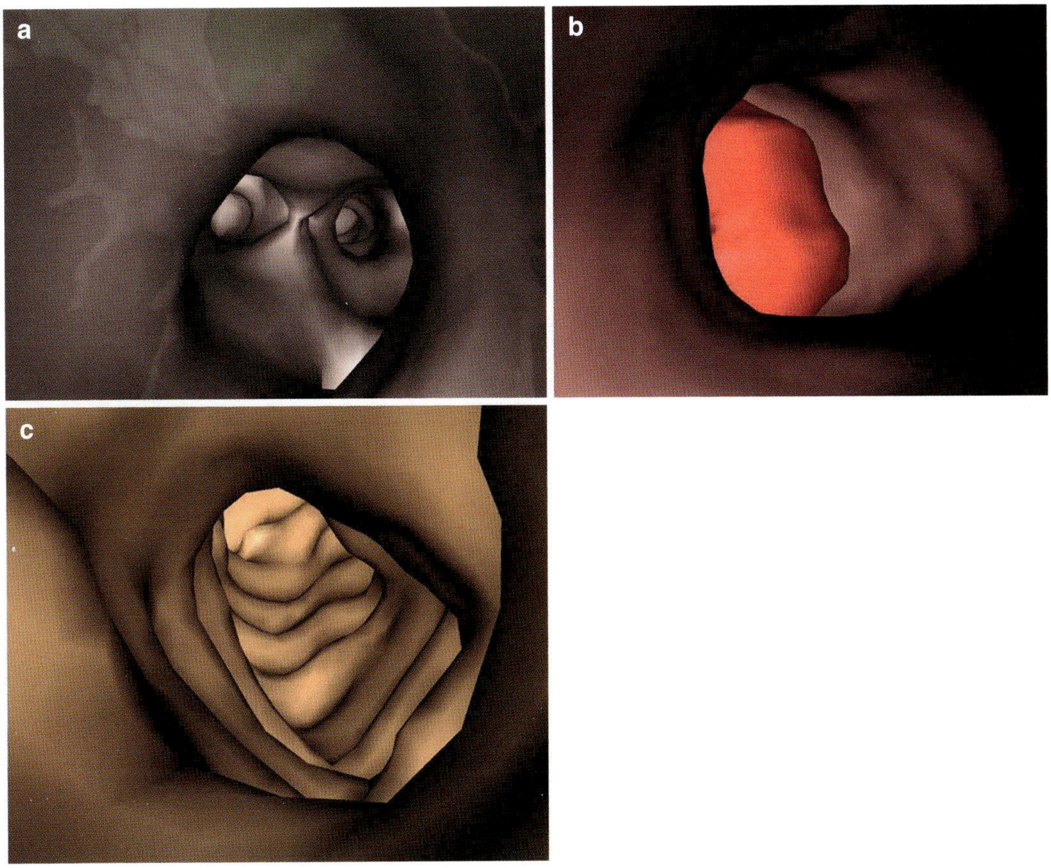

Fig. 31.3 Visible Patient Planning used for a virtual fibroscopy with transparency on bronchus tree allowing to see a tumor in *green* (**a**), a virtual gastroscopy with a *red* GIST detection (**b**), and a virtual coloscopy (**c**) from patient-specific 3D modelling

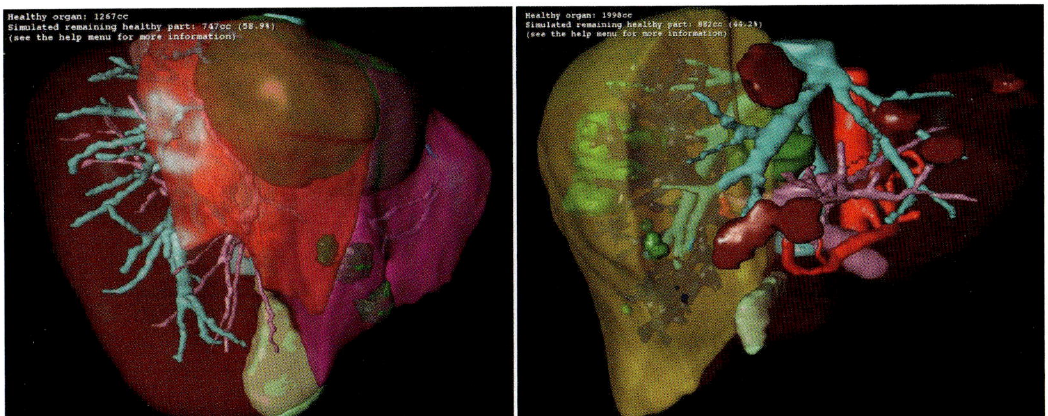

Fig. 31.4 Virtual left hepatectomy extended to segment 8 (*left*) and virtual right hepatectomy of a patient having several thermal ablations and a right embolization (*right*) using the clip applying function of Visible Patient Planning software

cient to ensure safety during the surgical procedure. Such an improvement can be provided by an intraoperative use of virtual reality through the augmented reality concept. Augmented reality consists in superimposing the preoperative 3D patient modelling onto the live intraoperative video view of the patient. Augmented reality can thus provide a transparency view of patients. Several kinds of augmented reality have been developed: interactive (IAR), semiautomatic (SemIAR), and fully automated (AAR).

Interactive augmented reality (IAR) is based on an interactive registration performed by an operator through an image overlay of the patient's model superimposed onto the patient's view, which can be direct (no camera) or indirect (with a camera). The patient's view can be external, to visualize his/her skin, or internal (e.g., in laparoscopic surgery) to display an organ. The registration is then guided by anatomical landmarks visible on the patient's view and on the patient's model through the image overlay. Four main image overlay techniques are available: direct projection of the patient model onto patient skin through a video projector [8, 9], direct visualization through a transparent screen placed between surgeons and the patient [10], indirect visualization using a camera to provide a patient view visualized on a screen that can overlay the virtual patient model [11], and specific display such as the robotic 3D view display of the da Vinci robot [12]. The indirect visualization using a camera is today the best available solution that provides the camera's point of view regardless of surgeon position or movement, which avoids the usual error linked to the detection of several points of view.

We have developed a two-step interactive augmented reality method [11, 12]. The first step consists in registering an external view of the real patient with a similar external view of the virtual patient. The second step consists in real-time positioning and correction of the virtual camera so that it is orientated similarly to the laparoscopic camera. Real video views are provided by two cameras inside the OR: the external real view of the patient is provided by the camera of the shadowless lamp or by an external camera, and the laparoscopic camera provides the internal image (see Fig. 31.5).

Both images are sent via a fiber-optic network and are visualized on two different screens by the independent operator in the video room. A third screen displays the view of the 3D patient rendering software working on a laptop equipped with a good 3D graphic card and controlled by the operator. The augmented reality view is then obtained by using a video mixer Panasonic MX 70, offering a merged view of both interactively selected screens. This system also gives the possibility to reduce the augmented reality effect to a limited part of the image as illustrated in Fig. 31.6. Visible Patient Planning software allows to realize any virtual views of the patient, from internal or external point of view as illustrated in Chap. 2. It is then used to provide the similar point of view of the real camera in the virtual world.

The technique used several anatomical landmarks chosen on the skin (such as the ribs, xiphoid process, iliac crests, and the umbilicus) and inside the abdomen (inferior vena cava and two laparoscopic tools). The resulting registration accuracy can immediately be checked by properly superimposing the virtual organs onto the real visible ones. This method would take a while to implement, and adjustment of the various external landmarks was sometimes imperfect. However, this method, evaluated during more than 50 procedures, always provided good results.

In the OR, the surgeon can see the laparoscopic view on a standard laparoscopic video screen, and, on a second screen, both resulting augmented reality images (internal or external view on Fig. 31.6) show the view selected by the independent operator from a remote site. If he/she uses the da Vinci robot, he/she can see both real and augmented reality laparoscopic views in picture of the Master part 3D screen of the robot. Due to camera movement, the augmented reality view has to be adjusted continuously by using the visible contours of anatomical structures as efficient landmarks.

We have tested with success this IAR on more than 50 surgical oncological procedures for liver,

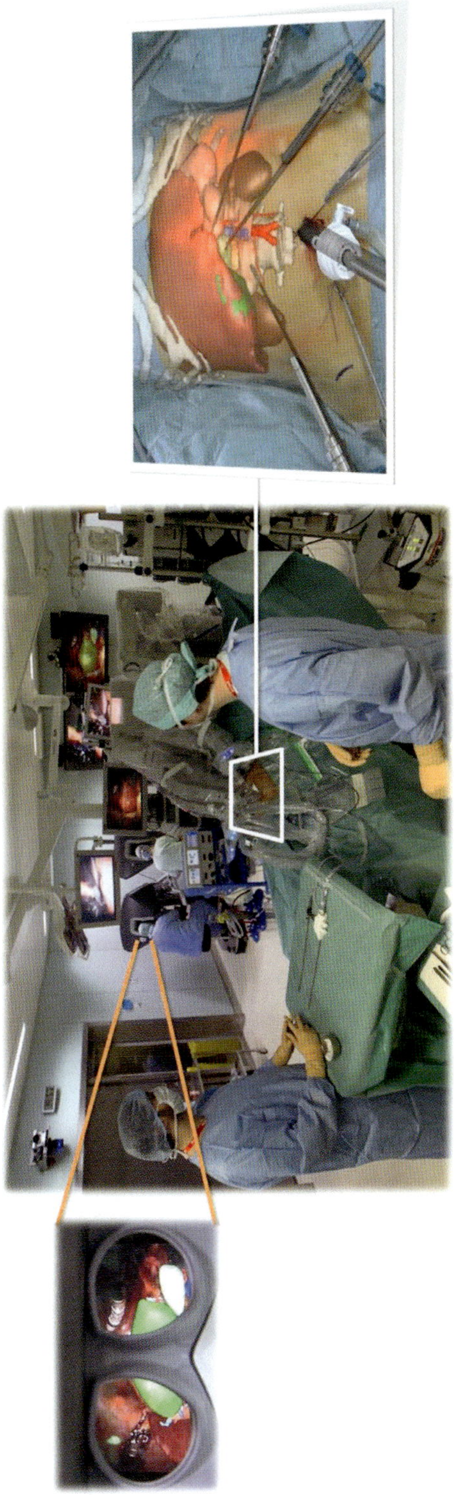

Fig. 31.5 Interactive augmented reality realized on the da Vinci robot providing an internal AR view in the Master Vision system (*left*) and an external AR view of the patient (*right*)

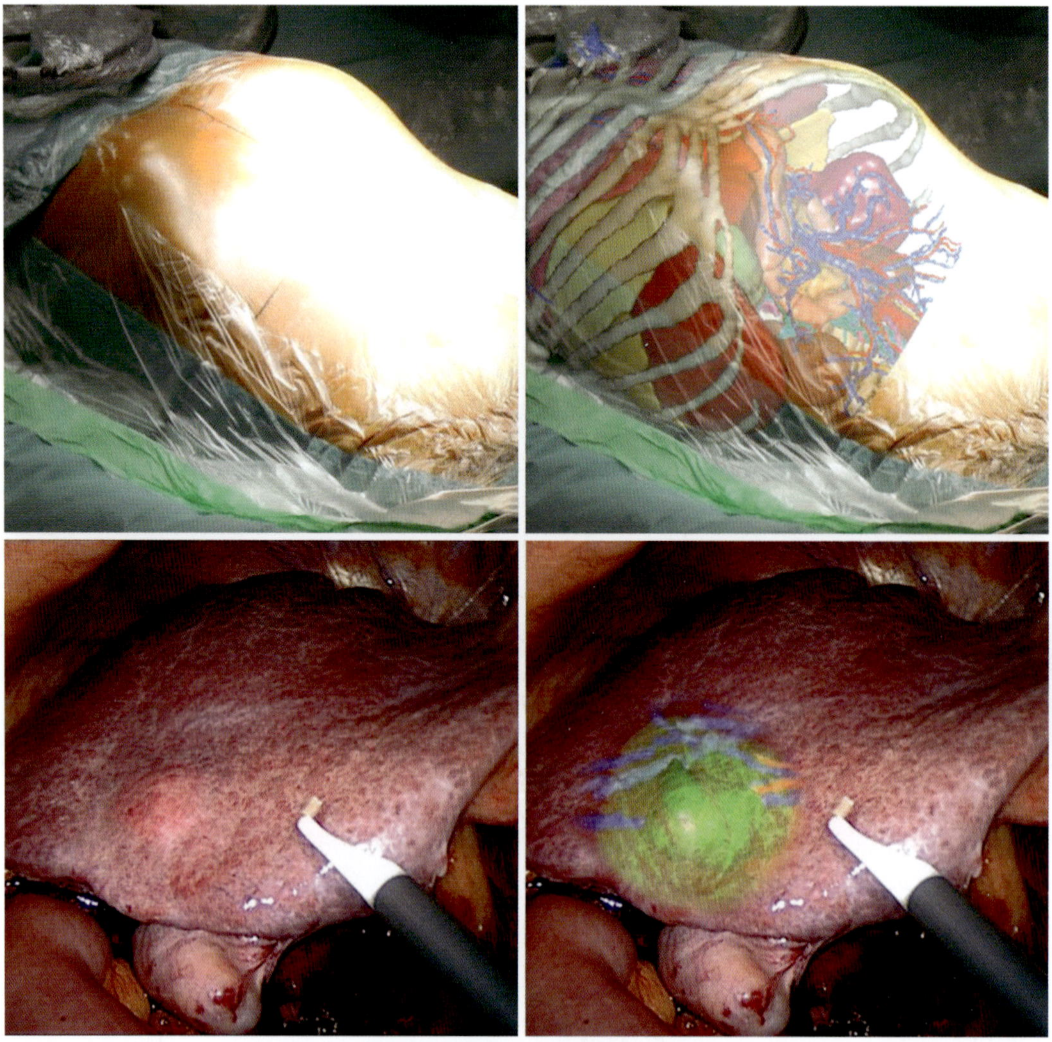

Fig. 31.6 External (*top*) and internal (*bottom*) interactive augmented reality views

adrenal gland, pancreas, and parathyroid tumor resection. The majority of our tests have been performed in the classical laparoscopic approach [6, 7, 11, 13], but more recently we have applied the same techniques in robotic surgery with the same success [12, 14]. Superimposition has been possible for each operation. Vascular control also showed the efficiency of the system despite the interaction required to make it work.

Although registration for the external view is efficient, it remains user dependent and is therefore not reproducible. Moreover, any movement of the external camera and/or of the patient after the first registration requires a new registration, which is time consuming and harder to implement during the surgical intervention. One of the main limits is caused by the system's inability to easily track the patient's natural movements (breathing, heartbeats). Moreover, since the system uses 3D rigid models, organs that are being deformed during the intervention cannot be deformed virtually.

31.4 Automated Augmented Reality

Automated augmented reality replaces user interaction by computer computation, the system being then no longer user dependent. Main user interaction in IAR laparoscopic surgery is achieved by registering a preoperative high-definition 3D model (e.g., segmentation from CT images or MRI) with the video display from the endoscopic camera. This proves to be a challenge, as the data to be registered may be very different due to several factors. First, the data often originates from different imaging modalities and dimensions (3D CT grayscale image vs. 2D RGB full HD endoscopic sequence). Second, patient anatomy may significantly differ between the preoperative and intraoperative acquisitions. The organs often shift due to a different position for the patient and the intra-abdominal gas insufflation which applies pressure on the viscera. Moreover, surgeon actions obviously affect the surgical scene as he mobilizes organs or resects tissues.

For the sake of accuracy, a laparoscopic AR system would have to take this deformation into account. Many different approaches have been proposed to solve this issue, but most require either some manual intervention from the surgeon or external tracking systems. Tracking will allow to compute tool positioning during surgery and must be a real-time system. A large number of systems exist allowing for automatic tracking of surgical tools. Such systems are usually based on optical tracking using two infrared cameras. Other common but more limited tracking methods are based on an electromagnetic system. Several commercial solutions exist, and such automation is today about to be solved for rigid tools. Normal infrared optic cameras and electromagnetic tracking systems provide only the position and shape of instruments or landmarks stuck on the patient that can be virtually visualized. These tracking systems remain expensive and are not user-friendly.

Registration will allow to compute the patient position in the same environment as 3D models. A perfect registration should take patient movements into account. There are three kinds of movements that have to be tracked and compensated for: if the patient moves altogether (e.g., sliding), local organ movement due to surgeon interaction, and deformation caused by physiological movements (breathing and heartbeat). Usually, registration of existing methods is done at the beginning of surgery without taking movement into account. If a single body-wide movement can be solved through a new intraoperative registration, other movements require complex algorithms based on nonrigid registration.

To solve such a problem, several approaches have been proposed [1]. The main one consists in segmenting real-time intraoperative medical images (US, MRI, or CT) providing the real shape of organs during the surgical procedure. In surgical practice, most of the work is based on intraoperative ultrasonography and MRI. However, one approach seems promising due to the popularization of intraoperative scanners (e.g., CBCT) in so-called "hybrid" operating rooms (OR). An acquisition from such a system can serve as an intermediary in the registration process between the preoperative scan and the endoscopic images and can help compensate for the deformation between the preoperative and intraoperative states.

We propose a new paradigm to automatically register the referential frame of the intraoperative model with that of the endoscopic camera, without any external tracking system [15]. By including the distal part of the endoscope within the intraoperative acquisition field and holding it with an articulated arm, we are able to estimate the direction of the optical axis and the position of the optical center in the reconstructed volume. This approach allows us to determine directly the correspondence between the endoscopic camera and the intraoperative scanner (in our case, an Artis Zeego by Siemens) and thus to register their data fully automatically (see Fig. 31.7).

Intraoperative medical images being registered with the intraoperative video view, it remains mandatory to nonrigidly register the preoperative 3D modelling of the patient, in order to take deformation into account. Our previous work [16] proposed an approach that computes a nonrigid registration of a preoperative patient model (including abdominal wall, visceral set, and liver) using information analysis of an intraoperative image of the patient. The adaptation of this method based on CT scan imaging to Dyna-CT imaging allowed us to obtain a fully automatic nonrigid registration of preoperative modelling onto the video view of the patient [17].

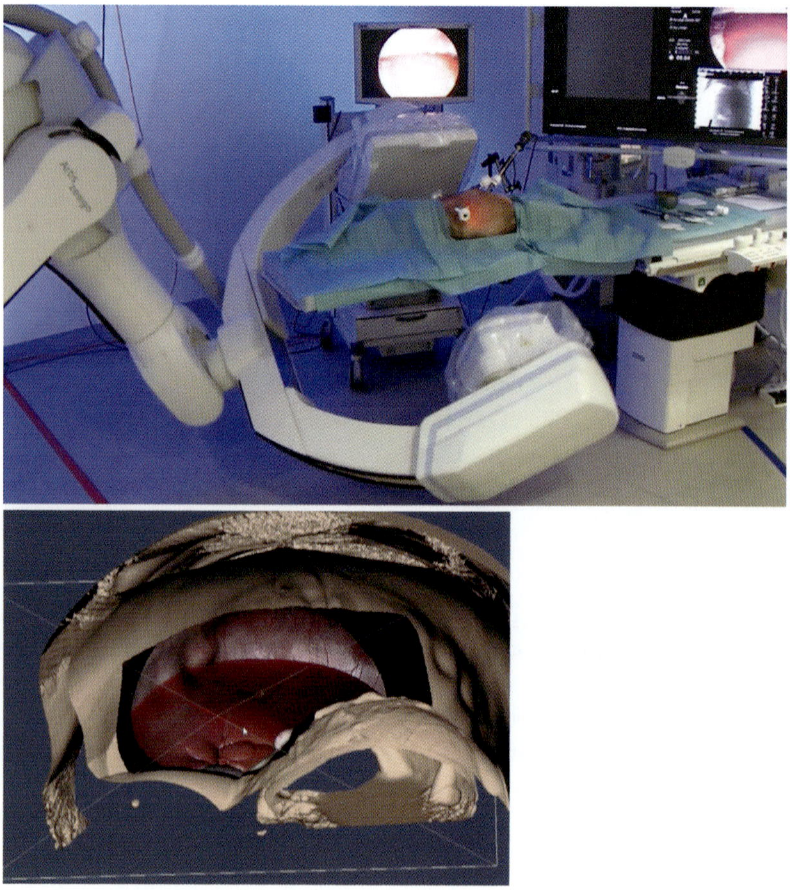

Fig. 31.7 The Dyna-CT images provided by the Artis Zeego (*top*) allow to detect the laparoscope position in the image and then to register video and medical image (*bottom*)

After this automatic initial nonrigid registration, the remaining problem consists in correcting in real time this nonrigid registration in order to take organ deformation due to breathing movement and surgeon interaction into account. To solve such a problem, our solution consists in a predictive real-time simulation of organ deformation by tracking tool movement and organ deformation in video images. As we showed for the physiological breathing movements [18], such an approach is feasible by preoperatively modelling the patient, along with his/her physiological movements, and by simulating these movements intraoperatively. The simulation is controlled by real patient information (skin surface) tracked and extracted in real time, thanks to an analysis of video images. Our results showed that this solution provides good results (2 mm of accuracy for real-time registration of deformable organs).

A similar idea can be applied to laparoscopic surgery, an analysis of stereo-laparoscopic video images replacing the external video image analysis. During abdominal surgery, tissue and organs are continuously deforming and the surgeon is free to move the laparoscopic camera. The objective of the temporal registration is then to modify the model shape and location of an organ in the same way as the real organ by tracking its deformation and movement in real time. Several methods have been developed based on real-time virtual organ surface reconstruction of the organ [19, 20], mechanical modelling of the organ [21, 22], and feature tracking. The resulting precision is currently limited around 5 mm, but it will be

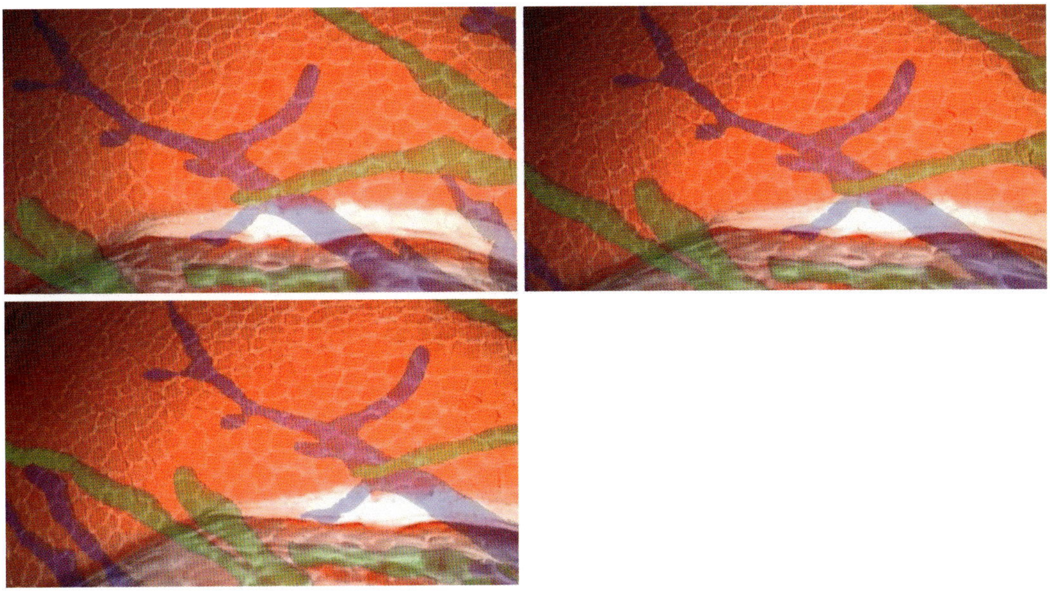

Fig. 31.8 Sample of temporal registration from Mountney et al. research work [20] allowing to correct in real time deformation of the liver due to breathing movement

improved progressively through the addition of patient-specific elasticity and viscosity modelling of organs, thanks to elastography [23] (Fig. 31.8).

Conclusions

We have presented research on computer-assisted minimally invasive surgery based on virtual and augmented reality. They allow to superimpose the virtual image of internal organs and pathologies onto the abdominal view of the patient. These systems, at an experimental stage, are progressively being tested clinically for minimally invasive surgery, with the objective of using them in clinical routine. First results show that the systems work very efficiently and that future solutions will combine predictive simulation and real-time medical image analysis in order to solve current limitations. To be efficient, patient-specific modelling will have to integrate more information than the geometric model only. Mechanical properties, functional anatomy, and biological modelling will gradually improve the quality of simulation and prediction which, combined with intraoperative image analysis, will provide the awaited accuracy.

This research also represents the first essential phase for surgical gesture automation, which will allow to reduce surgical mistakes. Indeed, procedure simulation will allow to identify the unnecessary or imperfect surgical moves, using it as a programming of the final gesture. These moves will then be transmitted to a surgical robot which, thanks to augmented reality and visual servoing, will be able to precisely reproduce the surgeon's optimized moves. Tomorrow's surgery is on its way.

References

1. Sielhorst T, Feuerstein M, Navab N (2008) Advanced medical displays: a literature review of augmented reality. J Display Technol 4(4):451–467
2. OsiriX Imaging Software. www.osirix-viewer.com
3. Lima M, Reinberg O, Ruggeri G, De Buys Roessingh AS, Gardano T, Soler L, Mogiatti M, Cantone N (2013) 3D virtual rendering before laparoscopic partial splenectomy in children. Journal of Pediatric Surgery 48(8):1784–1788
4. Destro F, Maffi M, Gargano T, Ruggeri G, Soler L, Lima M (2013) Thoracoscopic treatment of congenital malformation of the lung: preliminary experience with preoperative 3D virtual rendering. JEMIS 1:1–4

5. Bégin A, Martel G, Lapointe R, Belblidia A, Lepanto L, Soler L, Mutter D, Marescaux J, Vandenbroucke-Menu F (2014) Accuracy of preoperative automatic measurement of the liver volume by CT-scan combined to a 3D virtual surgical planning software. Surg Endosc 28(12):3408–3412
6. Soler L, Nicolau S, Pessaux P, Mutter D, Marescaux J (2014) Real-time 3D image reconstruction guidance in liver resection surgery. Hepatobiliary Surg Nutr 3(2):73–81
7. Mutter D, Soler L, Marescaux J (2010) Recent advances in liver imaging. Informa Healthc 4(5):613–621
8. Osorio A, Galan JA, Nauroy J, Lobato JJ, Dahdouh S, Navarro I, Donars P, Caballero JP, Frenoux E (2008) Planning and validating percutaneous nephrolithotomies in a non-classical patient's position using a new 3D augmented reality system. Int J CARS 3(1):S130–S132
9. Sugimoto M, Yasuda H, Koda K, Suzuki M, Yamazaki M, Tezuka T, Kosugi C, Higuchi R, Watayo Y, Yagawa Y, Uemura S, Tsuchiya H, Azuma T (2010) Image overlay navigation by markerless surface registration in gastrointestinal, hepatobiliary and pancreatic surgery. J Hepatobiliary Pancreat Sci 17(5):629–636
10. Masamune K, Fichtinger G, Deguet A, Matsuka D, Taylor R (2002) An image overlay system with enhanced reality for percutaneous therapy performed inside CT scanner. MICCAI 2002, LNCS 2489:77–84
11. Marescaux J, Rubino F, Arena M, Soler L (2004) Augmented reality assisted laparoscopic adrenalectomy. JAMA 292(18):2214–2215
12. Pessaux P, Soler L, Marzano E, Diana M, Piardi T, Mutter D, Marescaux J (2015) Towards cybernetic surgery: robotic and augmented reality-assisted liver segmentectomy. Langenbecks Arch Surg 400(3):381–385
13. Hallet J, Soler L, Diana M, Mutter D, Baumert TF, Habersetzer F, Marescaux J, Pessaux P (2015) Trans-thoracic minimally invasive liver resection guided by augmented reality. J Am Coll Surg 220(5):e55–e60
14. Pessaux P, Diana M, Soler L, Piardi T, Mutter D, Marescaux J (2014) Robotic duodenopancreatectomy assisted with augmented reality and real-time fluorescence guidance. Surg Endosc 28(8):2493–2498
15. Bernhardt S, Nicolau SA, Agnus V, Soler L, Doignon C, Marescaux J (2014) Automatic detection of endoscope in intraoperative CT image: application to AR guidance in laparoscopic surgery. IEEE international symposium on biomedical imaging (ISBI 2014), pp 563–567
16. Bano J, Hostettler A, Nicolau S, Cotin S, Doignon C, Wu HS, Huang MH, Soler L, Marescaux J (2012) Simulation of pneumoperitoneum for laparoscopic surgery planning. Proceedings of MICCAI, 2012, pp 91–98
17. Bano J, Nicolau SA, Hostettler A, Doignon C, Marescaux J, Soler L (2014) Registration of preoperative liver model for laparoscopic surgery from intraoperative 3d acquisition. In Augmented reality environments for medical imaging and computer-assisted interventions. Springer, Heidelberg New York Dordrecht London, LNCS 8198:201–210
18. Hostettler A, Nicolau SA, Marescaux J, Soler L (2010) A real-time predictive simulation of abdominal viscera position during quiet free breathing. Prog Biophys Mol Biol 103(2-3):169–184
19. Mountney P, Yang GZ (2010) Motion compensated slam for image guided surgery. In: Jiang T, Navab N, Pluim JPW, Viergever MA (eds) MICCAI 2010, Part II. LNCS, vol 6362. Springer, Heidelberg, pp 496–504
20. Mountney P, Fallert J, Nicolau S, Soler L, Mewes PW (2014) An augmented reality framework for soft tissue surgery. Med Image Comput Comput Assist Interv 17(1):423–431
21. Haouchine N, Dequidt J, Peterlik I, Kerrien E, Berger MO, Cotin S (2013) Image-guided simulation of heterogeneous tissue deformation for augmented reality during hepatic surgery. ISMAR 2013, pp 199–208
22. Plantefeve R, Peterlik I, Haouchine N, Cotin S (2016) Patient-specific biomechanical modeling for guidance during minimally-invasive hepatic surgery. Ann Biomed Eng 44(1):139–153
23. Vappou J, Hou G, Marquet F, Shahmirzadi D, Grondin J, Konofagou E (2015) Non-contact, ultrasound-based indentation method for measuring elastic properties of biological tissues using Harmonic Motion Imaging (HMI). Phys Med Biol 60(7):2853–2868

Index

M. Lima (ed.), *Pediatric Digestive Surgery*, DOI 10.1007/978-3-319-40525-4

R